Shoulder Arthritis across the Life Span

Augustus D. Mazzocca
Emilio Calvo · Giovanni Di Giacomo
Editors

Shoulder Arthritis across the Life Span

From Joint Preservation to Arthroplasty

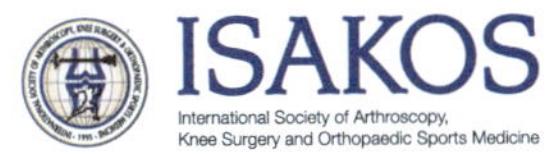

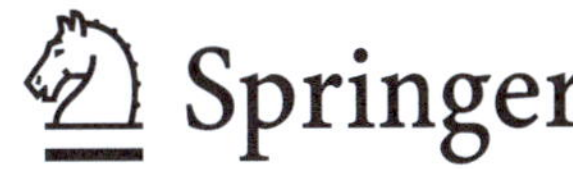

Editors
Augustus D. Mazzocca
Department of Orthopaedic Surgery
Massachusetts General Hospital
Boston, MA, USA

Giovanni Di Giacomo
Concordia Hospital
Rome, Italy

Emilio Calvo
Department of Orthopedic Surgery
and Traumatology
Fundacion Jimenez Diaz
Universidad Autonoma
Madrid, Spain

ISBN 978-3-031-33300-2   ISBN 978-3-031-33298-2   (eBook)
https://doi.org/10.1007/978-3-031-33298-2

This Springer imprint is published by the registered company Springer Nature Switzerland AG
The registered company address is: Gewerbestrasse 11, 6330 Cham, Switzerland

I would like to dedicate this book to my wife Jennifer who supports and challenges me to be the best, our wonderful children Augustus, Jillian, and Nicolo who are incredible members of society and have brought tremendous joy to us, my parents Gus and D'Ann who are incredible role models and teachers, and my sister Ann and her husband Tony who are caring and loving people.

Augustus D Mazzocca MS, MD, FAAOS, FAOA

I would like to acknowledge the many people involved in making this book possible. First, my wife, Rorres, and my lovely kids, Javier and Elena. Nothing would have been possible without their generous support. I love you. Second, my parents, Juliana and Emilio, who taught me the meaning of hard work, perseverance, and resiliency. Third, my co-editors and co-authors. Writing a book is hard work that requires a determined commitment to education critical for our patients' healthcare. Finally, I would like to thank ISAKOS and Springer for their continuous support throughout this project.

Emilio Calvo, MD, PhD, MBA

I want to dedicate this book to my daughter, Jacqueline, and her heart-warming smile; to the entire Concordia Hospital Team in Rome; and to all the patients who have entrusted us with their health and continue to do so.

Giovanni Di Giacomo

Contents

**Part V	Joint Replacement: Open Treatment in Elderly**

**Part VI	New Technologies in Shoulder Arthroplasty**

Part I

Joint Preservation: Conservative Non-operative Treatment

Physical Therapy and Exercise to Increase ROM and Decrease Pain

1

Hiroaki Ishikawa, Takayuki Muraki,
Ronaldo Alves Cunha, Benno Ejnisman,
and Eiji Itoi

1.1 Clinical Presentation

1.1.1 Pain

Patients with glenohumeral osteoarthritis (OA) typically present shoulder pain characterized by gradual onset. The pain is often localized posteriorly and deep within the glenohumeral joint [1–3]. The patients often complain of difficulty in falling asleep due to night pain [2]. This pain progressively aggravates over time and leads to decreased quality of life and mental health problems [4, 5].

The etiology of pain in patients with glenohumeral OA is complex because various factors affect the pain. Although articular cartilage damage is a key feature of glenohumeral OA, the articular cartilage is insensitive and may not be the source of pain. By contrast, the subchondral bone, synovia, ligaments, joint capsule, and muscles are richly innervated and can be the causes of rest pain due to inflammation [6, 7]. Motion pain in the midrange of motion may be associated with subacromial impingement or compressive stress on chondral lesions [8, 9]. At the end range of motion, tensile stress on the glenohumeral ligament and capsule and muscles surrounding the shoulder may cause the pain.

1.1.2 Shoulder ROM

In patients with glenohumeral OA, shoulder range of motion (ROM) is frequently limited in various directions rather than in specific directions. Jia et al. [10] reviewed the preoperative data of patients who underwent shoulder surgery for 13 years ($n = 1913$). In this study, mean active shoulder ROM in patients with glenohumeral OA was 86° of abduction, 49° of external rotation (ER) with the arm abducted 90°, and 14° of internal rotation (IR) with the arm abducted 90°. In addition, patients with glenohumeral OA had more severe ROM loss than other shoulder diseases (i.e., rotator cuff disease, shoulder instability, and SLAP lesions).

The loss of shoulder ROM in patients with glenohumeral OA can be caused by pain, decreased flexibility of soft tissues, and glenoid deformity related to the OA. To increase shoulder

H. Ishikawa · T. Muraki
Department of Rehabilitation, Tohoku University Hospital, Sendai, Japan

Department of Physical Medicine and Rehabilitation, Tohoku University Graduate School of Medicine, Sendai, Japan

R. A. Cunha · B. Ejnisman
Department of Sports Medicine, Federal University of São Paulo, São Paulo, Brazil
e-mail: cunha@unifesp.br

E. Itoi (✉)
Department of Orthopaedic Surgery, Tohoku Rosai Hospital, Sendai, Japan
e-mail: itoi-eiji@med.tohoku.ac.jp

© ISAKOS 2023
A. D. Mazzocca et al. (eds.), *Shoulder Arthritis across the Life Span*,
https://doi.org/10.1007/978-3-031-33298-2_1

ROM, physical therapy focuses mainly on improving the decreased flexibility of soft tissues, whereas surgical treatment focuses mainly on correcting the glenoid deformity.

1.1.3 Shoulder Muscle Function

Muscle weakness can occur by disuse due to pain in patients with glenohumeral OA. Previous studies evaluated muscle atrophy in patients with glenohumeral OA by comparing muscle area with healthy subjects [11, 12]. These studies showed that patients with glenohumeral OA had decreased muscle area of the supraspinatus [12], whereas no difference in the deltoid muscle area was found compared with the healthy subjects [11]. Based on these findings, glenohumeral OA is associated with supraspinatus atrophy, but the causation remains unknown. In addition, other previous studies compared the muscle area among different subgroups of glenohumeral OA [13, 14]. Aleem et al. [14] showed that patients with Walch type B had increased ratio of the posterior rotator cuff (i.e., the infraspinatus and teres minor) area to the anterior rotator cuff (i.e., the subscapularis) area compared with Walch type A. Moverman et al. [13] demonstrated that increased area of the posterior rotator cuff is independently associated with Walch type B (relative to Walch type A). The rotator cuff muscle imbalance in the transverse plane is one of the characteristic findings in patients with Walch type B.

1.1.4 Shoulder Kinematics

Alterations in shoulder kinematics are frequently observed in patients with glenohumeral OA [15–18]. Fayad et al. [18] examined the differences in scapulothoracic and glenohumeral motions during arm elevation between affected and unaffected shoulders in patients with glenohumeral OA. They found increased scapular external rotation and decreased glenohumeral elevation on the affected side. Lädermann et al. [15] demonstrated that scapular anterior tilt during internal rotation at 90° on the affected side was greater than that on the unaffected side in patients with Walch type B OA. Bruttel et al. [16] compared glenohumeral motion during activities of daily living (ADL), such as perineal care, washing the axilla, combing hair, and taking a book from a shelf, between patients with glenohumeral OA and healthy subjects. This study showed less glenohumeral elevation in patients with glenohumeral OA during all ADL. Roren et al. [17] demonstrated that scapular external rotation during hair combing on the affected side was greater than that on the unaffected side in patients with glenohumeral OA. These reports tell us that the abnormal scapular motions are most likely adaptive changes to the restricted glenohumeral motion.

1.2 Management Principles

There remains inconclusive evidence to support physical therapy for the initial treatment of glenohumeral OA [19, 20]. However, physical therapy may clinically benefit select patients with glenohumeral OA. Physical therapy for patients with glenohumeral OA is performed in order to (1) decrease pain, (2) increase shoulder ROM, and (3) protect the glenohumeral joint.

First, we should assess whether pain appears at rest or during shoulder motion. For the rest pain, medications and intra-articular injections rather than physical therapy can be effective because the cause of pain may be inflammation within the glenohumeral joint. If pain appears in the midrange of shoulder motion (particularly shoulder elevation), the cause of pain may be subacromial impingement or compressive stress on chondral lesions. These causes can be identified by physical examinations. Pain at the end range of shoulder motion may be attributed to tightness of the soft tissues surrounding the shoulder.

To improve shoulder ROM loss, we need to identify the soft tissues affecting the ROM loss. For instance, the tightness of the posterior capsule, infraspinatus, and teres minor causes loss of shoulder IR [21, 22]. However, the primary tissues responsible for decreased shoulder IR are different by arm position; the tightness of the posterior capsule (middle and inferior portions) restrains IR at 30° of shoulder elevation, whereas the infraspinatus and teres minor restrain IR at 90° of shoulder elevation. If improvement of IR at 90° of shoulder elevation is needed, we should perform stretching or relaxation of the infraspinatus and teres minor.

Muscle weakness and/or imbalance of the rotator cuff may contribute to increased glenoid deformity. Some previous studies demonstrated increased muscle area of the infraspinatus/teres minor relative to the subscapularis was associated with posterior glenohumeral subluxation and increased glenoid retroversion in patients with Walch type B [12, 14]. Based on these findings, it is speculated that an imbalanced force in the transverse plane changes the direction of the resultant force posteriorly, resulting in eccentric posterior wear. If the muscle weakness and/or imbalance of the rotator cuff are found, interventions to the muscles are recommended. However, excessive strengthening exercise should be avoided as it may cause exacerbation of symptoms.

1.3 Assessment

1.3.1 Physical Examination

Physical examinations such as palpation and special tests are useful for the identification of pain associated with glenohumeral OA. In patients with glenohumeral OA, palpation of the regions that correspond to the swollen synovium and the protruding bony osteophytes of the GH joint may provoke pain [3].

The compression-rotation test is conducted to identify the pain resulting from chondral lesions (Fig. 1.1) [23]. If there is pain during shoulder motion (particularly the midrange of motion) and the compression-rotation test is positive, the pain resulting from chondral lesions should be suspected. The Neer, Hawkins-Kennedy, painful arc, empty can, and external rotation resistance tests are used to identify subacromial impingement

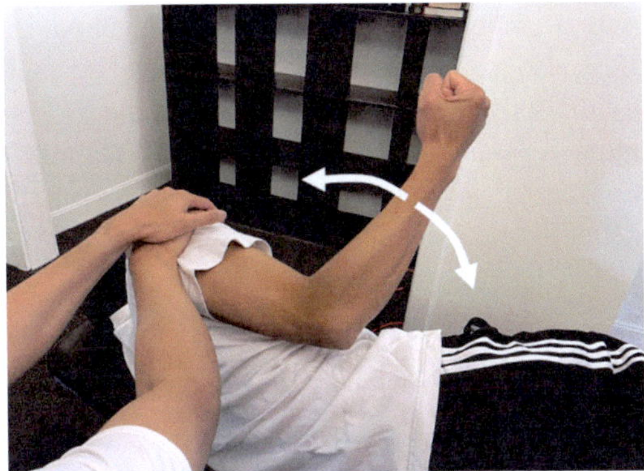

Fig. 1.1 Compression-rotation test. The patient is in a side-lying position on the unaffected side, with the affected arm at the side and the elbow flexed. The examiner compresses the arm into the glenoid. The patient is asked to rotate the arm internally and externally. The compression-rotation test is considered positive if pain occurs

[24]. The less than 3 positive of 5 rules out subacromial impingement [24].

1.3.2 Self-reported Functional Outcome

Generally, shoulder pain and function are evaluated using self-reported outcome measures such as disability of the shoulder and hand (DASH) and shoulder pain and disability index (SPADI). The Western Ontario Osteoarthritis of the Shoulder (WOOS) index is a disease-specific questionnaire for measurement of the quality of life (QOL) among patients with glenohumeral OA [25]. It provides scores on four domains (19 questions): (1) physical symptoms, (2) sport/recreation/work, (3) lifestyle, and (4) emotions. Each question is tested on a visual analog scale from 0 to 100, and the total score ranges from 0 to 1900.

1.3.3 ROM Measurement

Active and passive range of motion (ROM) for shoulder flexion, abduction, ER and IR, and horizontal abduction and adduction are measured with a goniometer or an inclinometer. Shoulder IR is also measured as the vertebral level reached by the fully extended thumb [26]. In the assessment of passive ROM, manual scapular stabilization in an appropriate manner is important to better isolate glenohumeral motion [27, 28].

1.3.4 Muscle Strength Testing

Muscle strengths of the shoulder girdle muscles are evaluated with manual muscle testing [29]. However, manual muscle testing is prone to interobserver variability [30]. Handheld dynamometer is a useful tool for clinicians to quantitatively evaluate muscle strength and verify intervention effect. The measurement technique using a dynamometer is shown to be reliable for detecting weakness in the shoulder [31, 32].

1.3.5 Assessment of Shoulder Kinematics

Several previous studies proposed reliable clinical assessment methods for scapular position/motion. The clinical methods are divided into visual observation and objective assessment.
1. Visual observation
Visible alterations in scapular position and motion patterns have been termed "scapular dyskinesis." The current recommendation for clinical assessment of scapular dyskinesis is the use of dynamic scapular dyskinesis test [33, 34]. Scapular dyskinesis is categorized into three types (Type I, increased scapular anterior tilt; Type II, increased scapular internal rotation; Type III, increased scapular elevation and upward rotation) [35]. For the scapular dyskinesis test, scapular motion during arm elevation is determined as "yes" (presence of scapular dyskinesis) or "no" (no presence).
2. Objective assessment
Objective assessment of scapular position and motion is conducted with a digital inclinometer. For the assessment of scapular upward

rotation, the inclination angle of the digital inclinometer aligned along the scapular spine is measured [36]. This method using a digital inclinometer is also useful for the assessment of scapulohumeral rhythm. The scapulohumeral rhythm is represented as the ratio of glenohumeral elevation to scapular upward rotation and calculated by measuring scapular upward rotation over the entire arc of arm elevation.

1.4 Management

1.4.1 ROM and Stretching Exercises

Active and passive shoulder ROM exercises aim at improving movement of the glenohumeral joint. The intensity of the exercises is based on the severity of shoulder pain. We start from performing active shoulder ROM exercise within no pain. If the pain becomes mild, we perform passive shoulder ROM exercise. Additionally, selective stretching exercises for the soft tissues affecting the shoulder ROM loss are performed.
1. Shoulder flexion/abduction
The pectoralis major and latissimus dorsi muscles are the primary tissues responsible for decreased shoulder flexion/abduction. For the pectoralis major muscle, the clavicular and sternal regions are stretched by passive shoulder horizontal extension at 90° of abduction, and the abdominal region is stretched by passive shoulder horizontal extension at 135° of abduction [37]. The latissimus dorsi muscle is stretched by passive contralateral rotation and bending of the trunk, with shoulder maximally elevated [38].
2. Shoulder extension/adduction
The anterior deltoid and supraspinatus muscles are the primary tissues responsible for decreased shoulder extension/adduction. The anterior deltoid muscle is considered to be stretched by passive shoulder extension. The supraspinatus muscle is stretched by passive shoulder adduction at shoulder extension [22].

3. Shoulder ER

The coracohumeral ligament and anterior inferior glenohumeral ligament (AIGHL) and subscapularis muscle are the primary tissues responsible for decreased shoulder ER. The coracohumeral ligament is stretched by passive shoulder ER at shoulder adduction [39]. The AIGHL is stretched by passive shoulder ER at 90° of shoulder abduction [40]. The subscapularis muscle (the inferior portion) is stretched by passive shoulder ER at 90° of shoulder flexion or abduction, or passive horizontal extension [41].

4. Shoulder IR

The posterior capsule and infraspinatus and teres minor muscles are the primary tissues responsible for decreased shoulder IR. For the posterior capsule, the superior portion of the posterior capsule is stretched by passive shoulder IR at 30° of shoulder extension, whereas the middle and inferior portions of the posterior capsule are stretched by passive shoulder IR at 30° of shoulder elevation [21]. For the infraspinatus and teres minor muscles, both muscles are stretched by passive shoulder IR at 90° of shoulder elevation [22].

The modified cross-body stretch and modified sleeper stretch are effective self-stretching techniques and widely used for improving flexibility of the infraspinatus and teres minor muscles (Fig. 1.2) [42, 43]. Particularly, the modified cross-body stretch is effective for the teres minor and the modified sleeper stretch for the infraspinatus muscles [43].

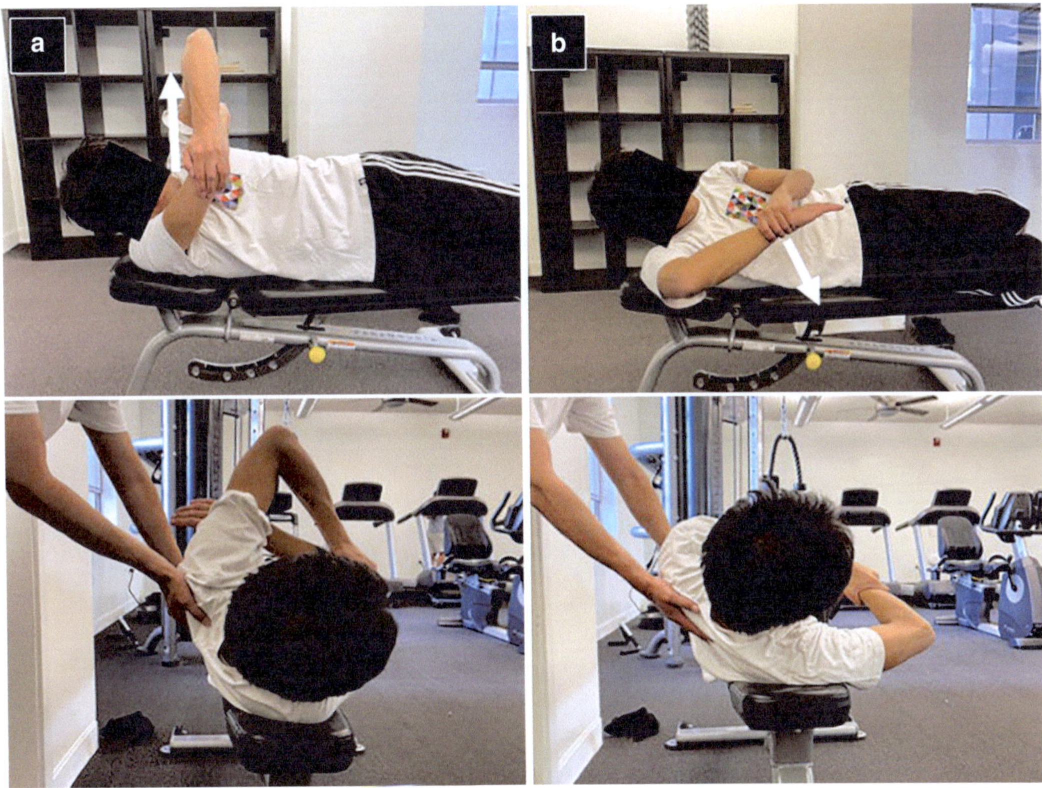

Fig. 1.2 Modified cross-body stretch and modified sleeper stretch. The patient is in the side-lying position on the affected side. For the modified cross-body stretch (**a**), external rotation is restricted via counterpressure of the opposite forearm, and then the humerus of the affected side is moved into horizontal flexion using the opposite arm. For the modified sleeper stretch (**b**), the humerus of the affected side is moved into shoulder internal rotation using the opposite arm

1.4.2 Joint Mobilization

Joint mobilization is a therapeutic approach to improve joint play and accessory motion, resulting in pain relief and increased ROM. A structured exercise program combined with joint mobilization has been shown to decrease pain and improve function in patients with various shoulder disorders [44].

Crowell et al. [45] reported a single-case study investigating therapeutic effect of exercise program (i.e., ROM and muscle strengthening exercises) combined with joint mobilization in patients with glenohumeral OA (a 38-year-old male military officer). The patient was treated for a total of five sessions over a period of 4 weeks. The two most common joint mobilization techniques (inferior and anterior-to-posterior glides) were used in this study (Fig. 1.3). After the 4-week intervention, SPADI scores decreased from 43 to 17%. The exercise and joint mobilization program for patients with glenohumeral OA can provide clinically meaningful short-term improvements in pain and function.

1.4.3 Muscle Strengthening Exercise

Strengthening exercises for the rotator cuff are important to stabilize the humeral head in the glenoid fossa and protect the glenohumeral joint.
1. Supraspinatus muscle
To strengthen the supraspinatus muscle, exercises to maximize supraspinatus activity while particularly minimizing deltoid activity are recommended in clinical practice. Full-can exercise and prone external rotation exercise

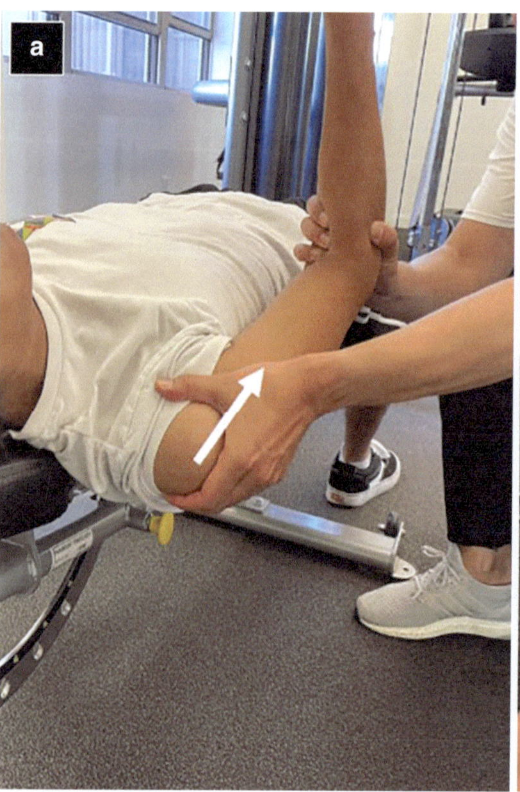
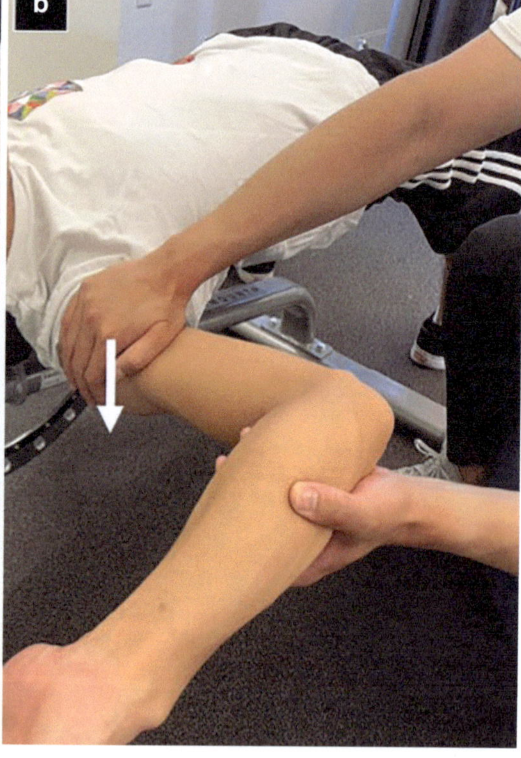

Fig. 1.3 Joint mobilization techniques (inferior and anterior-to-posterior glides). The patient is in a supine position. For the inferior glide (**a**), distal hand grasps the patient's elbow; proximal hand grasps the patient's humeral head; and then gentle inferior glide force is applied. For the anterior-to-posterior glide (**b**), distal hand grasps the patient's forearm; proximal hand grasps the patient's humeral head; and then gentle anterior-to-posterior glide force is applied with the arm in abduction and external rotation

are optimal to strengthen supraspinatus as these exercises produce high activity of the supraspinatus with less activity of the deltoid muscle [46, 47]. These exercises should be chosen depending on the patient's situation; for instance, prone external rotation exercise should be chosen if patients have pain during shoulder elevation.

2. Infraspinatus and teres minor muscles

Side-lying ER exercise has been used for strengthening the infraspinatus and teres minor muscles (Fig. 1.4a) [48]. In the side-lying ER exercise, the use of a towel roll between the elbow and side is recommended as deltoid activity during the exercise is more inhibited with a towel roll than without a towel roll [49]. In addition, low-load ER exercise (10% of maximum voluntary contraction) produced higher activity of the infraspinatus with less activity of the deltoid muscle compared with high-load exercise [50].

3. Subscapularis muscle

IR exercise in the belly-press test position is effective for strengthening the subscapularis muscle (Fig. 1.4b). Some previous studies demonstrated that the belly-press test produced high activity of the subscapularis while minimizing activities of other shoulder internal rotators (i.e., the pectoralis major, latissimus dorsi, and teres major muscles) [51].

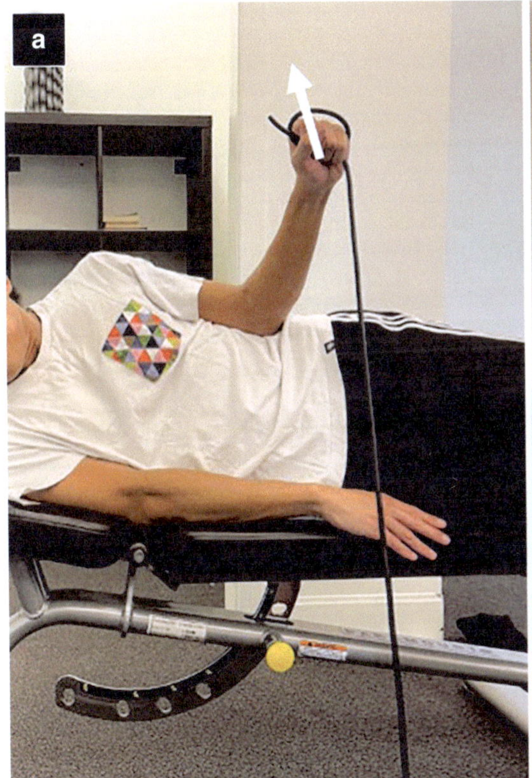
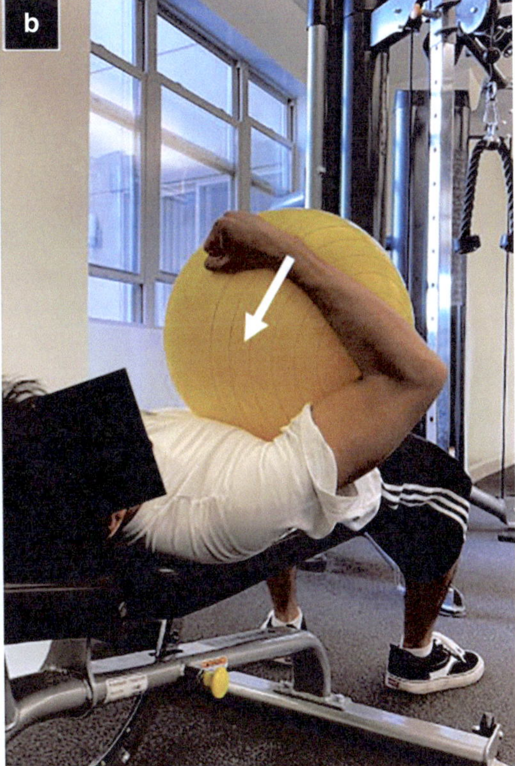

Fig. 1.4 Strengthening exercise for the infraspinatus, teres minor, and subscapularis. For the infraspinatus and teres minor strengthening exercise (**a**), the patient is in the side-lying position on the unaffected side and externally rotates the shoulder with the elbow at the side against resistance. For the subscapularis strengthening exercise (**b**), the patient is in a supine position and internally rotates the shoulder at 30° of shoulder abduction against resistance

References

1. Saltzman BM, Leroux TS, Verma NN, Romeo AA. Glenohumeral osteoarthritis in the young patient. J Am Acad Orthop Surg. 2018;26:e361–e70.
2. Ansok CB, Muh SJ. Optimal management of glenohumeral osteoarthritis. Orthop Res Rev. 2018;10:9–18.
3. Macias-Hernandez SI, Morones-Alba JD, Miranda-Duarte A, Coronado-Zarco R, Soria-Bastida MLA, Nava-Bringas T, et al. Glenohumeral osteoarthritis: overview, therapy, and rehabilitation. Disabil Rehabil. 2017;39:1674–82.
4. Cho CH, Song KS, Hwang I, Coats-Thomas MS, Warner JJP. Changes in psychological status and health-related quality of life following total shoulder arthroplasty. J Bone Joint Surg Am. 2017;99:1030–5.
5. Carter MJ, Mikuls TR, Nayak S, Fehringer EV, Michaud K. Impact of total shoulder arthroplasty on generic and shoulder-specific health-related quality-of-life measures: a systematic literature review and meta-analysis. J Bone Joint Surg Am. 2012;94:e127.
6. Dieppe PA, Lohmander LS. Pathogenesis and management of pain in osteoarthritis. Lancet. 2005;365:965–73.
7. Kidd BL, Photiou A, Inglis JJ. The role of inflammatory mediators on nociception and pain in arthritis. Novartis Found Symp. 2004;260:122–33; discussion 33–8, 277–9.
8. Chong PY, Srikumaran U, Kuye IO, Warner JJ. Glenohumeral arthritis in the young patient. J Shoulder Elbow Surg. 2011;20:S30–40.
9. Elser F, Braun S, Dewing CB, Millett PJ. Glenohumeral joint preservation: current options for managing articular cartilage lesions in young, active patients. Arthroscopy. 2010;26:685–96.
10. Jia X, Petersen SA, Khosravi AH, Almareddi V, Pannirselvam V, McFarland EG. Examination of the shoulder: the past, the present, and the future. J Bone Joint Surg Am. 2009;91(Suppl 6):10–8.
11. O'Neill DC, Christensen GV, Hillyard B, Kawakami J, Tashjian RZ, Chalmers PN. Glenoid retroversion associates with deltoid muscle asymmetry in Walch B-type glenohumeral osteoarthritis. JSES Int. 2021;5:282–7.
12. Chalmers PN, Beck L, Miller M, Stertz I, Henninger HB, Tashjian RZ. Glenoid retroversion associates with asymmetric rotator cuff muscle atrophy in those with Walch B-type glenohumeral osteoarthritis. J Am Acad Orthop Surg. 2020;28:547–55.
13. Moverman MA, Puzzitiello RN, Menendez ME, Pagani NR, Hart PJ, Churchill RW, et al. Rotator cuff fatty infiltration and muscle atrophy: relation to glenoid deformity in primary glenohumeral osteoarthritis. J Shoulder Elbow Surg. 2022;31:286–93.
14. Aleem AW, Chalmers PN, Bechtold D, Khan AZ, Tashjian RZ, Keener JD. Association between rotator cuff muscle size and glenoid deformity in primary glenohumeral osteoarthritis. J Bone Joint Surg Am. 2019;101:1912–20.
15. Lädermann A, Athwal GS, Bothorel H, Collin P, Mazzolari A, Raiss P, et al. Scapulothoracic alignment alterations in patients with Walch type B osteoarthritis: an in vivo dynamic analysis and prospective comparative study. J Clin Med. 2020;10:66.
16. Bruttel H, Spranz DM, Bülhoff M, Aljohani N, Wolf SI, Maier MW. Comparison of glenohumeral and humerothoracical range of motion in healthy controls, osteoarthritic patients and patients after total shoulder arthroplasty performing different activities of daily living. Gait Posture. 2019;71:20–5.
17. Roren A, Lefevre-Colau MM, Roby-Brami A, Revel M, Fermanian J, Gautheron V, et al. Modified 3D scapular kinematic patterns for activities of daily living in painful shoulders with restricted mobility: a comparison with contralateral unaffected shoulders. J Biomech. 2012;45:1305–11.
18. Fayad F, Roby-Brami A, Yazbeck C, Hanneton S, Lefevre-Colau MM, Gautheron V, et al. Three-dimensional scapular kinematics and scapulohumeral rhythm in patients with glenohumeral osteoarthritis or frozen shoulder. J Biomech. 2008;41:326–32.
19. Khazzam M, Gee AO, Pearl M. Management of glenohumeral joint osteoarthritis. J Am Acad Orthop Surg. 2020;28:781–9.
20. Izquierdo R, Voloshin I, Edwards S, Freehill MQ, Stanwood W, Wiater JM, et al. American academy of orthopaedic surgeons clinical practice guideline on: the treatment of glenohumeral joint osteoarthritis. J Bone Joint Surg Am. 2011;93:203–5.
21. Izumi T, Aoki M, Muraki T, Hidaka E, Miyamoto S. Stretching positions for the posterior capsule of the glenohumeral joint: strain measurement using cadaver specimens. Am J Sports Med. 2008;36:2014–22.
22. Muraki T, Aoki M, Uchiyama E, Murakami G, Miyamoto S. The effect of arm position on stretching of the supraspinatus, infraspinatus, and posterior portion of deltoid muscles: a cadaveric study. Clin Biomech (Bristol, Avon). 2006;21:474–80.
23. Ellman H, Harris E, Kay SP. Early degenerative joint disease simulating impingement syndrome: arthroscopic findings. Arthroscopy. 1992;8:482–7.
24. Michener LA, Walsworth MK, Doukas WC, Murphy KP. Reliability and diagnostic accuracy of 5 physical examination tests and combination of tests for subacromial impingement. Arch Phys Med Rehabil. 2009;90:1898–903.
25. Lo IK, Griffin S, Kirkley A. The development of a disease-specific quality of life measurement tool for osteoarthritis of the shoulder: the Western Ontario Osteoarthritis of the Shoulder (WOOS) index. Osteoarthritis Cartilage. 2001;9:771–8.
26. Edwards TB, Bostick RD, Greene CC, Baratta RV, Drez D. Interobserver and intraobserver reliability

of the measurement of shoulder internal rotation by vertebral level. J Shoulder Elbow Surg. 2002;11:40–2.

27. Wilk KE, Reinold MM, Macrina LC, Porterfield R, Devine KM, Suarez K, et al. Glenohumeral internal rotation measurements differ depending on stabilization techniques. Sports Health. 2009;1:131–6.

28. Boon AJ, Smith J. Manual scapular stabilization: its effect on shoulder rotational range of motion. Arch Phys Med Rehabil. 2000;81:978–83.

29. Kendall FP, McCreary EK, Provance PG. Muscles, testing and function: with posture and pain. 4th ed. Baltimore: Williams & Wilkins; 1993. 272–87 p.

30. Sapega AA. Muscle performance evaluation in orthopaedic practice. J Bone Joint Surg Am. 1990;72:1562–74.

31. Chamorro C, Arancibia M, Trigo B, Arias-Poblete L, Jerez-Mayorga D. Absolute reliability and concurrent validity of hand-held dynamometry in shoulder rotator strength assessment: systematic review and meta-analysis. Int J Environ Res Public Health. 2021;18:9293.

32. Michener LA, Boardman ND, Pidcoe PE, Frith AM. Scapular muscle tests in subjects with shoulder pain and functional loss: reliability and construct validity. Phys Ther. 2005;85:1128–38.

33. McClure P, Tate AR, Kareha S, Irwin D, Zlupko E. A clinical method for identifying scapular dyskinesis, part 1: reliability. J Athl Train. 2009;44:160–4.

34. Kibler WB, Ludewig PM, McClure PW, Michener LA, Bak K, Sciascia AD. Clinical implications of scapular dyskinesis in shoulder injury: the 2013 consensus statement from the 'Scapular Summit'. Br J Sports Med. 2013;47:877–85.

35. Kibler WB, Uhl TL, Maddux JW, Brooks PV, Zeller B, McMullen J. Qualitative clinical evaluation of scapular dysfunction: a reliability study. J Shoulder Elbow Surg. 2002;11:550–6.

36. Johnson MP, McClure PW, Karduna AR. New method to assess scapular upward rotation in subjects with shoulder pathology. J Orthop Sports Phys Ther. 2001;31:81–9.

37. Umehara J, Sato Y, Ikezoe T, Yagi M, Nojiri S, Nakao S, et al. Regional differential stretching of the pectoralis major muscle: an ultrasound elastography study. J Biomech. 2021;121:110416.

38. Asayama A, Tateuchi H, Ota M, Motomura Y, Yanase K, Komamura T, et al. Differences in shear elastic modulus of the latissimus dorsi muscle during stretching among varied trunk positions. J Biomech. 2021;118:110324.

39. Izumi T, Aoki M, Tanaka Y, Uchiyama E, Suzuki D, Miyamoto S, et al. Stretching positions for the coracohumeral ligament: strain measurement during passive motion using fresh/frozen cadaver shoulders. Sports Med Arthrosc Rehabil Ther Technol. 2011;3:2.

40. Urayama M, Itoi E, Hatakeyama Y, Pradhan RL, Sato K. Function of the 3 portions of the inferior glenohumeral ligament: a cadaveric study. J Shoulder Elbow Surg. 2001;10:589–94.

41. Muraki T, Aoki M, Uchiyama E, Takasaki H, Murakami G, Miyamoto S. A cadaveric study of strain on the subscapularis muscle. Arch Phys Med Rehabil. 2007;88:941–6.

42. Wilk KE, Hooks TR, Macrina LC. The modified sleeper stretch and modified cross-body stretch to increase shoulder internal rotation range of motion in the overhead throwing athlete. J Orthop Sports Phys Ther. 2013;43:891–4.

43. Yamauchi T, Hasegawa S, Nakamura M, Nishishita S, Yanase K, Fujita K, et al. Effects of two stretching methods on shoulder range of motion and muscle stiffness in baseball players with posterior shoulder tightness: a randomized controlled trial. J Shoulder Elbow Surg. 2016;25:1395–403.

44. Ho CY, Sole G, Munn J. The effectiveness of manual therapy in the management of musculoskeletal disorders of the shoulder: a systematic review. Man Ther. 2009;14:463–74.

45. Crowell MS, Tragord BS. Orthopaedic manual physical therapy for shoulder pain and impaired movement in a patient with glenohumeral joint osteoarthritis: a case report. J Orthop Sports Phys Ther. 2015;45:453–61, A1–3.

46. Reinold MM, Macrina LC, Wilk KE, Fleisig GS, Dun S, Barrentine SW, et al. Electromyographic analysis of the supraspinatus and deltoid muscles during 3 common rehabilitation exercises. J Athl Train. 2007;42:464–9.

47. Boettcher CE, Ginn KA, Cathers I. Which is the optimal exercise to strengthen supraspinatus? Med Sci Sports Exerc. 2009;41:1979–83.

48. Reinold MM, Wilk KE, Fleisig GS, Zheng N, Barrentine SW, Chmielewski T, et al. Electromyographic analysis of the rotator cuff and deltoid musculature during common shoulder external rotation exercises. J Orthop Sports Phys Ther. 2004;34:385–94.

49. Sakita K, Seeley MK, Myrer JW, Hopkins JT. Shoulder-muscle electromyography during shoulder external-rotation exercises with and without slight abduction. J Sport Rehabil. 2015;24:109–15.

50. Clisby EF, Bitter NL, Sandow MJ, Jones MA, Magarey ME, Jaberzadeh S. Relative contributions of the infraspinatus and deltoid during external rotation in patients with symptomatic subacromial impingement. J Shoulder Elbow Surg. 2008;17:87S–92S.

51. Ginn KA, Reed D, Jones C, Downes A, Cathers I, Halaki M. Is subscapularis recruited in a similar manner during shoulder internal rotation exercises and belly press and lift off tests? J Sci Med Sport. 2017;20:566–71.

Corticosteroids, Nonsteroidal Anti-inflammatory Drugs, Oral Vitamins and Naturopathic Remedies That Can Help in Shoulder Arthritis

2

Dominik Szymski and Andreas Voss

2.1 Introduction

Arthritis of the glenohumeral joint is a common reason for pain and functional limitations of the shoulder caused by characteristic pathological changes. Thereby in patients older than 60 years, a prevalence rate of up to 20% is reported [1, 2]. Next to hip and knee joint degeneration, the glenohumeral osteoarthritis is one of the most relevant degenerative joint diseases. In the population of patients aged over 80 years, this issue becomes more notable with a mean prevalence rate of over 85%. Demographic change will make this problem even more serious and relevant in the future. Depending on patients' symptoms and severity of the degeneration, nonsurgical treatment options remain the first choice for the initial therapy of shoulder osteoarthritis. Next to physical therapy, which was highlighted in the previous chapter, pharmacological therapy is an integral component in the joint preservation process in patients with glenohumeral osteoarthritis.

The pathogenesis of glenohumeral osteoarthritis is complex and affected by various factors. Either abnormal load on normal cartilage or normal stress on abnormal cartilage leads to increased joint degeneration. In parallel with increasing age, the anabolic activity of the cartilage seems to decrease and catabolic processes predominate [3]. While degeneration of cartilage takes place, periarticular tissues of the synovia and subchondral bone, which are richly innervated, react on increased intraarticular pressure and cartilage damage with massive pain [1, 4]. Cartilage damage and subsequent subchondral sclerosis were mainly found in the cranial 2/3 of the humeral head. This zone is at between 60- and 100-degree abduction in contact with the glenoid and explains the immobilizing pain and functional limitations [1, 5].

Nonsurgical treatment of shoulder arthritis focusses on these processes and tries to break this circulus vitiosus. While the aim of physiotherapy is to restore and maintain the functionality of the joint (see Chap. 1), pharmacological therapy aims to reduce pain and diminish the process of joint degeneration. This chapter summarizes pharmacological treatment options with corticosteroids, nonsteroidal anti-inflammatory

D. Szymski · A. Voss (✉)
Department of Trauma Surgery, University Medical Center Regensburg, Regensburg, Germany

Sporthopaedicum Regensburg, Regensburg, Germany
e-mail: dominik.szymski@ukr.de;
voss@sporthopaedicum.de

A. D. Mazzocca et al. (eds.), *Shoulder Arthritis across the Life Span*,
https://doi.org/10.1007/978-3-031-33298-2_2

drugs, oral vitamins and naturopathic remedies for patients with glenohumeral osteoarthritis. Biologics as further nonsurgical option are discussed in Chap. 3.

2.2 Corticosteroids

The most common use of corticosteroids in shoulder arthrosis is intraarticular injections. However, these injections are often applied for patients with shoulder pain of all etiologies to treat an acute state of inflammation in the joint. The effects of corticosteroid injection only last for 4 weeks and can therefore be used for acute inflammatory and painful states, but corticosteroid injections do not show any positive effect on the development of cartilage or joint degeneration [6]. Nevertheless, an injection of corticosteroids can affect the cartilage negatively and even hasten the progression of glenohumeral osteoarthritis [7]. Local anesthetics are usually injected simultaneously with corticosteroids. In a recent meta-analysis of randomized controlled trials, Shanthanna et al. (2020) demonstrated that injections with corticosteroids provide no additional benefit compared to injections consisting of only local anesthetic agents [8]. Also, when using intraarticular corticosteroid injections, different adverse effects must be taken into account. In particular for patients suffering diabetes, increased episodes of hyperglycaemia and growing intraocular pressure are described [9]. At the same time, the number of injections performed should be limited to a maximum of three to prevent an increased risk of infection and further side effects [10].

Besides intraarticular injections, the oral prescription of corticosteroids for the treatment of shoulder arthritis is also possible. While some positive effects on the reduction of symptoms in osteoarthritis were mentioned, there is no effect on the progress of joint degeneration [11]. The adverse effects of systemically taken corticosteroids are very diverse and extensive; therefore an oral prescription cannot be recommended [12]. Also, the American Academy of Orthopaedic Surgeons (AAOS) discourages in their guidelines published in 2020 the use of corticosteroids, both for intraarticular and oral administration [13].

2.3 Nonsteroidal Anti-inflammatory Drugs (NSAIDs)

The most commonly used pharmacological therapy is based on nonsteroidal anti-inflammatory drugs (NSAIDs). By inhibition of cyclooxygenase (COX)-1 and COX-2 enzymes, the synthesis of prostaglandins is reduced and leads to reduction of inflammatory processes with concomitant analgesic effects. An improvement of symptoms was reported by up to 67% of patients with shoulder pain [12]. Compared to acetaminophen (paracetamol), NSAIDs demonstrated an increased pain reduction in osteoarthritis [14]. Due to a poorer side effect profile of unselective COX inhibitors, selective COX-2 inhibitors (e.g. celecoxib) are used especially for elderly patients and patients with comorbidities. Besides the oral application, the usage of topical NSAIDs is also a common part of therapy. Although topical administration does not achieve identical blood levels as oral administration, patients with shoulder osteoarthritis show sufficient pain reduction after several weeks of application [15]. On account of their good pain reduction and anti-inflammatory effect, NSAIDs are recommended as first-line therapy in the conservative treatment of shoulder osteoarthritis [16].

Although acetaminophens' (paracetamol) adverse effect profile is quite safe, the missing anti-inflammatory effect and low impact on peripheral COX enzymes are a possible reason for the advantages of NSAIDs [14]. Due to a better safety profile in particular in elderly patients, acetaminophen should be preferred to paracetamol.

2.4 Oral Vitamins

The National Institute for Health and Care Excellence (NICE) UK guidelines report the administration of oral vitamins as optional part for the treatment of shoulder arthrosis [12]. In particular vitamin C (ascorbic acid) and vitamin D showed positive effects on the development of cartilage. The chondroprotective mechanism of vitamin C is based on the antioxidant impact and the reduction of apoptosis. Simultaneously the stimulation of aggrecan and collagen synthesis increases the regenerative potential of the cartilage [17, 18]. Wang et al. (2004) demonstrated a threefold decrease in osteoarthritis by administering 120–200 mg of vitamin C [19]. Also, a sufficient pain reduction in patients with knee or hip osteoarthritis after oral supplementation of vitamin C was shown [19]. To our knowledge there is no clear evidence for the effects of vitamin C on shoulder arthrosis; nevertheless recent results in hip and knee arthrosis can be adopted to the glenohumeral joint.

Another oral supplement with benefits on degenerative joints is vitamin D preparations. Clinical studies demonstrated a controversial pattern with some trials showing a benefit in function and pain release of osteoarthritis joints, while some others could not find any positive impact after the administration of vitamin D. Though there are in clinical trials controversial results, in vivo studies demonstrated a reduction of cartilage degeneration in animals with increased vitamin D intake [20]. Taking these results into account, it can be assumed that the application of vitamin D with adverse effects (headache, nausea, obstipation) under consideration offers a potential as additional part of pharmacological treatment and is generally recommended by surgical societies [17, 21–23].

2.5 Naturopathic Remedies

Naturopathic drugs are often requested by patients with scepticism towards conventional oral medication and can be used as additional therapeutic part in the treatment of glenohumeral osteoarthritis. Various remedies act via identical receptors as conventional drugs (e.g. NSAIDs), but do not reach identical potency. Two of the most common used remedies are *Boswellia serrata* preparations and avocado-soya bean unsaponifiables (ASU). *Boswellia serrata* remedies act via direct inhibition of 5-lipoxygenase, which is a key enzyme in the production of leukotrienes and thus has a direct influence on inflammatory mediators [24]. Compared to placebo a light improvement of pain and function in patients with osteoarthritis was reported [25]. Due to a low rate of adverse side effects and a slightly positive effect on symptoms and function in patients with glenohumeral osteoarthritis, the administration of *Boswellia serrata* seems a suitable additional part of conservative treatment. In particular for the short-term use, avocado-soya bean unsaponifiables showed as well sufficient results with reduction of pain by over 30 points on the VAS scale (range 0–100). However long-term results show weaker effects of ASU. Measurement of the joint space showed also no significant improvement compared to placebo [25]. Liu et al. (2018) showed in their systematic review a sufficient pain reduction with clinical importance by administration of collagen hydrolysate, passion fruit peel extract, *Curcuma longa* extract, *Boswellia serrata* extract, curcumin, Pycnogenol and L-carnitine. For other supplements, as the above-mentioned avocado-soya bean unsaponifiables, statistically relevant relief of pain was also demonstrated, but clinical impact was unclear. Although a short-term reduction in pain and, in some cases, an improvement in function have been noted for phototherapeutic remedies, long-term results have not yet been able to fully confirm the positive effect. Likewise, the quality of the available studies to date is often weak; therefore the quality of evidence here is also quite low [26].

In recent years, the use of cannabis in medicine has grown and is also used in the pain therapy of osteoarthritis. Although there is to our knowledge no publication concerning the use in shoulder osteoarthritis, the topical application of cannabis (cannabidiol (CBD)) in knee and hip osteoarthritis showed already good results and could be adopted for the degenerative shoulder [27].

2.6 Conclusion

In the conservative treatment of glenohumeral osteoarthritis, administration of pharmacological agents is one of the major parts next to physiotherapeutical applications. The main aim of medical treatment is the reduction of pain and diminution of inflammation in the joint. To achieve this aim, NSAIDs are the one if the recommended medications and showed in oral and topical application sufficient results. Additionally, the supplementation of oral vitamins as vitamins C and D can help to slow down cartilage degeneration, while in the group of naturopathic remedies, *Boswellia serrata* and avocado-soya bean unsaponifiables can help in the reduction of pain and inflammation (Table 2.1). Depending on the individual comorbidities and contraindications, sufficient medication with good pain reduction is thus possible for each patient. This should interrupt the chronic inflammatory state in the joint and enable pain-free physical therapy exercise.

Table 2.1 Overall recommendations of multiple societies for pharmacological treatment in osteoarthritis adopted by Apostu et al. (2019) according to recommendations of the Royal Australian College of General Practitioners (RACGP), United Rheumatology, The College of Family Physicians of Canada (CFPC), the American Academy of Orthopaedic Surgeons (AAOS), the National Institute for Health and Care Excellence (NICE), the Osteoarthritis Research Society International (OARSI), the American College of Rheumatology (ACR) and American Family Physician (AFP) [17]

Application form	Drug	Recommendation
Systematic	Acetaminophen (paracetamol)	Recommended
	NSAIDs	Recommended
	Opioids	Not recommended
	Duloxetine	Recommended
	Glucosamine	Not recommended
	Pine bark extract	Inconclusive
	Vitamin D	Not recommended
	Omega-3	Not recommended
	Avocado-soya bean unsaponifiable (ASU)	Inconclusive
	Boswellia serrata	Inconclusive
	Curcuma	Inconclusive
Topical	NSAIDs	Recommended
	Capsaicin	Inconclusive
Intraarticular	Corticosteroids	Recommended
	Hyaluronic acid	Inconclusive

References

1. Ibounig T, Simons T, Launonen A, Paavola M. Glenohumeral osteoarthritis: an overview of etiology and diagnostics. Scand J Surg. 2021;110(3):441–51.
2. Kruckeberg BM, Leland DP, Bernard CD, Krych AJ, Dahm DL, Sanchez-Sotelo J, et al. Incidence of and risk factors for glenohumeral osteoarthritis after anterior shoulder instability: a US population-based study with average 15-year follow-up. Orthop J Sports Med. 2020;8(11):2325967120962515.
3. Shane Anderson A, Loeser RF. Why is osteoarthritis an age-related disease? Best Pract Res Clin Rheumatol. 2010;24(1):15–26.
4. Dieppe PA, Lohmander LS. Pathogenesis and management of pain in osteoarthritis. Lancet. 2005;365(9463):965–73.
5. De Palma AF. Surgery of the shoulder. Philadelphia: Lippincott; 1983.
6. Thomas M, Bidwai A, Rangan A, Rees JL, Brownson P, Tennent D, et al. Glenohumeral osteoarthritis. Shoulder Elbow. 2016;8(3):203–14.
7. Kompel AJ, Roemer FW, Murakami AM, Diaz LE, Crema MD, Guermazi A. Intra-articular corticosteroid injections in the hip and knee: perhaps not as safe as we thought? Radiology. 2019;293(3):656–63.
8. Shanthanna H, Busse J, Wang L, Kaushal A, Harsha P, Suzumura EA, et al. Addition of corticosteroids to local anaesthetics for chronic non-cancer pain injections: a systematic review and meta-analysis of randomised controlled trials. Br J Anaesth. 2020;125(5):779–801.
9. Gross C, Dhawan A, Harwood D, Gochanour E, Romeo A. Glenohumeral joint injections: a review. Sports Health. 2013;5(2):153–9.
10. Denard PJ, Wirth MA, Orfaly RM. Management of glenohumeral arthritis in the young adult. J Bone Joint Surg Am. 2011;93(9):885–92.
11. Latourte A, Kloppenburg M, Richette P. Emerging pharmaceutical therapies for osteoarthritis. Nat Rev Rheumatol. 2020;16(12):673–88.
12. Al-Mohrej OA, Prada C, Leroux T, Shanthanna H, Khan M. Pharmacological treatment in the management of glenohumeral osteoarthritis. Drugs Aging. 2022;39(2):119–28.
13. Khazzam MS, Pearl ML. AAOS clinical practice guideline: management of glenohumeral joint osteoarthritis. J Am Acad Orthop Surg. 2020;28(19):790–4.
14. Pincus T, Koch G, Lei H, Mangal B, Sokka T, Moskowitz R, et al. Patient preference for placebo,

acetaminophen (paracetamol) or celecoxib efficacy studies (PACES): two randomised, double blind, placebo controlled, crossover clinical trials in patients with knee or hip osteoarthritis. Ann Rheum Dis. 2004;63(8):931–9.

15. Derry S, Conaghan P, Da Silva JAP, Wiffen PJ, Moore RA. Topical NSAIDs for chronic musculoskeletal pain in adults. Cochrane Database Syst Rev. 2016;2016(4):CD007400.

16. Machado GC, Abdel-Shaheed C, Underwood M, Day RO. Non-steroidal anti-inflammatory drugs (NSAIDs) for musculoskeletal pain. BMJ. 2021;372:n104.

17. Apostu D, Lucaciu O, Mester A, Oltean-Dan D, Baciut M, Baciut G, et al. Systemic drugs with impact on osteoarthritis. Drug Metab Rev. 2019;51(4):498–523.

18. Jerosch J. Effects of glucosamine and chondroitin sulfate on cartilage metabolism in OA: outlook on other nutrient partners especially Omega-3 fatty acids. Int J Rheumatol. 2011;2011:969012.

19. Wang Y, Prentice L, Vitetta L, Wluka A, Cicuttini F. The effect of nutritional supplements on osteoarthritis. Altern Med Rev. 2004;9:275–96.

20. Li S, Niu G, Wu Y, Du G, Huang C, Yin X, et al. Vitamin D prevents articular cartilage erosion by regulating collagen II turnover through TGF-β1 in ovariectomized rats. Osteoarthritis Cartilage. 2016;24(2):345–53.

21. Sanaei M, Banasiri M, Shafiee G, Rostami M, Alizad S, Ebrahimi M, et al. Calcium vitamin D3 supplementation in clinical practice: side effect and satisfaction. J Diabetes Metab Disord. 2015;15:9.

22. Ding C, Jin X, Wang X, Cicuttini F, Wluka A, Zhu Z, et al. Vitamin D supplementation for the management of knee osteoarthritis: a randomized controlled trial. Osteoarthritis and Cartilage. 2016;24:S49.

23. Arden NK, Cro S, Sheard S, Doré CJ, Bara A, Tebbs SA, et al. The effect of vitamin D supplementation on knee osteoarthritis, the VIDEO study: a randomised controlled trial. Osteoarthritis Cartilage. 2016;24(11):1858–66.

24. Safayhi H, Mack T, Sabieraj J, Anazodo MI, Subramanian LR, Ammon HP. Boswellic acids: novel, specific, nonredox inhibitors of 5-lipoxygenase. J Pharmacol Exp Ther. 1992;261(3):1143–6.

25. Cameron M, Chrubasik S. Oral herbal therapies for treating osteoarthritis. Cochrane Database Syst Rev [Internet]. 2014 [cited 2022 Jun 11];(5). https://www.cochranelibrary.com/cdsr/doi/10.1002/14651858.CD002947.pub2/full.

26. Liu X, Machado GC, Eyles JP, Ravi V, Hunter DJ. Dietary supplements for treating osteoarthritis: a systematic review and meta-analysis. Br J Sports Med. 2018;52(3):167–75.

27. Deckey DG, Lara NJ, Gulbrandsen MT, Hassebrock JD, Spangehl MJ, Bingham JS. Prevalence of cannabinoid use in patients with hip and knee osteoarthritis. J Am Acad Orthop Surg Glob Res Rev. 2021;5(2):e20.00172.

Biologics in the Treatment of Glenohumeral Arthritis

3

Nobuyuki Yamamoto and Eiji Itoi

3.1 Introduction

Rotator cuff tears and glenohumeral osteoarthritis (OA) are two of the most common etiologies in clinical practice. Population-based studies suggest that 16.1–20.1% of adults older than 65 years have radiographic evidence of glenohumeral OA [1]. The gold standard of surgical treatment for glenohumeral OA has been the anatomic total shoulder arthroplasty (TSA). However, OA in young patients is still problematic and there is no consensus on treatment. Although TSA have been recommended for OA in young patients by some surgeons, long-term revision risk casts doubt on indications in a highly active and functionally demanding population. Complication rates are reported to be 12–15% at 5 years [2–4]. Glenoid component loosening is a major concern, with revision rates up to 70% at 15 years [5, 6].

Standard conservative treatments include medication such as anti-inflammatories, physical therapy, and corticosteroid injections. Corticosteroid injections are reported to be effective in many cases, but there are concerns regarding tendon and chondral toxicity [7]. Until recently, the next step in treatment was believed to be surgical treatment such as arthroplasty. Biologic injections such as platelet-rich plasma (PRP) and medicinal signaling cells (MSCs) have gathered increased attention over the past two decades. In fact, newer therapeutic options are now being increasingly used. There are some early successes in the use of biologic therapies for knee joint. For example, different formulations obtained through centrifugation of blood (PRP) and bone marrow aspirate appear as promising alternatives. Furthermore, cells obtained from adipose tissue have been proposed [8]. In this chapter, we review the biologic treatments in the glenohumeral OA. The effectiveness of the biologic injections and their mechanisms are also described.

3.2 Platelet-Rich Plasma Injections: Basic Science

PRP consists of a sample of autologous blood with platelet concentrations, which has been produced through the separation of whole blood by centrifugation. The term "platelet-rich plasma" includes a wide spectrum of PRP preparation protocols and formulations. Although some authors have attempted to characterize the various techniques in terms of preparation, content,

N. Yamamoto
Department of Orthopaedic Surgery, Tohoku
University School of Medicine, Sendai, Japan
e-mail: koyomoe@med.tohoku.ac.jp

E. Itoi (✉)
Department of Orthopaedic Surgery, Tohoku Rosai
Hospital, Sendai, Japan
e-mail: itoi-eiji@med.tohoku.ac.jp

© ISAKOS 2023
A. D. Mazzocca et al. (eds.), *Shoulder Arthritis across the Life Span*,
https://doi.org/10.1007/978-3-031-33298-2_3

and applications, no consensus has been reached thus far among experts in the field. The proposed mechanism is that PRP initiates the body's own repair processes, modulates inflammation, delivers growth factors, and attracts and activates MSCs, which promote a healing environment and reduce shoulder pain [9]. Especially, platelets possess biologically active growth factors, which have the potential to reduce joint inflammation, decrease cartilage breakdown, and promote tissue repair. It is believed that such elevated concentrations of growth factors may induce tissue healing. These factors include TGF-β, insulin-like growth factor, platelet-derived growth factor, basic fibroblast growth factor, and vascular endothelial growth factor.

3.3 Platelet-Rich Plasma Injections: Clinical Outcomes

There have been not many clinical studies evaluating the use of PRP injections to treat glenohumeral OA. A systematic review was undertaken by Robinson et al. [10] to evaluate the available evidence for biologic use in rotator cuff and glenohumeral OA. They concluded that biologics offer a relatively safe management option with inconclusive evidence for or against its use for rotator cuff pathology. No studies on glenohumeral OA met the inclusion criteria. There is one paper by Eliasberg et al. [11] reporting complications following biologic injections. In their study, the most common injections were intra-articular knee injections (50%), followed by intra-articular shoulder injections (21.4%). The most common underlying diagnosis was OA (78.5%). Types of injections included umbilical cord blood, PRP, bone marrow aspirate, placental tissue, and unspecified "stem cell" injections. Complications included infection (50%), suspected sterile inflammatory response (42.9%), and a combination of both (7.1%). They demonstrated that serious complications can occur following biologic injections, including infections requiring multiple surgical procedures and inflammatory reactions.

3.4 Bone Marrow Aspirate Injections: Basic Science

Bone marrow aspirate injections are becoming increasingly popular as a treatment for glenohumeral OA since it is included among the limited number of approaches. Bone marrow aspirate contains cells with the perceived capability to differentiate into cells that regenerate tissue functionality following injury [12]. In the literature, lots of mechanisms have been proposed to explain how bone marrow aspirate may work for cartilage lesions. Secretion of cytokines and growth factors through a paracrine mechanism play a role in anti-inflammation [13]. This paracrine activity is thought to stimulate angiogenesis and have anti-inflammatory properties [14]. MSCs are harvested from bone marrow, adipose, umbilical, or placental tissue sources. In vitro studies have shown these cells to express growth factors such as transforming growth factor beta (TGFβ) and vascular endothelial growth factor (VEGF), which are known to stimulate soft tissue repair [13].

3.5 Bone Marrow Aspirate Injections: Clinical Outcomes

The number of studies on the use of cell-based therapies, especially autologous bone marrow aspirate injections, to treat symptomatic knee osteoarthritis recently has grown. On the other hand, clinical evidence regarding the use of the bone marrow aspirate injection to treat glenohumeral OA is not enough. In a study by Centeno et al., 102 patients were treated with autologous bone marrow concentrate injections for symptomatic OA [15]. They observed preliminarily encouraging results following bone marrow concentrate injections for shoulder OA. A significant improvement was observed in the three outcome scores. Further large randomized trials remain necessary to determine the effectiveness of bone marrow aspirate injections on glenohumeral OA.

3.6 Adipose-Drived Stem Cell Injections: Basic Science

Adipose tissue is another major source of cells, considering that it can be easily accessed and harvested and that few complications have been reported with the procedure. Multiple mechanisms have been proposed for how adipose-drived stem cells (ASCs) may improve shoulder pain and function. Immunomodulatory and anti-inflammatory properties secondary to a paracrine secretion of growth factors and cytokines likely contribute to pain relief [13]. In micro-fragmented adipose tissue, these trophic properties can be attributed to the undifferentiated cells which are isolated from adult harvested adipose tissue [16]. Additionally, tendon needling when treating rotator cuff tears can have pain-relieving properties [17].

3.7 Adipose-Drived Stem Cell Injections: Clinical Outcomes

In 2004, Lendeckel et al. [18] reported a case of a 7-year-old girl suffering from widespread calvarial defects after severe head injury. Due to the limited amount of autologous cancellous bone available from the iliac crest, autologous ASCs were processed simultaneously and applied to the calvarial defects in a single operative procedure. CT scans showed new bone formation and near complete calvarial continuity 3 months after the reconstruction. There are two studies reporting stromal vascular fraction (SVF) outcomes on shoulder pain via arthroscopy. Jo et al. [19] treated 19 patients with rotator cuff tears with varying doses of culture expanded SVF at the time of an arthroscopic examination. Significant improvement was found at 6 months for the mid- and high-dose groups. Kim et al. [20] compared outcomes of surgical repair alone for rotator cuff tears against repair coupled with injection of adipose-derived MSCs loaded in fibrin glue. They found decreased re-tear rates in the surgery plus adipose-derived MSC group, but no significant differences in pain outcomes. There are few reports investigating the effect of ASC injections on patients with glenohumeral OA. Robinson et al. [21] evaluated the safety and clinical outcomes of patients treated with micro-fragmented adipose tissue for shoulder pain secondary to glenohumeral OA and rotator cuff tears. They concluded that micro-fragmented adipose tissue may be helpful to improve pain and function in patients with glenohumeral OA and rotator cuff tears. No major complications were identified in their case series. Striano et al. [22] conducted a study to evaluate 18 patients with OA and refractory shoulder pain who were treated with micro-fragmented adipose tissue. Significant improvement was observed at the 1-year follow-up in the clinical scores. There were no reports indicating any postprocedural complications or serious adverse events.

3.8 Amniotic Membrane and Umbilical Cord

The amnion is a natural, biodegradable tissue that exhibits low immunogenicity and stimulates new vascularization. Amniotic membrane (AM) and umbilical cord (UC) are well known to have anti-inflammatory properties and have been shown to promote healing in various orthopedic indications. In Ackley's [23] case series, ten patients received injection of 50 mg AM/UC for partial rotator cuff tears. The subjects range of motion was 77.9% at baseline and increased to 99.9% at 6 months. Follow-up MRI scans did not demonstrate any significant change in rotator cuff tear size. No adverse events were noted. This small case series provides preliminary data for the use of cryopreserved AM/UC particulate matrix in patients with partial rotator cuff tears. Nash et al. [24] investigated the process of TSA using a stemless system and how to incorporate the use of amnion matrix and platelet-rich plasma into the surgical technique. The rotator cuff interval is closed and the subscapularis is repaired in a side-to-side fashion with sutures. An amnion matrix is then applied over the subscapularis repair and fixed using sutures with the epithelial layer facing up. They concluded that the use of the stemless system along with biological agents likely produces an optimal outcome for patients with adequate humeral bone stock.

3.9 Conclusion

Although a potential benefit has been observed for knee osteoarthritis in the literature, this finding is not demonstrated to be reproducible in shoulder joint yet.

There are still questions regarding the use, indication, safety, and efficacy of biologics. Further large-scale randomized clinical trials need to be undertaken to determine the effectiveness of biologic injections.

References

1. Ansok CB, Muh SJ. Optimal management of glenohumeral osteoarthritis. Orthop Res Rev. 2018;10:9–18.
2. Wirth MA, Rockwood CA Jr. Complications of total shoulder-replacement arthroplasty. J Bone Joint Surg Am. 1996;78(4):603–16.
3. Bohsali KI, Wirth MA, Rockwood CA Jr. Complications of total shoulder arthroplasty. J Bone Joint Surg Am. 2006;88(10):2279–92.
4. Chin PY, Sperling JW, Cofield RH, Schleck C. Complications of total shoulder arthroplasty: are they fewer or different? J Shoulder Elbow Surg. 2006;15(1):19–22.
5. Lazarus MD, Jensen KL, Southworth C, Matsen FA 3rd. The radiographic evaluation of keeled and pegged glenoid component insertion. J Bone Joint Surg Am. 2002;84(7):1174–82.
6. Young A, Walch G, Boileau P, Favard L, Gohlke F, Loew M, Molé D. A multicentre study of the long-term results of using a flat-back polyethylene glenoid component in shoulder replacement for primary osteoarthritis. J Bone Joint Surg Br. 2011;93(2):210–6.
7. Dean BJ, Franklin SL, Murphy RJ, Javaid MK, Carr A. Glucocorticoids induce specific ion-channel-mediated toxicity in human rotator cuff tendon: a mechanism underpinning the ultimately deleterious effect of steroid injection in tendinopathy? Br J Sports Med. 2014;48(22):1620–6.
8. Francis SL, Duchi S, Onofrillo C, Di Bella C, Choong PFM. Adipose-derived mesenchymal stem cells in the use of cartilage tissue engineering: the need for a rapid isolation procedure. Stem Cells Int. 2018;2018:8947548.
9. Pourcho AM, Smith J, Wisniewski SJ, Sellon JL. Intraarticular platelet-rich plasma injection in the treatment of knee osteoarthritis: review and recommendations. Am J Phys Med Rehabil. 2014;93(11):S108–21.
10. Robinson DM, Eng C, Makovitch S, Rothenberg JB, DeLuca S, Douglas S, Civitarese D, Borg-Stein J. Non-operative orthobiologic use for rotator cuff disorders and glenohumeral osteoarthritis: a systematic review. J Back Musculoskelet Rehabil. 2021;34(1):17–32.
11. Eliasberg CD, Nemirov DA, Mandelbaum BR, Pearle AD, Tokish JM, Baria MR, Millett PJ, Shapiro SA, Rodeo SA. Complications following biologic therapeutic injections: a multicenter case series. Arthroscopy. 2021;37(8):2600–5.
12. DeChellis DM, Cortazzo MH. Regenerative medicine in the field of pain medicine: Prolotherapy, platelet-rich plasma therapy, and stem cell therapy—theory and evidence. Techn Reg Anesth Pain Manag. 2011;15(2):74–80.
13. Freitag J, Bates D, Boyd R, Shah K, Barnard A, Huguenin L, Tenen A. Mesenchymal stem cell therapy in the treatment of osteoarthritis: reparative pathways, safety and efficacy—a review. BMC Musculoskelet Disord. 2016;17:230.
14. Hudetz D, Borić I, Rod E, Jeleč Ž, Kunovac B, Polašek O, Vrdoljak T, Plečko M, Skelin A, Polančec D, Zenić L, Primorac D. Early results of intra-articular micro-fragmented lipoaspirate treatment in patients with late stages knee osteoarthritis: a prospective study. Croat Med J. 2019;60(3):227–36.
15. Centeno CJ, Al-Sayegh H, Bashir J, Goodyear S, Freeman MD. A prospective multi-site registry study of a specific protocol of autologous bone marrow concentrate for the treatment of shoulder rotator cuff tears and osteoarthritis. J Pain Res. 2015;8:269–76.
16. Bembo F, Eraud J, Philandrianos C, Bertrand B, Silvestre A, Veran J, et al. Combined use of platelet rich plasma & microfat in sport and race horses with degenerative joint disease: preliminary clinical study in eight horses. Muscles Ligaments Tendons J. 2016;6(2):198–204.
17. Krey D, Borchers J, McCamey K. Tendon needling for treatment of tendinopathy: a systematic review. Phys Sports Med. 2015 [cited 2019 Sep 9];43(1):80–6.
18. Lendeckel S, Jödicke A, Christophis P, Heidinger K, Wolff J, Fraser JK, Hedrick MH, Berthold L, Howaldt HP. Autologous stem cells (adipose) and fibrin glue used to treat widespread traumatic calvarial defects: case report. J Craniomaxillofac Surg. 2004;32(6):370–3.
19. Jo CH, Chai JW, Jeong EC, Oh S, Kim PS, Yoon JY, et al. Intratendinous injection of autologous adipose tissue-derived mesenchymal stem cells for the treatment of rotator cuff disease: a first-in-human trial. Stem Cells. 2018;36(9):1441–50.
20. Kim YS, Sung CH, Chung SH, Kwak SJ, Koh YG. Does an injection of adipose-derived mesenchymal stem cells loaded in fibrin glue influence rotator cuff repair outcomes? A clinical and magnetic resonance imaging study. Am J Sports Med. 2017;45(9):2010–8.

21. Robinson DM, Eng C, Mitchkash M. Outcomes after micronized fat adipose transfer for Glenohumeral joint arthritis and rotator cuff pathology: a case series of 18 shoulders. Muscles Ligaments Tendons J. 2020;10(3):393–8.

22. Striano RD, Malanga AG, Bilbool N, Khatira A. Refractory shoulder pain with osteoarthritis, and rotator cuff tear, treated with microfragmented adipose tissue. J Orthop Spine Sports Med. 2018;2(1):014.

23. Ackley JF, Kolosky M, Gurin D, Hampton R, Masin R, Krahe D. Cryopreserved amniotic membrane and umbilical cord particulate matrix for partial rotator cuff tears: a case series. Medicine (Baltimore). 2019;98(30):e16569.

24. Nash HM, Trang G, Bryant SA, Mirvish AB, Gardner BB, Chakrabarti MO, McGahan PJ, Chen JL. Stemless total shoulder arthroplasty with orthobiologic augmentation. Arthrosc Tech. 2021;10(2):e531–8.

Glenohumeral Arthritis: Nonoperative Management

4

Joseph Noack, Eric McCarty, and Mary K. Mulcahey

4.1 Patient Education/Activity Modification

When managing an athlete with glenohumeral OA, one of the most important initial steps is to make sure that the patient is educated on the diagnosis. For many athletes, understanding OA can be challenging, and it is important to provide an explanation of both the arthritic process and the potential long-term outlook on their condition. This includes a discussion of how this diagnosis may impact their athletic career [1]. Educating patients can help them make decisions regarding their treatment options and set expectations for their symptoms and function.

Activity modification may alleviate some of the symptoms related to glenohumeral joint OA. It is important for the athlete to understand which shoulder positions and actions cause pain and attempt to modify how they use their arms to limit these positions. This may be a particular challenge for the overhead throwing athlete, as well as for athletes who use their upper extremi-

ties heavily for their sport. Complete immobilization of the shoulder can lead to adhesive capsulitis and should be avoided [2]; however, limiting positions that cause extremes of range of motion, as well as avoiding activities that cause weight-bearing in the upper extremity, can help prevent exacerbations of pain.

4.2 Physical Therapy

Physical therapy (PT) can be useful in the management of symptoms related to glenohumeral OA. In particular, patients with minor radiographic changes and limitations in range of motion and strength are the most likely to benefit [1]. These characteristics are likely to be found in many of the younger athletes with early glenohumeral OA.

Physical therapy programs should incorporate joint mobilization techniques (active, active-assisted, and passive), with assessment of patient tolerance, and progress slowly as the patient gains increased mobility [3]. The physical therapist should also initiate a stretching program involving the rotator cuff, surrounding musculature, as well as the joint capsule. Using aids such as canes or sticks to assist with movement and stretching can be helpful.

After improvements in mobility and stretching have been obtained, strength training can be added to a physical therapy regimen with a

J. Noack · E. McCarty
Department of Orthopaedic Surgery, University of Colorado, Denver, CO, USA
e-mail: JOSEPH.NOACK@cuanschutz.edu;
ERIC.MCCARTY@cuanschutz.edu

M. K. Mulcahey (✉)
Department of Orthopedic Surgery and Rehabilitation, Loyola University Medical Center, Maywood, IL, USA
e-mail: mary.mulcahey@lumc.edu

© ISAKOS 2023
A. D. Mazzocca et al. (eds.), *Shoulder Arthritis across the Life Span*,
https://doi.org/10.1007/978-3-031-33298-2_4

focus on deltoid, the scapular girdle, and scapular balance [3]. Utilizing both isotonic and isometrics and advancing to concentric strength exercises are important when developing a strength training regimen [4]. Incorporating an aerobic exercise program in addition to the shoulder-focused strengthening has been shown to be beneficial. Additionally, once an athlete completes the dedicated course of physical therapy, it is important that they continue the exercise program at home, the gym, or their training facility to help maintain the improved range of motion and strength they gained from physical therapy.

While the data regarding the benefits of physical therapy in patients with glenohumeral osteoarthritis is limited, one case series found that the majority of patients who had a combined multimodal treatment regimen, including PT, found the therapy to be overall helpful in the management of their symptoms [5]. The general consensus is that in young patients who elect to proceed with nonoperative options, as well as in older patients who are not surgical candidates, PT can be particularly helpful in optimizing function and managing symptoms [6].

4.3 Oral Analgesics

Oral analgesics can be a helpful adjunct in the management of symptoms of glenohumeral OA. Acetaminophen (maximum dose 3–4 g/day) and nonsteroidal anti-inflammatory drugs (NSAIDs) can both be effective at alleviating symptoms. Through inhibition of cyclooxygenase, NSAIDs can prevent the production of proinflammatory mediators such as thromboxanes, prostaglandins, and prostacyclins. Approximately 50–67% of patients with underlying OA can expect improvement in pain with the use of NSAIDs [7]. Unfortunately, side effects related to NSAID use can affect many parts of the body including gastrointestinal (gastric irritation, stomach ulcers, bleeding), cardiac, and renal (renal failure), so these medications should be used cautiously and only when needed [8]. A meta-analysis found that 1 g of acetaminophen

dosed three to four times per day reduced pain relative to placebo; however, NSAIDs were found to be preferred by patients and provided more pain relief relative to acetaminophen [9]. Opioid pain medications should be avoided, if possible, given the abuse potential and high-risk side effect profile. Additionally, the use of opioid-related medications prior to shoulder replacement has been shown to lead to poor outcomes postoperatively [6]. It is important to have a detailed discussion with patients to ensure proper use of these medications and avoid potential side effects.

4.4 Alternative Therapies

At this time, there is no reliable evidence demonstrating the efficacy of alternative therapies such as acupuncture, dry needling, capsaicin, cannabidiol (CBD) oil, glucosamine and chondroitin, cupping, and transcutaneous electrical nerve stimulation (TENS) in the management of glenohumeral osteoarthritis. A Cochrane review from 2005, looking at the use of acupuncture in various shoulder-related disorders including osteoarthritis, did not find any clear evidence to support its use in these conditions [10]. The other alternative therapies have either no studies looking specifically at shoulder arthritis or single case reports supporting their use. Given the lack of evidence, these medications and modalities should be used cautiously [6].

4.5 Corticosteroid Injections

Intra-articular corticosteroid injections (CSI) have long been utilized in the management of pain and functional limitations related to shoulder OA. This procedure is often performed on initial evaluation of a patient with glenohumeral joint OA to improve symptoms and to assist with participation in physical therapy. Intra-articular corticosteroids reduce pain and inflammation by reducing synovial blood flow, lowering local leukocyte counts and inflammatory mediators, and altering collagen synthesis [11].

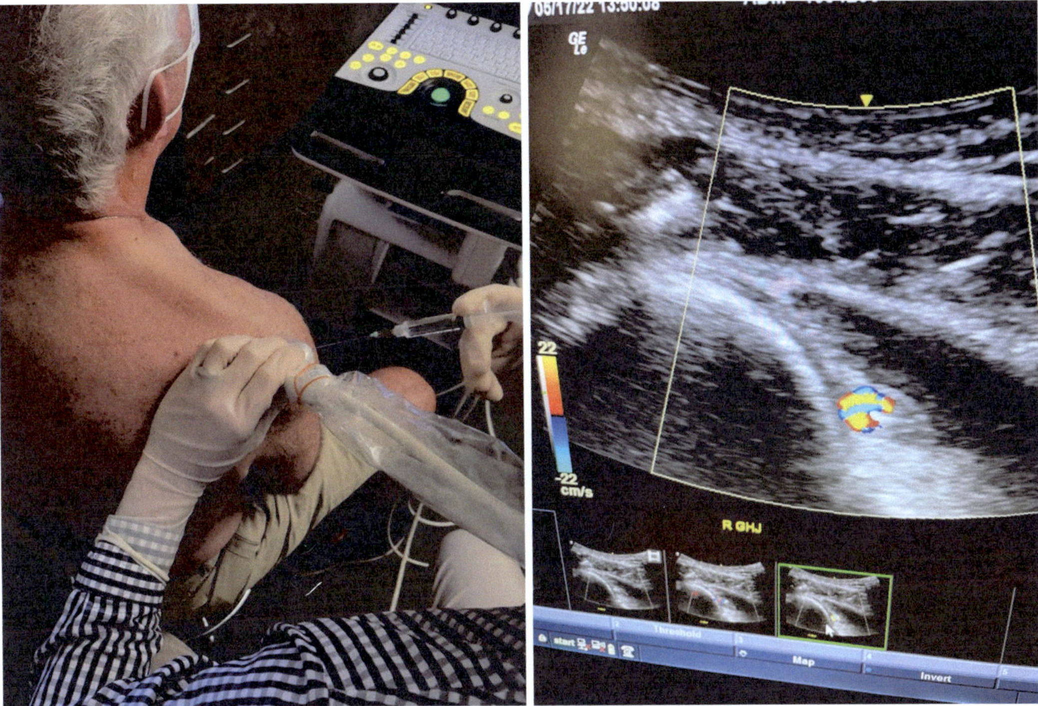

Fig. 4.1 Left: positioning for posterior approach to ultrasound-guided glenohumeral injection. Right: color flow Doppler confirming injection within the glenohumeral joint space

In 2021, Metzger et al. evaluated the efficacy of CSI in 30 patients with symptomatic glenohumeral OA [12]. The authors performed ultrasound-guided intra-articular corticosteroid injections and followed the patients for the next year evaluating pain and functional scores. They found that in the cohort of patients with more severe initial shoulder dysfunction, there were improvements in shoulder function up to 4 months after injection and pain improvement for up to 1 year, but it did not improve the time to surgery [12].

Using imaging guidance with either ultrasound or fluoroscopy has been shown to improve the accuracy of intra-articular glenohumeral joint injections (Fig. 4.1). In 2015, Aly et al. performed a meta-analysis evaluating the accuracy of landmark-based vs ultrasound-guided injections of the shoulder joint. They found that landmark-based injections had success rates of 72.5%, relative to 92.5% using an ultrasound-guided approach ($p = 0.025$) [13]. Patients with various shoulder conditions who underwent intra-articu-lar glenohumeral joint injections under image guidance with either ultrasound or fluoroscopy were also found to have improved outcomes relative to patients who underwent landmark-based injections [14]. Despite the potential benefit in symptom control from an intra-articular cortico-steroid injection, the physician must also balance this with the potential deleterious effects on carti-lage [15], in particular when treating the younger athlete.

4.6 Viscosupplementation

There have been numerous studies over the past 15 years evaluating the use of hyaluronic acid (HA) in the management of glenohumeral OA. Hyaluronic acid is a long polysaccharide chain that makes up a significant proportion of synovial fluid, and its content within the joint results in the viscoelasticity of synovial fluid. In an osteoarthritic knee, the concentration of HA is reduced by a factor of 2–3. This is related to both the inflammatory effusion, decreased production secondary to abnormal synoviocytes, and molecular fragmentation. This reduction can result in changes in the viscoelasticity of the synovial fluid, an alteration of the joint mechanics, and result in disruption of the underlying cartilage [16].

Initial, experimental studies showed promise as HA was noted to influence several key anti-inflammatory pathways within the synovium. In vitro and animal studies demonstrated that HA decreased mediators of inflammation such as prostaglandins and cAMP. HA was also demonstrated to have an analgesic effect on the synovium, related to both inhibition of nociceptors and decreasing synthesis of bradykinin and substance P [16, 17].

The use of hyaluronic acid in the treatment of arthritis was first described in the 1970s but was ultimately not approved by the FDA until 1997. Despite promising data for hyaluronic acid in other joints such as the knee, currently the American Academy of Orthopaedic Surgeons (AAOS) makes a strong recommendation against the use of hyaluronic acid injections in the treatment of glenohumeral OA. This recommendation is based on a few studies, which have failed to demonstrate a significant benefit of hyaluronic acid on the symptoms of glenohumeral OA [6].

In 2008, Blaine et al. performed a randomized control trial to determine the efficacy of hyaluronic acid in shoulder pain related to various etiologies [18]. The authors did not find any significant difference in pain scores between patients treated with HA and placebo; however in the subset of patients with underlying osteoarthritis, there was a noted statistical benefit in pain reduction at 6 months [18]. A recent meta-analysis regarding the use of HA for the management of glenohumeral OA evaluated 15 studies to determine the utility of HA in symptom and functional improvement [19]. The authors found an improvement in pain and functional outcomes in patients receiving intra-articular HA but also a similar improvement in the control groups indicating a strong placebo effect. They felt that while there was an improved functional outcome from baseline, it was not statistically different when compared to placebo or corticosteroid injection [19]. An additional recent review found no significant difference between HA and placebo or between HA and CSI when comparing functional and pain outcomes in adults with glenohumeral OA [20].

While intra-articular hyaluronic acid injections have shown intermittent promise with some improved outcomes when compared to baseline, overall, they have failed to show significant improvements when compared to placebo and at this time should not be routinely offered to athletes for the management of glenohumeral OA.

4.7 Biologic Therapies

The use of biologic options has become an area of increased focus in orthopedics in general over the past decade. While studies are gradually increasing and developing evidence suggesting benefit in numerous orthopedic conditions, their utility in treating osteoarthritis, and glenohumeral OA in particular, is relatively limited with only small retrospective studies and case studies supporting its use (Table 4.1) [21, 22].

Table 4.1 Biologic therapies available for the management of glenohumeral OA

Biologic therapy	Mechanism	Preparation time	Data in shoulder OA
Platelet-rich plasma	Growth factors reduce pro-inflammatory cytokines and slow catabolic pathways	~30 min	Limited, small studies and case reports
Alpha-2-microglobulin	Protease inhibitor reduces collagenases that can lead to cartilage catabolism	~30 min	None
Bone marrow aspirate concentrate	Recruits local progenitor cells and antagonizes local inflammatory mediators	~1 h	Limited, small studies
Mesenchymal stem cells	Anti-inflammatory and anti-catabolic effects through secretory process	~24 h	Limited, small studies

4.8 Platelet-Rich Plasma

Platelet-rich plasma (PRP) is autologous blood manipulated through centrifugation to produce an increased concentration of platelets. Through the specific preparation protocol used, the proportions of other cell components such as leukocytes and red blood cells can be manipulated. These include both leukocyte-rich (LR-PRP) and leukocyte-poor (LP-PRP) variations. The benefit of this preparation relies primarily on the components within the platelets themselves. The alpha granules within platelets contain high contents of proteins and growth factors, including platelet-derived growth factor (PDGF), TGF-B, and platelet factor 4, in addition to fibrinogen, albumin, and IgG [23, 24].

When platelets become activated, a large proportion of alpha granules are released, and the growth factors and other molecules within the platelets become active. The growth factors have the potential to reduce inflammation, decrease cartilage breakdown, and promote healing [25]. Through in vitro studies, these factors have been shown to promote a less inflammatory joint environment by reducing pro-inflammatory mediators such as cyclooxygenases and promoting the upregulation of anti-inflammatory mediators. Furthermore, PRP has shown an added benefit of slowing catabolic pathways within the joint. Through inhibition of matrix metalloproteinases (MMPs) such as MMP-3 and MMP-13, extracellular matrix protein degradation is prevented, and MMP catabolic effects are limited [23, 26, 27].

Despite a strong biochemical understanding of the theoretical benefits of PRP use in osteoarthritis, there is limited evidence evaluating the use of PRP in shoulder osteoarthritis. There is strong data in the literature demonstrating better outcomes with leukocyte-poor preparation (LP-PRP) in the treatment of knee OA, as opposed to the leukocyte-rich preparation of PRP [28]. With regard to data specifically examining outcomes in the shoulder, there is case report of a 62-year-old woman with pain related to underlying shoulder OA who underwent three ultrasound-guided LP-PRP injections into the glenohumeral joint over 3 consecutive weeks. The patient had improvement in pain and functional scores for the 42 weeks she was followed postinjection [21]. A recent retrospective study of patients with glenohumeral OA under age 50 found that LP-PRP improved pain in 86% of patients and that it was able to help delay arthroplasty in these patients [22].

4.9 Alpha-2-Microglobulin

A recently developed target for the management of osteoarthritis is alpha-2-microglobulin (A2M). This 720-kD protein complex is found primarily in the serum and acts as a protease inhibitor. The action of A2M is primarily through reduction in proteinases that can be harmful to underlying chondrocytes. Through in vitro as well as animal studies, A2M has been shown to inhibit MMP-13, reduce cytokine upregulation of collagenases, and decrease cartilage catabolism [29]. A recent study by Zhang et al. found that A2M variants inhibited cartilage degradation by up to 200% compared with wild-type A2M [30]. A2M is hypothesized to be a major contributor in the beneficial effects of PRP.

Intra-articular injections of A2M are currently being evaluated to determine if they have beneficial effects on the knee joint [29]. It is unclear if there are any current studies evaluating the potential effect of A2M in treating glenohumeral OA; however, if it is shown to be beneficial in clinical outcomes with regard to the knee, further evaluation in the shoulder may be warranted.

4.10 Cell Therapies

The two most common forms of cell therapies currently incorporated in orthopedic surgery are bone marrow aspirate concentrate (BMAC) and mesenchymal stem cells (MSCs).

The process of obtaining BMAC involves first harvesting the cell components through bone marrow aspiration (Fig. 4.2) and then undergoing a centrifugation process to separate the cell layers, which is overall similar to PRP. These layers include the primary cell lines of interest such as connective tissue stem and progenitor cells

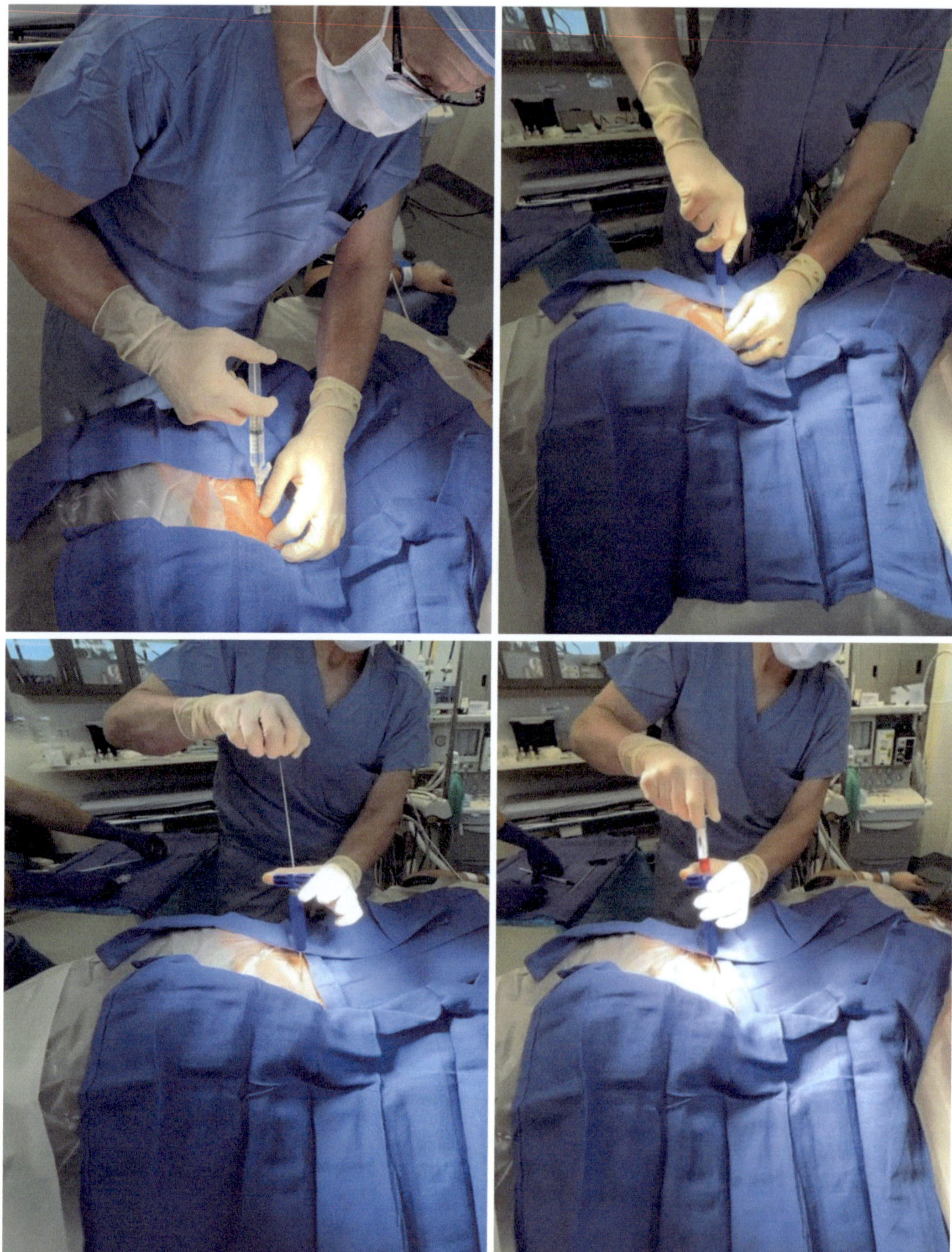

Fig. 4.2 Bone marrow aspiration technique from posterior iliac crest. Upper left: local anesthesia injected along the track to the iliac crest. Upper right: insertion of trocar needle and BMA cannula. Lower left: removal of trocar needle. Lower right: syringe attached to BMA cannula with aspiration of bone marrow from the iliac crest

and hematopoietic stem cells. The components of BMAC are hypothesized to result in tissue regeneration through stem cell and progenitor differentiation as well as recruitment of local progenitor cells and also limiting inflammation through high levels of IL-1 and IL-1B antagonism [21, 31].

Mesenchymal stem cells, on the other hand, are harvested through adipose tissue, primarily through liposuction at the abdominal fat pad. Adipose-derived stem cells (ADSCs) require a two-stage procedure, an initial aspiration followed by centrifugation and a period of incubation for 24–48 h prior to use. In comparison to BMAC, MSCs have been shown to have enhanced proliferative capacity and a longer retention of multipotency [32]. Similar to BMAC, MSCs have anti-inflammatory effects and influence the catabolic processes that take place within an osteoarthritic joint, primarily through a secretory effect [21].

There is limited data evaluating the use of these cell therapies for the management of glenohumeral OA. Studies examining both the use of BMAC and MSCs have been somewhat confounded by concomitant rotator cuff injuries in many of the patients studied. A study by Centeno et al. examining the use of image-guided intra-articular injection of BMAC for shoulder pathology found that patients with OA had significant improvement in pain outcome scores [33]. A more recent study compared a non-concentrated bone marrow aspirate injection to a corticosteroid injection for the management of glenohumeral OA. Although this was a small study (25 shoulders), the authors found significant differences in 3 of the 4 pain and functional outcomes studied in favor of BMAC [34]. In 2018, Striano et al. evaluated the efficacy of injecting ADSCs into the glenohumeral joint of patients and surrounding rotator cuff in patients with underlying shoulder pathology. A total of 95% of the patients in this study had shoulder OA on MRI. The authors found that the patients had improvement in pain and functional scores at various time points over the first year, however, a large proportion of these patients (75%) had rotator cuff pathology, and the study only included 20 patients [35]. Importantly, there were no serious adverse events related to ADSC injections noted during the study.

Over the past few years, several studies have been published evaluating the use of BMAC and MSCs in the management of knee OA and have shown promising results. However, the applicability of these studies to use in the treatment of glenohumeral OA remains to be seen, and more studies evaluating the use of these cell therapies in the shoulder are warranted, in order to better understand the potential beneficial effects.

4.11 Summary

Initial management of glenohumeral OA in athletes should focus on nonoperative options. A combined approach of activity modification and physical therapy can be effective. Oral medications such as acetaminophen and NSAIDs can provide patients with transient pain relief. Intra-articular corticosteroid injections may provide longer-term control of symptoms, but they must be used cautiously in athletes. There is mixed evidence for the efficacy of hyaluronic acid injections in the management of glenohumeral OA. Despite ongoing research related to the use of biologic modalities (PRP, A2M, BMAC, MSCs) in various orthopedic conditions, there is still limited evidence specifically regarding their use in glenohumeral OA. Further studies are necessary to determine the potential efficacy of these newer options.

References

1. Reineck JR, Krishnan SG, Burkhead WZ. Early glenohumeral arthritis in the competing athlete. Clin Sports Med. 2008;27(4):803–19.
2. Codsi M, Howe CR. Shoulder conditions: diagnosis and treatment guideline. Phys Med Rehabil Clin N Am. 2015;26(3):467–89.
3. Macías-Hernández SI, Morones-Alba JD, Miranda-Duarte A, Coronado-Zarco R, Soria-Bastida MD, Nava-Bringas T, Cruz-Medina E, Olascoaga-Gómez A, Tallabs-Almazan LV, Palencia C. Glenohumeral osteoarthritis: overview, therapy, and rehabilitation. Disabil Rehabil. 2017;39(16):1674–82.
4. Takamura KM, Chen JB, Petrigliano FA. Nonarthroplasty options for the athlete or active individual with shoulder osteoarthritis. Clin Sports Med. 2018;37(4):517–26.
5. Guo JJ, Wu K, Guan H, Zhang L, Ji C, Yang H, Tang T. Three-year follow-up of conservative treatments of shoulder osteoarthritis in older patients. Orthopedics. 2016;39(4):e634–41.
6. Khazzam MS, Pearl ML. AAOS clinical practice guideline: management of glenohumeral joint osteoarthritis. J Am Acad Orthop Surg. 2020;28(19):790–4.
7. Ansok CB, Muh SJ. Optimal management of glenohumeral osteoarthritis. Orthop Res Rev. 2018;10:9–18.

8. Nissen SE, Yeomans ND, Solomon DH, Lüscher TF, Libby P, Husni ME, Graham DY, Borer JS, Wisniewski LM, Wolski KE, Wang Q. Cardiovascular safety of celecoxib, naproxen, or ibuprofen for arthritis. N Engl J Med. 2016;(375):2519–29.

9. Zhang W, Jones A, Doherty M. Does paracetamol (acetaminophen) reduce the pain of osteoarthritis?: a meta-analysis of randomised controlled trials. Ann Rheum Dis. 2004;63(8):901–7.

10. Green S, Buchbinder R, Hetrick SE. Acupuncture for shoulder pain. Cochrane Database Syst Rev. 2005(2):CD005319.

11. Stephens MB, Beutler A, O'Connor FG. Musculoskeletal injections: a review of the evidence. Am Fam Physician. 2008;78(8):971–6.

12. Metzger CM, Farooq H, Merrell GA, Kaplan FT, Greenberg JA, Crosby NE, Peck KM, Hoyer RW. Efficacy of a single, image-guided corticosteroid injection for glenohumeral arthritis. J Shoulder Elbow Surg. 2021;30(5):1128–34.

13. Aly AR, Rajasekaran S, Ashworth N. Ultrasound-guided shoulder girdle injections are more accurate and more effective than landmark-guided injections: a systematic review and meta-analysis. Br J Sports Med. 2015;49(16):1042–9.

14. Soh E, Li W, Ong KO, Chen W, Bautista D. Image-guided versus blind corticosteroid injections in adults with shoulder pain: a systematic review. BMC Musculoskelet Disord. 2011;12(1):1–6.

15. Wernecke C, Braun HJ, Dragoo JL. The effect of intra-articular corticosteroids on articular cartilage: a systematic review. Orthop J Sports Med. 2015;3(5):2325967115581163.

16. Brockmeier SF, Shaffer BS. Viscosupplementation therapy for osteoarthritis. Sports Med Arthrosc Rev. 2006;14(3):155–62.

17. Ghosh P. The role of hyaluronic acid (hyaluronan) in health and disease: interactions with cells, cartilage and components of synovial fluid. Clin Exp Rheumatol. 1994;12(1):75–82.

18. Blaine T, Moskowitz R, Udell J, Skyhar M, Levin R, Friedlander J, Daley M, Altman R. Treatment of persistent shoulder pain with sodium hyaluronate: a randomized, controlled trial: a multicenter study. J Bone Joint Surg Am. 2008;90(5):970–9.

19. Zhang B, Thayaparan A, Horner N, Bedi A, Alolabi B, Khan M. Outcomes of hyaluronic acid injections for glenohumeral osteoarthritis: a systematic review and meta-analysis. J Shoulder Elbow Surg. 2019;28(3):596–606.

20. Tran K, Loshak H. Intra-articular hyaluronic acid for viscosupplementation in osteoarthritis of the hand, shoulder, and temporomandibular joint: a review of clinical effectiveness and safety.

21. Freitag JB, Barnard A. To evaluate the effect of combining photo-activation therapy with platelet-rich plasma injections for the novel treatment of osteoarthritis. BMJ Case Rep. 2013;2013:bcr2012007463.

22. Kany J, Benkalfate T, Favard L, Teissier P, Charousset C, Flurin PH, Coulet B, Hubert L, Garret J, Valenti P, Werthel JD. Osteoarthritis of the shoulder in under-50 year-olds: a multicenter retrospective study of 273 shoulders by the French Society for Shoulder and Elbow (SOFEC). Orthop Traumatol Surg Res. 2021;107(1):102756.

23. Rossi LA, Piuzzi NS, Shapiro SA. Glenohumeral osteoarthritis: the role for orthobiologic therapies: platelet-rich plasma and cell therapies. JBJS Rev. 2020;8(2):e0075.

24. Greenberg SM, Kuter DJ, Rosenberg RD. In vitro stimulation of megakaryocyte maturation by megakaryocyte stimulatory factor. J Biol Chem. 1987;262(7):3269–77.

25. Osterman C, McCarthy MB, Cote MP, Beitzel K, Bradley J, Polkowski G, Mazzocca AD. Platelet-rich plasma increases anti-inflammatory markers in a human coculture model for osteoarthritis. Am J Sports Med. 2015;43(6):1474–84.

26. Bendinelli P, Matteucci E, Dogliotti G, Corsi MM, Banfi G, Maroni P, Desiderio MA. Molecular basis of anti-inflammatory action of platelet-rich plasma on human chondrocytes: mechanisms of NF-κB inhibition via HGF. J Cell Physiol. 2010;225(3):757–66.

27. Kim HJ, Yeom JS, Koh YG, Yeo JE, Kang KT, Kang YM, Chang BS, Lee CK. Anti-inflammatory effect of platelet-rich plasma on nucleus pulposus cells with response of TNF-α and IL-1. J Orthop Res. 2014;32(4):551–6.

28. Riboh JC, Saltzman BM, Yanke AB, Fortier L, Cole BJ. Effect of leukocyte concentration on the efficacy of platelet-rich plasma in the treatment of knee osteoarthritis. Am J Sports Med. 2016;44(3):792–800.

29. Orhurhu V, Schwartz R, Potts J, Peck J, Urits I, Orhurhu MS, Odonkor C, Viswanath O, Kaye A, Gill J. Role of Alpha-2-microglobulin in the treatment of osteoarthritic knee pain: a brief review of the literature. Curr Pain Headache Rep. 2019;23(11):1–9.

30. Zhang Y, Wei X, Browning S, Scuderi G, Hanna LS, Wei L. Targeted designed variants of alpha-2-macroglobulin (A2M) attenuate cartilage degeneration in a rat model of osteoarthritis induced by anterior cruciate ligament transection. Arthritis Res Ther. 2017;19(1):1–1.

31. LaPrade RF, Geeslin AG, Murray IR, Musahl V, Zlotnicki JP, Petrigliano F, Mann BJ. Biologic treatments for sports injuries II think tank—current concepts, future research, and barriers to advancement, part 1: biologics overview, ligament injury, tendinopathy. Am J Sports Med. 2016;44(12):3270–83.

32. Burrow KL, Hoyland JA, Richardson SM. Human adipose-derived stem cells exhibit enhanced proliferative capacity and retain multipotency longer

than donor-matched bone marrow mesenchymal stem cells during expansion in vitro. Stem Cells Int. 2017;2017:2541275.

33. Centeno CJ, Al-Sayegh H, Bashir J, Goodyear S, Freeman MD. A prospective multi-site registry study of a specific protocol of autologous bone marrow concentrate for the treatment of shoulder rotator cuff tears and osteoarthritis. J Pain Res. 2015;8:269.

34. Dwyer T, Hoit G, Lee A, Watkins E, Henry P, Leroux T, Veillette C, Theodoropoulos J, Ogilvie-Harris D, Chahal J. Injection of bone marrow aspirate for glenohumeral joint osteoarthritis: a pilot randomized control trial. Arthrosc Sports Med Rehabil. 2021;3(5):e1431–40.

35. Striano RD, Malanga GA, Bilbool N, Azatullah K. Refractory shoulder pain with osteoarthritis, and rotator cuff tear, treated with micro-fragmented adipose tissue. Orthop Spine Sports Med. 2018;2(1):1–5.

Part II

Joint Preservation: Arthroscopic Management

Glenohumeral Osteoarthritis: Arthroscopic Management—Capsular Release, Chondroplasty, and Debridement

Christopher M. LaPrade, Mark E. Cinque, and Michael T. Freehill

5.1 Introduction

Glenohumeral osteoarthritis (GHOA) presents a challenging problem for young, active patients with Matsen et al. [1] reporting a significantly worsened quality of life and shoulder function. While arthroplasty may be an effective option for older patients, for younger patients, especially those with high demands, there is a concern of longevity following arthroplasty. In a systematic review of patients under 65 years undergoing total shoulder arthroplasty (TSA), Roberson et al. [2] reported a 17% revision rate and 54% rate of glenoid loosening at a mean of 9 years. These findings are similar to reports by Denard et al. [3] who reported the survivorship after TSA with a keeled glenoid implant was only 62.5% at 10 years in those under 55 years of age. These more recent reports build upon the previous studies showing poor long-term results in those undergoing hemiarthroplasty or TSA at a young age [4, 5].

Given these concerns for the longevity of arthroplasty, multiple studies have proposed arthroscopic procedures to provide relief to these young patients with GHOA [6–13]. A systematic review and meta-analysis by Sayegh et al. [14]

reported that arthroscopic debridement resulted in less complications than TSA or hemiarthroplasty with equal revision rate between the groups. In addition, they reported a similar satisfaction rating between TSA and arthroscopic debridement. This led the authors to conclude that arthroscopy may provide a safe short-term alternative to arthroplasty for younger patients with concern for arthroplasty [14]. Similarly, a Markov decision model was used by Spiegl et al. [15] to conclude that arthroscopic debridement was the preferred treatment for patients under 47 years with GHOA, while patients over 66 years would be more ideal for TSA. It should also be noted that young patients have a much lower incidence of primary GHOA with Saltzman et al. [16] reporting this number as low as 21% in those with a diagnosis of GHOA under the age of 50.

The purpose of this review is to first highlight the current literature regarding the treatment options for arthroscopic debridement for GHOA. This will include all reports including the use of arthroscopic debridement and lavage of the glenohumeral joint, oftentimes in conjunction with synovectomy, capsular releases, subacromial decompression, loose body removal, biceps tenotomy or tenodesis, or distal clavicle resection. Studies discussing comprehensive arthroscopic management (CAM) or those involving microfracture or cartilage transplantation will be discussed in separate chapters. We

C. M. LaPrade · M. E. Cinque · M. T. Freehill (✉)
Department of Orthopaedic Surgery and Sports Medicine, Stanford University,
Redwood City, CA, USA
e-mail: claprade@stanford.edu; Mec89@stanford.edu

© ISAKOS 2023
A. D. Mazzocca et al. (eds.), *Shoulder Arthritis across the Life Span*,
https://doi.org/10.1007/978-3-031-33298-2_5

will then illustrate the current clinical evidence for the arthroscopic debridement of GHOA.

5.2 Arthroscopic Treatment Options

After the exhaustion of nonoperative options, a surgical procedure to address GHOA may be required. A young patient with high demands may not be an ideal patient or even amenable to an arthroplasty procedure [2, 3, 14, 15, 17]. It is important to fully discuss the risks, benefits, and potential limitations of an arthroscopic procedure with a young patient emphasizing the goals of the procedure are to provide a period of improved function and relief of symptoms that may only be short-term [17–19].

Proper indications or contraindications are essential to the determination of the role of arthroscopy for a patient with GHOA. Studies have evaluated the results of arthroscopic debridement with other associated concomitant procedures and found worse results in those with high-grade (III or IV) Kellgren-Lawrence radiographic GHOA or intraoperative high-grade Outerbridge cartilage lesions [13, 20], cartilage lesions greater than 2 cm^2 [6], preoperative joint space narrowing less than 2 mm [12], bipolar cartilage lesions [6, 8, 12], and large osteophytes [12]. Grade IV Kellgren-Lawrence lesions included those with severe loss of joint space, osteophyte formation, and loss of concentricity between the humeral head and glenoid [13] (Table 5.1). Figure 5.1 demonstrates an example

Table 5.1 Indications and contraindications for arthroscopic debridement for glenohumeral osteoarthritis

Indications	Relative contraindications
Advanced symptomatic GH arthritis	Bipolar cartilage lesions
Young patient (<55 years)	<2 mm joint space on radiographs
Active or high-demand	Grade III or IV Kellgren-Lawrence
Failure of nonoperative treatment	Large humeral head osteophytes
Acceptance of potential short-term benefits	>2 cm^2 cartilage lesions

of radiographic and magnetic resonance imaging (MRI) from a patient that chose to undergo arthroscopic debridement, loose body removal, and open biceps tenodesis.

A recent review outlined the many different pathologies often seen in association with GHOA and the recommended procedures to perform in conjunction with arthroscopic debridement [17]. These associated procedures include (1) synovectomy for synovitis, (2) chondroplasty for cartilage fraying or fragmentation, (3) loose body removal, (4) capsular release for capsular tightness or decreased range of motion (ROM), (5) subacromial decompression for subacromial impingement, as well as more complex procedures such as microfracture or osteoplasty as indicated. In addition, a biceps tenotomy or tenodesis may be indicated if there is pathology of the long head of the biceps [7, 17, 21] or distal clavicle resection if concomitant acromioclavicular (AC) joint arthritis is present [7].

Williams et al. [19] performed a systematic review on the outcomes after arthroscopic debridement for GHOA. They included eight studies that fulfilled the requirements of describing the debridement procedure and reported on clinical outcomes following the procedures [19]. They classified the procedures into three categories of "escalating intervention."

The first category of three studies described largely "simple debridement procedures" [7, 8, 13] that described arthroscopic lavage, debridement of degenerative labral or cartilage lesions, loose body removal, partial synovectomy or osteophytectomy, distal clavicle resection, or subacromial decompression as indicated [19]. Henry et al. [7] also included debridement of partial tears of biceps up to 50% through the tendon, while tears more than 50% were treated with tenodesis or tenotomy. The debridement of degenerative chondral or labral lesions, as well as loose body removal, can help to improve mechanical symptoms [22, 23]. Studies have hypothesized that lavage may have a role in removing proinflammatory enzymes and proteins in the synovial fluid [13, 23]. The involvement of subacromial decompression or distal clavicle resec-

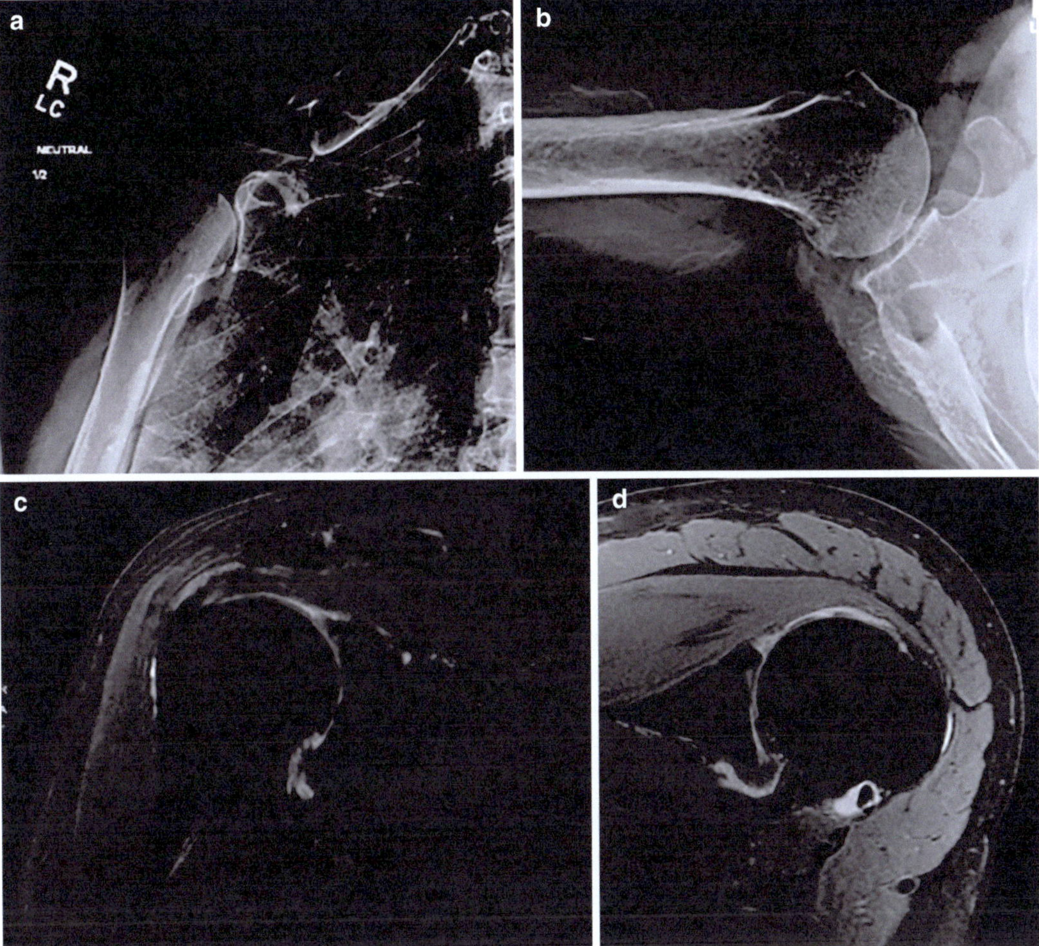

Fig. 5.1 Representative imaging from a patient who chose to undergo arthroscopic management of her right shoulder glenohumeral osteoarthritis (GHOA). Radiographic AP (**a**) and axillary (**b**) views demonstrating grade II Kellgren-Lawrence GHOA. Magnetic resonance imaging (MRI) further demonstrating the GHOA with T2 coronal (**c**) and axial (**d**) images

tion may help to additionally address concomitant sources of pain [7].

The next level of complexity involves the above arthroscopic debridement with additional releases including release of the rotator interval, release of middle or inferior glenohumeral ligaments, or anterior, posterior, or inferior capsular releases [6, 10, 11]. As theorized by Richards et al. [10], by releasing the capsule, there are decreased joint contact pressures through a greater range of motion. They stated that "capsular release may not prevent the osteoarthritic cascade, but it may provide a window of improved symptoms and function before deterioration of the joint leads to a more significant operation, especially in those younger patients with mild or moderate osteoarthritic changes with physically demanding occupations or vocations" [10].

Finally, the last level of complexity as described by Williams et al. [19] was the "most comprehensive treatments" further addressing bony, chondral, and soft tissue pathology. These included the addition of microfracture, fluoroscopically guided removal of humeral head osteophytes, and/or axillary nerve neurolysis [9, 12]. These more complex procedures, especially those involving microfracture and the CAM procedure, are beyond the scope of this article and will be discussed in the subsequent chapters.

The preferred arthroscopic technique for the senior author involves a systematic approach to addressing any potential sources of pain in the shoulder (Figs. 5.2 and 5.3). Similar to other reports, a careful consideration of all the possible sources of pain should be made [17, 22, 23]. We commonly perform an extensive debridement and edge stabilization of any cartilage or labral pathology to help improve mechanical symptoms in association with loose body removal and synovectomy. Given the known role of long head of the biceps tendon as a pain generator in the shoulder [24, 25], especially given its complex innervation of sensory sympathetic fibers that may play a role in pain [26], we will routinely perform a biceps tenodesis versus a tenotomy depending on patient-specific factors. We do believe that tenotomy is an acceptable option, especially given the systematic review and meta-analysis by Ahmed et al. [27] showing no significant differences between biceps tenodesis and tenotomy for clinical outcomes or supination strength. However, given the significantly higher risk of Popeye deformity after tenotomy [27], and our clinical experience of patient's dissatisfaction with this occurrence, we usually choose to perform a tenodesis. In addition, we will perform a subacromial decompression, as well as an AC joint resection if indicated. A capsular release is also a routine part of this procedure; however, this differs from the axillary neurolysis performed with the capsular releases as part of the CAM procedure [9, 17].

Lastly, if there are significant larger unipolar focal cartilage defects or humeral inferior osteophytes, we will consider progression to more complex procedures such as microfracture or the CAM procedure, both of which will be covered in subsequent chapters. In particular, we agree with Millett et al. [17] that arthroscopic debridement only would not be able to address the pain generator, that is, the large inferior humeral osteophyte, which may additionally require an axillary nerve neurolysis given the close proximity of the nerve to inferior humeral osteophytes.

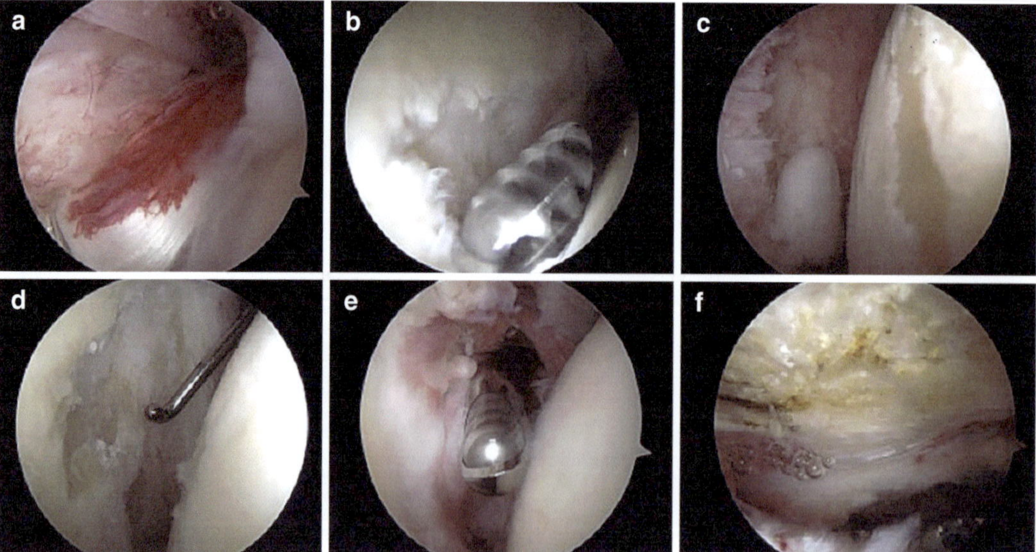

Fig. 5.2 Arthroscopic images from the same patient in Fig. 5.1 demonstrating (**a**) long head biceps tenosynovitis treated with an open subpectoral tenodesis, (**b**) chondroplasty for cartilage lesions, (**c**) grade 2–3 humeral head chondromalacia and a loose body that was removed, (**d**) grade 3–4 glenoid chondromalacia, (**e**) capsular release of the rotator interval (majority performed with radiofrequency and arthroscopic cutters), and (**f**) subacromial decompression

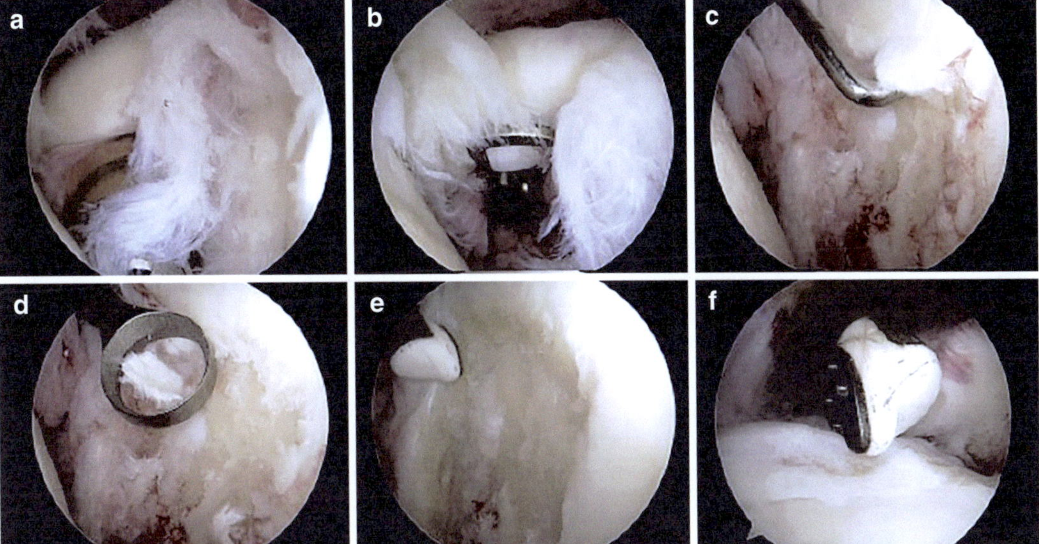

Fig. 5.3 Arthroscopic images demonstrating (**a**, **b**) significant degenerative fraying of the biceps and superior labrum treated with debridement and open biceps tenodesis after intra-articular tenotomy, (**c–e**) grade 3 chondromalacia of the glenoid treated with chondroplasty and edge stabilization, and (**f**) capsular releases of the rotator interval

The procedure can be performed in the lateral decubitus or beach chair position depending on surgeon comfort and familiarity.

5.3 Clinical Outcomes After Arthroscopic Debridement

Williams et al. [19] reported on a systematic review of all studies reporting on clinical outcomes after arthroscopic debridement of GHOA confirmed during arthroscopy. Of the eight studies included, one reported on the CAM procedure [9], while the other seven reported on arthroscopic debridement in combination with other concomitant procedures. All seven studies focusing on arthroscopic debridement were level IV with follow-up ranging from a mean of 13.7 months to 43.4 months [19]. The mean age in these studies ranged from 38 to 59 years of age [19].

Weinstein et al. [13] reported in 2000 on 25 patients treated with "lavage of the glenohumeral joint, debridement of labral tears and chondral lesions, loose body removal, and partial synovectomy and subacromial bursectomy." At a mean follow-up of 34 months, results were rated as excellent in 2 patients (8%), good in 19 patients (72%), and unsatisfactory in 5 (20%). They noted that 26% of patients with grade III or grade IV articular cartilage lesions during arthroscopy had unsatisfactory results. They categorized the results as excellent if the patients had "no pain, full use of the extremity, and essentially normal motion and strength" [13]. Kerr and McCarty [8] reported on a similar surgical protocol in 20 shoulders with arthroscopic debridement as well as other concomitant procedures including subacromial decompression with or without acromioplasty (65%), biceps tenotomy (25%), distal clavicle resection (10%), microfracture (10%), or SLAP repair (5%). They excluded those with rotator cuff pathology and had a mean follow-up of 20 months. The average Single Assessment Numeric Evaluation (SANE) score was 71% of normal shoulder function postoperatively [8]. They did not find any difference in clinical outcomes scores between those with grade 2 cartilage changes versus those with grade 3 or 4 lesions; however, they did report that those with bipolar lesions of the articular cartilage of the glenoid and humerus had significantly worse SANE, American Shoulder and Elbow Surgeons (ASES), and Western Ontario Osteoarthritis of the Shoulder (WOOS) scores than those with unipolar cartilage lesions [8]. Additionally, Henry et al. [7] reported on a similar technique with debridement and synovectomy in association with acromioplasty in 82%, distal clavicle resection in 57%, and biceps tenodesis or tenotomy in 7%. They reported on 56 patients with at least 2-year follow-up and excluded any patients with rotator cuff injury [7]. At 1- or 2-year follow-up, they reported statistically significant improvement in Constant and ASES scores, strength, and active pain-free ROM. However, at a mean of 26 months, 32% had planned or undergone arthroplasty. While there were no differences prior to debridement between those progressing to arthroplasty for age, symptom duration, or sex, the patients who progressed to arthroplasty had significantly worse Constant and ASES scores and pain-free ROM post-debridement [7].

In addition to arthroscopic debridement, there have been multiple studies that additionally included capsular releases to their surgical protocol [6, 10–12]. Cameron et al. [6] reported on 61 patients with grade IV osteochondral lesions at mean 34 months of follow-up. These patients underwent arthroscopic debridement with additional concomitant procedures of capsular release (36%), acromioplasty (30%), distal clavicle resection (15%), and rotator cuff debridement (5%). They reported a significant improvement in patient satisfaction after surgery with 87% indicating they would choose to undergo surgery again [6]. Pain relief occurred in 88% of patients with the average pain relief lasting 28 months. Patients without pain relief (12%) or with pain that returned (31%) were reported to have cartilage lesions greater than 2 cm^2 and bipolar cartilage lesions [6]. In the patients who underwent capsular release, there was a significant improvement in forward elevation and external rotation postoperatively [6]. Overall, 10% of patients underwent conversion to arthroplasty with these occurring at a mean of 16 months after debridement. Richards and Burkhart [10] reported on eight patients at a mean of 13 months after

arthroscopic debridement with the addition of releases of the rotator interval, anterior capsule, posterior capsule, and axillary recess. In addition, the authors also described a distal clavicle resection or subacromial decompression if indicated. They reported a ROM improvement postoperatively for forward elevation (21°), external rotation (17°), and internal rotation (31°) [10]. Van Thiel et al. [12] reported on 71 patients with a follow-up mean of 27 months undergoing arthroscopic debridement plus concomitant procedures of capsular releases (62%), subacromial decompressions (39), biceps tenodesis or tenotomy (20%), loose body or osteophyte removal (17%), and microfracture (15%). They excluded all concomitant labral or rotator cuff repairs [12]. The authors reported significantly improved visual analog scale (VAS), ASES, and Simple Shoulder Test (SST) scores, as well as ROM in flexion, abduction, and external rotation, after debridement, without any significant improvements in Short Form 12 scores after debridement [12]. They reported that 16% underwent arthroplasty at a mean 10 months after debridement. Those who underwent arthroplasty had significantly less joint space and larger humeral head osteophytes, in addition to all having grade IV articular cartilage damage and 88% having bipolar cartilage lesions [12].

Lastly, Skelley et al. [11] reported on 33 patients undergoing arthroscopic debridement and capsular release at a mean follow-up of 43.4 months. Their capsular releases included releases of the rotator interval, middle and inferior glenohumeral ligaments, and anterior and inferior capsule. In contrast to the above studies, this study excluded all patients who underwent concomitant procedures, such as subacromial decompression, rotator cuff repair, or distal clavicle resection [11]. The authors reported a satisfaction rate of only 40% with an initial significant improvement in VAS score and active external rotation and forward elevation at the first postoperative visit. At approximately 3 months, the VAS scores and ROM were not significantly improved from preoperative levels [11]. The authors also reported that 42% of patients underwent arthroplasty at a mean of 38 weeks after arthroscopic debridement [11]. The poor results in their study lead the authors to conclude that isolated arthroscopic debridement for GHOA without addressing other possible concomitant factors contributing to pain is unlikely to result in substantial benefit [11].

5.4   Conclusion

In young, active patients with high demands, shoulder arthroscopy with debridement may provide a short-term benefit to help delay performing an arthroplasty. The current literature lacks the level I or II evidence to definitively state the benefits of arthroscopic debridement, but it does seem to support that the debridement should be performed in conjunction with other indicated procedures, such as subacromial decompression, capsular releases, biceps tenodesis or tenotomy, or distal clavicle excision. Even in conjunction with these procedures, it should be emphasized in discussion with patients the likely need for eventual arthroplasty. Additionally, it is unclear whether the addition of more complex procedures, such as microfracture or osteoplasty for osteophyte resection, is beneficial. We recommend future studies to compare the addition of these procedures to the arthroscopic debridement discussed in this chapter.

References

1. Matsen FA 3rd, Ziegler DW, DeBartolo SE. Patient self-assessment of health status and function in glenohumeral degenerative joint disease. J Shoulder Elbow Surg. 1995;4(5):345–51.
2. Roberson TA, Bentley JC, Griscom JT, Kissenberth MJ, Tolan SJ, Hawkins RJ, Tokish JM. Outcomes of total shoulder arthroplasty in patients younger than 65 years: a systematic review. J Shoulder Elbow Surg. 2017;26(7):1298–306.
3. Denard PJ, Raiss P, Sowa B, Walch G. Mid- to long-term follow-up of total shoulder arthroplasty using a keeled glenoid in young adults with primary glenohumeral arthritis. J Shoulder Elbow Surg. 2013;22(7):894–900.
4. Deshmukh AV, Koris M, Zurakowski D, Thornhill TS. Total shoulder arthroplasty: long-term survivorship, functional outcome, and quality of life. J Shoulder Elbow Surg. 2005;14(5):471–9.
5. Sperling JW, Cofield RH, Rowland CM. Minimum fifteen-year follow-up of Neer hemiarthroplasty and total shoulder arthroplasty in patients aged fifty years or younger. J Shoulder Elbow Surg. 2004;13(6):604–13.
6. Cameron BD, Galatz LM, Ramsey ML, Williams GR, Iannotti JP. Non-prosthetic management of grade IV osteochondral lesions of the glenohumeral joint. J Shoulder Elbow Surg. 2002;11(1):25–32.
7. Henry P, Razmjou H, Dwyer T, Slade Shantz JA, Holtby R. Relationship between probability of future shoulder arthroplasty and outcomes of arthroscopic debridement in patients with advanced osteoarthritis of glenohumeral joint. BMC Musculoskelet Disord. 2015;16:280.
8. Kerr BJ, McCarty EC. Outcome of arthroscopic debridement is worse for patients with glenohumeral arthritis of both sides of the joint. Clin Orthop Relat Res. 2008;466(3):634–8.
9. Mitchell JJ, Warner BT, Horan MP, Raynor MB, Menge TJ, Greenspoon JA, Millett PJ. Comprehensive arthroscopic management of glenohumeral osteoarthritis: preoperative factors predictive of treatment failure. Am J Sports Med. 2017;45(4):794–802.
10. Richards DP, Burkhart SS. Arthroscopic debridement and capsular release for glenohumeral osteoarthritis. Arthroscopy. 2007;23(9):1019–22.
11. Skelley NW, Namdari S, Chamberlain AM, Keener JD, Galatz LM, Yamaguchi K. Arthroscopic debridement and capsular release for the treatment of shoulder osteoarthritis. Arthroscopy. 2015;31(3):494–500.
12. Van Thiel GS, Sheehan S, Frank RM, Slabaugh M, Cole BJ, Nicholson GP, Romeo AA, Verma NN. Retrospective analysis of arthroscopic management of glenohumeral degenerative disease. Arthroscopy. 2010;26(11):1451–5.
13. Weinstein DM, Bucchieri JS, Pollock RG, Flatow EL, Bigliani LU. Arthroscopic debridement of the shoulder for osteoarthritis. Arthroscopy. 2000;16(5):471–6.
14. Sayegh ET, Mascarenhas R, Chalmers PN, Cole BJ, Romeo AA, Verma NN. Surgical treatment options for glenohumeral arthritis in young patients: a systematic review and meta-analysis. Arthroscopy. 2015;31(6):1156–1166.e8.
15. Spiegl UJ, Faucett SC, Horan MP, Warth RJ, Millett PJ. The role of arthroscopy in the management of glenohumeral osteoarthritis: a Markov decision model. Arthroscopy. 2014;30(11):1392–9.
16. Saltzman MD, Mercer DM, Warme WJ, Bertelsen AL, Matsen FA 3rd. Comparison of patients undergoing primary shoulder arthroplasty before and after the age of fifty. J Bone Joint Surg Am. 2010;92(1):42–7.
17. Millett PJ, Fritz EM, Frangiamore SJ, Mannava S. Arthroscopic management of glenohumeral arthritis: a joint preservation approach. J Am Acad Orthop Surg. 2018;26(21):745–52.
18. Denard PJ, Wirth MA, Orfaly RM. Management of glenohumeral arthritis in the young adult. J Bone Joint Surg Am. 2011;93(9):885–92.

19. Williams BT, Beletsky A, Kunze KN, Polce EM, Cole BJ, Verma NN, Chahla J. Outcomes and survivorship after arthroscopic treatment of glenohumeral arthritis: a systematic review. Arthroscopy. 2020;36(7):2010–21.
20. Guyette TM, Bae H, Warren RF, Craig E, Wickiewicz TL. Results of arthroscopic subacromial decompression in patients with subacromial impingement and glenohumeral degenerative joint disease. J Shoulder Elbow Surg. 2002;11(4):299–304.
21. Pitta M, Davis W 3rd, Argintar EH. Arthroscopic management of osteoarthritis. J Am Acad Orthop Surg. 2016;24(2):74–82.
22. Chong PY, Srikumaran U, Kuye IO, Warner JJ. Glenohumeral arthritis in the young patient. J Shoulder Elbow Surg. 2011;20(2 Suppl):S30–40.
23. Saltzman BM, Leroux TS, Verma NN, Romeo AA. Glenohumeral osteoarthritis in the young patient. J Am Acad Orthop Surg. 2018;26(17):e361–70.
24. Ahrens PM, Boileau P. The long head of biceps and associated tendinopathy. J Bone Joint Surg Br. 2007;89(8):1001–9.
25. Nho SJ, Strauss EJ, Lenart BA, Provencher MT, Mazzocca AD, Verma NN, Romeo AA. Long head of the biceps tendinopathy: diagnosis and management. J Am Acad Orthop Surg. 2010;18(11):645–56.
26. Alpantaki K, McLaughlin D, Karagogeos D, Hadjipavlou A, Kontakis G. Sympathetic and sensory neural elements in the tendon of the long head of the biceps. J Bone Joint Surg Am. 2005;87(7):1580–3.
27. Ahmed AF, Toubasi A, Mahmoud S, Ahmed GO, Al Ateeq Al Dosari M, Zikria BA. Long head of biceps tenotomy versus tenodesis: a systematic review and meta-analysis of randomized controlled trials. Shoulder Elbow. 2021;13(6):583–91.

Emilio Calvo, Carlos Rebollon Guardado,
and Vanesa Lopez Fernandez

6.1 Introduction

Osteoarthritis (OA) of the glenohumeral joint is a common and disabling condition characterized by symptoms of weakness, pain, sleep disturbance, and decreased range of motion [1]. Currently, nonoperative modalities including activity and/or occupation modifications, physical therapy, pharmacotherapy with nonsteroidal anti-inflammatory medications, steroid injections, and viscosupplementation are the first-line treatment of choice as they are capable of reducing symptoms improving quality of life [2–4]. When standard nonsurgical methods are unsuccessful, total shoulder arthroplasty (TSA) provides predictable clinical outcomes with low revision rates and high patient satisfaction in elderly or low-demand population. However, although glenohumeral OA typically manifest after sixth decade of life [5], younger patients may also suffer from this affection. In those

patients who are symptomatic but radiographically show less advanced disease, or those who maintain demanding lifestyles, TSA may not be the best option because it has shown undesirable outcomes with decreased component survival [6–8].

As arthroscopic technique has evolved, more recent evidence suggests that carefully selected patients with glenohumeral osteoarthritis may benefit from it, providing pain relief and delaying the need for arthroplasty, which is why this technique has been included in the low-risk management options [9, 10]. In 2011 Millet and colleagues [11] described the CAM procedure, an acronym for comprehensive arthroscopic management. It is a joint-preserving arthroscopic approach for young, active patients with advanced shoulder osteoarthritis that addresses the different pain generators and pathoanatomic features that lead to functional deficits in glenohumeral osteoarthritis [12]. The CAM procedure includes classic arthroscopic debridement features such as synovectomy, loose body removal, subacromial decompression, chondroplasty, and microfractures but also involves an extensive capsular release, biceps tenotomy or tenodesis, and humeral osteoplasty or osteophyte excision (goat's beard removal) to reshape the humeral head. Onc aspect described as unique of the CAM procedure is the axillary nerve decompression. It can be done indirectly by osteophyte excision or directly by nerve neurolysis when

E. Calvo (✉)
Department of Orthopedic Surgery and
Traumatology, Fundacion Jimenez Diaz, Universidad
Autonóma, Madrid, Spain

C. R. Guardado
Centro Ortopédico Panamá Clinic, The Panama
Clinic, Panama City, Panama

V. L. Fernandez
Department of Orthopedic Surgery and
Traumatology, Hospital Rey Juan Carlos,
Madrid, Spain

© ISAKOS 2023
A. D. Mazzocca et al. (eds.), *Shoulder Arthritis across the Life Span*,
https://doi.org/10.1007/978-3-031-33298-2_6

scarring is observed [12–15]. The purpose of this chapter is to describe the CAM procedure as a joint-preserving technique for glenohumeral osteoarthritis.

6.2 Patient Selection

Identifying predictive factors of early failure is cardinal to proper patient selection and critical to achieving successful outcomes [16, 17]. This technique provides predictable results in young and active patients with advanced glenohumeral osteoarthritis who wish to delay TSA.

Patients with mild or asymptomatic OA, complete irreparable rotator cuff tears, bipolar lesions with diffuse flattening of the humeral head, or severe joint incongruity on radiographs are not suitable for the CAM procedure. Some other factors have been defined as associated with failure of the technique [14] like narrow joint space (less than 2 mm), more severe arthritis according to the Kellgren-Lawrence classification [18], and Walch type B2 or C glenoid shapes [19]. Age is also something to consider. Mitchell et al. [14] found that age older than 50 years is associated with worse outcomes. A recent Markov decision analysis published by Spiegl and colleagues [16] concluded that arthroscopic management of glenohumeral OA was the preferred treatment strategy for patients younger than 47 years, while TSA was for patients older than 66 years. Between 47 and 66 years of age, they did not find clear advantage for one technique over the other, requiring individualized treatments in this age group [16].

6.3 Surgical Technique

Following the insertion of an interscalene catheter, which will provide analgesia during the immediate postoperative period and initial rehabilitation, general anesthesia allows the surgeon to perform a complete intraoperative examination of the range of motion of both shoulders. This is defined as crucial to identify the specific angles at which shoulder mobility restrictions occur.

The next step is the placement of sterile drapes with the patient in a beach chair position and including the fluoroscopic C-arm in the surgical field.

Through the standard posterior arthroscopic portal and using a 30° arthroscope, a complete arthroscopic glenohumeral inspection is performed to identify intra-articular injuries. Areas of synovitis are treated with either a mechanical oscillating shaver or a radiofrequency device (Fig. 6.1), loose bodies are removed (Fig. 6.2), and degenerative labral tissue and articular sur-

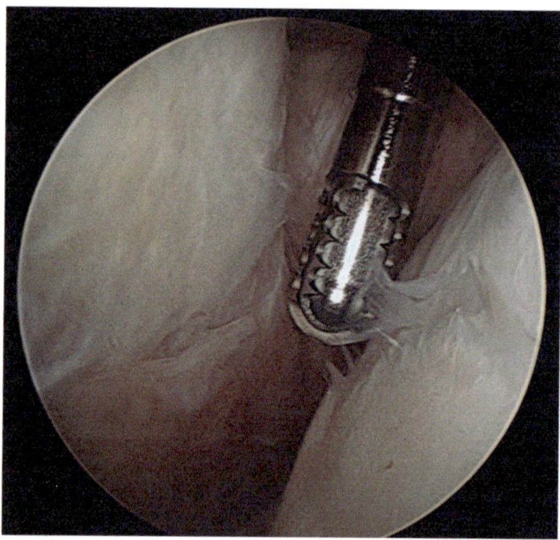

Fig. 6.1 Debridement of humeral head cartilage fibrillation using a motorized full radius synoviotome

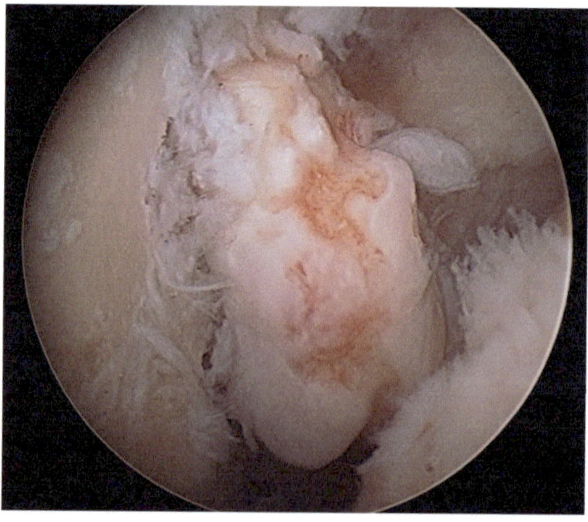

Fig. 6.2 Arthroscopic imaging of glenohumeral loose body

faces are debrided and stabilized with the shaver. Outerbridge grade IV chondral injuries can be addressed with microfractures. The long head of the biceps tendon is also examined.

At this point, anterior and posterior capsule and the rotator interval must be completely released (Fig. 6.2). In our experience, performing a full rotator interval opening, as well as anterior and posterior capsular releases before osteophyte removal, provides greater mobility of the shoulder and allows easier intra-articular excursion of arthroscopic instruments, facilitating osteophyte removal (Fig. 6.3). The subscapularis recess is inspected for loose bodies. Some authors perform the anterior and posterior capsular releases after C-arm-assisted removal of the osteophytes.

Since previous literature concluded that the inferior osteophyte (goat's beard) may affect the course of the axillary nerve and contribute to pain, its removal is essential. To visualize this osteophyte, the inferior capsule, the axillary pouch, and the axillary nerve, a posteroinferior or 7-o'clock portal is established by the use of a spinal-needle localization technique.

Spur excision and humeral osteoplasty are done with a high-speed shaver and a high-speed burr (Fig. 6.4). We usually use a curved curette and a rasp to aid in the removal of the osteophyte and the contouring of the humerus. Internal and external rotation under the C-arm visualization is

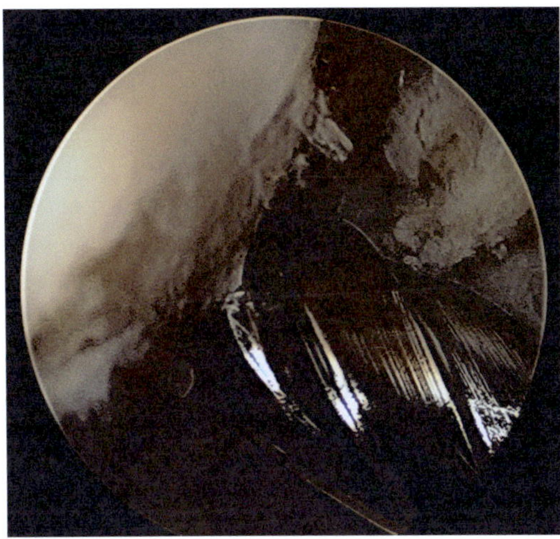

Fig. 6.4 Imaging of the posterior aspect of the right glenohumeral joint. A motorized burr is used to remove the inferior osteophyte

useful to aid in the excision of the osteophyte and to verify its complete resection.

The inferior capsule helps protect the axillary nerve, so its release with arthroscopic scissors or a monopolar radiofrequency probe can be only performed after the resection of the inferior osteophyte.

If preoperative magnetic resonance images or symptoms consistent with axillary nerve impingement are found, axillary nerve neurolysis and decompression can be performed. Symptoms may include posterior and lateral shoulder pain, atrophy of the teres minor or posterior deltoid, and weakness in external rotation without the presence of a rotator cuff tear. The nerve should be carefully decompressed from proximal to distal with a blunt probe and arthroscopic punches, taking great care to identify and preserve all arborizing branches. In our experience, axillary nerve neurolysis is not necessary if the inferior osteophyte is completely removed.

With the arthroscope inserted through the lateral portal, subacromial and subcoracoid decompressions can be performed. Bursectomy and resection of subacromial adhesions are mandatory and useful because they help examine the rotator cuff and facilitate postoperative shoulder mobility, and acromioplasty is only performed if a Bigliani type III acromion or an impingement

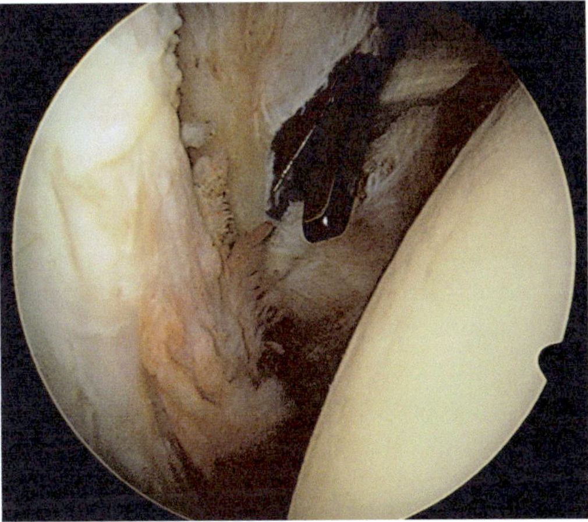

Fig. 6.3 Anterior capsulotomy performed using arthroscopic scissors

lesion (fraying or scuffing of coracoacromial ligament) is noticed.

If an injury, degeneration, or instability of the long head of the biceps had been noticed during the first steps of the technique, it must be treated because it can act as a pain generator. Therefore, it is released at its origin, and, depending on patient-specific characteristics, a tenotomy or an arthroscopic suprapectoral biceps tenodesis with an interference screw may be performed.

The glenohumeral joint is gently manipulated to maximize range of motion, portals are closed in standard fashion, and the arm is placed in a sling.

6.4 Postoperative Management

Rehabilitation during the early postoperative period is vital to prevent scarring, maintain shoulder motion achieved at surgery, and improve shoulder kinematics. So, it starts after just 1 or 2 days using the sling. During the first 4–6 weeks, the priority is immediate active and passive range of motion. Nonsteroidal anti-inflammatory drugs are also used to help reduce swelling during this early postoperative period. After week 6 to about week 12, rehabilitation focuses on strengthening the rotator cuff and periscapular musculature. Finally, at week 12, the central point is the progressive return of the patient to their normal activities, including sports. Maximum recovery is expected between 4 and 6 months.

6.5 Results of the CAM Procedure

Mitchell et al. published the midterm outcomes at a minimum 5-year follow-up [13]. They concluded that this procedure showed reasonable results with patients reported a high mean satisfaction of 9 out of 10 and significant pain relief, documented using the visual analogue scale (VAS). American Shoulder and Elbow Surgeons (ASES), Single Assessment Numeric Evaluation (SANE), and Quick Disabilities of the Arm, Shoulder, and Hand (QuickDASH) scores not only improved but also remained stable over time. It should be noted that older patients (with a positive correlation) had improved results at a minimum 5-year follow-up. Twenty-four percent of the patients needed to undergo a TSA. Preoperative joint space narrowing (less than 2 mm) and Walch type B2 or C glenoid shapes were found to be associated with failure of the technique and progression to TSA. Survivorship for the CAM procedure, with the analysis performed using Kaplan-Meier survival curves, was reported around 96% at 1 year, 87% at 3 years, and 77% at 5 years.

In 2021, similar outcomes have been reported in a long-term study at minimum 10-year follow-up [15]. Median patient satisfaction was 7.5 out of 10 and ASES and SANE scores improved significantly. 60.5% of patients did not need to undergo TSA. Survivorship, with its analysis performed using Kaplan-Meier survival curves, was 63.2% at 10 years, and they found that CAM failure is significantly associated with greater humeral head incongruity and humeral head spur size. Recently Lopez-Fernandez et al have reported the results of the CAM procedure in a series of 25 patients. After a mean follow-up of 42 months all objective and subjective scores analysed showed significant improvements. The authors demonstrated that axillary nerve release and subacromial decompression are not necessary to achieve satisfactory results [20].

6.6 Risks and Complications

The main surgical risks and potential complications can be avoided if the procedure is performed systematically following a meticulous surgical technique. There is a potential risk of damaging the axillary nerve and its branches during inferior capsular release and during neurolysis because they are often difficult to see during the arthroscopy. Inferior osteophyte resection should be performed prior to inferior capsular release to prevent fluid extravasation and protect the nerve. The inferior capsular scar tissue that often develops postoperatively can involve the axillary nerve, which can lead to recurrent posterior and lateral shoulder pain. An early rehabilitation program and thorough surgical hemostasis will help to avoid recurrent scarring, stiffness, and contracture.

The subscapularis tendon is also at risk during surgery and care must be taken to avoid its injury.

6.7 Conclusion

The CAM procedure is an effective procedure for glenohumeral osteoarthritis, especially in young patients who want to stay active improving their quality of life because it decreases shoulder pain and, at the same time, improves shoulder function and delays the need for prosthetic replacement. The survivorship is around 76.9% and 63.2% at 5- and 10-year follow-up, respectively.

Patients who underwent the CAM procedure demonstrate significant improvements in ASES, SANE, and VAS scores. It is a safe technique with no significant complications, and moreover, if the technique fails to relieve symptoms, it does not compromise any future surgical treatment.

However, it should be known that some features are related to worse outcomes, such as Walch type B2 or C glenoid morphology, narrower preoperative joint space, and glenohumeral incongruity.

References

1. Matsen FA 3rd, Ziegler DW, DeBartolo SE. Patient self-assessment of health status and function in glenohumeral degenerative joint disease. J Shoulder Elbow Surg. 1995;4(5):345–51.
2. Cole BJ, Yanke A, Provencher MT. Nonarthroplasty alternatives for the treatment of glenohumeral arthritis. J Shoulder Elbow Surg. 2007;16(5 Suppl):S231–40.
3. Denard PJ, Wirth MA, Orfaly RM. Management of glenohumeral arthritis in the young adult. J Bone Joint Surg Am. 2011;93(9):885–92.
4. Silverstein E, Leger R, Shea KP. The use of intra-articular hylan G-F 20 in the treatment of symptomatic osteoarthritis of the shoulder: a preliminary study. Am J Sports Med. 2007;35(6):979–85.
5. Nakagawa Y, et al. Epidemiologic study of glenohumeral osteoarthritis with plain radiography. J Shoulder Elbow Surg. 1999;8(6):580–4.
6. Sperling JW, Cofield RH, Rowland CM. Neer hemiarthroplasty and Neer total shoulder arthroplasty in patients fifty years old or less. Long-term results. J Bone Joint Surg Am. 1998;80(4):464–73.
7. Saltzman MD, et al. Comparison of patients undergoing primary shoulder arthroplasty before and after the age of fifty. J Bone Joint Surg Am. 2010;92(1):42–7.
8. Schoch B, et al. Shoulder arthroplasty in patients younger than 50 years: minimum 20-year follow-up. J Shoulder Elbow Surg. 2015;24(5):705–10.
9. Bishop JY, Flatow EL. Management of glenohumeral arthritis: a role for arthroscopy? Orthop Clin North Am. 2003;34(4):559–66.
10. Kerr BJ, McCarty EC. Outcome of arthroscopic debridement is worse for patients with glenohumeral arthritis of both sides of the joint. Clin Orthop Relat Res. 2008;466(3):634–8.
11. Millett PJ, Gaskill TR. Arthroscopic management of glenohumeral arthrosis: humeral osteoplasty, capsular release, and arthroscopic axillary nerve release as a joint-preserving approach. Arthroscopy. 2011;27(9):1296–303.
12. Millett PJ, et al. Comprehensive arthroscopic management (CAM) procedure: clinical results of a joint-preserving arthroscopic treatment for young, active patients with advanced shoulder osteoarthritis. Arthroscopy. 2013;29(3):440–8.
13. Mitchell JJ, et al. Survivorship and patient-reported outcomes after comprehensive arthroscopic management of glenohumeral osteoarthritis: minimum 5-year follow-up. Am J Sports Med. 2016;44(12):3206–13.
14. Mitchell JJ, et al. Comprehensive arthroscopic management of glenohumeral osteoarthritis: preoperative factors predictive of treatment failure. Am J Sports Med. 2017;45(4):794–802.
15. Arner JW, et al. Survivorship and patient-reported outcomes after comprehensive arthroscopic management of glenohumeral osteoarthritis: minimum 10-year follow-up. Am J Sports Med. 2021;49(1):130–6.
16. Spiegl UJ, et al. The role of arthroscopy in the management of glenohumeral osteoarthritis: a Markov decision model. Arthroscopy. 2014;30(11):1392–9.
17. Millett P, Greenspoon JA, Warth RJ. The comprehensive arthroscopic management (CAM) procedure for young patients with glenohumeral osteoarthritis. In: Kelly IV JD, editor. Elite techniques in shoulder arthroscopy: new frontiers in shoulder preservation. Cham: Springer; 2016. p. 129–37.
18. Kellgren JH, Lawrence JS. Radiological assessment of osteo-arthrosis. Ann Rheum Dis. 1957;16(4):494–502.
19. Walch G, et al. Morphologic study of the glenoid in primary glenohumeral osteoarthritis. J Arthroplasty. 1999;14(6):756–60.
20. Vanesa, Lopez-Fernandez Gonzalo, Luengo-Alonso María, Valencia Natalia, Martínez-Catalán Antonio María, Foruria Emilio, Calvo. Comprehensive arthroscopic management without axillary nerve release or subacromial decompression achieves satisfactory and durable results in young patients with glenohumeral osteoarthritis Knee Surgery Sports Traumatology Arthroscopy. 2023;31(8):3565–71. https://doi.org/10.1007/s00167-023-07377-0.

Microfracture for Cartilage Lesions on the Glenoid and Humerus

Ivan Wong and Jose Castillo de la Peña

7.1 Introduction

Articular cartilage is the connective tissue that covers the contact surfaces of diarthrodial joints [1]. The main component is extracellular matrix, which comprises 95% of the volume, while chondrocytes constitute only 2% [2]. Chondrocytes have mesenchymal cell lineage; they produce the extracellular matrix and work in an anaerobic environment [2]. Survival of these highly specialized cells depends on mechanical loads, hydrostatic pressures, piezo-electric forces, etc. [2].

On the microscopic level, the articular cartilage is comprised of four different layers, each one with a different configuration and properties as seen in Fig. 7.1 [2]. The more superficial layer, called the lamina splendens, has a tight configuration of type II and IX collagen fibers parallel to the articular surface, combined with flattened chondrocytes that provide shear resistance [1–3]. The intermediate or transitional layer is composed of spherical chondrocytes, and collagen fibers in this layer are obliquely oriented to provide more compression resistance [1–3]. In the deep layer, both collagen fibers and

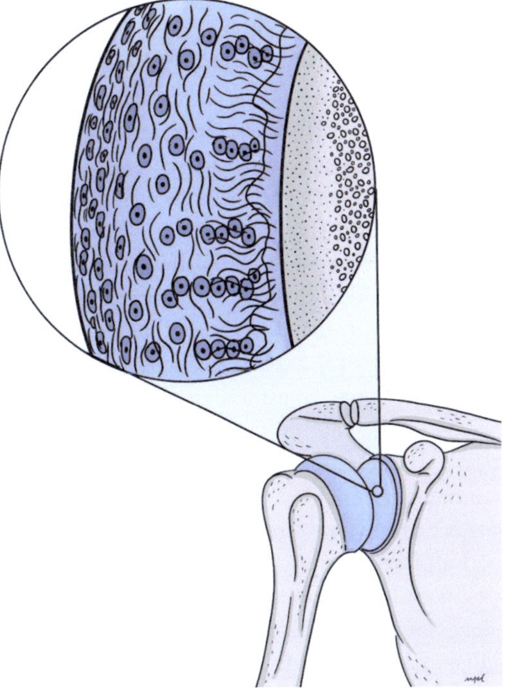

Fig. 7.1 Cartilage diagram. Representation of collagen fiber disposition and cellular configuration in the articular cartilage. (Illustration by Melissa Peñuelas Rodriguez)

chondrocytes are perpendicular to the surface, giving even more compressive resistance [1–3]. The deep zone is the calcified layer, which provides the adhesion to the subchondral bone [1–3].

The thickness of the articular cartilage varies in every joint [1]. In the glenohumeral joint, both

I. Wong (✉) · J. Castillo de la Peña
Division of Orthopaedic Surgery, Department of Surgery, Dalhousie University, Halifax, NS, Canada
e-mail: iw@drivanwong.com

© ISAKOS 2023
A. D. Mazzocca et al. (eds.), *Shoulder Arthritis across the Life Span*,
https://doi.org/10.1007/978-3-031-33298-2_7

surfaces have a different thickness distribution [4, 5]. The glenoid has a mean thickness of 1.88 mm, with a thicker layer on the periphery as compared to the center (bare area) [4, 5]. The humeral head has a mean thickness of 1.24 mm, being thicker in the center [4–6].

7.2 Glenohumeral Cartilage Injuries

Hyaline articular cartilage preservation is one of the principles, if not the most important mainstay, of orthopedic treatment. It is widely known that once the cartilage is injured, there is nothing to bring it back as it was before. Cartilage's lack of blood vessels and its complex structure limit the intrinsic capacity for healing and repair [1]. Decades of research have shown multiple treatment options, but none of them are the same as native cartilage.

Injuries, generating partial-thickness or small lesions, produce changes in microscopic structure with decreased stiffness and increased water permeability [2]. These situations lead to increased force transmission which begins a vicious cycle that produces cartilage degeneration [2]. The absence of bleeding in these pure cartilaginous injuries doesn't lead to an inflammatory or reparative response [2].

Full-thickness injuries involving the subchondral bone have a higher repair capacity in theory, since they produce bleeding and activate the inflammatory cascade that ends with the formation of fibrocartilage [2, 7, 8]. Unfortunately, this reparative tissue has different mechanical properties compared with the native tissue, less stiffness, and decreased wear resistance [1, 2, 8].

Chondral injuries have been widely studied in other joints such as the knee [9, 10], hip [11, 12], and ankle [13, 14], where they have a higher prevalence. These injuries are also present in the glenohumeral joint and can be a source of pain, theoretically leading to osteoarthritis (OA) [15–18].

7.3 Etiology

Cartilage lesions in the shoulder have diverse etiologies and most of the time they are not the main surgical indication [4, 19]. These injuries have been associated with shoulder instability [20, 21], superior labrum anterior to posterior (SLAP) tears [22], rotator cuff tears [23], osteochondritis dissecans [24], and iatrogenic injuries [25] but can also be present as the main entity as a post-traumatic cartilage injury [26].

7.4 Classification

The typical classification systems used for other joints are also applied in the shoulder since glenohumeral hyaline cartilage has the same four histological layers [2]. Two main classification techniques are widely used, the first one described by Outerbridge in 1961 [27] for chondromalacia patellae and the other one described by the International Cartilage Repair Society [28].

7.5 Clinical Evaluation

In the shoulder, symptomatic cartilage lesions should be an exclusion diagnosis and most of the time they present with concomitant pathology, requiring a thorough interrogation and physical examination [15]. Presence of cartilage injuries should be suspected in the setting of prior trauma, instability, mechanical symptoms, etc. [15].

The patient can present with nonspecific symptoms like crepitus, pain, weakness, limited range of motion, etc. [15]. If a cartilage injury is suspected, a compression-rotation test can be applied; for this test the shoulder is abducted to 90°, and axial load is applied while the patient actively performs internal and external rotation; the test is positive if it reproduces the symptoms [29]. A lidocaine subacromial injection can be performed prior to the test to improve the accuracy [29].

7.6   Imaging

Diagnostic imaging should be requested to determine grade of cartilage lesion, location, grade of osteoarthritis, and concomitant pathology. A set of plain X-rays of the involved shoulder including a true anteroposterior (AP) view and Y-scapular view and axillary projection are recommended to determine grade of arthritis (joint space, osteophytes, subchondral sclerosis, subchondral cysts, acromion acetabularization), loose bodies, superior humeral head migration, etc. [30].

Advanced imaging is highly recommended with magnetic resonance imaging (MRI) having a sensitivity of 87.2% and a specificity of 80.6% to detect cartilage lesions in the glenohumeral joint [31]. Cartilage-specific sequences (T2-weighted with or without fat suppression and a T1-weighted with fat suppression) in a 1.5 to 3 Tesla strength study should be obtained to estimate cartilage lesion grade, location, and involvement of the subchondral plate [4, 32, 33]. Computed tomography (CT) has a limited utility in the diagnosis of chondral lesions but is helpful in the setting of advanced osteoarthritis and is key in pre-surgical evaluation in the setting of joint replacement, which will be discussed in further chapters.

7.7   Treatment

The goals of treatment are improvement of function, decrease in pain, and avoiding or slowing progression of arthritis. Partial-thickness lesions (i.e., grades I and II) usually benefit from nonoperative treatment which has been discussed in previous chapters. On the other hand, grade III and IV lesions have shown better outcomes with operative treatment. Surgical options are divided into four main categories: palliative, reparative, restorative, and reconstructive [4].

Microfracture is considered a reparative technique. It is based on the perforation of the subchondral bone of a contained full-thickness cartilage lesion, resulting in the release of blood and mesenchymal cells from the bone marrow. This induces a reparative response which results in the formation of fibrocartilage (mainly type I collagen) within the defect [34, 35]. This treatment modality has multiple benefits. It can be performed arthroscopically as a single-stage procedure with a low cost. It has a low surgical morbidity, is not technically demanding, and affects surgical time minimally. It has been widely used for several years in other joints, providing good pain relief and function improvement at the midterm [19, 36, 37].

Microfractures are indicated in the setting of symptomatic full-thickness cartilage defects, preferably of small diameter. The literature is limited in the shoulder, and a precise defect size hasn't been determined. In the knee, different factors are related with improved outcomes: lesions smaller than 4 cm^2 in size, duration of symptoms less than 12 months, age less than 40 years, body mass index less than 30 kg/m^2, Tegner score greater than 4, and microfracture in the primary setting [35, 38]. Microfractures are not recommended in patients with involvement of the subchondral bone (osteochondral lesions), bipolar/kissing lesions (articulating defects on the glenoid and humeral head), or advanced and generalized osteoarthritis [35, 38].

In 2003, Siebold et al. published a prospective case series of five patients that underwent open shoulder surgery with microfracture plus a periosteal flap [18]. All of the cartilage lesions in this population were in the humeral head, with an average size of 311 mm^2 [18]. After an average follow-up of 25.8 months, the patients had a significant improvement in Constant score (CS), preservation of ROM, OA progression in two patients, and no complications [18].

A retrospective case series of 31 eligible shoulders after arthroscopic surgery were published in 2009 [39]. Most of the population underwent concomitant procedures such as stabilization, subacromial decompression, biceps tenodesis/tenotomy, capsular release, etc. [39]. After a minimum 2-year follow-up, they showed decreased pain and improved function and American Shoulder and Elbow Surgeons (ASES) score [39]. Lower scores were reported in patients who underwent more than two concomitant procedures and had a prior surgery and patients with bipolar and glenoid side defects, as well as big lesions [39].

Short- and long-term outcomes of the same cohort were published in two separate papers [17, 19]. Of the 15 eligible shoulders, 66% underwent concomitant procedures (subacromial decompression, biceps tenodesis/tenotomy, capsular release, etc.) [17, 19]. After a 10.2-year mean follow-up, they found significant improvement in ASES, visual analog scale (VAS), and Simple Shoulder Test (SST) scores, with no difference between short- and long-term follow-up [17]. In contrast with other papers, the size and location of the lesions were not related with differences in patient-reported outcomes (PROs) [17].

Hünnebeck et al. published their long-term outcomes in a paper including 32 patients, with a mean follow-up of 105 months [40]. Interestingly, they compared the PROs with the non-operated shoulder at the end of follow-up and not with pre-operative measurements, which resulted in no significant difference between groups [40]. When compared with pre-surgery measurements, they showed preservation of ROM and radiographic progression of OA in 57% of the patients [40].

Another long-term follow-up case series was published by Frank et al. Of the 16 eligible patients, 43.8% underwent concomitant procedures (subacromial decompression, acromioclavicular joint resection, tendinous calcium deposit removal, biceps tenodesis/tenotomy, etc.) [41]. After a mean follow-up of 122 months, they showed significant improvement in PROs including CS, Oxford Shoulder Score (OSS), and Subjective Shoulder Value (SSV) [41]. No differences could be found between bipolar and unipolar lesions. Radiographic progression of OA was observed in 16.7% of the patients [41].

7.8 Technique

7.8.1 Setup and Positioning

The surgical setup is established for a routine shoulder arthroscopy. The procedure can be performed both in the beach chair and the lateral

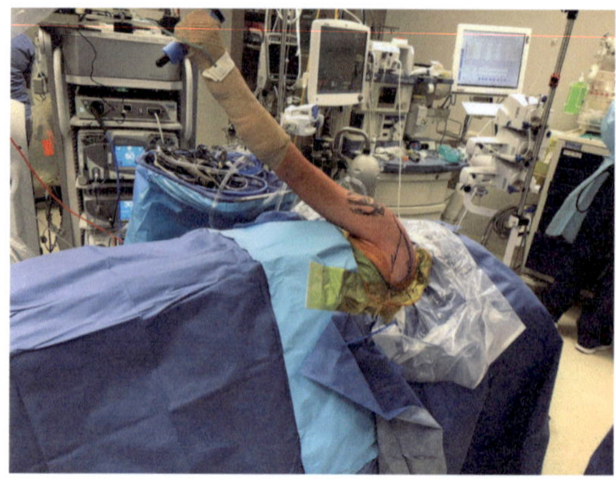

Fig. 7.2 Setup and patient positioning. According to surgeon's preferences, the patient can be positioned in lateral decubitus or beach chair position. A sterile ring curette and microfracture awl should be available in any shoulder arthroscopy

decubitus positions. As a personal preference, a lateral decubitus position is used with a vacuum beanbag beneath the patient and a pneumatic arm positioner as seen in Fig. 7.2.

7.8.2 Diagnostic Arthroscopy and Portal Placement

A routine diagnostic arthroscopy following the 15-point routine described by Snyder et al. is performed through standard posterior and anterior portals [42]. Concomitant pathologies are identified, and portal placement is planned according to the procedures needed. If the defect can be approached in an appropriate angle with one of the prior established portals, no extra portals are needed. If the defect can't be reached, a spinal needle can be used to estimate the ideal location.

7.8.3 Debridement

Once an ideal portal is established, the cartilage defect is inspected with a probe looking for unstable cartilage flaps. An arthroscopic shaver can be used to debride any cartilage remnants and unstable flaps. A curette is used to obtain vertical walls of stable healthy cartilage surrounding the

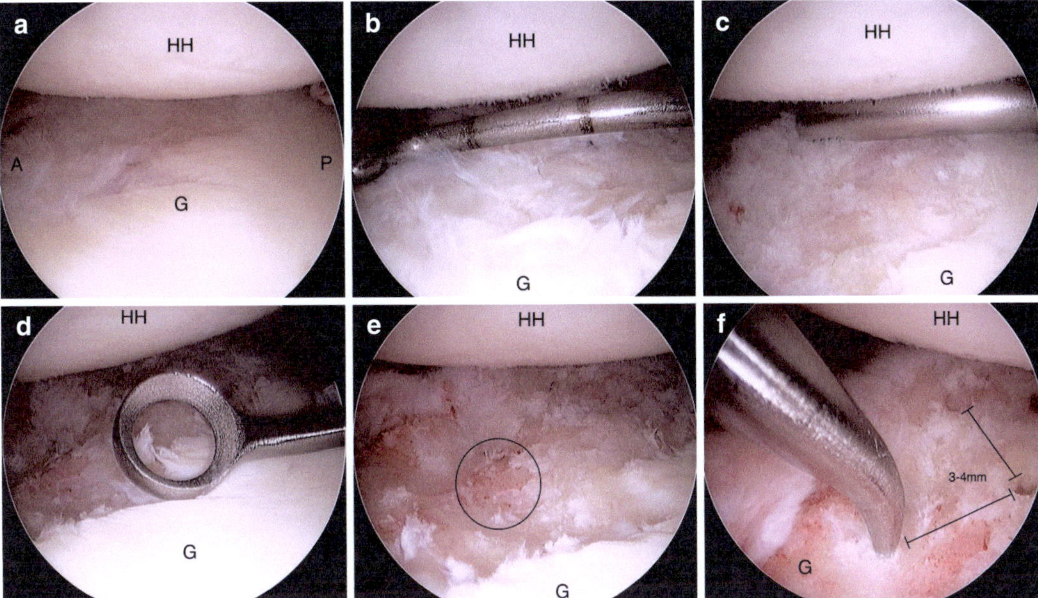

Fig. 7.3 Glenoid cartilage lesion microfracture. Arthroscopic view of a right shoulder, using a 30° lens from the anterosuperior portal. (**a**) Diagnostic arthroscopy shows a grade III–IV cartilage injury of the anteroinferior quadrant of the glenoid face. (**b**) Measuring anteroposterior and superolateral dimension of the defect with a calibrated probe. (**c**) Debridement of unstable cartilage flaps using a shaver from the posterior portal. (**d**) A ring curette is used to obtain vertical walls of stable cartilage; it is recommended to work from both the posterior and anterior portals. (**e**) The ring curette is used to remove the calcified layer, preserving the subchondral layer. (**f**) Microfractures starting from the periphery and moving to the center of the lesion, 3–4 mm bridge between perforations

defect, as seen in the sequence in Fig. 7.3d. It's recommended to debride the calcified layer that lies over the subchondral bone.

complete, the pressure of the pump can be decreased to see the marrow elements emerging from the holes.

7.8.4 Microfracture

To perform the microfractures, two different types of instruments can be utilized: awls or microdrilling devices. The regular set of awls has different angulations, usually 45°, 60°, and 90°; we recommend using either 45° or 60° for better control. The microfractures should progress from the periphery to the center of the lesion, with a space between holes of 3–4 mm, each one with an ideal depth of 4–6 mm. Once the procedure is

7.9 Rehabilitation

The rehabilitation program is usually guided by the concomitant procedures performed. If microfracture is the only procedure, the patient follows a stage protocol containing four phases as described in Table 7.1. Literature shows controversial evidence regarding the use of continuous passive motion (CPM); in our own experience, it is not regularly used since these patients can begin with pendulum exercises same day of surgery [16, 30, 43, 44].

Table 7.1 Rehabilitation protocol

Phase	Week	Exercises	Goals
1—protection	0–2	Pendulum 600–800 cycles Full passive ROM Active scapula-thoracic, elbow, and wrist exercises Cryotherapy Abandon sling as soon as tolerated	Pain and inflammation control Full passive ROM
2—active ROM and basic strengthening	2–6	Progress active-assisted to active ROM Resistance band rotator cuff exercises Scapulothoracic control/strengthening	Full active ROM Nearly normal scapular position
3—advanced strengthening	6–12	Open chain progressed to closed chain exercises. Advanced resistance for rotator cuff strength and scapular control Proprioceptive neuromuscular training Basic functional activities	Pain-free full ROM Normal scapular position and control 4/5 to 4+/5 rotator cuff strength
4—activity/sport-specific activities	>12	Progress strengthening, resistance and endurance Continue open and closed chain program Plyometric strengthening Occupational therapist intervention Sport-specific program	5/5 rotator cuff strength Normal scapular control Pain-free workout routine

7.10 Conclusions

Results in the literature are promising, demonstrating improvement of clinical outcomes, preservation of range of motion both at short and long term. Unfortunately, the evidence supporting this is of low level (level III–IV), and in most of the case series, a big proportion of the population underwent concomitant procedures that could explain the improvement in clinical outcomes on their own.

As an expert opinion, we recommend using microfractures in grade IV, symptomatic, focal, monopolar cartilage injuries with a diameter between 5 and 10 mm in the glenoid and between 10 and 15 mm in the humeral head.

Conflict of Interest The authors don't have conflicts of interest related to this chapter.

References

1. Sophia Fox AJ, Bedi A, Rodeo SA. The basic science of articular cartilage: structure, composition, and function. Sports Health. 2009;1:461–8.
2. Alford JW, Cole BJ. Cartilage restoration, part 1: basic science, historical perspective, patient evaluation, and treatment options. Am J Sports Med. 2005;33:295–306.
3. Buckwalter JA, Mankin HJ. Articular cartilage: tissue design and chondrocyte-matrix interactions. Instr Course Lect. 1998;47:487.
4. Saltzman BM, Leroux T, Cole BJ. Management and surgical options for articular defects in the shoulder. Clin Sports Med. 2017;36:549–72.
5. Yeh LR, Kwak S, Kim YS, Chou DSW, Muhle C, Skaf A, et al. Evaluation of articular cartilage thickness of the humeral head and the glenoid fossa by MR arthrography: anatomic correlation in cadavers. Skeletal Radiol. 1998;27:500.
6. Fox JA, Cole BJ, Romeo AA, Meininger AK, Williams JM, Glenn RE, et al. Articular cartilage thickness of the humeral head: an anatomic study. Orthopedics. 2008;31:216.
7. Goldberg VM, Caplan AI. Biologic restoration of articular surfaces. Instr Course Lect. 1999;48:623.
8. Armiento AR, Alini M, Stoddart MJ. Articular fibrocartilage—why does hyaline cartilage fail to repair? Adv Drug Deliv Rev. 2019;146:289.
9. Bekkers JEJ, Inklaar M, Saris DBF. Treatment selection in articular cartilage lesions of the knee: a systematic review. Am J Sports Med. 2009;37:148.
10. Bedi A, Feeley BT, Williams RJ. Management of articular cartilage defects of the knee. J Bone Joint Surg Am. 2010;92:994.
11. Chahla J, la Prade RF, Mardones R, Huard J, Philippon MJ, Nho S, et al. Biological therapies for cartilage lesions in the hip: a new horizon. Orthopedics. 2016;39:e715.
12. Mardones R, Larrain C. Cartilage restoration technique of the hip. J Hip Preserv Surg. 2016;3:30–6.
13. O'Loughlin PF, Heyworth BE, Kennedy JG. Current concepts in the diagnosis and treatment of osteochondral lesions of the ankle. Am J Sports Med. 2010;38:392.

14. van Bergen CJA, Baur OL, Murawski CD, Spennacchio P, Carreira DS, Kearns SR, et al. Diagnosis: history, physical examination, imaging, and arthroscopy: proceedings of the international consensus meeting on cartilage repair of the ankle. Foot Ankle Int. 2018;39(1_suppl):3S–8S.

15. Elser F, Braun S, Dewing CB, Millett PJ. Glenohumeral joint preservation: current options for managing articular cartilage lesions in young, active patients. Arthroscopy. 2010;26:685–96.

16. DePalma AA, Gruson KI. Management of cartilage defects in the shoulder. Curr Rev Musculoskelet Med. 2012;5:254–62.

17. Wang KC, Frank RM, Cotter EJ, Davey A, Meyer MA, Hannon CP, et al. Long-term clinical outcomes after microfracture of the glenohumeral joint: average 10-year follow-up. Am J Sports Med. 2018;46:786–94.

18. Siebold R, Lichtenberg S, Habermeyer P. Combination of microfracture and periosteal-flap for the treatment of focal full thickness articular cartilage lesions of the shoulder: a prospective study. Knee Surg Sports Traumatol Arthrosc. 2003;11:183–9.

19. Frank RM, van Thiel GS, Slabaugh MA, Romeo AA, Cole BJ, Verma NN. Clinical outcomes after microfracture of the glenohumeral joint. Am J Sports Med. 2010;38:772–81.

20. Tischer T, Vogt S, Kreuz PC, Imhoff AB. Arthroscopic anatomy, variants, and pathologic findings in shoulder instability. Arthroscopy. 2011;27:1434–43.

21. Nourissat G, Hardy MB, Garret J, Mansat P, Godenèche A. Glenoid cartilage lesions compromise outcomes of surgical treatment for posterior shoulder instability. Orthop J Sports Med. 2020;8:2325967119898124.

22. Patzer T, Lichtenberg S, Kircher J, Magosch P, Habermeyer P. Influence of SLAP lesions on chondral lesions of the glenohumeral joint. Knee Surg Sports Traumatol Arthrosc. 2010;18:982–7.

23. Gartsman GM, Taverna E. The incidence of glenohumeral joint abnormalities associated with full-thickness, reparable rotator cuff tears. Arthroscopy. 1997;13:450.

24. Gill J, Tytherleigh-Strong G. Osteochondritis dissecans with associated secondary chondromatosis in an adolescent shoulder. Shoulder Elbow. 2019;11:275–81.

25. Hogan CJ, Diduch DR. Progressive articular cartilage loss following radiofrequency treatment of a partial-thickness lesion. Arthroscopy. 2001;17:E24.

26. Ruckstuhl H, de Bruin ED, Stussi E, Vanwanseele B. Post-traumatic glenohumeral cartilage lesions: a systematic review. BMC Musculoskelet Disord. 2008;9:107.

27. Outerbridge RE. The etiology of chondromalacia patellae. J Bone Joint Surg Br. 1961;43-B:752–7.

28. Brittberg M, Winalski CS. Evaluation of cartilage injuries and repair. J Bone Joint Surg Am. 2003;85:58.

29. Ellman H, Harris E, Kay SP. Early degenerative joint disease simulating impingement syndrome: arthroscopic findings. Arthroscopy. 1992;8:482–7.

30. Salata MJ, Kercher JS, Bajaj S, Verma NN, Cole BJ. Glenohumeral microfracture. Cartilage. 2010;1:121–6.

31. Hayes ML, Collins MS, Morgan JA, Wenger DE, Dahm DL. Efficacy of diagnostic magnetic resonance imaging for articular cartilage lesions of the glenohumeral joint in patients with instability. Skeletal Radiol. 2010;39:1199.

32. Saxena V, D'Aquilla K, Singh A, Gordon JA, Fenty M, Carey JL, et al. T1ρ magnetic resonance imaging to assess cartilage damage after primary shoulder dislocation. Orthop J Sports Med. 2015;3:2325967115S0002.

33. Lazik-Palm A, Kraff O, Rietsch SHG, Ladd ME, Kamminga M, Beck S, et al. 7-T clinical MRI of the shoulder in patients with suspected lesions of the rotator cuff. Eur Radiol Exp. 2020;4:10.

34. Alford JW, Cole BJ. Cartilage restoration, part 2: techniques, outcomes, and future directions. Am J Sports Med. 2005;33:443–60.

35. Douleh D, Frank RM. Marrow stimulation: microfracture, drilling, and abrasion. Oper Techn Sports Med. 2018;26:170.

36. Orth P, Gao L, Madry H. Microfracture for cartilage repair in the knee: a systematic review of the contemporary literature. Knee Surg Sports Traumatol Arthrosc. 2020;28:670.

37. Weber AE, Locker PH, Mayer EN, Cvetanovich GL, Tilton AK, Erickson BJ, et al. Clinical outcomes after microfracture of the knee: midterm follow-up. Orthop J Sports Med. 2018;6:2325967117753572.

38. Mithoefer K, Mcadams T, Williams RJ, Kreuz PC, Mandelbaum BR. Clinical efficacy of the microfracture technique for articular cartilage repair in the knee: an evidence-based systematic analysis. Am J Sports Med. 2009;37:2053.

39. Millett PJ, Huffard BH, Horan MP, Hawkins RJ, Steadman JR. Outcomes of full-thickness articular cartilage injuries of the shoulder treated with microfracture. Arthroscopy. 2009;25:856–63.

40. Hünnebeck SM, Magosch P, Habermeyer P, Loew M, Lichtenberg S. Knorpelschäden des Schultergelenks: Langzeiteffekte der Mikrofrakturierung. Obere Extremitat. Dr. Dietrich Steinkopff Verlag GmbH and Co. KG; 2017;12:165–170.

41. Frank JK, Heuberer PR, Laky B, Anderl W, Pauzenberger L. Glenohumeral microfracturing of contained glenohumeral defects: mid- to long-term outcome. Arthrosc Sports Med Rehabil. 2020;2:e341–6.

42. Snyder S, Karzel R, Getelman M, Burns J, Bahk M, Auerbach D, et al. Shoulder arthroscopy. 3rd ed. Philadelphia: Lippincott Williams & Wilkins; 2014.

43. Slabaugh MA, Frank RM, Cole BJ. Resurfacing of isolated articular cartilage defects in the glenohumeral joint with microfracture: a surgical technique & case report. Am J Orthop (Belle Mead NJ). 2010;39:326–32.

44. Hensley CP, Sum J. Physical therapy intervention for a former power lifter after arthroscopic microfracture procedure for grade iv glenohumeral chondral defects. Int J Sports Phys Ther. 2011;6:10–26.

Fresh Osteochondral Allograft Transplantation in the Shoulder

8

Andrew Vega and Raffy Mirzayan

Focal chondral and osteochondral lesions of the glenohumeral joint can be debilitating, particularly in shoulders with otherwise pristine anatomy. Osteochondral allograft transplantation to correct focal articular cartilage lesions has been well-established; however, the majority of our knowledge and practice of this technique have been centered on chondral defects in the knee [1]. Unlike the joints of the lower extremity which experience higher impact loading forces as weight-bearing articulations in support of the axial skeleton, these lesions do not occur as frequently in the glenohumeral joint, with an annual incidence of 5–17% [2, 3]. Furthermore, the natural history of these isolated, full-thickness chondral lesions is less clear than those of the knee or ankle. Individuals with manual labor occupations, athletes who bear significant loads overhead, and young to middle-aged patients with associated glenohumeral pathologies are most often those who present with these articular lesions [4]. Patients generally present with non-localizing complaints and physical examination findings similar to other shoulder diagnoses, par-

ticularly impingement syndromes [5]. Pain due to osteochondral defects is of a dull quality and is exacerbated with increased activity [6]. These lesions can cause mechanical symptoms with active range of motion, which may be indicative of joint surface irregularity and possible chondral damage.

Osteochondral lesions occur as isolated pathology or, more commonly, in concert with other internal derangements of the glenohumeral joint. They may be caused by trauma, infection, osteonecrosis, osteochondritis dissecans, osteoarthritis, inflammatory arthritides, idiopathic chondrolysis, rotator cuff arthropathy, recurrent instability, or iatrogenic injury secondary to the effects of intra-articular pain pumps, radiofrequency devices, and prominent surgical implants [7, 8]. Of these, shoulder instability is most often quoted to be associated with these lesions. In a case series by Krych et al. [9], 64% of shoulders undergoing arthroscopic stabilization for shoulder instability demonstrated evidence of focal articular cartilage defects. Those with a history of prior dislocation with closed reduction were significantly associated with focal articular cartilage lesions of the glenoid. Moreover, chondral lesion grade was directly proportional to the number of dislocations sustained. This association between instability and chondral damage is also seen in patients with superior labrum anterior to posterior (SLAP) tears. In a prospective observational study by Patzer et al. [10], chondral lesions

A. Vega
Department of Orthopaedic Surgery, USC Keck School of Medicine, Los Angeles, CA, USA

R. Mirzayan (✉)
Department of Orthopaedic Surgery, Kaiser Permanente Southern California,
Baldwin Park, CA, USA
e-mail: Raffy.mirzayan@kp.org

© ISAKOS 2023
A. D. Mazzocca et al. (eds.), *Shoulder Arthritis across the Life Span*,
https://doi.org/10.1007/978-3-031-33298-2_8

occurred at a rate of 20% at the humerus, 18% at the glenoid, and 14% on both chondral surfaces in patients with SLAP tears. These lesions often localized beneath the biceps tendon on the humeral side and along the anterior half of the glenoid. In a large series of full-thickness rotator cuff tears, Gartsman et al. [11] identified focal cartilage lesions in 13% of shoulders. Humeral lesions were all located on the posterior aspect of the articular surface, were circular, and averaged 250 mm². The glenoid lesions averaged 200 mm².

Osteonecrosis of the humeral head affects patients at younger ages, and many cases are not detected until advanced stages when collapse occurs, resulting in focal chondral damage [12]. Lesions due to osteochondritis dissecans, although rare in the shoulder, have been described in young male patients in the anterosuperior aspect of the humeral head [13]. Glenohumeral chondrolysis has been seen after routine shoulder arthroscopy, with ablative thermal energy implicated as a causative factor [14]. Moreover, numerous studies have demonstrated the cytotoxic effects of local anesthetics on articular chondrocytes [15]. Finally, prominent or malpositioned hardware, such as suture anchors or intra-articular screw penetration following osteosynthesis of the humeral head, can destroy the chondral surface.

Diagnosis is often difficult. These defects are often found incidentally during arthroscopic or open surgical management of other glenohumeral pathologies. Plain radiographs of the shoulder, including anteroposterior view, scapular Y-view, and axillary view, are first-line. West Point and Stryker notch views may be obtained to evaluate for glenoid bone loss and Hill-Sachs lesions, respectively. These films should also be evaluated for the presence of any concurrent degenerative processes that may change management. When chondral injury is suspected, magnetic resonance imaging (MRI) is the diagnostic study of choice for further evaluation. MRI also allows for the evaluation of concurrent soft tissue pathologies, including tendinous and labral disease. T2-weighted sequences and T1-weighted, fat-suppressed, cartilage-sensitive sequences, such as fast spin echo, are used to assess articular cartilage. In an MRI study of the glenohumeral joint, Carroll et al. described these focal osteochondral lesions as contour deformities about the articular margin with areas of abnormal signal intensity [16]. Humeral head cartilage defects were often located in the posterosuperior portion of the humeral head, medial to the expected location of a typical Hill-Sachs lesion. In overhead athletes, the lesions were located near the rotator cuff insertion. Subchondral bone marrow edema may also be seen in those with an acute or subacute presentation and may imply a traumatic etiology or be suggestive of a full-thickness defect [16]. However, MRI as well as magnetic resonance arthrography (MRA) can fail to demonstrate these focal lesions, as has been shown in multiple studies, with rates as high as 45% misdiagnosis of grade IV lesions [17, 18]. In patients with anterior shoulder instability, MRI is quoted to have a 60% accuracy and 87% sensitivity for diagnosing focal osteochondral lesions of the humeral head [19]. Lastly, computed tomography (CT) is used to assess glenohumeral alignment, glenoid bone loss, glenoid version, and glenoid inclination to aid in preoperative planning for those undergoing joint-preserving or reconstructive procedures.

The Outerbridge classification system, originally described in relation to chondromalacia of the patella, is utilized to categorize these lesions as no specific classification system has been developed specific to the glenohumeral joint [20]. Grade 0 signifies normal cartilage. Grade I is characterized by chondral softening and swelling. Grade II lesions are partial-thickness chondral defects with fissures that do not exceed 1 cm in diameter or reach subchondral bone. Grade III lesions involve fissuring of the cartilage surface with a diameter greater than 1 cm with an area reaching subchondral bone, and grade IV lesions demonstrate full-thickness articular cartilage loss down to subchondral bone. Moreover, size and degree of peripheral containment are descriptive characteristics that are also utilized to document these lesions and should be employed to facilitate surgical planning.

Because of the lower forces typically sustained by the glenohumeral joint, most of these lesions are well-tolerated or even asymptomatic [21]. However, focal lesions that then become symptomatic can be challenging to manage. Because of a lack of direct vascular perfusion as well as access to pluripotent progenitor cells, these lesions are limited in their native healing capacity. Initial management of isolated chondral defects of the glenohumeral joint is nonsurgical. The mainstays of activity modification, physical therapy, nonsteroidal anti-inflammatory drugs, and corticosteroid injections remain first-line [22]. Although there are no studies to date which assess the clinical outcomes of these nonsurgical interventions with respect to isolated chondral defects of the glenohumeral joint, they should be prescribed for patients in an effort to avoid more invasive procedures if possible. Moreover, those with limitations in active range of motion, either due to pain from these focal defects or due to a concomitant pathology, would benefit from pre-operative rehabilitation to maximize clinical benefit when surgical intervention is undergone. Physical therapy should aim to improve glenohumeral as well as scapulothoracic stability, mobility, and strength.

For those who fail nonoperative management, several surgical options are available to provide pain relief, create reparative biology, and restore the articular surface, including arthroscopic debridement, microfracture, matrix-induced autologous chondrocyte implantation, particulated juvenile allograft cartilage, osteochondral autograft transplantation, and fresh osteochondral allograft transplantation. In a systematic review, Gross et al. reported high patient satisfaction rates for these procedures, ranging from 66 to 100% [21]. No firm consensus yet exists on the most appropriate operative treatment among them, as comparative data is lacking. However, these joint-preserving procedures are of particular importance in younger, more active patients with focal osteochondral lesions to evade joint reconstruction, including anatomic and reverse total shoulder arthroplasty, which bear a limited life span and may inflict activity limitations. Survivorship has been quoted to be as low as 61% at 10 years in a series of 33 shoulders in patients with a mean age of 46 at the time of

arthroplasty [23]. Thus, joint reconstructive procedures should be reserved for those with more diffuse, degenerative disease of the glenohumeral joint, more commonly seen in those in later decades of life. Contraindications to these joint salvage procedures include infection, immunosuppression, musculoskeletal neoplasm, and inflammatory arthritides. Positive prognostic factors predictive of statistically significant functional improvements following these procedures include unipolar lesions, lesions of a lower grade, lesions isolated to the humeral head, and lesions less than 2 cm^2 in size. Negative prognostic factors included bipolar lesions, lesions greater than 2 cm^2 in size, and a history of surgical intervention in the operative shoulder [21].

Osteochondral allograft transplantation shows promise as a joint-preserving procedure within the glenohumeral joint, particularly in young and more active populations. The procedure resembles osteochondral autograft transplantation but benefits from decreased surgical time and avoids the morbidity associated with harvesting of autograft plugs. In addition, allograft allows for treatment of larger, full-thickness lesions that may not be adequately treated with available autograft sources. The disadvantages of osteochondral allograft transplantation include potential immunogenic response, potential infectious disease transmission, and cost [24]. Although an uncommon technique overall, osteochondral allograft transplantation has been used to correct engaging Hill-Sachs lesions, bone defects of the proximal humerus secondary to neoplastic resection, and glenoid bone loss in the setting of recurrent instability with encouraging results [25].

Osteochondral allografts contain viable chondrocytes, chondrogenic growth factors, and extracellular matrix proteins to promote cartilage repair [26]. They are available in fresh, fresh-frozen, or cryopreserved preparations. Fresh osteochondral allografts have the highest percentage of viable chondrocytes but suffer from a shelf life of approximately 30 days and require precise preoperative sizing. In contrast, fresh-frozen allografts have minimal viable chondrocytes. Fresh-frozen grafts are essentially acellular because of the freeze-thaw process. Cryopreserved osteochondral allografts are reported to have up to a 2-year shelf life and may maintain up to 70.5% of viable chondrocytes [27]; however, they are limited to treat defects up to 20 by 25 mm in size. Several allograft sources have been considered and utilized. Humeral head and femoral head allografts are commonly transplanted for humeral-sided lesions; however, glenoid allografts are not commonly used to treat glenoid lesions. In a cadaveric study comparing radial head, scaphoid fossa of the distal radius, lunate fossa of the distal radius, medial tibial plateau, and lateral distal tibial osteochondral allografts, Dehaan et al. demonstrated that lateral distal tibial osteochondral allografts were most congruent to the glenoid's radius of curvature and fit best when used for glenoid augmentation in the setting of critical bone loss and recurrent glenohumeral instability [28]. However, medial tibial plateau and other commercially available and pre-shaped allograft options are available for glenoid allograft transplantation [29, 30].

It is imperative that osteochondral allograft plugs match the articular surface geometry of their recipient to ensure a congruent articular surface and normalize articular contact pressures; however, the anatomy of the glenohumeral joint can make this challenging [31]. The chondral surface of the humeral head is thickest at its center, approximately 1.2 mm, and thins to less than 1 mm along its periphery [32]. In contrast, the chondral surface of the glenoid is thickest along its periphery and thins toward its center at the bare area where no articular cartilage exists [33]. Moreover, the glenoid is approximately 1.5° retroverted and 4.2° superiorly inclined; its radius of curvature is within 2–3 mm of the humeral head. Gebhart et al. analyzed several anthropometric measurements and found that patient height, maximum humeral length, epicondylar width, and sex were most predictive of humeral head curvature [34]. Tissue banks can use these parameters to improve donor and recipient geometric matching to aid surgeons in anatomic restoration of the articular osteochondral surface and rebalance glenohumeral biomechanics.

Osteochondral allograft transplantation is most commonly performed through an open deltopectoral or deltoid-splitting approach; however, arthroscopic and arthroscopic-assisted techniques have also been described [35, 36]. The most common technique employed for osteochondral allograft transplantation is the press-fit circular plug technique, which allows for a precise graft fit and decreases the need for supplemental internal fixation. The lesion is first inspected to define its margins. Surrounding nonviable cartilage and bone are debrided. Then, the size of the osteochondral allograft is estimated using the commercially available cannulated, cylindrical sizing guides. Each guide is positioned to encompass the defect, sequentially increasing in size, thereby determining the optimal plug diameter. It is imperative that the guide sit flush with the surrounding normal articular surface to ensure proper restoration of articular geometry. Once the lesion is sized, it is critical to ensure that the available allograft can accommodate the harvesting of such a size. If the available allograft is too narrow to accommodate a graft of appropriate diameter, then two individual press-fit plugs may be placed in overlapping fashion via "snowman" technique. A guide wire is placed through the cylindrical, cannulated sizing guide perpendicular to the articular surface. The cartilage surface is scored, and a cannulated counter-bore reamer is used to remove the articular cartilage and subchondral bone until healthy, bleeding bone is obtained. Typically, approximately 8–10 mm of depth needs to be resected for osteochondral lesions. The guide wire is then removed, the 12 o'clock position is determined, and depth measurements are recorded at the 3, 6, 9, and 12 o'clock positions of the recipient site. Attention is then turned to allograft plug harvesting. The available allograft is first scrutinized to determine which part of the articular surface best matches the geometry of the recipient site. The donor graft is then secured to the allograft workstation, and the appropriate diameter cylindrical, cannulated sizing guide is positioned and secured perpendicular to the articular surface of the graft at the desired location utilizing a bushing attached to the workstation. The sizing guide is then removed, and the appropriate size coring reamer is passed through the bushing and advanced through the graft at a depth greater than that needed for the recipient site. The graft is then removed as a long cylindrical plug, utilizing an oscillating saw to release the plug from the surrounding allograft inferior to the desired depth of the plug. The 12 o'clock position of the plug is determined, the previously measured depths of the recipient site are marked out on the plug using a skin marker, and the plug is cut 1–2 mm less than the measured depth of the socket. A rongeur can be utilized to bevel the edges of the osseous side of the plug in order to facilitate initial press-fit. It is critical that blood and marrow elements are copiously irrigated off the plug with a pulse lavage in an effort to decrease the risk of a host immune response [37]. The recipient site is irrigated, and demineralized bone matrix or similar adjunctive, commercially available preparations can be placed into the base of the recipient site prior to allograft transplantation. The donor plug is then oriented over the recipient site with the 12 o'clock positions aligned and pressed into place under manual pressure. If there remains resistance to insertion, an oversized tamp can be used to dilate the recipient site. Gentle tamping with the cylindrical, cannulated sizing guide can be performed to fully seat the graft, but excessive loading should be avoided to prevent damaging the graft or subsidence of the graft beneath the surrounding articular surface. The final plug position should sit flush relative to the surrounding articular surface with minimal to no step-off to prevent asymmetric loading and premature wear. At this time, graft stability is assessed. If necessary, small cortical bone screws, headless compression screws, bioabsorbable screws, or plastic screws can be placed; however, a stable press-fit technique without additional internal fixation is preferred as the additional hardware has the potential to become symptomatic. If utilizing the "snowman" technique for multiple allograft plugs, it is critical to stabilize the first graft with a small Kirschner wire to prevent dislodgement during preparation of the second overlapping site; this wire is then removed once all plugs are seated. After final irrigation, the shoulder is reduced and carried through passive range of motion to ensure a stable and congruent arc of motion without bony block prior to closure in standard fashion.

A typical postoperative course includes initial sling immobilization for less than 1 week with passive and active-assisted range of motion exercises beginning on postoperative day 1. If a subscapularis tenotomy has been performed, care should be taken to avoid active internal rotation or excessive external rotation to not jeopardize the repair. At 3 weeks, active range of motion is allowed, and strengthening may begin at the 5-week mark. Overhead sports may be introduced at the 4- to 6-month mark if symptoms have resolved. Early complications may include arthrofibrosis, surgical site infection, and recurrent sterile effusions [38]. Early graft failure with fragmentation or collapse, delayed union, nonunion, and immunogenic reaction are extremely rare but can occur, particularly in patients with poor subchondral bone stock and with the use of larger allograft plugs. Late complications may include graft failure with fragmentation, collapse, and resorption. Progression of underlying disease processes may result in recurrent or persistent symptoms regardless of ultimate graft viability.

Humeral head osteochondral allograft transplantation has primarily been employed for recurrent glenohumeral instability in the setting of a large Hill-Sachs defect. In a case report, Kropf and Sekiya introduced this concept in the treatment of a 19-year-old US Navy SEAL man [39]. Osteochondral allograft transplantation in this setting not only recreates articular surface congruency but also restores stability to the glenohumeral joint by preventing engagement of "off-track" osteochondral lesions with the glenoid rim. Large humeral head osteochondral lesions that comprise at least 37.5% of the articular surface significantly increase the risk of recurrent instability and can be addressed with this technique to restore the stabilizing concavity-compression effect of glenohumeral biomechanics [40]. In a systematic review by Saltzman et al., the authors reported improvements in shoulder range of motion and functional outcome scores as well as low dislocation rates following humeral head allograft transplantation [41]. In a case series by Diklic et al. treating chronic, locked, posterior shoulder dislocations due to large humeral head defects comprising 25–50% of the articular surface, 9 of 13 total patients (69%) had no pain or restrictions of activities of daily living at final follow-up of 54 months [42]. The mean Constant-Murley shoulder score was 86.8, and no patient endorsed symptoms of instability. In a series of 20 patients, Riff et al. reported a 5-point improvement in VAS score, a 41-point improvement in the Simple Shoulder Test score, a 37-point improvement in the American Shoulder and Elbow Surgeons score, and a 10-point improvement in the Medical Outcome Study 12-Item Short Form physical component summary score at final follow-up of 24 months following osteochondral allograft transplantation of humeral head osteochondral defects [43]. Humeral head osteochondral allograft transplantation has a reported 20–30% complication rate, including a 26% reoperation rate. In a series of five patients with anterior shoulder instability, DiPaola et al. reported loss of 23 degrees of forward flexion, 8 degrees of external rotation, and two vertebral levels of internal rotation on average when compared to the contralateral shoulder despite improvements in the ASES and UCLA shoulder scores at 28 months of follow-up [44]. Moreover, 50% of shoulders required conversion to a total shoulder arthroplasty at 5-year follow-up [41]. Despite substantial complication and reoperation rates, studies report high rates of return to work and patient satisfaction. At least one study reports inferior patient satisfaction in patients with a history of intra-articular pain pump use [43].

Osteochondral allograft transplantation for glenoid deficiency has primarily been employed in the setting of recurrent instability and represents an alternative, adjunctive, or salvage procedure to traditional arthroscopic stabilization and coracoid transfer techniques. The prevalence of anteroinferior glenoid deficiency is reportedly up to 70% in cases of recurrent instability and is more commonly seen in those who sustain a high-energy mechanism or dislocate with minimal force [45, 46]. In those with greater than 25% glenoid bone loss, arthroscopic Bankart repair has been shown to have a 67% recurrence rate [47, 48]. Glenoid bone loss decreases the articular arc length and depth of articular conformity to the humeral head, causing glenohumeral mismatch and loss of the stabilizing concavity-compression effect [49, 50]. Moreover, there is an increase in the shear forces born by the capsulolabral static stabilizers as glenoid bone loss approaches 15% [48]. At 30%, glenohumeral contact pressures can increase by up to 400% [51]. In comparison to coracoid transfer, glenohumeral contact pressures are significantly improved following distal tibial allograft reconstruction of glenoid defects [52]. Therefore, a glenoid deficiency of more than 20% indicates the need for osteochondral augmentation [46]. Osteochondral allograft transplantation supersedes these aforementioned techniques in that it can restore the congruity of the glenoid radius of curvature with an articular cartilage interface, not only restoring glenohumeral stability but also preventing early degenerative changes and instability arthropathy that can manifest following glenoid rim augmentation with non-chondral surfaces. The depth of glenoid bone stock has caused some concern regarding osteochondral grafting. The glenoid can support grafts up to 20 mm in diameter and 4 mm in depth at its center, covering 52% of the glenoid articular surface on average [53]. Three-dimensional CT should be utilized as routine preoperative planning to better assess glenoid bone stock prior to osteochondral transplantation.

Several preparations have been popularized for osteochondral allograft reconstruction of the glenoid, including distal tibial allograft and glenoid allograft. In a cadaveric study, lateral distal tibial osteochondral allograft has been shown to fit more anatomically than other allograft sources, other than glenoid allograft [54]. Provencher et al. first introduced the use of lateral distal tibial allograft [55]. The distal tibia is composed of dense, cortical, and metaphyseal cancellous bone with associated cartilaginous layer that is highly congruent to the glenoid radius of curvature and fits nearly anatomically on the distal two thirds of the glenoid, allowing for normalization of glenohumeral articular contact pressures [31]. In a systematic review involving eight level IV studies assessing the clinical and radiographic outcomes following osteochondral allograft reconstruction for glenoid bone loss, the authors demonstrated excellent clinical outcomes, reduced incidence of recurrent instability, and low rates of graft resorption [56]. The Rowe score, a validated clinical assessment of shoulder instability, improved by 57.5 points, with a mean final score of 90.6 points. One hundred percent of shoulders achieved bony integration of the graft at 44.5 months of follow-up without signs of graft resorption. Only 7.1% of shoulders had recurrence of glenohumeral instability. More than 90% of patients experienced pain improvement or complete resolution, and 93% percent of patients were satisfied with the outcome of their surgery. In a case report of a 25-year-old former multisport athlete who had failed extensive nonoperative management of a large glenoid defect, Camp et al. reported significant improvements in the subjective shoulder value score, from 40 to 99%, QuickDASH score, from 36 to 2, and the ASES score, from 46 to 92, following osteochondral allograft transplantation using a medial tibial plateau allograft at 1-year follow-up [57]. Moreover, radiographs obtained at 3 months and MRI obtained at 6 months postoperatively demonstrated articular surface congruity restoration and graft incorporation into surrounding subchondral bone. Thus, osteochondral allograft transplantation proves to be a viable option in the management of glenoid bone loss and focal osteochondral lesions, but there remains a need for long-term outcome data to support its efficacy and widespread adoption.

Combinations of these techniques have been employed to treat bipolar osteochondral lesions of the glenohumeral joint with varying success (Fig. 8.1). In a care series by Familiari et al., osteochondral glenoid allograft combined with humeral head hemiarthroplasty resulted in three early failures and only one satisfactory clinical outcome; however, their sole success was associated with severe glenoid erosion [58]. Giannini et al. introduced the technique of bipolar fresh osteochondral allograft of the shoulder in a case report [59]. At 30 months of follow-up, the patient had full, painless range of motion and was asymptomatic. The Constant score increased from 40 to 78, the DASH disability/symptom score decreased from 64 to 10, and the DASH work module score decreased from 94 to 0. At 5 months, graft integration was evident on radiographs; however, partial resorption with some degenerative changes was evident at final follow-up. Interestingly, immunohistochemical analysis demonstrated viable cartilage with high type II collagen expression at 19 months. In a follow-up case series, Giannini et al. again demonstrated patients having full, painless range of motion and being asymptomatic at final follow-up of 34 months [59]. All transplanted allografts demonstrated signs of integration on CT at 4 months postoperatively, and all shoulders demonstrated a congruent cartilage layer at 6 months postoperatively. Provencher et al. reported a case of distal tibial allograft reconstruction of the glenoid with humeral head allograft reconstruction of the humerus following postsurgical glenohumeral anchor arthropathy [60]. At 16 months of follow-up, the patient had symptomatic resolution, excellent range of motion, full strength, and high satisfaction with his clinical outcome.

Limitations in tissue access and logistics have constrained the widespread application of osteochondral allograft transplantation. Under the American Association of Tissue Banks guidelines, osteochondral allograft tissue undergoes thorough microbiologic and serologic testing in a 14-day screening period [61]. Because chondrocyte viability drops precipitously after 28 days, only approximately 2 weeks remains to allow for donor and recipient matching and transplantation [62]. Innovations in logistics and biologics are being investigated in an effort to improve allograft storage and preserve chondrocyte viability to allow for greater accessibility and widespread use of this technique [63].

Focal articular cartilage lesions of the glenohumeral joint remain a challenging pathology. It is imperative to obtain a thorough workup of the patient, including lesion grade, lesion size, patient activity level, and severity of symptoms to develop a treatment plan. Although most studies in the literature have demonstrated favorable

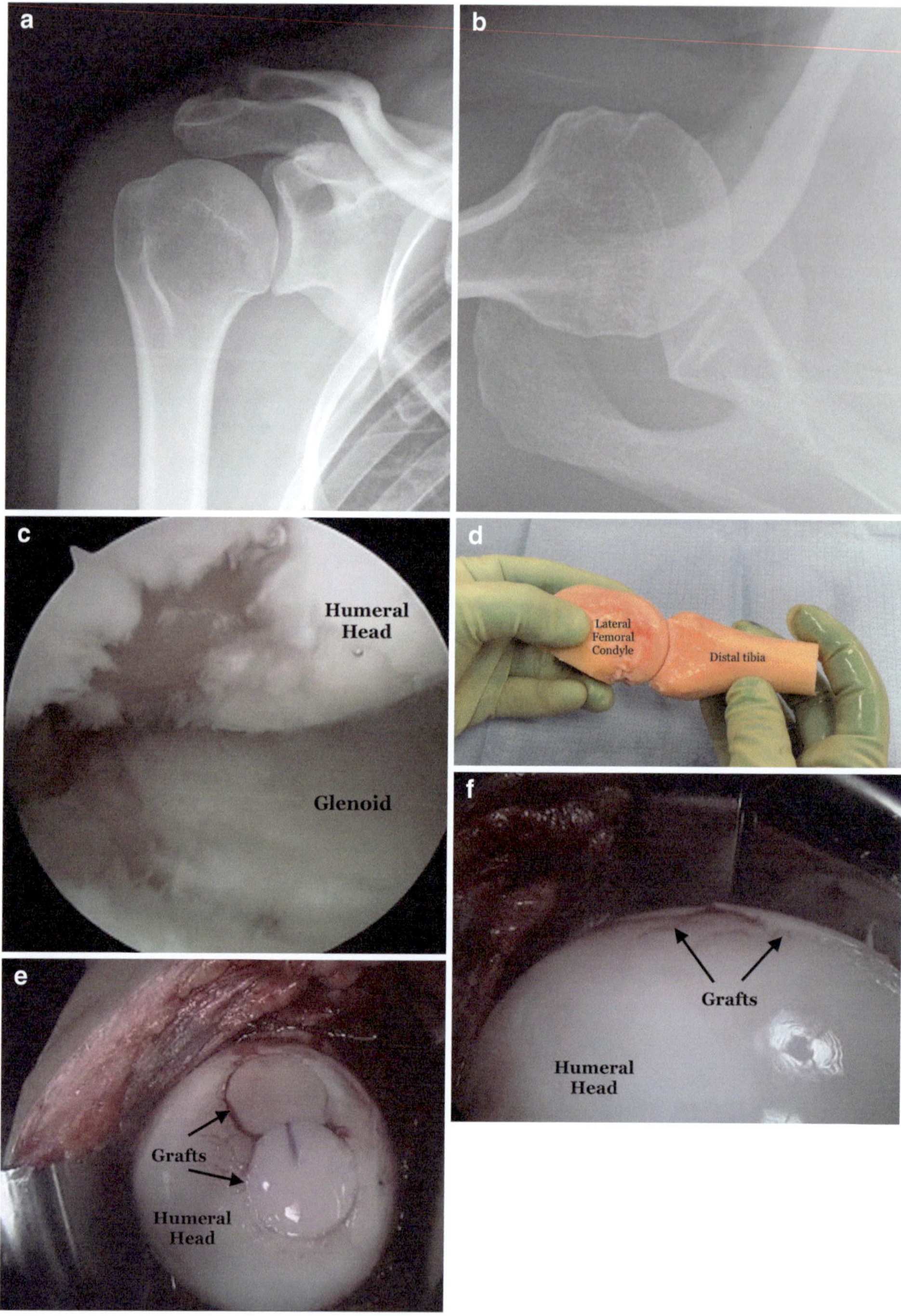

Fig. 8.1 34-year-old male warehouse worker fell off a ladder 12 years prior to presentation. He has had over 15 redislocations. He presented with pain and instability without locking or catching. He had full range of motion and strength and no ligamentous laxity, with positive apprehension and relocation signs. (**a**) AP and (**b**) lateral radiographs. (**c**) Arthroscopy demonstrating significant glenoid bone loss anteriorly and grade IV chondromalacia in the central humeral head. (**d**) A lateral femoral condyle and distal tibial allograft were used to restore the humeral head and glenoid, respectively. (**e**) Humeral head after two osteochondral allograft plugs is inserted in a "Mastercard" technique; (**f**) side view of the grafts demonstrating restoration of the radius of curvature; (**g**) 6-month and (**h**) 5-year postoperative CT scan of the glenoid demonstrating anatomic reconstruction on anterior glenoid and graft incorporation. (**i**) 5-year clinical follow-up demonstrating patient with full range of motion, being stable, and without pain or limitations

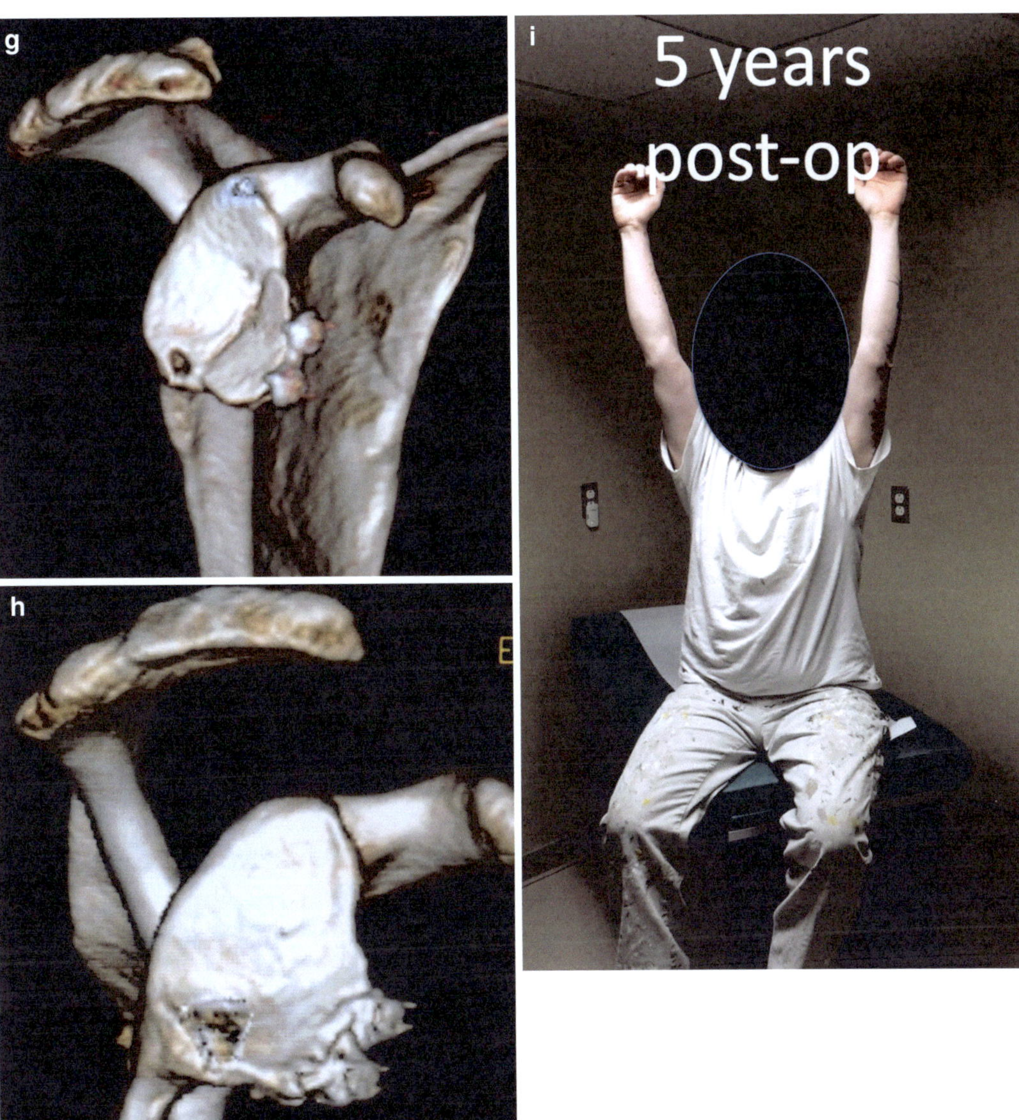

Fig. 8.1 (continued)

results, the evidence available for the use of osteochondral allograft transplantation is low. Decision-making about operative management of these lesions should be tailored to the individual patient as long-term data and high-quality randomized trials are undertaken to better define the efficacy, indications, and comparative nature of this procedure in relation to other available treatment modalities.

References

1. Sherman SL, Garrity J, Bauer K, Cook J, Stannard J, Bugbee W. Fresh osteochondral allograft transplantation for the knee: current concepts. J Am Acad Orthop Surg. 2014;22(2):121–33.
2. Frank RM, Van Thiel GS, Slabaugh MA, Romeo AA, Cole BJ, Verma NN. Clinical outcomes after microfracture of the glenohumeral joint. Am J Sports Med. 2010;38(4):772–81.
3. O'Brien J, Grebenyuk J, Leith J, Forster BB. Frequency of glenoid chondral lesions on MR arthrography in patients with anterior shoulder instability. Eur J Radiol. 2012;81(11):3461–5.
4. Slabaugh MA, Frank RM, Cole BJ. Resurfacing of isolated articular cartilage defects in the glenohumeral joint with microfracture: a surgical technique & case report. Am J Orthop (Belle Mead NJ). 2010;39(7):326–32.
5. Ellman H, Harris E, Kay SP. Early degenerative joint disease simulating impingement syndrome: arthroscopic findings. Arthroscopy. 1992;8(4):482–7.
6. Salata MJ, Kercher JS, Bajaj S, Verma NN, Cole BJ. Glenohumeral microfracture. Cartilage. 2010;1(2):121–6.
7. Provencher MT, Navaie M, Solomon DJ, Smith JC, Romeo AA, Cole BJ. Joint chondrolysis. J Bone Joint Surg Am. 2011;93(21):2033–44.
8. Shin JJ, Mellano C, Cvetanovich GL, Frank RM, Cole BJ. Treatment of glenoid chondral defect using micronized allogeneic cartilage matrix implantation. Arthrosc Tech. 2014;3(4):e519–22.
9. Krych AJ, Sousa PL, King AH, Morgan JA, May JH, Dahm DL. The effect of cartilage injury after arthroscopic stabilization for shoulder instability. Orthopedics. 2015;38(11):e965–9.
10. Patzer T, Lichtenberg S, Kircher J, Magosch P, Habermeyer P. Influence of SLAP lesions on chondral lesions of the glenohumeral joint. Knee Surg Sports Traumatol Arthrosc. 2010;18(7):982–7.
11. Gartsman GM, Taverna E. The incidence of glenohumeral joint abnormalities associated with full-thickness, reparable rotator cuff tears. Arthroscopy. 1997;13(4):450–5.
12. Mont MA, Maar DC, Krackow KA, Jacobs MA, Jones LC, Hungerford DS. Total hip replacement without cement for non-inflammatory osteoarthrosis in patients who are less than forty-five years old. J Bone Joint Surg Am. 1993;75(5):740–51.
13. Hamada S, Hamada M, Nishiue S, Doi T. Osteochondritis dissecans of the humeral head. Arthroscopy. 1992;8(1):132–7.
14. Levine WN, Clark AM Jr, D'Alessandro DF, Yamaguchi K. Chondrolysis following arthroscopic thermal capsulorrhaphy to treat shoulder instability. A report of two cases. J Bone Joint Surg Am. 2005;87(3):616–21.
15. Chu CR, Antoniou J, Donley BG, Frick SL, Hilibrand AS, Ricci WM, et al. The 2007 ABC traveling fellowship: building international orthopaedic bridges. J Bone Joint Surg Am. 2008;90(3):672–4.
16. Carroll KW, Helms CA, Speer KP. Focal articular cartilage lesions of the superior humeral head: MR imaging findings in seven patients. AJR Am J Roentgenol. 2001;176(2):393–7.
17. Guntern DV, Pfirrmann CW, Schmid MR, Zanetti M, Binkert CA, Schneeberger AG, et al. Articular cartilage lesions of the glenohumeral joint: diagnostic effectiveness of MR arthrography and prevalence in patients with subacromial impingement syndrome. Radiology. 2003;226(1):165–70.
18. Cameron BD, Galatz LM, Ramsey ML, Williams GR, Iannotti JP. Non-prosthetic management of grade IV osteochondral lesions of the glenohumeral joint. J Shoulder Elbow Surg. 2002;11(1):25–32.
19. Denti M, Monteleone M, Trevisan C, De Romedis B, Barmettler F. Magnetic resonance imaging versus arthroscopy for the investigation of the osteochondral humeral defect in anterior shoulder instability. A double-blind prospective study. Knee Surg Sports Traumatol Arthrosc. 1995;3(3):184–6.
20. Outerbridge RE. The etiology of chondromalacia patellae. J Bone Joint Surg Br. 1961;43-B:752–7.
21. Gross CE, Chalmers PN, Chahal J, Van Thiel G, Bach BR Jr, Cole BJ, et al. Operative treatment of chondral defects in the glenohumeral joint. Arthroscopy. 2012;28(12):1889–901.
22. Elser F, Braun S, Dewing CB, Millett PJ. Glenohumeral joint preservation: current options for managing articular cartilage lesions in young, active patients. Arthroscopy. 2010;26(5):685–96.
23. Sperling JW, Antuna SA, Sanchez-Sotelo J, Schleck C, Cofield RH. Shoulder arthroplasty for arthritis after instability surgery. J Bone Joint Surg Am. 2002;84(10):1775–81.
24. Gross AE, Kim W, Las Heras F, Backstein D, Safir O, Pritzker KP. Fresh osteochondral allografts for posttraumatic knee defects: long-term followup. Clin Orthop Relat Res. 2008;466(8):1863–70.
25. DeGroot H, Donati D, Di Liddo M, Gozzi E, Mercuri M. The use of cement in osteoarticular allografts for proximal humeral bone tumors. Clin Orthop Relat Res. 2004(427):190–197.
26. Becerra J, Andrades JA, Guerado E, Zamora-Navas P, Lopez-Puertas JM, Reddi AH. Articular cartilage: structure and regeneration. Tissue Eng Part B Rev. 2010;16(6):617–27.
27. Geraghty S, Kuang JQ, Yoo D, LeRoux-Williams M, Vangsness CT Jr, Danilkovitch A. A novel, cryopreserved, viable osteochondral allograft designed to augment marrow stimulation for articular cartilage repair. J Orthop Surg Res. 2015;10:66.
28. Dehaan A, Munch J, Durkan M, Yoo J, Crawford D. Reconstruction of a bony bankart lesion: best fit based on radius of curvature. Am J Sports Med. 2013;41(5):1140–5.

29. Rios D, Jansson KS, Martetschlager F, Boykin RE, Millett PJ, Wijdicks CA. Normal curvature of glenoid surface can be restored when performing an inlay osteochondral allograft: an anatomic computed tomographic comparison. Knee Surg Sports Traumatol Arthrosc. 2014;22(2):442–7.

30. Smucny M, Miniaci A. Pre-shaped allograft for glenoid reconstruction in anterior shoulder instability. Arthrosc Tech. 2018;7(4):e343–8.

31. Ghodadra N, Gupta A, Romeo AA, Bach BR Jr, Verma N, Shewman E, et al. Normalization of glenohumeral articular contact pressures after Latarjet or iliac crest bone-grafting. J Bone Joint Surg Am. 2010;92(6):1478–89.

32. Fox JA, Cole BJ, Romeo AA, Meininger AK, Williams JM, Glenn RE Jr, et al. Articular cartilage thickness of the humeral head: an anatomic study. Orthopedics. 2008;31(3):216.

33. Yeh LR, Kwak S, Kim YS, Chou DS, Muhle C, Skaf A, et al. Evaluation of articular cartilage thickness of the humeral head and the glenoid fossa by MR arthrography: anatomic correlation in cadavers. Skeletal Radiol. 1998;27(9):500–4.

34. Gebhart JJ, Miniaci A, Fening SD. Predictive anthropometric measurements for humeral head curvature. J Shoulder Elbow Surg. 2013;22(6):842–7.

35. Gobezie R, Lenarz CJ, Wanner JP, Streit JJ. All-arthroscopic biologic total shoulder resurfacing. Arthroscopy. 2011;27(11):1588–93.

36. Skendzel JG, Sekiya JK. Arthroscopic glenoid osteochondral allograft reconstruction without subscapularis takedown: technique and literature review. Arthroscopy. 2011;27(1):129–35.

37. Hunt HE, Sadr K, Deyoung AJ, Gortz S, Bugbee WD. The role of immunologic response in fresh osteochondral allografting of the knee. Am J Sports Med. 2014;42(4):886–91.

38. Kainer MA, Linden JV, Whaley DN, Holmes HT, Jarvis WR, Jernigan DB, et al. Clostridium infections associated with musculoskeletal-tissue allografts. N Engl J Med. 2004;350(25):2564–71.

39. Kropf EJ, Sekiya JK. Osteoarticular allograft transplantation for large humeral head defects in glenohumeral instability. Arthroscopy. 2007;23(3):322.e1–5.

40. Sekiya JK, Wickwire AC, Stehle JH, Debski RE. Hill-Sachs defects and repair using osteoarticular allograft transplantation: biomechanical analysis using a joint compression model. Am J Sports Med. 2009;37(12):2459–66.

41. Saltzman BM, Riboh JC, Cole BJ, Yanke AB. Humeral head reconstruction with osteochondral allograft transplantation. Arthroscopy. 2015;31(9):1827–34.

42. Diklic ID, Ganic ZD, Blagojevic ZD, Nho SJ, Romeo AA. Treatment of locked chronic posterior dislocation of the shoulder by reconstruction of the defect in the humeral head with an allograft. J Bone Joint Surg Br. 2010;92(1):71–6.

43. Riff AJ, Yanke AB, Shin JJ, Romeo AA, Cole BJ. Midterm results of osteochondral allograft trans-plantation to the humeral head. J Shoulder Elbow Surg. 2017;26(7):e207–15.

44. DiPaola MJ, Jazrawi LM, Rokito AS, Kwon YW, Patel L, Pahk B, et al. Management of humeral and glenoid bone loss—associated with glenohumeral instability. Bull NYU Hosp Jt Dis. 2010;68(4):245–50.

45. Rowe CR, Sakellarides HT. Factors related to recurrences of anterior dislocations of the shoulder. Clin Orthop. 1961;20:40–8.

46. Provencher MT, Bhatia S, Ghodadra NS, Grumet RC, Bach BR Jr, Dewing CB, et al. Recurrent shoulder instability: current concepts for evaluation and management of glenoid bone loss. J Bone Joint Surg Am. 2010;92(Suppl 2):133–51.

47. Burkhart SS, De Beer JF. Traumatic glenohumeral bone defects and their relationship to failure of arthroscopic Bankart repairs: significance of the inverted-pear glenoid and the humeral engaging Hill-Sachs lesion. Arthroscopy. 2000;16(7):677–94.

48. Itoi E, Lee SB, Berglund LJ, Berge LL, An KN. The effect of a glenoid defect on anteroinferior stability of the shoulder after Bankart repair: a cadaveric study. J Bone Joint Surg Am. 2000;82(1):35–46.

49. Piasecki DP, Verma NN, Romeo AA, Levine WN, Bach BR Jr, Provencher MT. Glenoid bone deficiency in recurrent anterior shoulder instability: diagnosis and management. J Am Acad Orthop Surg. 2009;17(8):482–93.

50. Lazarus MD, Sidles JA, Harryman DT 2nd, Matsen FA 3rd. Effect of a chondral-labral defect on glenoid concavity and glenohumeral stability. A cadaveric model. J Bone Joint Surg Am. 1996;78(1):94–102.

51. Greis PE, Scuderi MG, Mohr A, Bachus KN, Burks RT. Glenohumeral articular contact areas and pressures following labral and osseous injury to the anteroinferior quadrant of the glenoid. J Shoulder Elbow Surg. 2002;11(5):442–51.

52. Bhatia S, Van Thiel GS, Gupta D, Ghodadra N, Cole BJ, Bach BR Jr, et al. Comparison of glenohumeral contact pressures and contact areas after glenoid reconstruction with Latarjet or distal tibial osteochondral allografts. Am J Sports Med. 2013;41(8):1900–8.

53. Cvetanovich GL, Chalmers PN, Yanke AB, Gupta AK, Klosterman EL, Verma NN, et al. Feasibility of an osteochondral allograft for biologic glenoid resurfacing. J Shoulder Elbow Surg. 2014;23(4):477–84.

54. DeHaan AM, Groat T, Priddy M, Ellis TJ, Duwelius PJ, Friess DM, et al. Salvage hip arthroplasty after failed fixation of proximal femur fractures. J Arthroplasty. 2013;28(5):855–9.

55. Provencher MT, Ghodadra N, LeClere L, Solomon DJ, Romeo AA. Anatomic osteochondral glenoid reconstruction for recurrent glenohumeral instability with glenoid deficiency using a distal tibia allograft. Arthroscopy. 2009;25(4):446–52.

56. Sayegh ET, Mascarenhas R, Chalmers PN, Cole BJ, Verma NN, Romeo AA. Allograft reconstruction for glenoid bone loss in glenohumeral instability: a systematic review. Arthroscopy. 2014;30(12):1642–9.

57. Camp CL, Barlow JD, Krych AJ. Transplantation of a tibial osteochondral allograft to restore a large glenoid osteochondral defect. Orthopedics. 2015;38(2):e147–52.

58. Familiari F, Hochreiter B, Gerber C. Unacceptable failure of osteochondral glenoid allograft for biologic resurfacing of the glenoid. J Exp Orthop. 2021;8(1):111.

59. Giannini S, Buda R, Cavallo M, Ruffilli A, Grigolo B, Fornasari PM, et al. Bipolar fresh osteochondral allograft for the treatment of glenohumeral posttraumatic arthritis. Knee Surg Sports Traumatol Arthrosc. 2012;20(10):1953–7.

60. Provencher MT, LeClere LE, Ghodadra N, Solomon DJ. Postsurgical glenohumeral anchor arthropathy treated with a fresh distal tibia allograft to the glenoid and a fresh allograft to the humeral head. J Shoulder Elbow Surg. 2010;19(6):e6–e11.

61. Gortz S, Bugbee WD. Fresh osteochondral allografts: graft processing and clinical applications. J Knee Surg. 2006;19(3):231–40.

62. Wang T, Wang DX, Burge AJ, Pais M, Kushwaha B, Rodeo SA, et al. Clinical and MRI outcomes of fresh osteochondral allograft transplantation after failed cartilage repair surgery in the knee. J Bone Joint Surg Am. 2018;100(22):1949–59.

63. Cook JL, Stoker AM, Stannard JP, Kuroki K, Cook CR, Pfeiffer FM, et al. A novel system improves preservation of osteochondral allografts. Clin Orthop Relat Res. 2014;472(11):3404–14.

Autologous Cartilage Implantation (ACI) for Lesions on the Glenoid and Humerus

9

Daniel P. Berthold and Andreas B. Imhoff

9.1 Introduction

Focal cartilage defects in the glenohumeral joint remain challenging in both diagnostic and therapeutic management, especially in the young and active patients. In contrast to the knee, ankle, or hip joint, symptomatic focal cartilage lesions in the shoulder joint seem to be an under-investigated entity but relatively common [1]. When scanning current literature, the incidence of cartilage defects has been reported to be as high as 13–17% in patients with rotator cuff tears and overhead throwing athletes [2, 3]. Moreover, Guntern et al. reported in 2003 that 29% of patients undergoing arthroscopy for subacromial impingement had humeral cartilage lesions [4], while glenoid cartilage lesions were present in 15% of the cases. Interestingly, patients with cartilage defects in either glenoid or humerus present with a vast variety of symptoms including constant deep shoulder pain or sharp pain, crepitation, or generalized achiness during activity [5–8]. However, from our clinical practice, there are also a considerable number of patients who remain asymptomatic and do not require conservative or operative treatment. The etiology of focal carti-

lage defects often includes trauma (especially shoulder dislocations), previous surgery, osteochondritis dissecans, progressive shoulder instability, rotator cuff injuries, avascular necrosis, and others such as inflammatory arthritis [2].

When conservative treatment fails, current literature reports on a variety of surgical options including joint-preserving interventions and prosthetic joint replacement [2, 9, 10]. This chapter is focusing on joint-preserving options for patients, who are deemed too young for more invasive joint replacement, including autologous chondrocyte implantation (ACI). Other minimal-invasive procedures, such as micro fracturing, osteochondral autograft transfer (OAT), and osteochondral allograft (OCA) transplantation, have been discussed in previous chapters.

9.2 Autologous Chondrocyte Implantation

9.2.1 Indications

As adult hyaline cartilage has poor capacity for intrinsic healing, efforts have been made to augment cartilage repair and regeneration in order to help the intrinsic capacity for hyaline cartilage restoration [9]. While smaller symptomatic cartilage defects are reserved for bone marrow stimulation techniques such as micro fracturing or subchondral drilling [10], autologous chondrocyte

D. P. Berthold
Department of Orthopaedic Sports Medicine,
Technical University of Munich, Munich, Germany

A. B. Imhoff (✉)
Technical University of Munich, Munich, Germany
e-mail: imhoff@tum.de

© ISAKOS 2023
A. D. Mazzocca et al. (eds.), *Shoulder Arthritis across the Life Span*,
https://doi.org/10.1007/978-3-031-33298-2_9

implantation may be a viable option for larger defects. To date, ACI, a cell-based therapy, has been mainly used in the knee or ankle, where it represents a safe two-step minimal-invasive procedure with good long-term outcomes. However, its use in the shoulder joint has been limited to a few small investigations. Consequently, considering the lack of evidence for ACI in the shoulder joint, the criteria used in knee surgery, whereas ACI is indicated for full-thickness cartilage defects with intact subchondral bone (2–3 cm^2), may be directly translated to shoulder surgery [5]. Identifying the exact cause of shoulder pain in patients with both cartilage lesions and rotator cuff tears, long head of the bicep's lesions or disruptions of the labrum remain highly challenging, even for experienced shoulder surgeons. Consequently, we feel that concomitant shoulder pathologies should be addressed first, and small cartilage defects (<2 cm^2) are best treated with one-step bone marrow stimulation techniques or debridement. If isolated symptomatic large cartilage defects (>2 cm^2) are present, ACI as a two-step procedure may be considered [5]. Similarly, when concomitant injuries are present, especially an unstable shoulder where Ruckstuhl et al. showed a 57% incidence of glenoid cartilage lesions [11], these injuries should be treated first. If the cartilage defect is deemed symptomatic, ACI may be a viable option to prevent worsening of the cartilage damage and progression of osteoarthritis.

9.2.2 Patient-Reported Outcomes

A recent systematic review from Fiegen et al. revealed that between January 1996 and November 2018, only one study reported on ACI in five patients with focal cartilage defects in the glenohumeral joint [2]. Since then, only one other study was published in 2020. Recently, Boehm et al. reported on seven patients, who were treated for a focal cartilage defect of the humeral head with a mean follow-up of 2.7 years [12]. Although significant improvements were noted in subjective shoulder value (SSV) scores,

this study remains limited for its small sample size. Interestingly, four out of five patients had to undergo second-look arthroscopy, where no relapse of focal chondral defect was noted. Similarly, in 2013, Buchmann et al. reported on four male patients (range 21–36 years), who underwent ACI for focal cartilage defects on the humeral head ($n = 3$) and the glenoid ($n = 1$) [5]. Of interest, the Magnetic Resonance Observation of Cartilage Repair Tissue (MOCART) score was indicative of satisfactory defect coverage showing signs of fibrocartilaginous repair tissue. Similarly, at final follow-up (mean 41.3 ± 24.9 months), the mean visual analog scale (VAS) score was 0.3, the mean unweighted Constant score was 83.3 ± 9.9, and the mean American Shoulder and Elbow Surgeons index was 95.3 ± 8.1, showing that patients undergoing ACI for chondral defects can expect satisfactory clinical outcomes.

9.2.3 Complications

When it comes to complications, none of the studies reported direct intraoperative or complication to the cartilage repair itself [5, 12]. However, as ACI is a two-step procedure requiring an open approach, subscapularis insufficiency may occur. Consequently, careful detachment and stable insertion should be performed [5]. Also, patients need to be informed that ACI may fail and osteoarthritis progression occurs. However, in our hands, in the young and active patient, joint-preserving interventions should be favored over prosthetic replacement. Besides, even if ACI fails, it does not destroy the path for future interventions.

9.2.4 Technique

In summary, the procedure is performed in the beach chair position under general anesthesia. Before ACIs, diagnostic arthroscopy is performed and the cartilage defect is debrided. Care should be taken to not open the subchondral layer.

Cartilage biopsy can be either performed from macroscopic healthy cartilage at the border of the defect or at the anterosuperior humeral head close to the cartilage-bone transition zone [5]. Then, the probe is sent for cellular proliferation at a specialized facility. After 3–6 weeks of cellular proliferation, the second operation is performed through a standard deltopectoral approach with detachment of the subscapularis. Again, the lesion is debrided to its base using a ringed curette without opening the subchondral bone plate. This step is of importance to gain stable 90° walls perpendicular to its base. The defect is measured and transferred to the type I/III collagen-based membrane to be sized accordingly. The membrane is undergoing cell seeding intraoperatively, while a minimum density of 10^6 cells/cm^2 is reached. After 10 min of incubation, the chondrocyte membrane is now transferred into the defect, while circumferential no 6.0 absorbable sutures are placed adjacent to the articular cartilage. Fibrin glue can be used to achieve supplemental fixation. Finally, the capsule is closed, while the subscapularis tendon is refixed to the lesser tuberosity using transosseous sutures.

9.2.5 Rehabilitation

Starting from the first postoperative day, passive mobilization of the shoulder can be performed, while flexion and abduction are limited to 90° for 6 weeks. Consequently, a shoulder brace is used for 6 weeks. Active exercise is allowed starting from the seventh week, while return to sports is allowed after 6 weeks.

9.3 Conclusion

Focal cartilage defects in the glenohumeral joint remain challenging in both diagnostic and therapeutic management, especially in the young and active patients. As the incidence of cartilage defects in the shoulder joint is high, joint-preserving approaches such as ACI should be considered, as satisfactory outcomes and a fibrocartilaginous repair tissue can be expected. However, ACI is a two-step procedure requiring an open approach with detachment of an intact subscapularis tendon. As such, meticulous refixation of the subscapularis has to be performed to avoid subscapularis insufficiency in the young and active patient. Future investigations should be focused on long-term outcomes and minimal-invasive procedures.

Conflict of Interest ABI is a consultant for Arthrex, Arthrosurface, and Medi Bayreuth. DPB has nothing to declare.

References

1. Gartsman GM, Taverna E. The incidence of glenohumeral joint abnormalities associated with full-thickness, reparable rotator cuff tears. Arthroscopy. 1997;13(4):450–5.
2. Fiegen A, Leland DP, Bernard CD, et al. Articular cartilage defects of the glenohumeral joint: a systematic review of treatment options and outcomes. Cartilage. 2021;13(1_suppl):401S–13S.
3. Paley KJ, Jobe FW, Pink MM, Kvitne RS, ElAttrache NS. Arthroscopic findings in the overhand throwing athlete: evidence for posterior internal impingement of the rotator cuff. Arthroscopy. 2000;16(1):35–40.
4. Guntern DV, Pfirrmann CW, Schmid MR, et al. Articular cartilage lesions of the glenohumeral joint: diagnostic effectiveness of MR arthrography and prevalence in patients with subacromial impingement syndrome. Radiology. 2003;226(1):165–70.
5. Buchmann S, Salzmann GM, Glanzmann MC, Wörtler K, Vogt S, Imhoff AB. Early clinical and structural results after autologous chondrocyte transplantation at the glenohumeral joint. J Shoulder Elbow Surg. 2012;21(9):1213–21.
6. Johnson DL, Warner JJ. Osteochondritis dissecans of the humeral head: treatment with a matched osteochondral allograft. J Shoulder Elbow Surg. 1997;6(2):160–3.
7. Park T-S, Kim T-S, Cho J-H. Arthroscopic osteochondral autograft transfer in the treatment of an osteochondral defect of the humeral head: report of one case. J Shoulder Elbow Surg. 2006;15(6):e31–6.
8. Provencher MT, LeClere LE, Ghodadra N, Solomon DJ. Postsurgical glenohumeral anchor arthropathy treated with a fresh distal tibia allograft to the glenoid and a fresh allograft to the humeral head. J Shoulder Elbow Surg. 2010;19(6):e6–e11.

9. Condron NB, Kester BS, Tokish JM, et al. Nonoperative and operative soft-tissue, cartilage, and bony regeneration and orthopaedic biologics of the shoulder: an Orthoregeneration Network (ON) foundation review. Arthroscopy. 2021;37(10):3200–18.

10. Porcellini G, Cecere AB, Giorgini A, Micheloni GM, Tarallo L. The GLAD lesion: are the definition, diagnosis and treatment up to date? A systematic review. Acta Biomed. 2020;91(Suppl 14):e2020020.

11. Ruckstuhl H, de Bruin ED, Stussi E, Vanwanseele B. Post-traumatic glenohumeral cartilage lesions: a systematic review. BMC Musculoskelet Disord. 2008;9(1):1–8.

12. Boehm E, Minkus M, Scheibel M. Autologous chondrocyte implantation for treatment of focal articular cartilage defects of the humeral head. J Shoulder Elbow Surg. 2020;29(1):2–11.

Guillermo Arce, Marcos Deimundo, and Pablo Adelino Narbona

10.1 Background

In treating patients with shoulder instability, the main objective of the surgical treatment is to recover joint stability and allow the patients to return to active life and sports without dislocations or subluxations. Most of the literature focuses on the dislocation recurrence rate as the primary treatment end goal [1–6].

Regarding the techniques to achieve these goals, there are "anatomic repairs" such as labrum repair, arthroscopic Bankart repair (ABR), and others called "not anatomic," like bone blocks or the Latarjet procedure. The general thought is that the "anatomic repairs" such as ABR produce less or no shoulder arthritis and the bone blocks, including the Latarjet, generate more joint deterioration [7–11].

However, after a relatively long follow-up, shoulder osteoarthritis (OA) is common in patients suffering shoulder instability with or without surgical treatment. This is a devastating complication in young or middle-aged patients [12–14].

This situation is also a significant challenge for the attending physicians. They usually face many dilemmas. What is the reason for these degenerative changes in this young patient? How has this happened? What can I do to improve the patient's symptoms? Is there any way to prevent this joint deterioration?

This chapter aims to (1) review the possible causes or risk factors of shoulder osteoarthritis in the unstable shoulder, (2) evaluate the role of the arthroscopic Bankart repair (ABR) in this problem, and (3), after reaching a global consensus among the members of the ISAKOS Shoulder Committee, suggest guidelines or best practices to decrease the incidence of this severe complication.

10.2 The Unstable Shoulder and Arthritis

The relationship between shoulder instability and joint deterioration is well established. When the first-time dislocation results from high-energy trauma, such as in collision sports, the impact produces labrum avulsions with glenoid fragments and a posterior impaction fracture at the humeral head. These lesions, called bony Bankart and Hill-Sachs, respectively, are approached with different surgical techniques, but the associated articular cartilage damage is seldom evaluated [15, 16].

Multiple dislocation episodes produce considerable damage to the glenoid and humeral articu-

G. Arce (✉) · M. Deimundo
Instituto Argentino de Diagnóstico y Tratamiento (IADT), Buenos Aires, Argentina

P. A. Narbona
Sanatorio Allende, Córdoba, Argentina

© ISAKOS 2023
A. D. Mazzocca et al. (eds.), *Shoulder Arthritis across the Life Span*,
https://doi.org/10.1007/978-3-031-33298-2_10

lar cartilage. The complete dislocations, subluxations, and abnormal biomechanics deteriorate the joint.

The "dislocation arthropathy" is defined as cartilage deterioration, joint narrowing, and osteophyte formation after symptomatic shoulder instability with or without shoulder stabilization procedures [17–23].

The cartilage wear and osteophyte growth decrease the range of motion, improving the joint stability, but pain and stiffness rapidly increase with time [24–26].

The classifications for shoulder arthritis help determine the grade of articular damage and define the options for surgical treatment. Most published data are based on the Samilson and Prieto classification [17, 27].

Regarding the natural history of dislocation arthropathy without surgical treatment, Hovelius et al. reported an incidence of 29% mild, 9% moderate, and 17% severe (56% in total) after 25 years of follow-up of patients with at least one dislocation [18–21].

Novakofski et al. recently reported a group of 254 patients (73% male) followed for at least 10 years (mean follow-up of 17 years) due to symptomatic instability and dislocations. Fifty-eight percent of the patients have pain, and 12.2% have OA with symptoms [23].

The published findings of OA in patients suffering shoulder instability without surgical treatment are summarized in Table 10.1.

Briefing the published data, around 50% of the patients with symptomatic shoulder instability without any surgical treatment may suffer pain, and 30% have some degree of shoulder arthritis in the long term.

Table 10.1 Reported data about osteoarthritis after shoulder instability with conservative treatment without surgery [18–21, 23, 24]

Author	OA without surgery	Follow-up in years
Hovelius L et al. JBJS 1996	Mild 11% Moderate 9% Total: 20%	10
Hovelius L et al. J Shoulder Elb Surg 2009	39%	25
Novakofski K J Shoulder Elb Surg 2020	58% pain 12.2% OA	17
Kruckeberg B OJSM 2020	17% OA	15.2

10.3 Shoulder Arthritis After Arthroscopic Bankart Repair

Facing symptomatic shoulder instability with multiple dislocation episodes, the patient is already at risk of developing arthritis. After undergoing an ABR, they can expect a good result regarding the recurrences. Still, the cartilage deterioration and osteoarthritis changes will continue after surgery and may worsen in many cases [24, 28].

The incidence of OA after ABR is summarized in Table 10.2.

Reviewing the data in Tables 10.1 and 10.2, it seems that (1) many of the patients already have mild or moderate OA before the ABR, (2) the OA appears or becomes worse after the ABR and an extended follow-up, and (3) it is difficult to define if the high postoperative OA grade is triggered by the operation or just a consequence of the previous instability and a long sequel.

Table 10.2 Reported data about osteoarthritis after arthroscopic Bankart repair (ABR) [1–3, 27–35]

Authors	OA before surgery	OA after surgery	Procedure	Mean follow-up: years
Buscayret F et al. AJSM 2004	9.2%	19.7%	ABR	6.5
Franceschi F et al. AJSM 2011		4% mild 14% moderate 4% severe Total: 22%	ABR	8
Larsen Van Gastel M et al. KSSTA 2019	9.8%	49% mild 7.3% moderate 3.6% severe Total: 60%	ABR	13.1
Plath J et al. AJSM 2015		41% mild 16% moderate 12% severe Total: 69%	ABR	13
Castagna A et al. AJSM 2010		29% mild 10% moderate Total: 39%	ABR	10.9
Murphy A et al. JSES 2019		35.4% mild 8.8% moderate 1.7% severe Total: 59.4%	ABR	10
Privitera D et al. AJSM 2012		20% mild 25% moderate 15% severe Total: 60%	ABR	13.5
Aboalata M et al. AJSM 2016		12%	ABR	13
Elmlund et al. KSSTA 2012		24% mild 18% moderate	ABR	7.9
Zaffagnini S et al. KSSTA 2012		37%	ABR	14.7
Kruckeberg B et al. OJSM 2020		28%	ABR	15.2
Rosenberg B et al. AJSM 1995		42% mild 9% moderate 3% severe 54% total	BR	15
Ono Y et al. JSES 2019		36.8% moderate to severe	ABR	10

The dislocation episodes may produce a critical glenoid bone loss. Also, in other cases, the bone loss appears after many subluxation episodes as attritional bone loss. In any of these settings, when the glenoid bone loss is over 13.5%, most surgeons prefer to indicate a bony reconstruction procedure like an allograft, an autograft bone block, or the Latarjet technique. These bone blocks may also produce OA in the long term [7, 9–11].

10.4 Contributing Risk Factors to Develop Osteoarthritis After ABR

During the ABR, there are some operative factors that, even though they increase stability and decrease the recurrence rate, may have the negative connotation of producing arthritis. These factors are anchors, knots, and postoperative stiffness. Other risk factors contributing to developing OA are older age at the first episode, glenoid rim fractures, and the number of preoperative dislocations [27, 36].

The risk factors for developing osteoarthritis after ABR are briefed in Table 10.3.

To recover the labrum bumper effect, some authors recommended placing the anchors on the glenoid face about 2 mm from the glenoid edge. Even though this location may positively impact stability, avoiding medial labrum healing at the glenoid neck could negatively affect the articular cartilage. Hirose T. et al. recently reported less glenoid rim erosion locating the anchors at the glenoid rim [37].

The number and location of anchors and knots seem critical to preserving or damaging the articular cartilage. The anchor eyelet below the cartilage level but out of the bone produces a devastating joint deterioration [32]. A thorough evaluation of the anchors' positions is essential for all the patients reporting pain after ABR (Fig. 10.1).

Nonabsorbable sutures and big knots are other frequent findings in shoulders with arthritis after ABR. These knots scuff the cartilage during the shoulder motion and contribute to OA development (Fig. 10.2).

Another risk factor for developing OA is shoulder stiffness. The so-called anatomic repairs reduce the labrum to its original native location to regain shoulder stability. However, they can partially restrict the range of motion for at least a few months after the index procedure.

The plastic elongation of the capsule due to dislocation episodes or the patient's primary laxity is also challenging to quantify. The surgeon must repair the labrum to treat these unstable shoulders and tighten or plicate the capsule in different amounts. This reduction of the capsular volume has been described as one of the keys to a successful treatment but may produce biomechanical changes and overloading of the joint. The increase of the contact shearing forces on the cartilage generates arthritis [13, 14].

The humeral head has an average of 30 degrees of retroversion. After surgery and postoperative rehabilitation, any patient who doesn't recover at least 30 degrees of external rotation cannot center their humeral head at the glenoid. This stiffness

Table 10.3 Risk and contributing factors to develop osteoarthritis after ABR [27, 36]

Risk factors in developing shoulder arthritis after ABR
1. Osseous glenoid rim lesions
2. Older age at the first episode, >23 years old
3. The number of dislocations. Delayed surgery
4. The number of anchors and knots
5. Postoperative decrease in external rotation

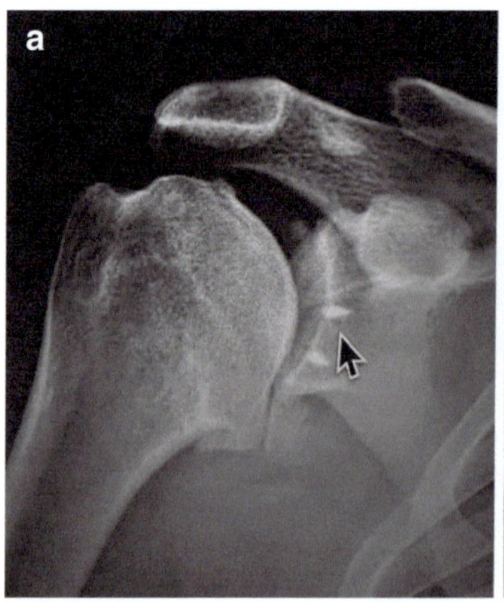
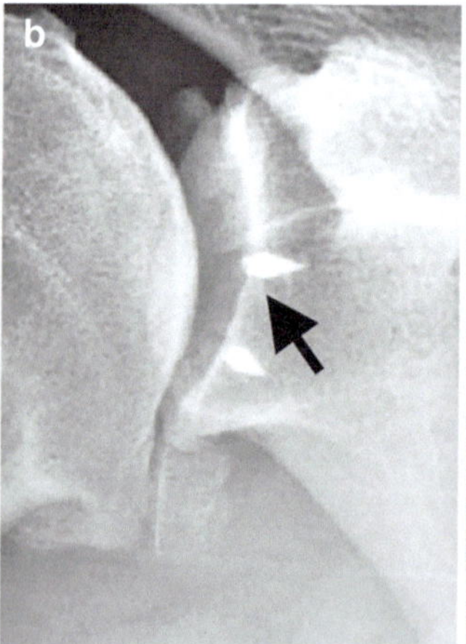
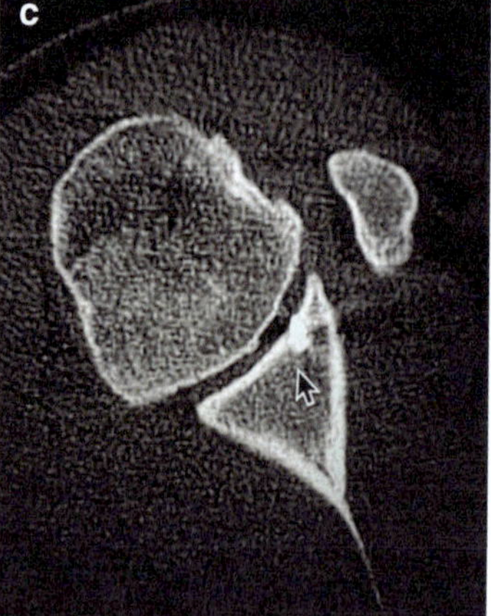

Fig. 10.1 Advanced osteoarthritis 9 years after arthroscopic Bankart repair. Right shoulder. Imaging evaluation of degenerative changes and anchors' placement. (**a**) Regular X-ray. The anchors' placement looks adequate. (**b**) A closer look at the X-ray suggests one of the anchors may have the eyelet out of the bone. (**c**) The CT scan confirms that the anchor eyelet is below the cartilage but out of the bone

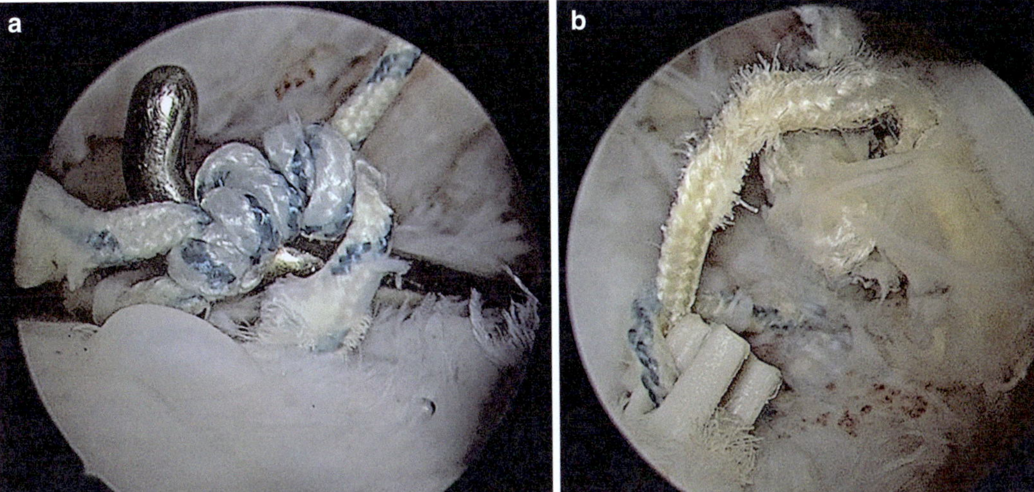

Fig. 10.2 Arthroscopic findings at second-look arthroscopies after Bankart repair. (**a**) Nonabsorbable sutures and big knots producing cartilage damage. (**b**) Anchor eyelet out of the bone leads to devastating joint deterioration

after ABR for anterior shoulder instability produces a posterior translation of the center of rotation and secondary articular damage [27, 29].

The "remplissage" is indicated to treat the humeral bone defect. This French term means "filling." A part of the posterior capsule and the infraspinatus tendon is introduced into the posterior humeral head bone defect (Hill-Sachs lesion) to prevent engaging and dislocations. This procedure is commonly used to enhance shoulder stability during an ABR but also changes shoulder biomechanics and can reduce the range of motion-producing OA [38, 39].

10.5   What Can Prevent OA After Arthroscopic Bankart Repair (ABR)?

Patients complaining about pain and stiffness more than 3 months after ABR should be deeply evaluated. Good-quality X-rays, 2-D or 3-D CT scans, and an MRI should be obtained to recognize the origin of the pain and the loss of external rotation. The anchors' placement should be determined when osteoarthritis changes appear early after the index procedure.

Six months after the ABR, the patients should be asymptomatic. If pain and stiffness persist, a second-look arthroscopy is warranted to rule out intra-articular problems that can damage the cartilage. In this setting, all causes of pain and stiffness are checked. Any anchor at the articular cartilage and knots contacting the joint surfaces must be removed.

In situations where the external rotation loss is critical, a conservative capsular release can be done by pie-crusting the capsule to increase the range of motion without compromising the previous labrum repair [36].

The comprehensive arthroscopic management (CAM) procedure described by Mook and Millet et al. is indicated in patients with mild to moderate OA changes (Samilson and Prieto grades A to C) with more than 2 mm joint space and an inferior osteophyte at the humeral head [40].

A joint debridement, loose body removal, long head of the biceps tenotomy or tenodesis, capsular releases, chondroplasty, and osteophyte removal are performed. After surgery, a complete rehabilitation program is recommended to increase the range of motion, strength, and scapula control (Figs. 10.3 and 10.4).

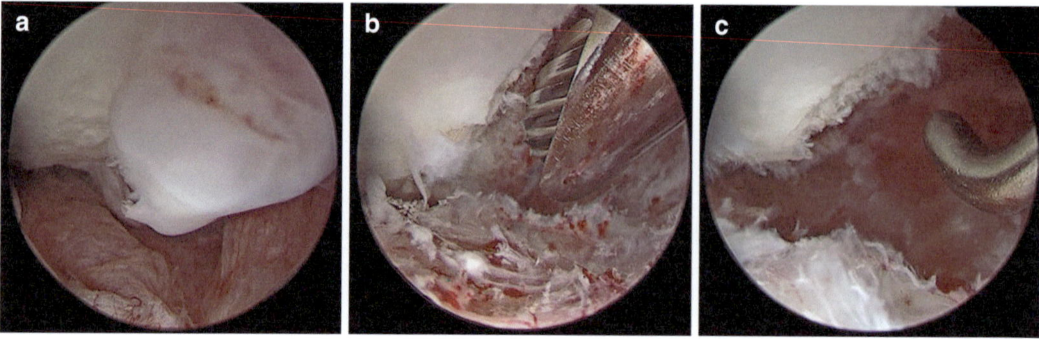

Fig. 10.3 Right shoulder. Comprehensive arthroscopic management. Arthroscopic views from the posterior portal. (**a**) Inferior humeral osteophyte before resection. (**b**) Osteophyte resection with burr from the posterior-inferior portal. (**c**) Final arthroscopic control after adequate osteophyte removal

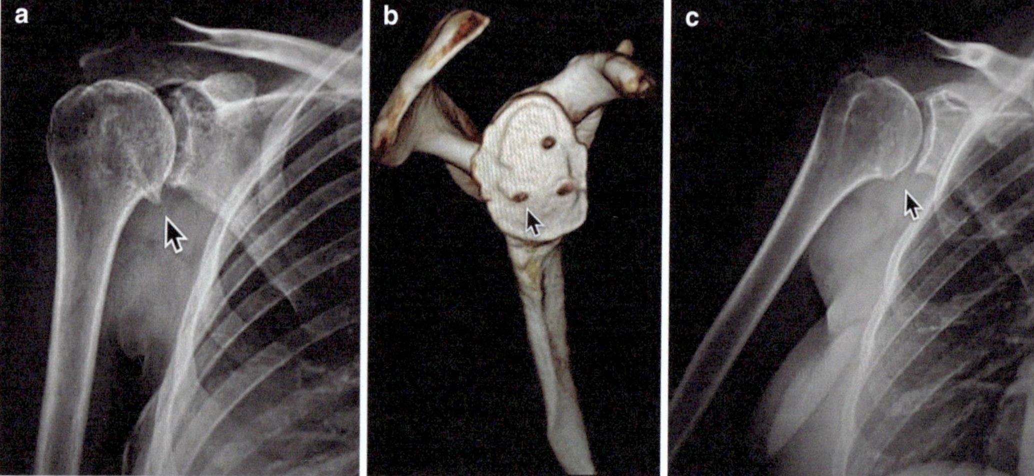

Fig. 10.4 Images of shoulder arthritis after Bankart repair. (**a**) Preoperative AP X-ray showing a grade III humeral osteophyte. (**b**) Tridimensional CT scan. Anchors at the glenoid face produce joint deterioration. (**c**) Postoperative AP X-ray after CAM procedure demonstrates adequate humeral bone spur resection

10.6   Final Thoughts

The ISAKOS Shoulder Committee, during its Consensus Meeting in Madrid, extensively discussed the reported causes of OA after ABR. After reviewing the published data, the level V experts' experience was added to consent about the best practices to prevent OA after ABR. These suggestions are summarized in Table 10.4.

The progression of osteoarticular damage and osteoarthritis before and after arthroscopic Bankart repair is a devastating complication and

Table 10.4 Five best practices to prevent osteoarthritis after ABR

1	Decrease the number of preoperative dislocations
2	Place the anchors at the glenoid rim—anchors' eyelets inside the bone—knots and sutures at the capsule side, not near the cartilage
3	Tailored capsular plication to avoid postoperative stiffness
4	All patients with pain or decreased external rotation after ABR warrant detailed X-rays, CT scans, and MRI evaluations
5	Patients with pain and stiffness 6 months after ABR justify a second-look arthroscopy to prevent cartilage damage by anchors or knots

could be worse than the recurrence of dislocations. The surgeons must be aware of these concepts to explain the problem to the patients and their families before the operation. Then, perform the best technique to avoid instability without increasing the degenerative changes.

From the ISAKOS Shoulder Committee, we hope this chapter will help the readers to be aware of these critical complications and improve their decision-making and techniques to achieve better long-term results for patients suffering from shoulder instability.

References

1. Larsen van Gastel M, Willigenburg N, Dijksman L, Lindeboom R, van den Bekerom M, van der Hulst V, et al. Ten percent re-dislocation rate 13 years after the arthroscopic Bankart procedure. Knee Surg Sports Traumatol Arthrosc. 2019;27(12):3929–36.
2. Murphy A, Hurley E, Hurley D, Pauzenberger L, Mullett H. Long-term outcomes of the arthroscopic Bankart repair: a systematic review of studies at 10-year follow-up. J Shoulder Elbow Surg. 2019;28(11):2084–9.
3. Aboalata M, Plath J, Seppel G, Juretzko J, Vogt S, Imhoff A. Results of arthroscopic Bankart repair for anterior-inferior shoulder instability at 13-year follow-up. Am J Sports Med. 2016;45(4):782–7.
4. Harris J, Gupta A, Mall N, Abrams G, McCormick F, Cole B, et al. Long-term outcomes after Bankart shoulder stabilization. Arthroscopy. 2013;29(5):920–33.
5. Bottoni C, Johnson J, Zhou L, Raybin S, Shaha J, Cruz C, et al. Arthroscopic versus open anterior shoulder stabilization: a prospective randomized clinical trial with 15-year follow-up with an assessment of the glenoid being "on-track" and "off-track" as a predictor of failure. Am J Sports Med. 2021;49(8):1999–2005.
6. Berendes TD, Wolterbeek R, Pilot P, Verburg H, Slaa RL. The open modified Bankart procedure: outcome at follow-up of 10 to 15 years. J Bone Joint Surg. 2007;89:1064–8.
7. Menon A, Fossati C, Magnani M, Boveri S, Compagnoni R, Randelli P. Low grade of osteoarthritis development after Latarjet procedure with a minimum 5 years of follow-up: a systematic review and pooled analysis. Knee Surg Sports Traumatol Arthrosc. 2021;30:2074–83.
8. Kavaja L, Pajarinen J, Sinisaari I, Savolainen V, Björkenheim J, Haapamäki V, et al. Arthrosis of glenohumeral joint after arthroscopic Bankart repair: a long-term follow-up of 13 years. J Shoulder Elbow Surg. 2012;21(3):350–5.
9. Rollick N, Ono Y, Kurji H, Nelson A, Boorman R, Thornton G, et al. Long-term outcomes of the Bankart and Latarjet repairs: a systematic review. Open Access J Sports Med. 2017;8:97–105.
10. Zimmermann S, Scheyerer M, Farshad M, Catanzaro S, Rahm S, Gerber C. Long-term restoration of anterior shoulder stability: a retrospective analysis of arthroscopic Bankart repair versus open Latarjet procedure. J Bone Joint Surg. 2016;98(23):1954–61.
11. Ernstbrunner L, De Nard B, Olthof M, Beeler S, Bouaicha S, Gerber C, et al. Long-term results of the arthroscopic Bankart repair for recurrent anterior shoulder instability in patients older than 40 years: a comparison with the open Latarjet procedure. Am J Sports Med. 2020;48(9):2090–6.
12. Komnos G, Banios K, Liantsis A, Alexiou K, Varitimidis S, Bareka M, et al. Results of arthroscopic Bankart repair in recreational athletes and laborers: a retrospective study with 5 to 14 years of follow-up. Orthop J Sports Med. 2019;7(11):232596711988164.
13. Zink S, Pfeiffenberger T, Müller A, Krisam R, Unglaub F, Pötzl W. The arthroscopic Bankart operation: a 10-year follow-up study. Arch Orthop Trauma Surg. 2022;142:3367.
14. Bock J, Buckup J, Reinig Y, Zimmermann E, Colcuc C, Hoffmann R, et al. The arthroscopic Bankart repair procedure enables complete quantitative labrum restoration in long-term assessments. Knee Surg Sports Traumatol Arthrosc. 2018;26(12):3788–96.
15. Cameron M, Kocher M, Briggs K, Horan M, Hawkins R. The prevalence of glenohumeral osteoarthrosis in unstable shoulders. Am J Sports Med. 2003;31(1):53–5.
16. Lu Y, Pareek A, Wilbur R, et al. Understanding anterior shoulder instability through machine learning. New models that predict recurrence, progression or surgery, and development of arthritis. Orthop J Sports Med. 2021;9(11):232596712110533.
17. Samilson R, Prieto V. Dislocation arthropathy of the shoulder. J Bone Joint Surg Am. 1983;65:456–60.
18. Hovelius L, Augustini BG, Fredin H, et al. Primary anterior dislocation of the shoulder in young patients: a ten-year prospective study. J Bone Joint Surg. 1996;78:1677–84.
19. Hovelius LK, Sandström BC, Rösmark DL, et al. Long-term results with the Bankart and Bristow-Latarjet procedures: recurrent shoulder instability and arthropathy. J Shoulder Elbow Surg. 2001;10:445–52.
20. Hovelius L, Sandström B, Saebö M. One hundred eighteen Bristow-Latarjet repairs for recurrent anterior dislocation of the shoulder prospectively followed for fifteen years: study II—the evolution of dislocation arthropathy. J Shoulder Elbow Surg. 2006;15:279–89.
21. Hovelius L, Saeboe M. Arthropathy after primary anterior shoulder dislocation; 223 shoulders prospectively followed up for twenty-five years. J Shoulder Elbow Surg. 2009;18(3):339–47.
22. Brophy R, Marx R. Osteoarthritis following shoulder instability. Clin Sports Med. 2005;24(1):47–56.
23. Novakofski K, Melugin H, Leland D, Bernard C, Krych A, Camp C. Nonoperative management of anterior shoulder instability can result in high rates of

recurrent instability and pain at long-term follow-up. J Shoulder Elbow Surg. 2022;31(2):352–8.

24. Kruckeberg BM, Leland DP, Bernard CD, Krych AJ, Dahm DL, Sanchez-Sotelo J, Camp CL. Incidence of and risk factors for glenohumeral osteoarthritis after anterior shoulder instability: a US population-based study with average 15-year follow-up. Orthop J Sports Med. 2020;8(11):232596712096251.

25. Coifman I, Brunner UH, Scheibel M. Dislocation arthropathy of the shoulder. J Clin Med. 2022;11(7):2019–20.

26. Cerciello S, Corona K, Morris B, et al. Shoulder arthroplasty to address the sequelae of anterior instability arthropathy and stabilization procedures: systematic review and meta-analysis. Arch Orthop Trauma Surg. 2020;140(12):1891–900.

27. Buscayret F, Bradley T, Szabo I, Adeleine P, Coudane H, Walch G. Glenohumeral arthrosis in anterior instability before and after surgical treatment incidence and contributing factors. Am J Sports Med. 2004;32(5):1165–72.

28. Plath J, Aboalata M, Seppel G, Juretzko J, Waldt S, Vogt S, et al. Prevalence of and risk factors for dislocation arthropathy. Am J Sports Med. 2015;43(5):1084–90.

29. Franceschi F, Papalia R, Del Buono A, Vasta S, et al. Glenohumeral osteoarthritis after arthroscopic Bankart repair for anterior instability. Am J Sports Med. 2011;39:1654–9.

30. Castagna A, Markopoulos N, Conti M, Rose GD, Papadakou E, Garofalo R. Arthroscopic Bankart suture anchor repair: radiological and clinical outcomes at minimum 10 years of follow-up. Am J Sports Med. 2010;38:2012–6.

31. Privitera DM, Bisson LJ, Marzo JM. Minimum 10-year follow-up of arthroscopic intra-articular Bankart repair using bioabsorbable tacks. Am J Sports Med. 2012;40:100–7.

32. Elmlund AO, Ejerhed L, Sernert N, Rostgard LC, Kartus J. Dislocation arthropathy and drill hole appearance in a mid- to long-term follow-up study after arthroscopic Bankart repair. Knee Surg Sports Traumatol Arthrosc. 2012;20:2156–62.

33. Zaffagnini S, Marcheggiani Muccioli GM, Giordano G, et al. Long-term outcomes after repair of recurrent posttraumatic anterior shoulder instability: comparison of arthroscopic transglenoid suture and open Bankart reconstruction. Knee Surg Sports Traumatol Arthrosc. 2012;20:816–21.

34. Rosenberg B, Richmond J, Levine W. Long-term followup of Bankart reconstruction. Am J Sports Med. 1995;23(5):538–44.

35. Ono Y, Dávalos Herrera D, Woodmass J, Lemmex D, Carroll M, Yamashita S, et al. Long-term outcomes following isolated arthroscopic Bankart repair: a 9- to 12-year follow-up. JSES Open Access. 2019;3(3):189–93.

36. Vezeridis P, Ishmael C, Jones K, Petrigliano F. Glenohumeral dislocation Arthropathy: etiology, diagnosis and management. J Am Acad Orthop Surg. 2019;27:227–35.

37. Hirose T, Nakagawa S, Uchida R, et al. On-the-edge anchor placement may be protective against glenoid rim erosion after arthroscopic Bankart repair compared to on-the-face anchor placement. Arthroscopy. 2021;38:1099.

38. Ding Z, Cong S, Xie Y, Feng S, Chen S, Chen J. Location of the suture anchor in Hill-Sachs lesion could influence glenohumeral cartilage quality and limit range of motion after arthroscopic Bankart repair and Remplissage. Am J Sports Med. 2020;48(11):2628–37.

39. Argintar E, Heckmann N, Wang L, Tibone JE, Lee TQ. The biomechanical effect of shoulder remplissage combined with Bankart repair for the treatment of engaging Hill-Sachs lesions. Knee Surg Sports Traumatol Arthrosc. 2016;24(2):585–92.

40. Mook W, Petri M, Greenspoon J, Millett P. The comprehensive arthroscopic management procedure for treatment of glenohumeral osteoarthritis. Arthroscopy Tech. 2015;4(5):435–41.

Part III

Joint Replacement Open Treatment in the Young Patient

Daniel P. Berthold, Paulo J. Llinas-Hernandez, and Andreas B. Imhoff

11.1 Partial Humeral Head Resurfacing

11.1.1 Introduction

Large full-thickness cartilage defects of the proximal humeral are known to be a cause for severe shoulder pain, mostly in patients of younger age. The early diagnosis of cartilage defect remains challenging, mainly as they are often overseen in primary diagnostic and detected delayed during shoulder arthroscopy. Consequently, shoulder surgeons have to decide whether to neglect these injuries or if cartilage restoration procedures are indicated. If conservative or prior joint preserving treatment fails, resurfacing of the humeral head may be seen as a treatment option to restore full shoulder function and relieve pain. To date, the two most commonly used implants are the Partial Eclipse implant (Arthrex, Naples, FL, USA) and the HemiCAP implant (Arthrosurface, Franklin, MA, USA) [1]. Historically, the Arthrosurface prosthesis is implanted in an open fashion, whereas the Eclipse implant was designed to be implanted via a minimal-invasive procedure. However, both implants are similar in design, and both provide inlay resurfacing [1]. The advantage of the minimal-invasive procedure is full preservation of the subscapularis tendon and the possibility of early postoperative mobilization, while positioning of the implant requires a high learning curve. Besides, reduced visualization and preparation of the cartilage defect can also be challenging, while peripheral defects of the humerus are seen as a contraindication for all-arthroscopic procedures.

When compared to total arthroplasty, in partial resurfacing, the glenoid is not affected intraoperatively; as such, all revision options on the glenoid side remain available during revision surgery. Consequently, partial resurfacing of the humeral head should be reserved for younger patients, who may have a higher probability to undergo future revision procedures. Besides, humeral head resurfacing may better preserve the native biomechanics, maintaining a more anatomic center of rotation, with less eccentric loading of the glenoid [2, 3].

As described below, partial resurfacing of the humeral head should be reserved for full-thickness focal cartilage defects, while more diffuse chondral lesions or osteoarthritis should be reserved for anatomic total shoulder arthroplasty [1, 4, 5].

D. P. Berthold · A. B. Imhoff (✉)
Department of Orthopaedic Sports Medicine,
Technical University of Munich, Munich, Germany
e-mail: imhoff@tum.de

P. J. Llinas-Hernandez
Valle del Lili Foundation University Hospital, ICESI
University, Cali, Colombia

© ISAKOS 2023
A. D. Mazzocca et al. (eds.), *Shoulder Arthritis across the Life Span*,
https://doi.org/10.1007/978-3-031-33298-2_11

11.1.1.1 Indications

Historically, the true indication for partial humeral head resurfacing included osteoarticular pathology, especially in younger patients who showed a preserved rotator cuff or were deemed too young for total shoulder arthroplasty or hemiarthroplasty. However, as limited data is available for joint preserving approaches in patients with large cartilage defects, partial humeral head resurfacing has emerged as a potential surgical solution in this challenging patient cohort. Advantages of this technique include preservation of the remaining healthy cartilage and bone stock, which may be beneficial, if revision surgery requiring total shoulder arthroplasty is needed. Besides, native biomechanics including neck-shaft angle, humeral offset, and center of rotation are maintained [6]. By maintaining the humeral offset and the radius of curvature, shoulder range of motion can be maintained. Interestingly, small changes in ROC were shown to change shoulder ROM significantly. This can be noted in current literature, whereas several authors reported improvements in ROM after partial resurfacing, even in external rotation [7, 8].

Indications for partial resurfacing include large focal humeral head defects in young and/or active patients, mostly resulting from avascular necrosis, trauma, instability, or idiopathic chondrolysis [9]. Moreover, patients with large, mostly engaging Hill-Sachs lesions may benefit from partial resurfacing to prevent further engaging or progression of osteoarthritis [10, 11].

11.1.1.2 Outcomes

In current literature, only a few studies are reporting patient-reported outcomes of partial humeral head resurfacing in patients with focal cartilage defects, while most of the studies report on patients with the open HemiCAP implant, and only one study dealt with the arthroscopic Partial Eclipse implant [12]. Bessette et al. reported on 16 patients (mean age 32.3 years) who underwent HemiCAP partial resurfacing for Hill-Sachs defects [10]. Thirteen patients (81%) returned to the preinjury activity level, while one patient had postoperative stiffness, and another patient had a

sensation of instability, which did not require further intervention. Similarly, in 2015, Sweet et al. reported on 19 patients (mean age: 48.9 years) undergoing HemiCAP for AVN ($n = 4$) or osteoarthritis ($n = 16$) [8]. All patient reported satisfactory outcomes including mean American Shoulder and Elbow Surgeons (ASES) score, simple shoulder test (SST) score, and visual analog scale (VAS) score as well as improvements in forward flexion (from 100° to 129°) and external rotation (from 23° to 43°). Of interest, there was no radiographic evidence for periprosthetic fracture, component loosening, or failure. Similarly, Uribe et al. prospectively reported 12 patients with HemiCAP for advanced stage AVN with a mean age of 56 years [11]. Overall, forward flexion improved significantly from 94° to 142°, while Constant score also improved from 23 to 60. Recently, Holschen et al. reported mid-term results on 18 patients with focal Outerbridge grade IV cartilage defects of the proximal humerus and subsequent partial resurfacing of the humeral head [1]. Of those, 13 patients were treated with a partial humeral head prosthesis in an open technique, while 5 patients received a partial humeral head prosthesis in an arthroscopic technique. At mean follow-up, the mean Constant score rated 79.5 and the mean ASES score 85.5 points, while the mean VAS score was low with 0.7 points. When compared between the groups, the open groups had slightly lower scores (CS 75.3; ASES 83) than the arthroscopic group (CS 88.8 and ASES 92.6). Only one patient was converted to total shoulder arthroplasty due to progressive glenohumeral osteoarthritis, while 50% of the patients showed progressive glenohumeral osteoarthritis. However, according to the authors, this radiographic observation does not affect the clinical outcomes.

11.1.1.3 Complications

Only a few studies reported on complications following resurfacing of the humerus. However, no implant-related complications such as aseptic loosening, infection, and incorrect implant placement were reported, indicating that partial resurfacing is a safe procedure. Overall, when compared to conventional shoulder arthroplasty, revision rates and periprosthetic fractures are low [9], but osteoarthritis progression may not be delayed. The Australian National Joint Replacement Registry reported a revision rate of only 0.6 per 100 observed implant-years. As stated by Holschen et al. [1], careful patient selection is mandatory for successful outcomes, as patients with signs of general osteoarthritis on standardized radiographs should not be indicated for this procedure. Otherwise, concomitant pathology or prior surgery has been associated with worse clinical outcomes and higher revision rates [4].

11.1.1.4 Surgical Technique

Surgery starts with the patient in beach chair position and diagnostic shoulder arthroscopy via a standard posterior portal. Exact localization and size of the defect as well as any concomitant injuries are detected.

Partial Eclipse Implant

If the focal cartilage defect is located centrally, the Partial Eclipse implant is indicated via all-arthroscopic approach. First, the defect is debrided using a shaver. Consequently, a drill guide is inserted to determine the size of the focal cartilage defect, which should not widely exceed 25 mm. A 2.4 mm guide pin is drilled through the drill guide from the lateral proximal humerus into the joint. Subsequently, after removing the drill guide, the guide pin is now over-drilled using a 4 mm cannulated drill. A guide sleeve is inserted through the transhumeral canal, while the guide pin is exchanged to a retro pin. This pin is then connected to a reamer, which is introduced to the joint via anterior portal. Consequently, retrograde reaming of the cartilage defect is performed to prepare the bed for the implant. Then, the retro pin is removed and a cannulated screwdriver is inserted into the guide sleeve. The Eclipse implant is inserted into the joint using a nonabsorbable suture. If the implant is now placed correctly, the implant is fixed using a screw at the humeral head (Figs. 11.1, 11.2, and

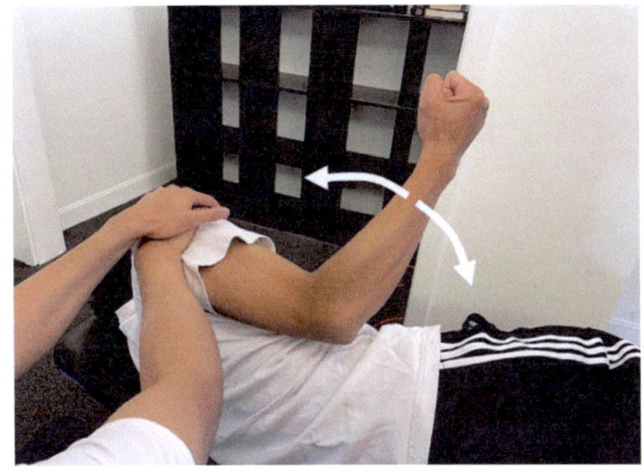

Fig. 11.1 Anteroposterior view of an Eclipse implant in a patient with a large, focal cartilage defect of the humeral head

11.3). Surgery ends with consecutive wound closure.

HemiCAP Implant

If the focal cartilage defect is located eccentrically, an open approach using the HemiCAP implant may be indicated. To do so, a standard deltopectoral approach is used with detachment of the subscapularis tendon. The humeral head is now dislocated and the cartilage defect debrided using a curette. The defect is measured and a pin is inserted through a drill guide into the center of the cartilage lesion. The pin is over-drilled using a cannulated drill, while a tap is inserted to prepare the thread for the taper post. Consequently, the taper post is introduced and the guide pin can be removed. The next step is of importance: to determine the implant's size and its convexity, a contact probe is used by measuring offsets at four different points. Subsequently, reaming is performed by placing it over the guide pin to prepare the bed. A trial component is inserted to confirm the correct form and the correct depth of the implant. If the healthy cartilage surface is matched, the definitive articular surface implant is introduced into the taper post. Surgery ends with a reconstruction of the subscapularis tendon with nonabsorbable sutures and consecutive wound closure.

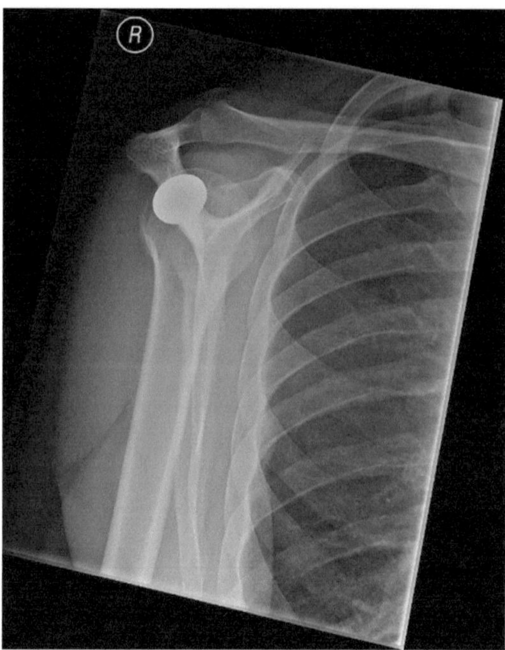

Fig. 11.2 Y-view or transscapular view of an Eclipse implant in a patient with a large, focal cartilage defect of the humeral head

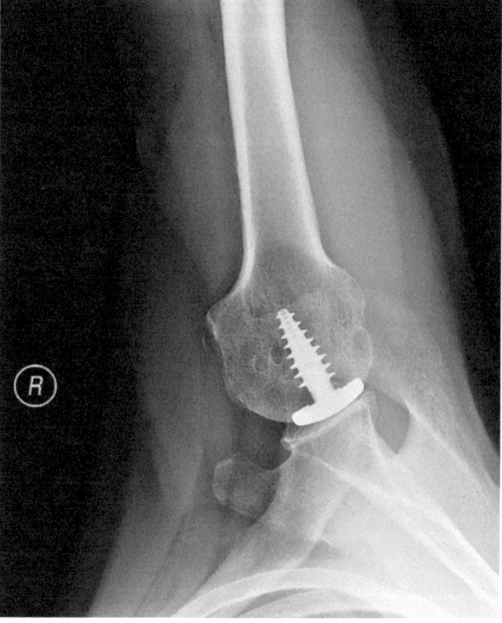

Fig. 11.3 Axial view of an Eclipse implant in a patient with a large, focal cartilage defect of the humeral head

11.1.2 Rehabilitation

If an all-arthroscopic approach is used, physiotherapy starts immediately after surgery with no restriction in range of motion or resistance. An arm sling can be used but is not mandatory. When choosing the open approach, patients are placed in an abduction pillow for 3 weeks, with limited passive external rotation and active internal rotation for 3 more weeks to protect the subscapularis tendon.

11.1.3 Conclusion

If conservative or prior joint preserving treatment fails, resurfacing of the humeral head may be seen as a treatment option to restore full shoulder function and relieve pain. Both implants, the Arthrosurface and the Eclipse implant, are similar in design, and both provide inlay resurfacing. When compared to conventional total shoulder arthroplasty, humeral head resurfacing may better preserve the native biomechanics, maintaining a more anatomic center of rotation, with less eccentric loading of the glenoid. In current literature, only a few studies are reporting patient-reported outcomes of partial humeral head resurfacing in patients with focal cartilage defects, while most of the studies report on patients using the HemiCAP implant. However, good clinical outcomes, restoration of range of motion, and low revision rates can be expected.

11.2 Total Humeral Head Resurfacing

11.2.1 Introduction

Glenohumeral osteoarthritis in young and active patients does currently not have an ideal solution. Typically, this pathology occurs in older patients due to genetic causes or as a result of rotator cuff injuries. However, in the young and athletic population, it mostly develops as a consequence of arthropathy due to instability, trauma, overuse, or avascular or postsurgical necrosis. Conservative treatment, consisting of modification in sports activity, physiotherapy, infiltrations, and anti-inflammatory medication, may often not be satisfactory, generating an inability to return to sports and day-to-day activities. In this group of patients with high demands and expectations, arthroscopic surgery offers less invasive procedures which include debridement, chondroplasty, loose body removal, biceps tenodesis, axillary nerve neurolysis, acromioplasty, capsular releases, osteophyte removal, and humeral osteoplasty gathered in the concept of comprehensive arthroscopic management (CAM) described by Millet [13].

In cases of diffuse lesions, humeral head resurfacing (HHR) is an option to avoid the problems associated with the glenoid and humeral stems, which may come along with unacceptably high rates of early loosening in young patients. [14–17] At the 10-year follow-up, the failure rate of total shoulder arthroplasty (TSA) in young patients can reach up to 62.5% [18, 19].

HHR is designed to avoid humeral osteotomy, which leads to advantages when compared to traditional stems: bone stock savings by preserving the neck and >50% of the humeral head, neck-diaphyseal angle, version, inclination, center of original rotation and offset [20]. There is evidence showing that humeral resurfacing does not alter any of these values and that anatomical restoration is seen as an important factor [14, 20–24]. In theory, by not modifying the original anatomy of the proximal humerus, resurfacing revision surgery can be done with conventional replacements, which, in young patients, is a clear advantage in saving time in the scenario of possible failure.

The first resurfacing procedures on the humerus were done with implants originally developed for the hip in the 1970s. The radius of curvature was then modified to adapt them more precisely to the humeral head, cementing them in all cases and without any procedure on the glenoid [25]. Simultaneously, Copeland developed cementless resurfacing prostheses that had a central pin anchored to the proximal metaphysis and a screw

fixated to the lateral cortex, combined with a polyethylene glenoid component that was also secured with a pin [26]. Due to the high rate of early loosening of these designs, it was modified using hydroxyapatite covers and the cortical fixation screw was removed [25]. Current components have pegs of various shapes, sizes, and lengths. Most are made of cobalt-chromium or titanium alloys, with a porous hydroxyapatite coating, uncemented and with "press-fit" fixation.

When scanning current literature, the gold standard for the management of advanced glenohumeral osteoarthritis remains anatomical TSA. However, young patients come along with a totally different scenario; consequently, TSA may not be an ideal solution for this challenging patient cohort, given the complications in the short and medium term: glenohumeral instability, periprosthetic fractures, loosening, and loss of bone stock. Logically, complications are found more frequent in younger patients with greater functional and sports demand. This is particularly true for glenoid cemented components in which the medium- and long-term loosening percentage is up to 39% [18]. In recent decades, resurfacing arthroplasty has subsequently become a popular alternative in young patients. In contrast to conventional anatomical prostheses, which require resecting the entire humeral head and placing a humeral stem, proximal humeral resurfacing consists of scarifying the proximal portion of the humeral head and inserting a metal alloy cap over it. The theoretical advantage, in addition to those mentioned above, is to maintain the bone stock, making a revision surgery easier in case it is required in the future.

11.2.1.1 Indications

Humeral head resurfacing procedure is indicated for patients under 50 years of age with primary, postsurgical (Fig. 11.4), or post-traumatic osteoarthritis, extensive full-thickness focal lesions, and avascular necrosis of the humeral head. Another typical indication is patients with proximal metaphyseal deformities from trauma where a humeral stem is difficult or impossible to insert.

The sine qua non condition is not having an irreparable rotator cuff injury. In this regard, the

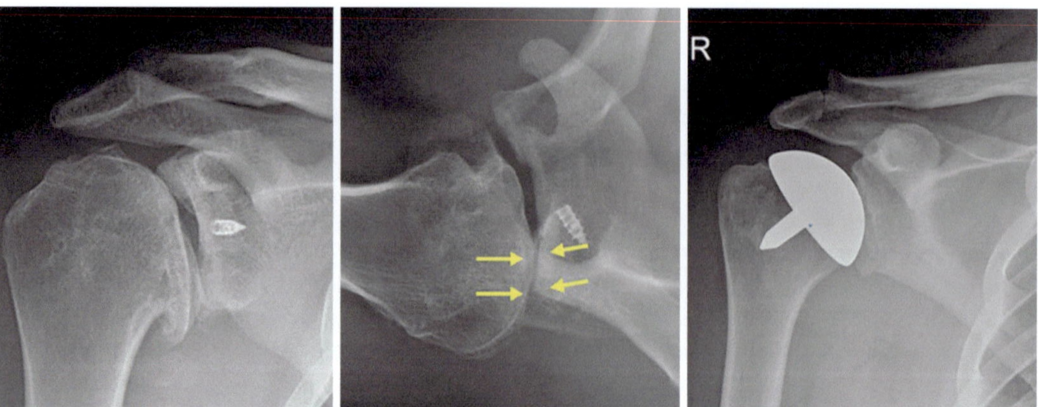

Fig. 11.4 Post-surgical glenohumeral osteoarthritis

integrity of the rotator cuff components should be carefully assessed with MRI. Particular attention must be paid to the integrity or reparability of the subscapularis tendon, since it plays a fundamental role in anterior stability and final mobility [27].

The CT scan allows to assess the congruence of the glenoid and its eccentric wear, which are risk factors in early failure for HHR. Additionally, the bone stock of the humerus must be at least 60%, which is important to evaluate in avascular necrosis and large Hill-Sachs lesions [22].

11.2.2 Surgical Technique

Patients can be admitted the same day of surgery and discharged on an outpatient basis. A combination of first-generation cephalosporin and vancomycin is administered 1 hour before surgery. General anesthesia plus interscalene block under ultrasound guidance is administered to all patients. The patient is placed on a surgical table in the supine position, with an auxiliary table to support the upper limb. A deltopectoral approach is used with preservation of the pectoralis major tendon and the circumflex brachial vessels. The subscapularis peel technique is done and repaired with nonabsorbable sutures for posterior reattachment (Fig. 11.5a). Aggressive soft tissue releases of the subscapularis and the anterior and inferior aspects of the capsule are performed when necessary to improve tendon excursion. These include a 360° release of the subscapularis tendon (the coracohumeral ligament and the rotator interval, the inferior and anterior aspects of the capsule, and any anterior subcoracoid adhesions). Tenodesis of the long head of the biceps is done routinely in all patients to avoid postsurgical tenosynovitis. The biceps is repaired with nonabsorbable suture to the surrounding rotator cuff tissue at its entrance into the joint at the end of the procedure. The intra-articular portion of the biceps tendon is released from the superior aspect of the labrum and was excised. The humeral head is dislocated and fully exposed, removing all peripheral osteophytes. This step is particularly important to fully expose the anatomical humeral neck and define the correct size of the implant. Head sizing is confirmed using the humeral head sizers (Fig. 11.5b). Marking the center of the humeral head is decisive since the final position depends on this. Landmarks are made on the upper, lower, and anterior borders with the electrocautery, and lines are drawn to intersect these marks (Fig. 11.5c). Once the center of the humeral head is located, a pin is placed up to the lateral cortex, for greater fixation and to avoid migration in the cancellous bone, which serves as a guide to start the reamers (Fig. 11.5c). Using the humeral head gauge, the diameter and

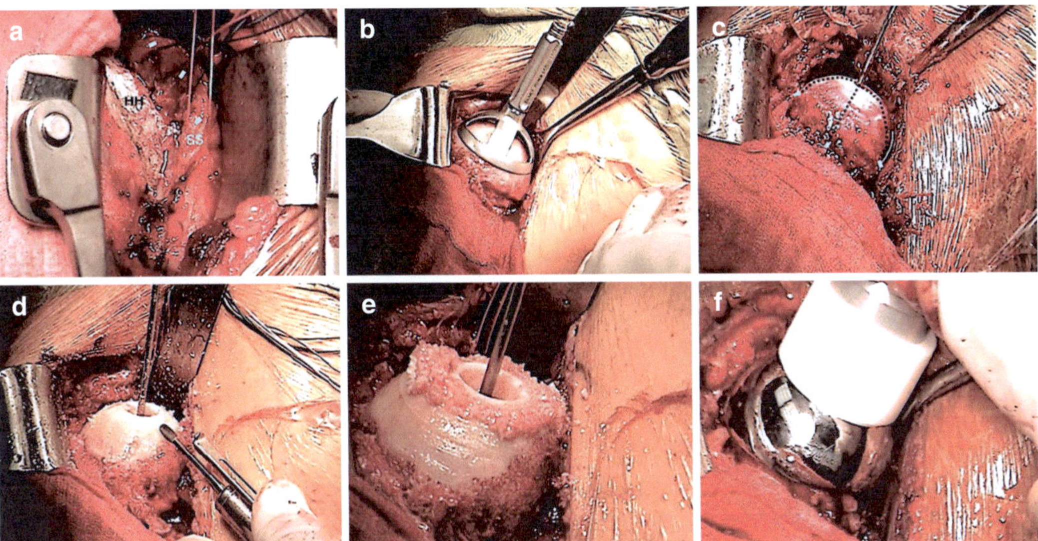

Fig. 11.5 (**a**) Subscapularis peel (**b**) Humeral head (HH) sizers (**c**) Landmark to find the center of the HH (**d**) Reamed to regularize the HH (**e**) Perforation of the central peg (**f**) Head impactor tool to completely seat the implant with a mallet

thickness of the humeral head are confirmed. The plane of the head sizer rim is parallel with the plane of the anatomical neck of the native humerus. Once the appropriate size is chosen, the head is regularized with the corresponding reamer, until the metaphyseal bone is exposed (Fig. 11.5d). The redundant bone is preserved to put it in the final cup, favoring integration (Fig. 11.5e). Reaming should cease before the sharp-toothed edge of the reamer damages the insertion of the superior capsule. When the reamer gets to this point, don't delve any further. The trial component is placed, ensuring coaptation of the bone to the inferior surface. According to the brand of prosthesis used, a perforation of the central peg with the corresponding shape is made (Fig. 11.5e). Use the head impactor tool to completely seat the implant with a mallet, until complete bone-prosthesis contact is ensured (Fig. 11.5f). Reposition the head in the glenoid fossa and verify that the laxity of the shoulder is adequate. The subscapularis is reattached with nonabsorbable sutures. Closure of the deltopectoral interval is performed in a routine fashion. No drains are used.

11.2.3 Outcomes

The results of the HHR should be evaluated in terms of revision rates/time, loosening failures, glenoid erosion, humeral head elevation due to rotator cuff damage, and return to sports activities. In general, the failures should be much higher compared to traditional shoulder prostheses, since the indications for HHR are young patients with a higher level of activity and demand.

When comparing the results of TSA versus HHR (37 vs. 37 patients) at 2-year follow-up, there are no significant differences in both groups in terms of static centering status of the humeral head, acromiohumeral distance, or signs of loosening between the two groups [28]. Fourman et al. [29] compared a series of 106 HHR versus 47 hemiarthroplasties (HA) with 8-year follow-up, finding better functional results in the HHR group. The ASES pain subscore was significantly worse in the HA group (25.2 ± 29.5 vs. 38.5 ± 12.7 after HHR, $p < 0.0001$). Contrary to these findings, in a review of the Nordic Arthroplasty Register Association, Rasmussen et al. [30]

found that HHR (n = 1923) and HA with stems (n = 1587) had an increased risk of failure compared with TSA (n = 2340) at 10-year follow-up (0.85, 0.93, and 0.96, respectively). For patients below 55 years, the 10-year cumulative survival rates were 0.75 (HHR n = 354), 0.81 (HA n = 146), and 0.87 (TSA n = 201). Regardless of the prosthesis used, younger patients had worse outcomes. Chillemi et al. [31] reported revision rates of 16% in a series of 25 patients with osteoarthritis and avascular necrosis. The patients had a mean age of 67.2 years and were evaluated at 7.5 years.

The return to sports activities has been scarcely evaluated in HHR. Bailie et al. [14] reported the return to sports in 36 patients with a minimum follow-up of 2 years. Thirty of the 36 patients returned to their sports activity level as that prior to surgery. In a survey of 310 members of the American Shoulder and Elbow Surgeons, the return to sports after humeral resurfacing compared with HA and TSA was the highest, at 92.0% of the respondents [32]. Most surgeons recommend low-impact or non-collision sports; however, in the authors' experience, with HHR, return to sports is recommended without limitation of the type of activity that was previously practiced.

11.2.4 Complications

The incidence of fractures and intraoperative complications is significantly lower when patients undergo HHR compared to those who are undergoing TSA (RR = 0.42 (CI 0.24–0.73) and 0.08 (CI 0.02–0.32), respectively) [33]. Early complications are associated with pain secondary to impingement (25%) [34], arthrofibrosis (8.3%) [34], rotator cuff tears [14], and hematomas. According to the Shoulder Arthroplasty New Australia register [35], the two main late complications that require revision are associated with glenoid erosion in 25.8% and pain in 22.6%. Rotator cuff insufficiency (11.5%), instability/dislocation (10.1%), and loosening (9.7%) followed in frequency. In our experience, the main

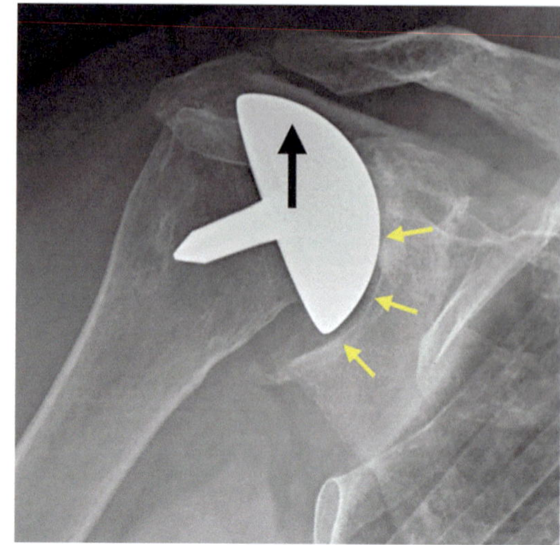

Fig. 11.6 Eight years post-HHR with glenoid erosion (yellow arrows) and humeral head elevation due to rotator cuff damage

causes of failure are pain and glenoid erosion (Fig. 11.6).

11.2.5 Rehabilitation

The patients are immobilized with an abduction pillow for 4 weeks. Passive and active mobility of the elbow and forearm is started the following day in a free manner. At 4 weeks, a progressive program is started to regain full range of motion of the shoulder and muscle strengthening is initiated. Sports activity is allowed to begin 6 months after surgery.

11.2.6 Conclusion

Early osteoarthritis in young and active patients remains difficult to treat. When all conservative and preventive management measures have failed, HHR may be seen as a potential alternative, especially in this challenging patient cohort. The results in the medium and short term are comparable with anatomical TSA; however, the advantages of bone preservation and nonmodification of the patient's own anatomy may be seen as favorable. Additionally, in case of future revision surgery, surgery may be technically easier, while conversion to conventional anatomical prosthesis is still possible.

Conflict of Interest ABI is a consultant for Arthrex, Arthrosurface, and Medi Bayreuth. DPB and PJL have nothing to declare.

References

1. Holschen M, Berg D, Schulte T, Bockmann MB, Witt KA, Steinbeck J. Arthroscopic and open partial arthroplasty for the treatment of focal grade IV cartilage defects of the humeral head. Arch Orthop Trauma Surg. 2021;141(9):1455–62. https://doi.org/10.1007/S00402-020-03552-X.
2. Bixby EC, Sonnenfeld JJ, Alrabaa RG, Trofa DP, Jobin CM. Partial humeral head resurfacing for avascular necrosis. Arthrosc Tech. 2019;9(1):e185–9. https://doi.org/10.1016/J.EATS.2019.09.025.
3. Giles JW, Elkinson I, Ferreira LM, et al. Moderate to large engaging Hill-Sachs defects: an in vitro biomechanical comparison of the remplissage procedure, allograft humeral head reconstruction, and partial resurfacing arthroplasty. J Shoulder Elbow Surg. 2012;21(9):1142–51. https://doi.org/10.1016/J.JSE.2011.07.017.
4. Delaney RA, Freehill MT, Higgins LD, Warner JJP. Durability of partial humeral head resurfacing. J Shoulder Elbow Surg. 2014;23(1):e14–22. https://doi.org/10.1016/J.JSE.2013.05.001.
5. Schnetzke M, Wittmann T, Raiss P, Walch G. Short-term results of a second generation anatomic short-stem shoulder prosthesis in primary osteoarthritis. Arch Orthop Trauma Surg. 2019;139(2):149–54. https://doi.org/10.1007/s00402-018-3039-1.
6. Hammond G, Tibone JE, McGarry MH, Jun BJ, Lee TQ. Biomechanical comparison of anatomic humeral head resurfacing and hemiarthroplasty in functional glenohumeral positions. J Bone Joint Surg Am. 2012;94(1):68–76. https://doi.org/10.2106/JBJS.I.00171.
7. Ranalletta M, Bertona A, Tanoira I, Rossi LA, Bongiovanni S, Maignón GD. Results of partial resurfacing of humeral head in patients with avascular necrosis. Rev Esp Cir Ortop Traumatol (Engl Ed). 2019;63(1):29–34. https://doi.org/10.1016/j.recot.2018.08.001.
8. Sweet SJ, Takara T, Ho L, Tibone JE. Primary partial humeral head resurfacing: outcomes with the HemiCAP implant. Am J Sports Med. 2015;43(3):579–87. https://doi.org/10.1177/0363546514562547.
9. Miniaci A, Scarcella MJ. Shoulder resurfacing for treatment of focal defects and diffuse osteoarthritis. Orthopade. 2021;50(2):112–8. https://doi.org/10.1007/S00132-020-04055-8.
10. Bessette MC, Frisch NC, Kodali P, Jones MH, Miniaci A. Partial resurfacing for humeral head defects associated with recurrent shoulder instability. Orthopedics. 2017;40(6):e996–e1003. https://doi.org/10.3928/01477447-20171012-01.
11. Uribe JW, Botto-van BA. Partial humeral head resurfacing for osteonecrosis. J Shoulder Elbow Surg. 2009;18(5):711–6. https://doi.org/10.1016/j.jse.2008.10.016.
12. Anderl W, Kriegleder B, Neumaier M, Laky B, Heuberer P. Arthroscopic partial shoulder resurfacing. Knee Surg Sports Traumatol Arthrosc. 2015;23(5):1563–70. https://doi.org/10.1007/s00167-014-2981-x.
13. Millett PJ, Horan MP, Pennock AT, Rios D. Comprehensive arthroscopic management (CAM) procedure: clinical results of a joint-preserving arthroscopic treatment for young, active patients with advanced shoulder osteoarthritis. Arthroscopy. 2013;29:440–8. https://doi.org/10.1016/j.arthro.2012.10.028.
14. Bailie DS, Llinas PJ, Ellenbecker TS. Cementless humeral resurfacing arthroplasty in active patients less than fifty-five years of age. J Bone Joint Surg Am. 2008;90(1):110–7. https://doi.org/10.2106/JBJS.F.01552.
15. Merolla G, Bianchi P, Lollino N, Rossi R, Paladini P, Porcellini G. Clinical and radiographic mid-term outcomes after shoulder resurfacing in patients aged 50 years old or younger. Musculoskelet Surg. 2013;97 Suppl 1:23–9. https://link.springer.com/article/10.1007/s12306-013-0261-4. Accessed 8 May 2022.
16. Muh SJ, Streit JJ, Shishani Y, Dubrow S, Nowinski RJ, Gobezie R. Biologic resurfacing of the glenoid with humeral head resurfacing for glenohumeral arthritis in the young patient. J Shoulder Elbow Surg. 2014;23(8):1–6. https://doi.org/10.1016/j.jse.2013.11.016.
17. Murthi AM, Cox RM, Strelzow JA, Athwal GS, Tashjian RZ, Abboud JA. Glenohumeral arthritis in young patients: scope, arthroplasty, interposition, arthrodesis, and resurfacing. Instr Course Lect. 2018;67:99–113. http://www.ncbi.nlm.nih.gov/pubmed/31411405. Accessed 22 May 2022.
18. Bohsali KI, Wirth MA, Rockwood CA. Complications of total shoulder arthroplasty. 2006;88:2279.
19. Sperling JW, Cofield RH, Rowland CM. Neer hemiarthroplasty and Neer total shoulder arthroplasty in patients fifty years old or less. Long-term results. J Bone Joint Surg Am. 1998;80(4):464–73. https://doi.org/10.2106/00004623-199804000-00002.
20. Thomas SR, Sforza G, Levy O, Copeland SA. Geometrical analysis of Copeland surface replacement shoulder arthroplasty in relation to normal anatomy. J Shoulder Elbow Surg. 2005;14(2):186–92. https://doi.org/10.1016/J.JSE.2004.06.013.
21. Buchner M, Eschbach N, Loew M. Comparison of the short-term functional results after surface replacement and total shoulder arthroplasty for osteoarthritis of the shoulder: a matched-pair analysis. Arch

Orthop Trauma Surg. 2008;128(4):347–54. https://doi.org/10.1007/s00402-007-0404-x.

22. Copeland S. The continuing development of shoulder replacement: "reaching the surface". J Bone Joint Surg Am. 2006;88(4):900–5. https://doi.org/10.2106/JBJS.F.00024.

23. Levy O, Copeland SA. Cementless surface replacement arthroplasty of the shoulder 5-to 10-year results with the Copeland Mark-2 prosthesis. J Bone Joint Surg Br. 2001;83(2):213–34.

24. Levy O, Funk L, Sforza G, Copeland SA. Copeland surface replacement arthroplasty of the shoulder in rheumatoid arthritis. J Bone Joint Surg Am. 2004;86(3):512–8. https://doi.org/10.2106/00004623-200403000-00008.

25. Burgess DL, McGrath MS, Bonutti PM, Marker DR, Delanois RE, Mont MA. Shoulder resurfacing. J Bone Joint Surg Am. 2009;91(5):1228–38. https://doi.org/10.2106/JBJS.H.01082.

26. Copeland S, Levy O, Brownlow H. Resurfacing arthroplasty of the shoulder. Obstet Gynecol. 2003;4(4):199–210.https://doi.org/10.1097/00132589-200312000-00007.

27. Collin P, Matsumura N, Lädermann A, Denard PJ, Walch G. Relationship between massive chronic rotator cuff tear pattern and loss of active shoulder range of motion. J Shoulder Elbow Surg. 2014;23(8):1195–202. https://doi.org/10.1016/J.JSE.2013.11.019.

28. Glanzmann MC, Kolling C, Schwyzer HK, Flury M, Audigé L. Radiological and functional 24-month outcomes of resurfacing versus stemmed anatomic total shoulder arthroplasty. Int Orthop. 2017;41(2):375–84. https://doi.org/10.1007/s00264-016-3310-4.

29. Fourman MS, Beck A, Gasbarro G, Irrgang JJ, Rodosky MW, Lin A. Humeral head resurfacing is associated with less pain and clinically equivalent functional outcomes compared with stemmed hemiarthroplasty at mid-term follow-up. Knee Surg Sports Traumatol Arthrosc. 2019;27(10):3203–11. https://doi.org/10.1007/s00167-019-05382-w.

30. Rasmussen JV, Hole R, Metlie T, et al. Anatomical total shoulder arthroplasty used for glenohumeral osteoarthritis has higher survival rates than hemiarthroplasty: a Nordic registry-based study. Osteoarthritis Cartilage. 2018;26(5):659–65. https://doi.org/10.1016/j.joca.2018.02.896.

31. Chillemi C, Paglialunga C, de Giorgi G, Proietti R, Carli S, Damo M. Outcome and revision rate of uncemented humeral head resurfacing: mid-term follow-up study. World J Orthop. 2021;12(6):403–11. https://doi.org/10.5312/wjo.v12.i6.403.

32. Golant A, Christoforou D, Zuckerman JD, Kwon YW. Return to sports after shoulder arthroplasty: a survey of surgeons' preferences. J Shoulder Elbow Surg. 2012;21(4):554–60. https://doi.org/10.1016/j.jse.2010.11.021.

33. Cowling PD, Holland P, Kottam L, Baker P, Rangan A. Risk factors associated with intraoperative complications in primary shoulder arthroplasty: a study using the England, Wales and Northern Ireland National Joint Registry dataset. Acta Orthop. 2017;88(6):587–91. https://doi.org/10.1080/17453674.2017.1362155.

34. Beck A, Lee H, Fourman M, et al. Preoperative comorbidities and postoperative complications do not influence patient-reported satisfaction following humeral head resurfacing: mid- to long-term follow-up of 106 patients. J Shoulder Elb Arthroplast. 2019;3:247154921983028. https://doi.org/10.1177/2471549219830284.

35. Australian Orthopaedic Association National Joint Replacement Registry. 2020. https://aoanjrr.sahmri.com/annual-reports-2020.

Hemiarthroplasty in the Young Patient with Post-traumatic AVN and Malunion

12

Benno Ejnisman, Paulo Henrique Schmidt Lara,
Paulo Santoro Belangero,
and Carlos Vicente Andreoli

12.1 Introduction

Hemiarthroplasty of the shoulder entails resurfacing the humeral head while leaving the glenoid intact. This operation was pioneered by Neer in the 1950s [1]. Once an extremely common operation with broad indications, hemiarthroplasty has become more rarely performed, as clinical studies have shown that a total shoulder arthroplasty (TSA) has outperformed hemiarthroplasty in pain relief, function, and revision rate in patients with primary glenohumeral (GH) osteoarthritis. Although these advantages of TSA are well known, there remain concerns for later glenoid implant loosening in young, physically active patients. Post-traumatic osteonecrosis presents a difficult challenge, as there are often tuberosity malunion and scar formation that make shoulder replacement difficult. Previous studies that have evaluated arthroplasty following traumatic osteonecrosis have had mixed results.

12.2 Hemiarthroplasty in the Young Patient with Post-traumatic Avascular Necrosis

Humeral head osteonecrosis accounts for approximately 7% of all osteonecrosis patients [2]. Osteonecrosis is the interruption of the normal blood supply to bone leading to cell death [3, 4]. An ascending branch of the anterior circumflex artery on the anterolateral aspect of the humeral head has been identified as providing a consistent supply to the humeral head. This ascending branch of the anterior circumflex artery enters the proximal humerus at the superior end of the bicipital groove or by way of its branches into the adjacent great and small tuberosities [5]. Once intraosseous, it continues its trajectory below the epiphysis with a tortuous course [6].

The humeral head is also perfused, to a lesser degree, by a posterior circumflex artery branch. The existence of only one principal artery and the extreme tortuousness of the subchondral arterioles make the vascularity of the humeral head exceptionally vulnerable to trauma and thromboembolic events [7]. The four-part fracture associated with dislocation has the highest incidence of osteonecrosis, varying from 15 to 30%. Open reduction and internal fixation of these fractures may impair the head blood supply even further, thus increasing the risk of osteonecrosis [8].

B. Ejnisman · P. H. S. Lara (✉) · P. S. Belangero
C. V. Andreoli
Centro de Traumatologia do Esporte da Escola
Paulista de Medicina, São Paulo, Brazil

© ISAKOS 2023
A. D. Mazzocca et al. (eds.), *Shoulder Arthritis across the Life Span*,
https://doi.org/10.1007/978-3-031-33298-2_12

Post-traumatic osteonecrosis presents a difficult challenge, as there are often tuberosity malunion and scar formation that make shoulder replacement difficult. Previous studies that have evaluated arthroplasty following traumatic osteonecrosis have had mixed results. Classification in the humeral head is based on a modification of the Ficat-Arlet system for the femoral head, originally described in 1968 and modified in 1980. Cruess et al. [9] adapted this classification to the humeral head, which has since become the most widely used system. Early osteonecrosis of the humeral head is characterized by increased subchondral sclerosis along the superior, central portion of the humeral head with evidence of bony remodeling and focal subchondral osteolysis. As the disease progresses, there are fracture of the subchondral plate, deformity of the humeral head, and, finally, erosion of the glenoid surface and secondary degenerative joint disease [10].

Archer et al. [11] found that time to surgery (less than or greater than 72 h) and patient age did not correlate with development of AVN after proximal humerus fracture. Notably, the number of fracture fragments did influence the rate of AVN identified in patients with proximal humerus fractures ($p = 0.002$).

If collapse of the humeral head has occurred, shoulder hemiarthroplasty is a good surgical option. Results are encouraging using hemiarthroplasty for patients with a normal glenoid on radiographs. If glenoid cartilage damage is present or if there is associated joint space narrowing on radiographs, total shoulder arthroplasty is likely a better treatment option [12–15].

The literature shows that the use of partial arthroplasty for the surgical treatment of osteonecrosis is effective for pain relief, increased shoulder mobility, and patient satisfaction, even when compared to total arthroplasty results [12, 14, 16, 17]. Pain relief and improved range of motion can be expected in the patient with osteonecrosis, but patients must be counseled that glenoid cartilage wear over time can result in return of symptoms and eventual revision [14, 18, 19].

It has been well demonstrated that post-traumatic necrosis resulted in inferior outcomes than primary avascular necrosis of the humeral head [12, 14, 20]. Hattrup et al. [13] found significantly less flexion and abduction in patients with a history of trauma, as well as a lower ASES score compared to steroid-induced osteonecrosis. Feeley et al. [12] reported the outcomes for 37 patients treated with hemiarthroplasty and 27 treated with total shoulder arthroplasty (TSA) for osteonecrosis. The TSA group was significantly older (mean age 71 vs. 59 years, $p < 0.05$). A comparable improvement in the ASES and L'Insalata scores was observed between the groups. In the TSA group, range of motion (ROM) was slightly less in flexion ($p = 0.07$), with no difference in internal and external rotation. Hattrup et al.'s [13] study reported the outcomes of 71 hemiarthroplasties and 56 TSAs, but only 88 patients' data were available at the last follow-up. The mean postoperative ASES scores were comparable in both groups (63 vs. 62 points), and in terms of ROM, no significant differences were reported ($p = 0.33$ for flexion, $p = 0.95$ for abduction, and $p = 0.47$ for external rotation). Furthermore, the outcomes were divided by etiology (steroid vs. trauma), showing a greater improvement in the ASES score in the subjects who were taking corticosteroid medication.

Hattrup et al. [13] compared total arthroplasty and hemiarthroplasty in AVN, and after a mean follow-up of 8.9 years, functional outcomes were similar with the two procedures, although survival was better with total arthroplasty. A study with a shorter follow-up of 4.8 years found no clinical differences between the two procedures but showed a 22% complication rate after total arthroplasty compared to only 8% after hemiarthroplasty [12].

Prosthesis survival after shoulder hemiarthroplasty is important to consider and is even crucial for patients younger than 50 years of age. In a study of patients younger than 50 years with a mean follow-up of 16.2 years, total arthroplasty was superior over hemiarthroplasty, with 10-year survival rates of 97% and 84%, respectively [21]. Gadea et al. [22] found a 94% survival rate after 10 years of hemiarthroplasty in AVN. The authors conclude that AVN is the best indication for hemiarthroplasty. Smith et al. [19] found a 95% survival rate after 15 years of hemiarthroplasty in AVN, but the cases were associated with steroid use.

Miyazaki et al. [23] analyzed long-term functional and radiographic results of partial shoulder replacement for humeral head osteonecrosis: 61.5% of the cases were post-traumatic (8/13), and the mean age of the patients at last assessment was 71 years. They found that glenoid erosion increased over time significantly ($p < 0.05$). Paradoxically, all active shoulder movements also improved ($p < 0.05$), while UCLA scores remained the same. Radiographic deterioration was not correlated with clinical function. They had an 84.7% survival rate for arthroplasties after a mean time of 16 years.

Ristow et al. [24] demonstrated that regarding the cohorts based on etiology (trauma, corticosteroid, sickle cell, and unknown), the shoulders in the trauma causal group trended toward higher outcome scores in three of the four scoring methods (Simple Shoulder Test, modified Constant score, UCLA Shoulder Rating Scale, and ASES score) and greater improvement in all four scoring methods than the other three etiologic groups. However, none of the differences were statistically significant in any of the four scoring methods ($P > 0.05$). A patient with humeral head osteonecrosis submitted to partial shoulder replacement is shown in Fig. 12.1.

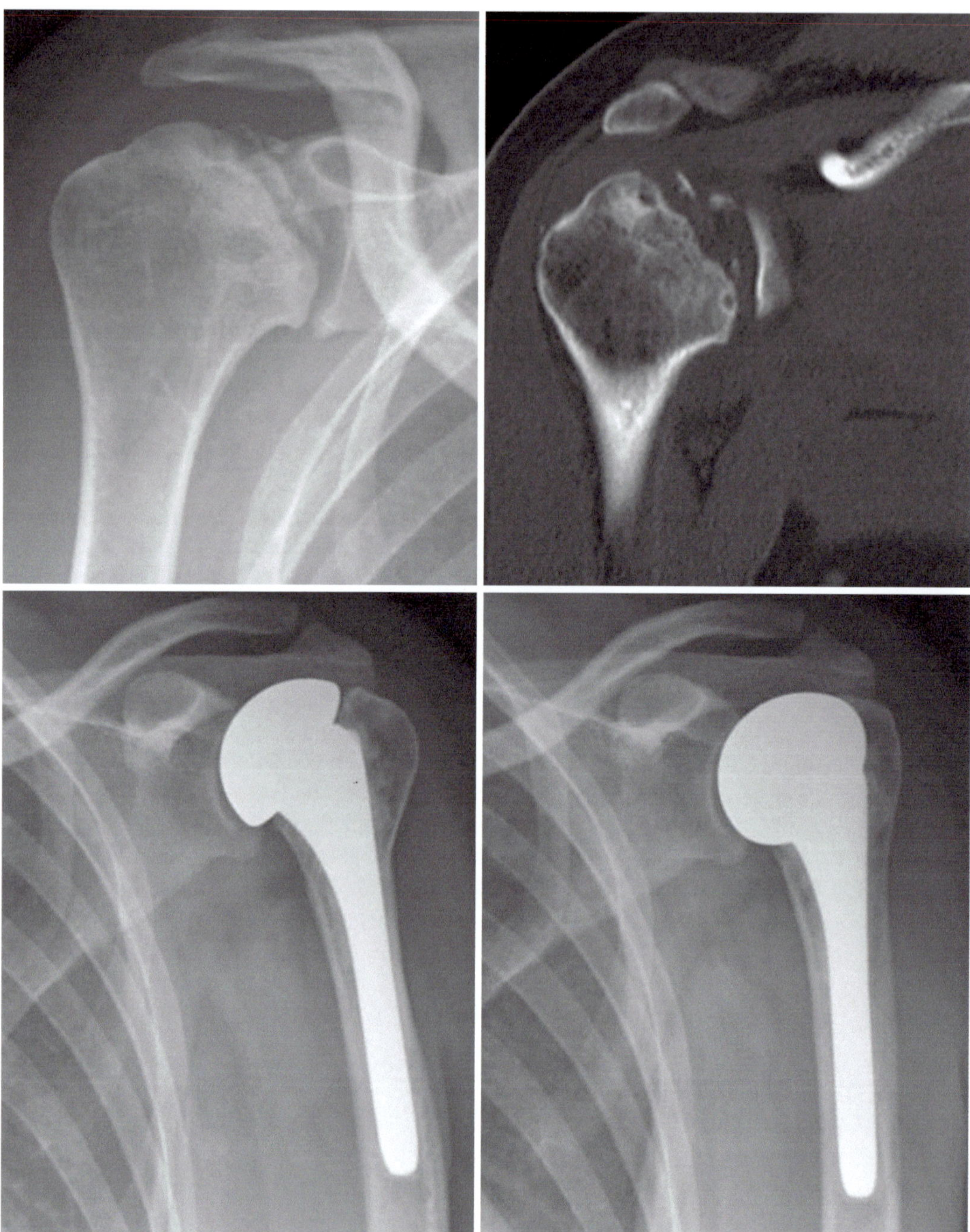

Fig. 12.1 Patient with humeral head osteonecrosis submitted to partial shoulder replacement

12.3 Hemiarthroplasty in the Young Patient with Malunion of the Proximal Humerus

The management of proximal humerus fractures has evolved quickly over the past few years. The predominance of impacted, non-displaced surgical neck fractures and conservative treatment no longer systematically corresponds to most of the complex, displaced fractures in osteoporotic bone. The ageing population has greatly contributed to an increase in the malunion rate, which is estimated at 4–20% [25]. No proximal humerus fracture treatment method (conservative treatment, internal fixation, etc.) is immune to the risk of malunion; even primary shoulder arthroplasty performed in fracture cases has the risk of periprosthetic malunion [26].

The overall results of patients with old trauma are inferior to the results currently obtained in patients with primary osteoarthritis or with recent four-part fractures who are treated initially with humeral head replacement [27–29]. Very little has been written on the results of shoulder arthroplasty for management of sequelae of proximal humeral fractures [29–39]. By definition, malunion of the proximal humerus corresponds to the healing of a fractured bone in a nonanatomical position. The misalignment and/or remodeling of the humeral head results in joint incongruity, which does not provide optimal mechanical conditions; this can lead to stiffness due to the retraction of capsule and ligament structures. Thus the joint is at risk, as is the bone [25].

The prognosis for surgical treatment of the sequelae of proximal humerus fractures has improved because of the classification proposed by Beredjiklian et al. [30] and Boileau et al. [40]. Tuberosity osteotomy has long been recognized as the main predictor for poor outcomes in cases of secondary arthroplasty [31, 36, 40–42]. The classification system for proximal humeral malunions proposed by Beredjiklian [30] and colleagues includes three types: type 1, malposition of the tuberosities; type 2, incongruity of articular surface; and type 3, articular fragment malposition. The authors emphasize that soft tissue pathology plays a major role in the functional impairment and stiffness seen in proximal humeral malunions. Both the bone and soft tissue pathology need to be corrected at the time of surgery to optimize outcome.

One of the leading causes of poor shoulder function in patients with malunion of the proximal humerus is varus angulation of the humeral head in relation to the shaft. This may be related to the acceptance of unsuccessful closed reduction or imperfect open reduction internal fixation. Varus deformity of the proximal humerus causes limitations in active forward elevation and abduction caused by impingement of the greater tuberosity. The subacromial space is decreased in these shoulders, and the proximity of the greater tuberosity to the coracoacromial arch makes it prone to impingement. The sliding surface between the humeral head and the glenoid is also decreased. In addition, the proximity between the supraspinatus origin and insertion decreases its lever arm, affecting shoulder function. Although some older patients are willing to accept functional limitations of shoulder elevation, many younger patients find this to be unacceptable. The results in patients with old trauma are inferior to the results currently obtained in patients with primary osteoarthritis or those with four-part fractures treated in the acute setting. Pain relief is more reliably achieved postoperatively than motion. Mansat et al. [42] reported on 28 patients with sequelae of proximal humeral fractures treated with shoulder arthroplasty. Based on the

Neer criteria, the results were satisfactory in only 64%. Mean active elevation was 107°, and 85% of patients reported no or slight pain. The final result was positively influenced by the integrity of the rotator cuff. Also, patients with acromio-humeral distances of greater than 8 mm had better results than those who did not. The authors conclude that the malunion of the greater tuberosity can be tolerated if it does not compromise acceptable positioning of the humeral component. However, if an osteotomy needs to be performed because of major displacement, results are unpredictable. All three patients who required a greater tuberosity osteotomy at the time of arthroplasty had an unsatisfactory result.

Similarly, Boileau et al. [31] reported 42% good to excellent results in 71 patients who underwent shoulder arthroplasty for sequelae of proximal humeral fractures. They reported a 27% complication rate, including four diaphyseal fractures, one metaphyseal fracture, two cases of deep infection, one return to the operating room for acromioplasty, and one failure of fixation of the greater tuberosity. The most significant factor affecting results was the need for greater tuberosity osteotomy. All patients who underwent a greater tuberosity osteotomy were not able to regain active elevation above 90. The authors emphasize that arthroplasty for the treatment of sequelae of proximal humeral fractures should be performed without a greater tuberosity osteotomy when possible. They believe that devascularization of the greater tuberosity, leading to tuberosity nonunion, migration, and resorption, is probably the reason for these poor results.

Antuna et al. [43] and Beredjiklian et al. [30] have reported similar results. Antuna et al. reported that 10 of 24 of their patients who had greater tuberosity osteotomy had a complication related to tuberosity nonunion, malunion, or resorption. Implantation of the humeral component in slight varus or valgus was not associated with an increased incidence of humeral component loosening. Humeral components with a modified curvature in the stem have been used with success in their experience. When the tuberosity is displaced 1.5 cm, it may be necessary to reposition it to avoid impingement. Beredjiklian et al. reported similar results but emphasized that malunion of the proximal humerus often is accompanied by some soft tissue abnormality, such as soft tissue contracture, a tear of the rotator cuff, or subacromial impingement, in addition to distortion of the bony anatomy. Both osseous and soft tissue abnormalities need to be corrected at the time of surgery to improve the chances of a satisfactory result. A patient with malunion of the proximal humerus is shown in Fig. 12.2.

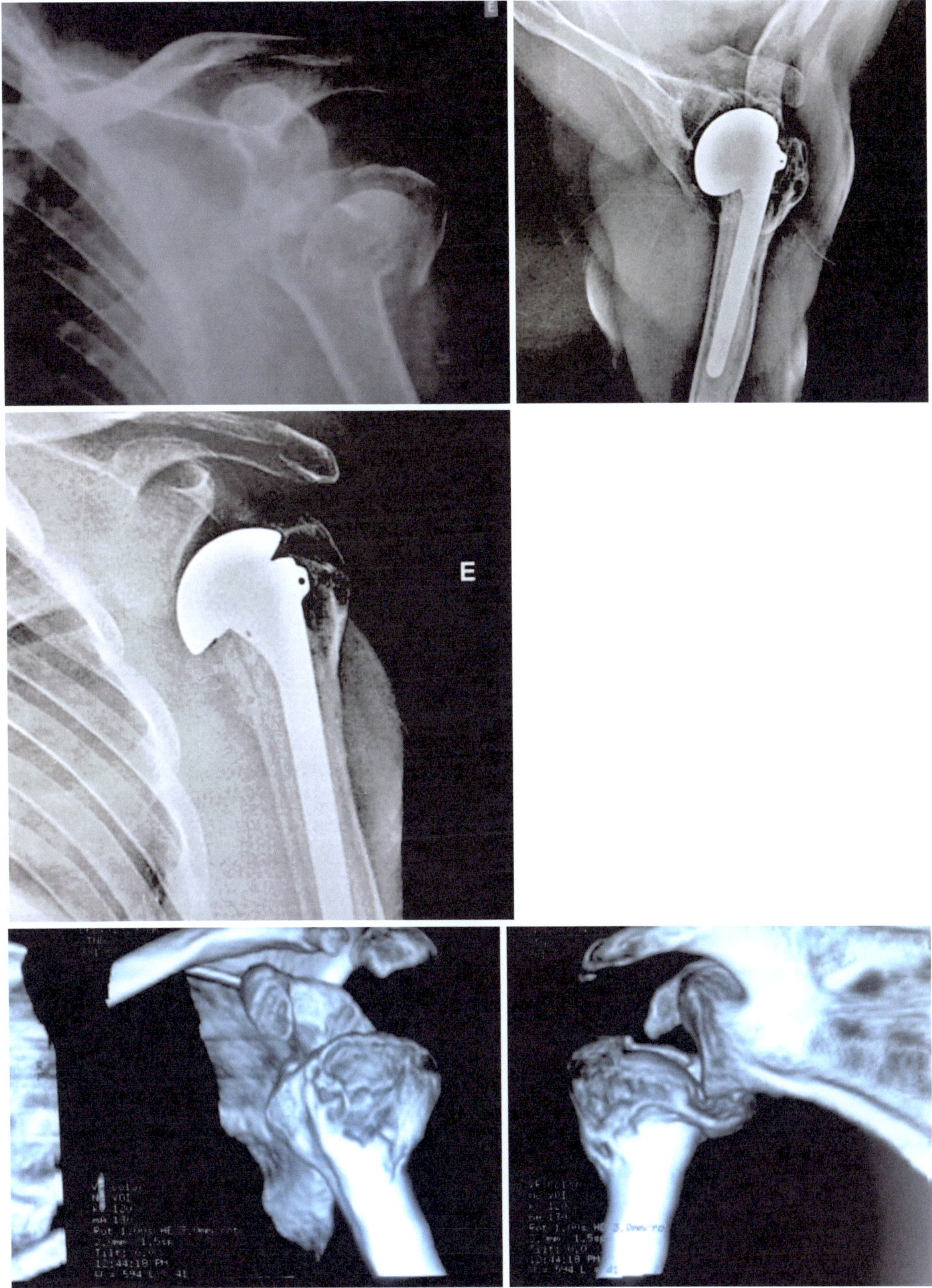

Fig. 12.2 Patient with malunion of the proximal humerus submitted to partial shoulder replacement with satisfactory result

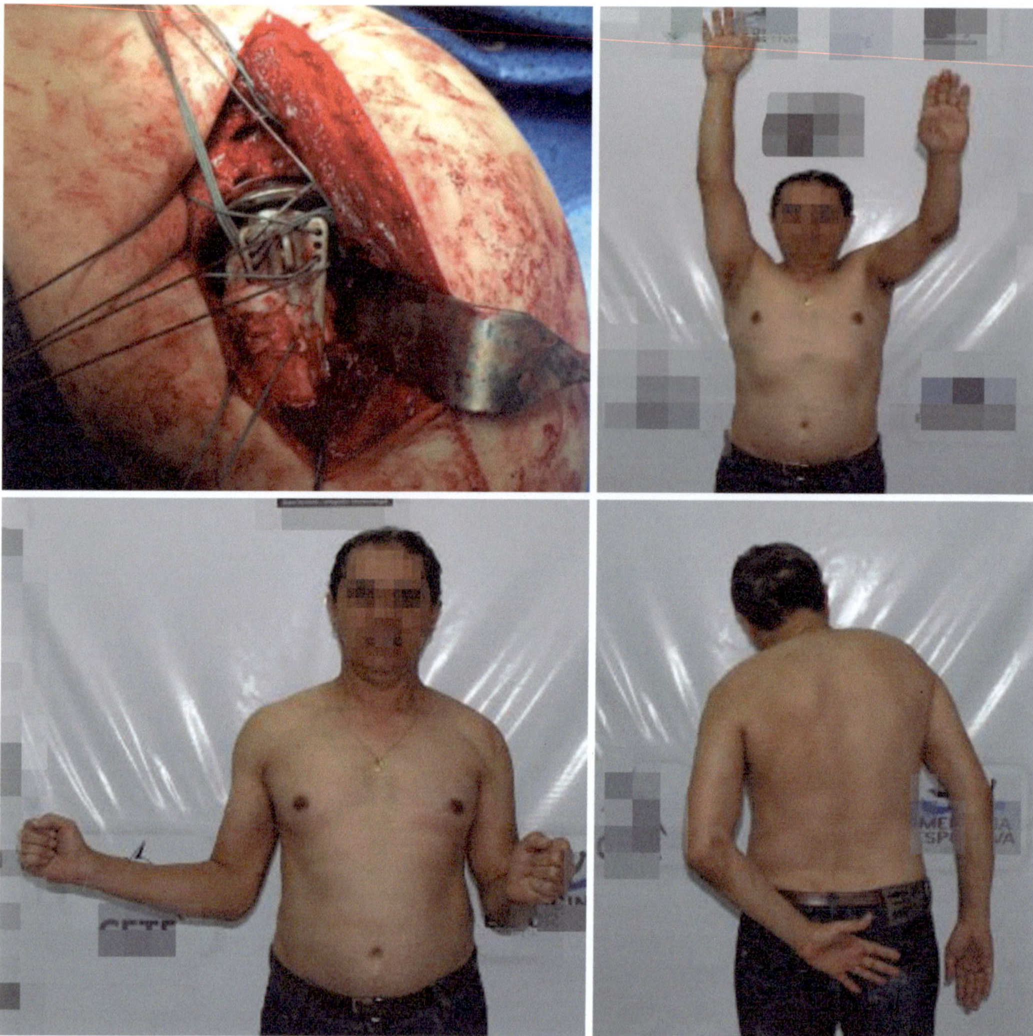

Fig. 12.2 (continued)

References

1. Neer CS. Articular replacement for the humeral head. J Bone Joint Surg Am. 1955;37:215–28.
2. Mont MA, Payman RK, Laporte DM, Petri M, Jones LC, Hungerford DS. Atraumatic osteonecrosis of the humeral head. J Rheumatol. 2000;27:1766–73.
3. Kahlstrom SC, Burton CC, Phemister DB. Aseptic necrosis of bone. II. Infarction of bone of undetermined etiology resulting in encapsulated and calcified areas in diaphyses and in arthritis deformans. Surg Gynecol Obstet. 1939;68:631–4.
4. Mankin HJ, Rosenthal DI, Xavier R. Gaucher disease: new approaches to an ancient disease. J Bone Joint Surg Am. 2001;83:748–63.
5. Gerber C, Schneeberger A, Vinh T. The arterial vascularization of the humeral head. An anatomical study. J Bone Joint Surg Am. 1990;72:1486–94.
6. Cushner MA, Friedman RJ. Osteonecrosis of the humeral head. J Am Acad Orthop Surg. 1997;5:339–46.
7. Friedman RJ. Arthroplasty of the shoulder. 1st ed. Portland: Thieme Medical Publishers; 1994.
8. Neer CS 2nd. Displaced proximal humeral fractures. II. Treatment of three-part and four-

part displacement. J Bone Joint Surg Am. 1970;52:1090–103.

9. Cruess RL. Experience with steroid-induced avascular necrosis of the shoulder and etiologic considerations regarding osteonecrosis of the hip. Clin Orthop Relat Res. 1978:86–93.

10. L'Insalata JC, Pagnani MJ, Warren RF, Dines DM. Humeral head osteonecrosis: clinical course and radiographic predictors of outcome. J Shoulder Elbow Surg. 1996;5:355–61.

11. Archer LA, Furey A. Rate of avascular and time to surgery in proximal humerus fractures. Musculoskelet Surg. 2016;100(3):213–6.

12. Feeley BT, Fealy S, Dines DM, Warren RF, Craig EV. Hemiarthroplasty and total shoulder arthroplasty for avascular necrosis of the humeral head. J Shoulder Elbow Surg. 2008;17(5):689–94.

13. Hattrup SJ, Cofield RH. Osteonecrosis of the humeral head: results of replacement. J Shoulder Elbow Surg. 2000;9(3):177–82.

14. Orfaly RM, Rockwood CA, Esenyel CZ, Wirth MA. Shoulder arthroplasty in cases with avascular necrosis of the humeral head. J Shoulder Elbow Surg. 2007;16(3 Suppl):27–32.

15. Smith RG, Sperling JW, Cofield RH, Hattrup SJ, Schleck CD. Shoulder hemiarthroplasty for steroid associated osteonecrosis. J Shoulder Elbow Surg. 2008;17(5):685–8.

16. Neer CS. Glenohumeral arthroplasty. In: Shoulder reconstruction. Philadelphia: W.B. Saunders; 1990. p. 143–227.

17. Schoch BS, Barlow JD, Schleck C, Cofield RH, Sperling JW. Shoulder arthroplasty for post-traumatic osteonecrosis of the humeral head. J Shoulder Elbow Surg. 2016;25(3):406–12.

18. Harreld KL, Marulanda GA, Ulrich SD, Marker DR, Seyler TM, Mont MA. Small-diameter percutaneous decompression for osteonecrosis of the shoulder. Am J Orthop (Belle Mead NJ). 2009;38(7):348–54.

19. Smith RG, Sperling JW, Cofield RH, Hattrup SJ, Schleck CD. Shoulder hemiarthroplasty for steroid-associated osteonecrosis. J Shoulder Elbow Surg. 2008;17:685–8.

20. Sowa B, Thierjung H, Bülhoff M, Loew M, Zeifang F, Bruckner T, Raiss P. Functional results of hemi- and total shoulder arthroplasty according to diagnosis and patient age at surgery. Acta Orthop. 2017;88:310–4.

21. Sperling J, Cofield R, Rowland C. Neer hemiarthroplasty and Neer total shoulder arthroplasty in patients fifty years old or less. Long-term results. J Bone Joint Surg Am. 1998;80:464–73.

22. Gadea F, Alami G, Pape G, Boileau P, Favard L. Shoulder hemiarthroplasty: outcomes and long-term survival analysis according to etiology. Orthop Traumatol Surg Res. 2012;98(6):659–65.

23. Miyazaki AN, Sella GDV, da Silva LA, Checchia CS, Lemos FC. Humeral head osteonecrosis: outcomes of hemiarthroplasty after minimum 10-year follow-up. Rev Bras Ortop. 2021;56(1):91–7.

24. Ristow JJ, Ellison CM, Mickschl DJ, Berg KC, Haidet KC, Gray JR, et al. Outcomes of shoulder replacement in humeral head avascular necrosis. J Shoulder Elbow Surg. 2019;28(1):9–14.

25. Siegel JA, Dines DM. Proximal humerus malunions. Orthop Clin North Am. 2000;31(1):35–49.

26. Duparc F, Muller JM, Freger P. Arterial blood supply of the proximal humeral epiphysis. Surg Radiol Anat. 2001;23:185–90.

27. Cofield RH. Total shoulder arthroplasty with the Neer prosthesis. J Bone Joint Surg Am. 1984;66:899–906.

28. Mansat M, Blazy O, Mansat P. Omarthroses centrées. Rev Chir Orthop Reparatrice Appar Mot. 1995;81(Suppl II):106–8.

29. Neer CS II, Watson KC, Stanton FJ. Recent experience in total shoulder replacement. J Bone Joint Surg Am. 1982;64:319–37.

30. Beredjiklian PK, Iannotti JP, Norris TR, Williams GR. Operative treatment of malunion of a fracture of the proximal aspect of the humerus. J Bone Joint Surg Am. 1998;80:1484–97.

31. Boileau P, Trojani C, Walch G, et al. Shoulder arthroplasty for the treatment of the sequelae of fractures of the proximal humerus. J Shoulder Elbow Surg. 2001;10:299–308.

32. Bosch U, Skutek M, Fremerey RW, Tscherne H. Outcome after primary and secondary hemiarthroplasty in elderly patients with fractures of the proximal humerus. J Shoulder Elbow Surg. 1998;7:479–84.

33. Dines DM, Warren RF, Altchek DW, Moeckel B. Posttraumatic changes of the proximal humerus: malunion, nonunion, and osteonecrosis. Treatment with modular hemiarthroplasty or total shoulder arthroplasty. J Shoulder Elbow Surg. 1993;2:11–21.

34. Frich LH, Sojbjerg JO, Sneppen O. Shoulder arthroplasty in complex acute and chronic proximal humeral fractures. Orthopedics. 1991;9:949–54.

35. Habermeyer P, Schweiberer L. Corrective interventions subsequent to humeral head fractures. Orthopade. 1992;21:148–57.

36. Huten D, Duparc J. Prosthetic arthroplasty in recent and old complex injuries of the shoulder [in French]. Rev Chir Orthop Reparatrice Appar Mot. 1986;72:517–529.

37. Norris TR, Green A, McGuigan FX. Late prosthetic shoulder arthroplasty for displaced proximal humerus fractures. J Shoulder Elbow Surg. 1995;4:271–80.

38. Postel JM, Tamames M, Lenoble E, Goutallier D. Les arthroses post-traumatiques. Rev Chir Orthop Reparatrice Appar Mot. 1995;81(Suppl II):111–5.

39. Tanner MW, Cofield RH. Prosthetic arthroplasty for fractures and fracture-dislocations of the proximal humerus. Clin Orthop. 1983;179:116–28.

40. Boileau P, Gabrion A, Neyton L, Trojani C. Sequelae of proximal humerus fractures: classification and treatment indications. In: Mansat P, editor. The sequelae of trauma to the glenohumeral joint. Monograph of the GEEC [book in French]. Montpellier: Sauramps Médical; 2006. p. 27–40.

41. Boileau P, Trojani C, Walch G, Sinnerton R, Habermayer P. Sequelae of fractures of the proximal humerus: results of shoulder arthroplasty with greater tuberosity osteotomy. In: Walch G, Boileau P, editors. Shoulder arthroplasty. Berlin: Springer; 1999. p. 372–9.
42. Mansat P, Guity MR, Bellumore Y, Mansat M. Shoulder arthroplasty for late sequelae of proximal humeral fractures. J Shoulder Elbow Surg. 2004;13(3):305–12.
43. Antuna SA, Sperling JW, Sanchez-Sotelo J, et al. Shoulder arthroplasty for proximal humeral nonunions. American Shoulder and Elbow Surgeon. J Shoulder Elbow Surg. 2002;11:114–21.

Alternatives to Glenoid Prosthesis in Young Patients: Arthroscopic Glenoid Resurfacing with Fascia Lata for Treatment of Shoulder Arthritis in Young Patients

Pablo Adelino Narbona [ID] and Guillermo Arce

13.1 Introduction

Glenohumeral arthritis (GA) may result in considerable disability condition in young patients and represents a major challenging problem in active population that may severely affect quality of life. Young adults with glenohumeral arthritis often have a more complex etiology especially secondary causes such us previous trauma, previous surgeries, or chondrolysis which might contribute to a worse surgical outcome [1]. Saltzman et al. reported an incidence of shoulder osteoarthritis of 21% of patients under the age of 50 [2]. However, in adults under the age of 60, and particularly in those under 50, traditional arthroplasty is usually not ideal, because outcomes are less predictable, due to higher activity levels, greater functional expectations, and implant longevity [1]. The main purpose of the surgical treatment of young adults with glenohumeral arthritis and an intact rotator cuff is to possibly relieve pain and improve active and passive range of motion while preserving the joint [3]. In addition to minimizing the major complication rate (infection or loosening), prevent lifetime work or recreational activities restriction, are important in the treatment decision to avoid shoulder prosthesis. This has led to exploring alternative treatment options. Arthroscopic joint preservation with arthroscopic glenoid resurfacing (AGR) for shoulder arthritis is an all-arthroscopic procedure that does not violate the subscapularis tendon and allows to treat the concomitant pathology while performing the interposition arthroplasty. The goal of this procedure is to manage the mechanical causes of pain and functional limitation associated with glenohumeral arthritis to reduce pain, improve function, and delay as an interim procedure or even avoid shoulder arthroplasty.

13.2 Pathophysiology and Production

Shoulder osteoarthritis in young patients is a rare condition and usually secondary to Bankart repair, trauma, stiffness or glenohumeral chondrolysis due to thermal injury, continuous infusion of intra-articular anesthetics, and more frequently the mispositioning of anchors or suture knots on the articular surface. Screw cutout and joint protrusion after proximal humerus fracture fixation can lead to accelerated joint degeneration [4–6]. Even bioabsorbable anchors, if proud, cause cartilage damage. Loss of the normal gliding surface and increased friction may play a role in rapid progression of the disease [7].

P. A. Narbona (✉)
Shoulder Department at Sanatorio Allende, Córdoba, Argentina

G. Arce
Instituto Argentino de Diagnóstico y Tratamiento (IADT), Buenos Aires, Argentina

© ISAKOS 2023
A. D. Mazzocca et al. (eds.), *Shoulder Arthritis across the Life Span*,
https://doi.org/10.1007/978-3-031-33298-2_13

Post-arthroscopic glenohumeral chondrolysis (PAGCL) is a term that has been applied to shoulders that have developed rapid, destructive degenerative changes after arthroscopic surgery. PAGCL differs from primary glenohumeral osteoarthritis because it typically develops symptoms within months of cartilage injury and generally affects young patients, while osteoarthritis can take years to become problematic [4]. Pre-existing cartilage damage as a result of multiple recurrent instability episodes may further play a role in the development of chondrolysis. Increased patient age, elapsed time from initial instability episode to surgery, and sign of osteoarthritis have been shown to increase the probability of chondral damage at the time of arthroscopic stabilization [8, 9]. Another reason for rapid joint degeneration in young patients is the overtightening of the capsule during instability surgery. Specifically, "capsulorrhaphy arthropathy" refers to the rapid posterior chondral wear due to overtightening of the anterior capsule and resultant compressive joint forces and loss of external rotation [10].

13.3 Clinical Assessment

Patient with shoulder pain and symptoms of osteoarthritis should be questioned about the quality, timing, localization, and aggravating factors of shoulder pain. Questions about the history of joint trauma, contact or collision sports, shoulder instability, previous shoulder surgeries, and timing of onset of pain can help distinguish the cause of joint degeneration. Stiffness, shoulder pain in the morning and with weather changes, or pain with increased activity are common complaints. Patients usually suffer chronic shoulder pain, discomfort to sleep at night, and global loss of motion. Physical examination demonstrates limited mobility, mostly in passive range of motion, typically in forward flexion and external rotation [5, 11, 12]. Crackles or mechanical symptoms such as a blockage and painful range of motion could be due to intra-articular loose bodies or loss of joint space with osteophytes. Mild muscle atrophy around their shoulder is possible to find due to limited range of motion and decrease muscle activation. As the arthritic process advances, patients progressively lose their ability to perform sports or leisure activities [13, 14].

13.4 Imaging

In X-rays, the West Point and apical oblique views offer visualization of the anteroinferior glenoid, whereas the Stryker notch and axillary views visualize the glenohumeral joint in three planes which help diagnose arthritis and eliminate alternative diagnoses. Glenohumeral arthritis is classically characterized by asymmetric joint narrowing, subchondral sclerosis, cyst formation, and osteophytes, although the latter may not be present in rapidly progressive arthritis as seen in chondrolysis [5, 13, 14]. Computed tomography scans may be more accurate than radiographs to assess glenoid version and are particularly valuable if glenoid erosion is a concern allowing excellent visualization of bony lesions and the architecture of the shoulder, especially the 3D reconstruction that allows more precise bony assessment and preoperative planning. Magnetic resonance imaging (MRI) is necessary to do a detailed evaluation of the rotator cuff and the articular cartilage. However, the thin cartilage thickness in the shoulder provides a challenge for accurate assessment. MRI had a high sensitivity (87.2%) and specificity (80.6%); however, the gold standard to diagnose chondral lesions is the arthroscopy [6, 15, 16] (Fig. 13.1).

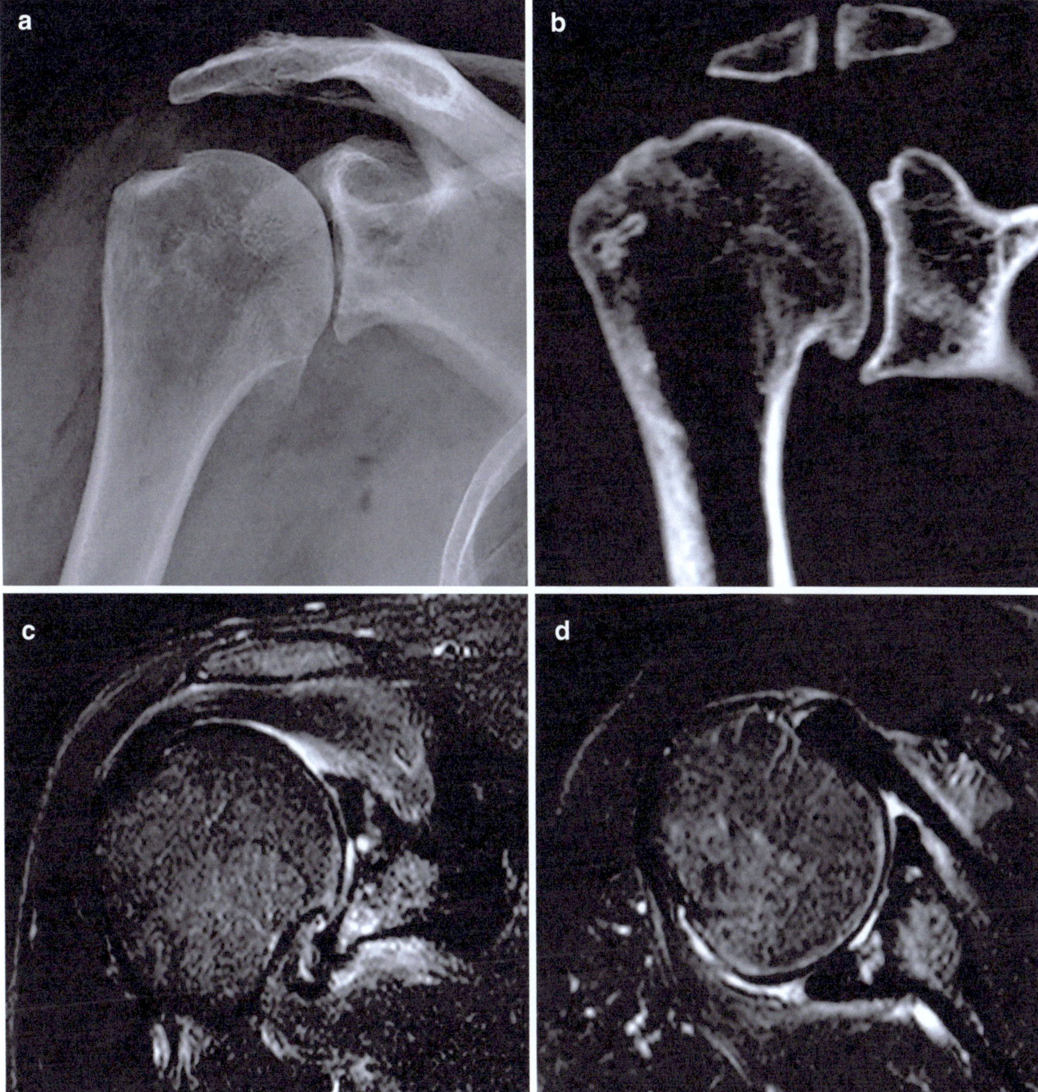

Fig. 13.1 (**a**) AP radiograph, (**b**) CT scan, (**c**) MRI coronal and (**d**) axial view. Findings typical of a young individual with right-sided glenohumeral osteoarthritis demonstrating fine bony and cartilage detail of subchondral cyst formation, sclerosis, joint space narrowing, and osteophyte formation

13.5   Classification

The Samilson and Prieto [17] classification system can be used to describe the degree of arthritis change in young. This classification has been expanded in its application to arthritis of varying etiology. Mild arthrosis is indicated by evidence on the anteroposterior radiograph of an inferior humeral or glenoid spur that measures less than 3 mm. Spur measuring between 3 and 7 mm and slight glenohumeral joint irregularity indicate moderate arthritis. Severe arthrosis is indicated by spurs measuring more than 7 mm and narrowing of the glenohumeral and sclerosis.

13.6 Treatment

13.6.1 Conservative Treatment

Nonoperative treatment options have been discussed in previous chapters. We do not recommend surgery in young patients as a primary treatment before standard conservative measures have been attempted.

13.6.2 Surgical Treatment

13.6.2.1 Surgical Indication

Different treatment options for glenohumeral arthritis in young range from debridement to biologic and nonbiologic replacement. We should consider in the surgical decision patient age, occupation, duration of symptoms, activity level, sports participation, radiographic stage of osteoarthritis, concomitant shoulder pathology, previous surgical procedures, and patient expectations [6]. The ideal indications for AGR are young patients with shoulder osteoarthritis without significant bone loss and with focal, large, or high degree of cartilage lesions not amenable to simple debridement or microfracture or young patients who are not good candidates for shoulder arthroplasty due to activity level or desire to avoid major surgery (Fig. 13.2) [3]. Advantages of arthroscopic surgery for shoulder arthritis include a low rate of complications, the joint and soft tissue preservation, and the avoidance of postoperative activity restrictions.

Problems: Problems include small case series available with high failure rate, progression radiographically of arthritis with mechanical damage and failure, and donor-site morbidity in autograft use.

Contraindications for AGR included osteoarthritis with severe bone loss or incongruous joint space and inflammatory arthritis. A preoperative joint space of <2 mm on true AP radiographs, bipolar cartilage lesions, and asymmetric glenoid have been shown to be associated with early failure of arthroscopic treatment [3].

13.6.2.2 Authors' Preferred Technique

The authors' preferred technique is to combine the Millett et al. [18, 19] proposed technique, called comprehensive arthroscopic management (CAM) procedure, with arthroscopic biologic glenoid resurfacing with a biologic graft interposition [3, 20–22], preferably preferred by those using fascia lata autograft. The authors choose double fascia lata autograft because it has been used successfully for many years for the reconstruction of human connective tissue in orthopedic surgical procedures [23].

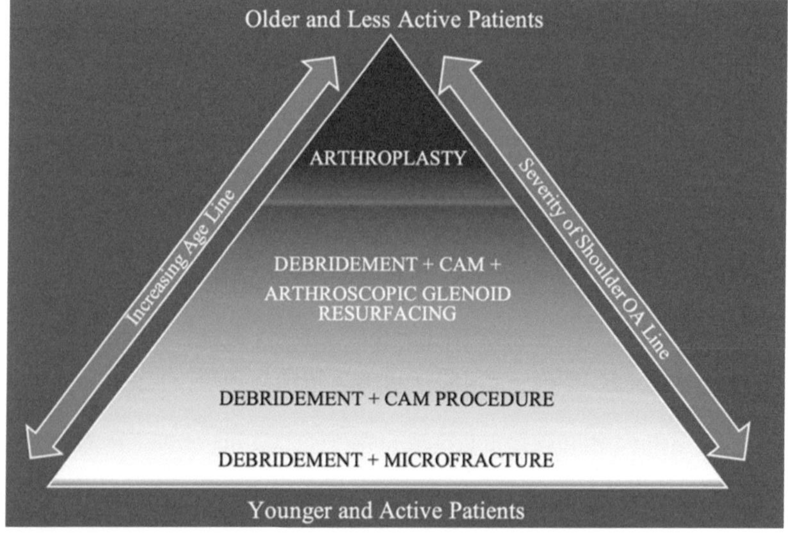

Fig. 13.2 Surgical recommendation of shoulder osteoarthritis according to age, activities, and severity of shoulder OA. In older, low-demand patients with more severe arthritis, we recommend shoulder arthroplasty, and in young high-demand patients with less severe arthritis, we recommend a joint preservation procedure

Arthroscopy Glenoid Resurfacing: Surgical Technique with Fascia Lata Autograft

Graft Harvesting

Fascia lata harvest is done with the patient in lateral decubitus position and general anesthesia. Trochanteric zone is prepared in sterile fashion and draped in standard fashion, a 5 cm longitudinal skin incision is made over the greater trochanter of the femur, and a 3 by 8–9 cm graft of fascia lata is harvested (Fig. 13.3). After closing the remaining fascia lata and surgical wound, we position the patient in beach chair position.

Diagnostic Arthroscopy, Footprint Preparation, and Measurement

We perform arthroscopic glenoid resurfacing in beach chair position with a Trimano (Arthrex Inc., Naples, Florida) arm holder, under general anesthesia and a supplementary interscalene nerve block, with the arm in 20°–30° of abduction and 10°–20° of forward flexion. The arm is prepared in sterile fashion and draped in standard fashion, and appropriate antibiotic prophylaxis is administered before incision. We use a standard posterior viewing portal to do a diagnostic arthroscopy with a 4 mm arthroscope with a 30° angled lens and an arthroscopic pump pressure at 40–60 mmHg. We create the anterior-superior lateral and anterior-inferior working portal, and an 8.25 mm cannula (Arthrex Inc., Naples, Florida) is inserted. We always do a biceps tenotomy or tenodesis. Then we complete the CAM procedure described by Millet et al. [18, 19]. The coexisting pathology can be addressed at the time of the arthroscopic debridement procedures. The capsular release is performed using radiofrequency devices and cutting instruments, with sequential release of the rotator interval; anterior, posterior, and inferior capsular release; synovectomy; humeral osteoplasty with excision of the goat's beard osteophyte from anterior to posterior; debridement of the labrum and chondral flaps; and removal of loose bodies to eliminate mechanical symptoms (Fig. 13.4). After this, glenoidplasty is performed which includes removal

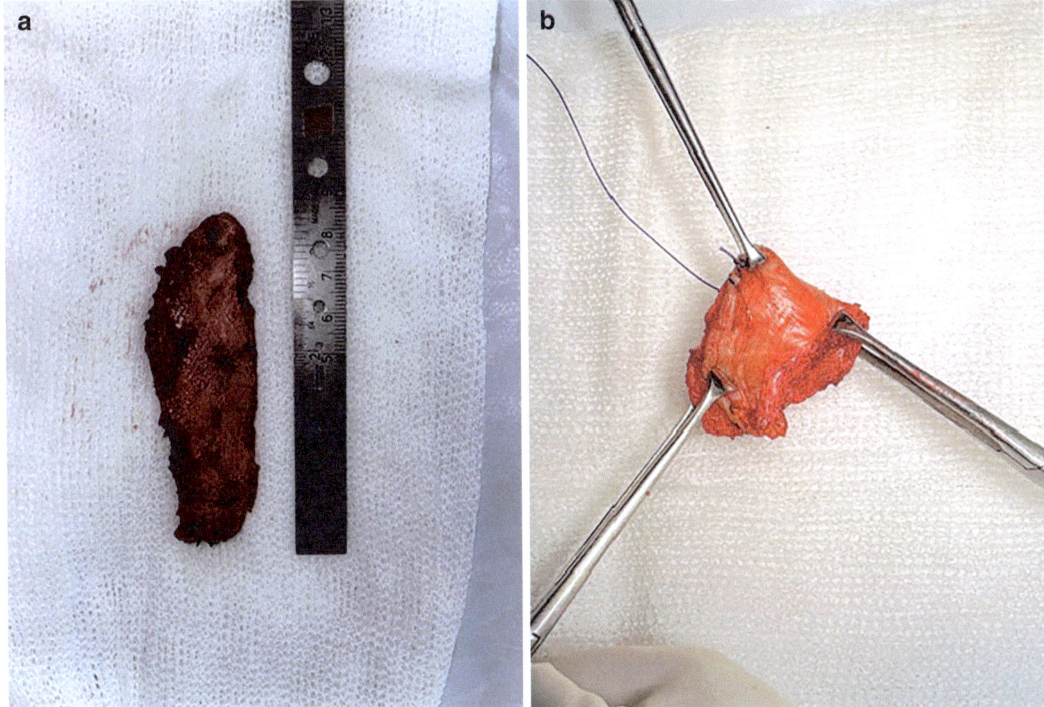

Fig. 13.3 (**a**) Harvested fascia lata. (**b**) Folded once to create a double fascia lata autograft

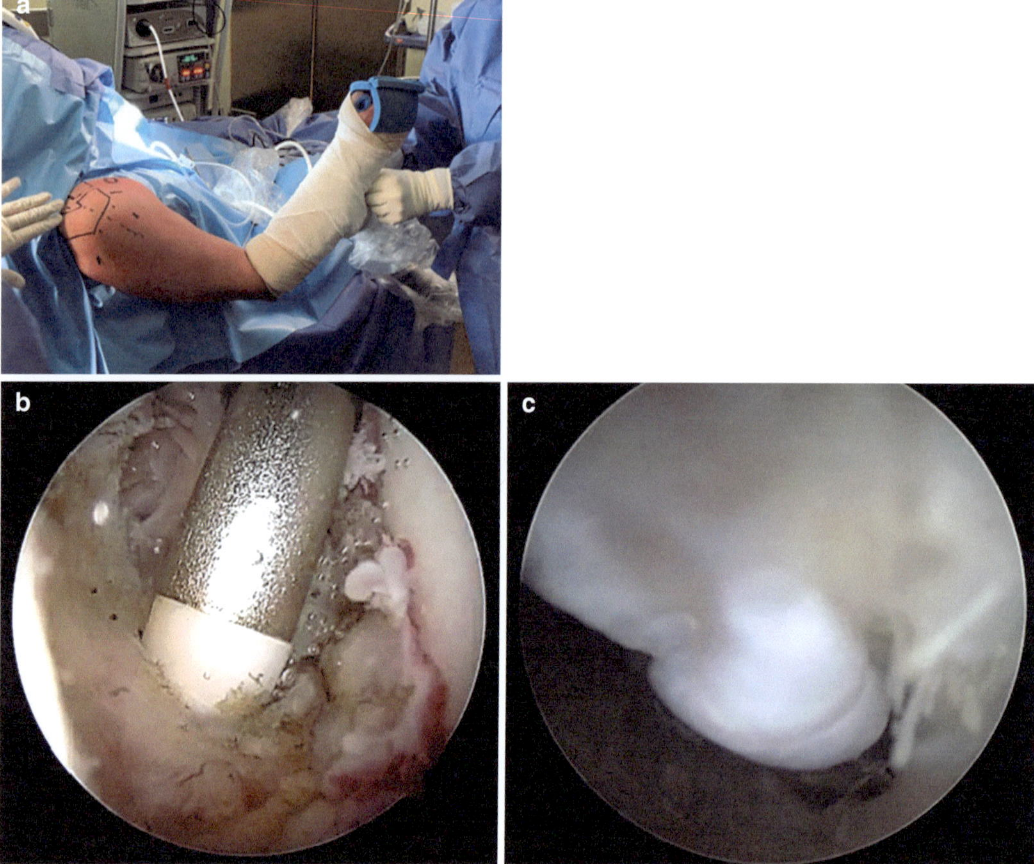

Fig. 13.4 (a) Right shoulder in beach chair position with a Trimano arm holder. (**b**) Sequential release of the rotator interval and anterior, posterior, and inferior capsular release. (**c**) The goat's beard osteophyte before humeral osteoplasty

of remaining cartilage and soft tissue to lightly decorticate the articular surface with a ring curette and burr to have a bleeding subchondral bone and correction of the abnormal biconcavity of the glenoid. Then microfracture is useful to generate a marrow-stimulated bleeding to deliver pluripotential cells to improve healing and graft incorporation. Then the glenoid dimensions are measured using measuring probes from anterior to posterior and from superior to inferior to prepare the graft (Fig. 13.5).

Graft Preparation

First, the graft is cut in the appropriate dimension according to previous arthroscopic measurement, to recreate the glenoid shape; then the graft is folded once to create a double fascia lata autograft. The edge of the graft is sutured around its periphery to be able to hold the stay sutures (Fig. 13.6).

Graft Delivery and Glenoid Graft Fixation

Using the posterior portal as a viewing portal, we first do the circumferential glenoid anchor placement for tissue fixation. We use 3 mm BioComposite SutureTac with FiberWire (Arthrex Inc., Naples, Florida), placing three anterior, two posterior, and two superior anchors. One limb from each anchor is retrieved out the anterosuperior portal. The anterior superolateral

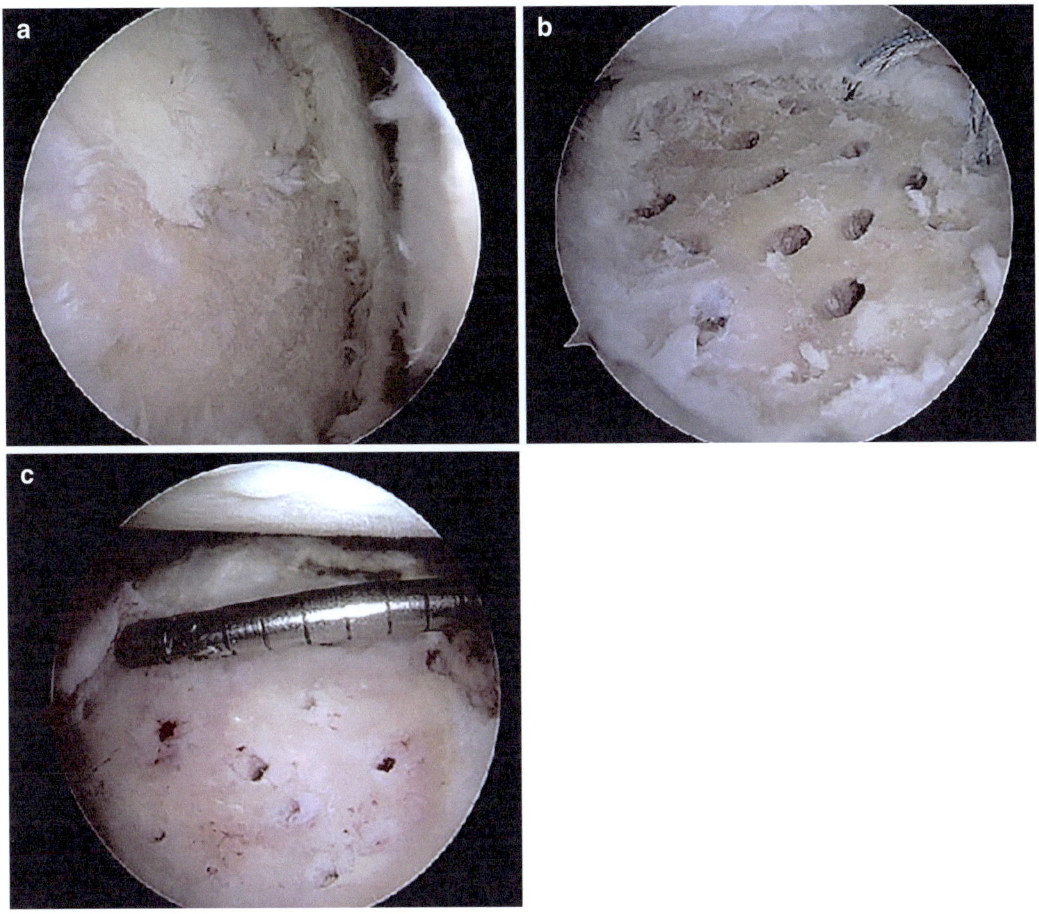

Fig. 13.5 Arthroscopic view of right shoulder with patient in beach chair position. (**a**) Osteochondral defects of the glenoid. (**b**) Glenoidplasty and microfracture to generate a marrow-stimulated bleeding to deliver pluripo-tential cells to improve healing and graft incorporation. (**c**) Glenoid dimension measurement from posterior portal

cannula must be removed and the portal is then slightly extended for an easy passage of the graft into the joint. The sutures are then passed through the graft with the FastPass Scorpion suture passer (Arthrex Inc., Naples, Florida) in the corresponding situation and secured with mulberry knots tied on the joint side of the graft (Fig. 13.7). At this point it is important to maintain gentle tension on the sutures to prevent tangling; then the graft is shuttled down into the joint through the anterosuperior portal while doing traction on the other limb of each suture. These sutures are then tied to get fixation of the graft. We close the knot from posteroinferior to anteroinferior and finally superior to complete the procedure. Circumferential graft fixation with a minimum of six points anchor fixation completes the operation [3, 22] (Fig. 13.8). At the final results, we can compare the preoperative XR with the 1-year follow-up XR (Fig. 13.9).

Ream and Run Technique

Another option to address the glenoid is the "ream and run" technique, which is used to restore a concentric glenohumeral joint while preserving the glenoid bone stock and avoiding

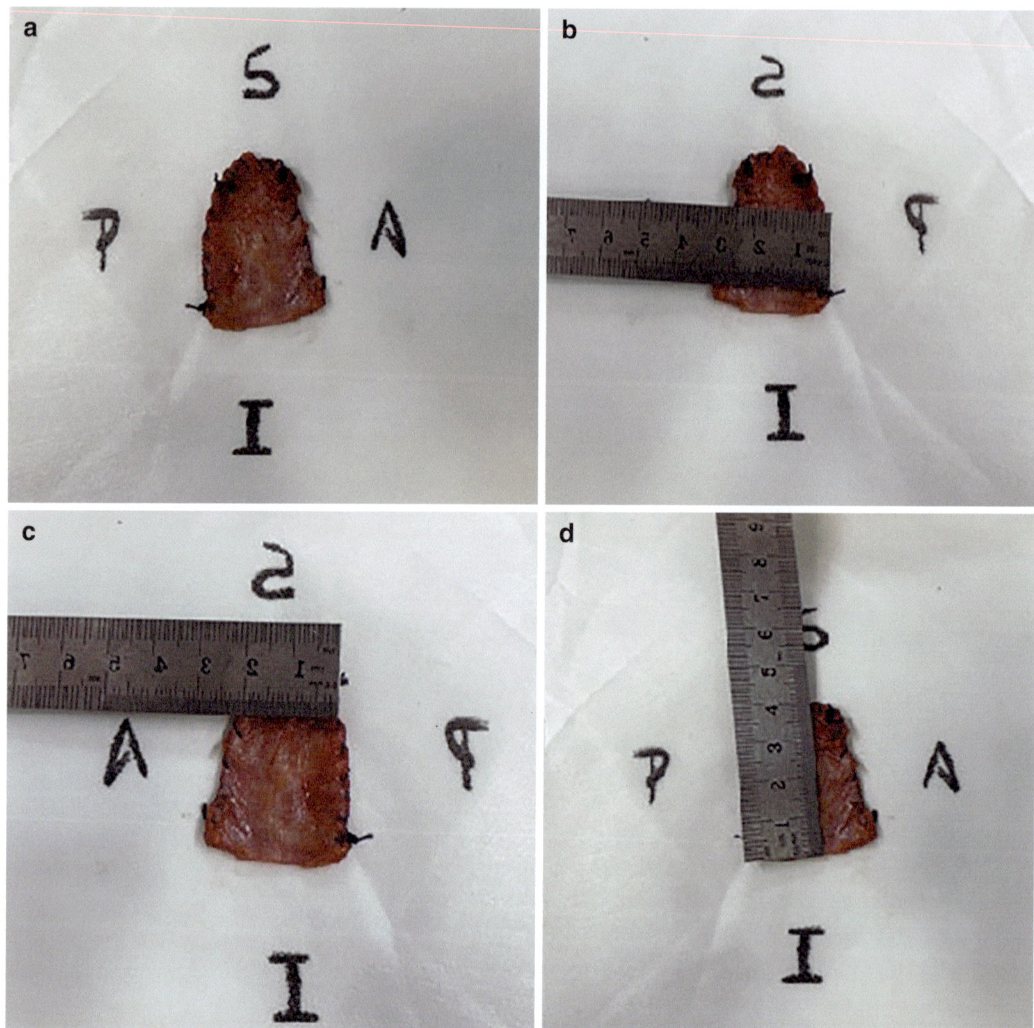

Fig. 13.6 Graft prepared according to previous arthroscopic measurement to recreate the glenoid shape. The graft is folded once to create a double fascia lata autograft. (**a**) The edge of the graft is sutured around its periphery. (**b**) Bottom length corresponding to the inferior AP length of the glena. (**c**) Top length corresponding to the superior AP length of the glena. (**d**) Upper lower length corresponding from top to bottom length of the glena

risks of polyethylene component wear or the complexities of soft tissue interposition. Saltzman et al. [24] have popularized a combination of hemiarthroplasty with concentric reaming of the glenoid as a potential option for patients with GH arthritis. This allows centering of the humeral component on the glenoid, to create a smooth fibrocartilaginous surface on which the component sits. Encouraging results have been documented. Results, of ream and run in combination with hemiarthroplasty in the young patients population, are not very hopeful with up to 14% revision in relatively short-term follow-up [24].

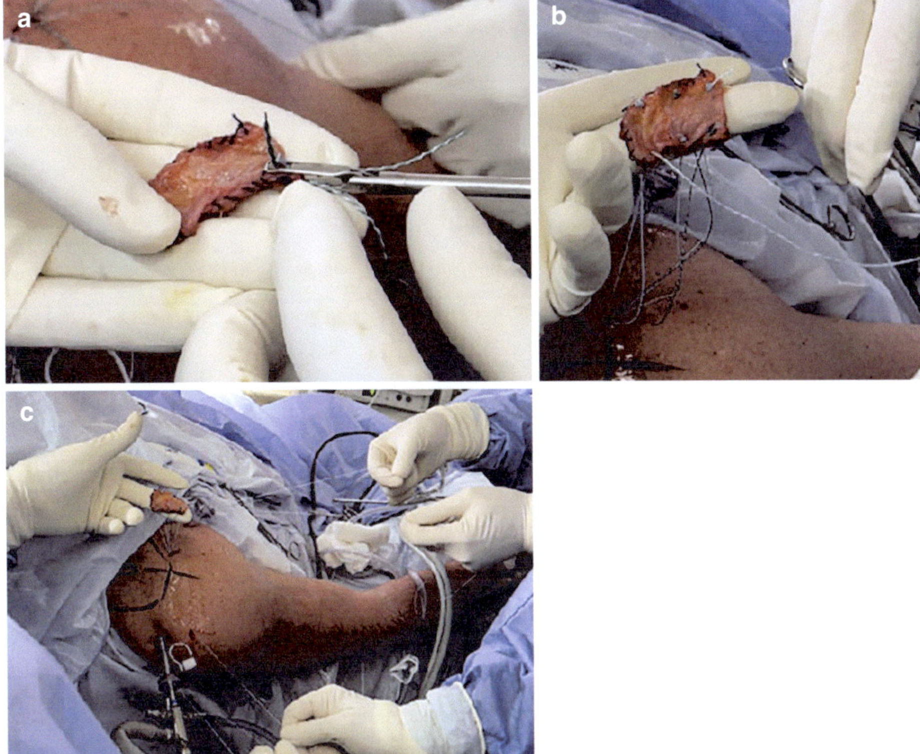

Fig. 13.7 (**a**) The sutures are passed through the graft with the FastPass Scorpion suture passer in the corresponding situation. (**b**) Secured with mulberry knots tied on the joint side of the graft. (**c**) To maintain gentle tension on the sutures to prevent tangling, the graft is shuttled down into the joint through the anterosuperior portal while doing traction on the other limb of each suture

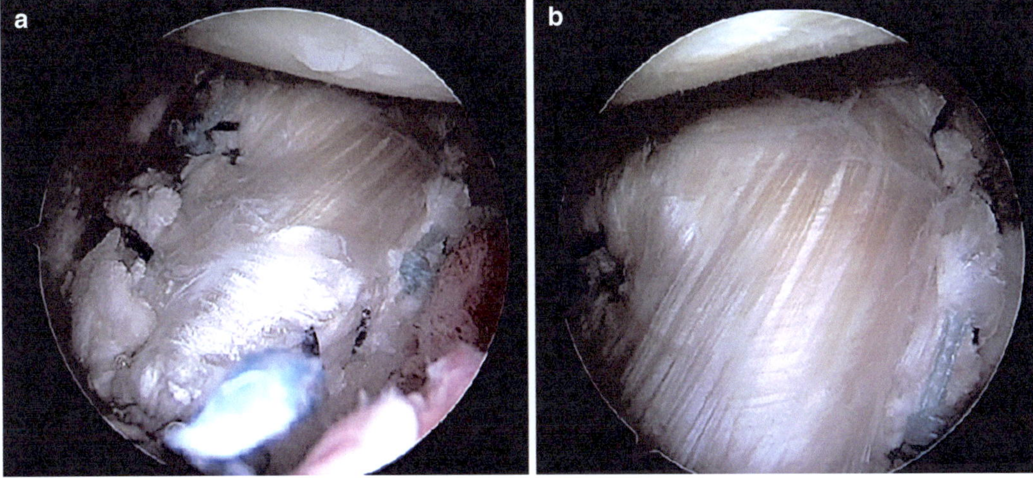

Fig. 13.8 Arthroscopic view of right shoulder in a patient who underwent arthroscopic biologic shoulder resurfacing with fascia lata autograft. (**a, b**) Circumferential graft fixation with a minimum of six points anchor fixation to complete the operation

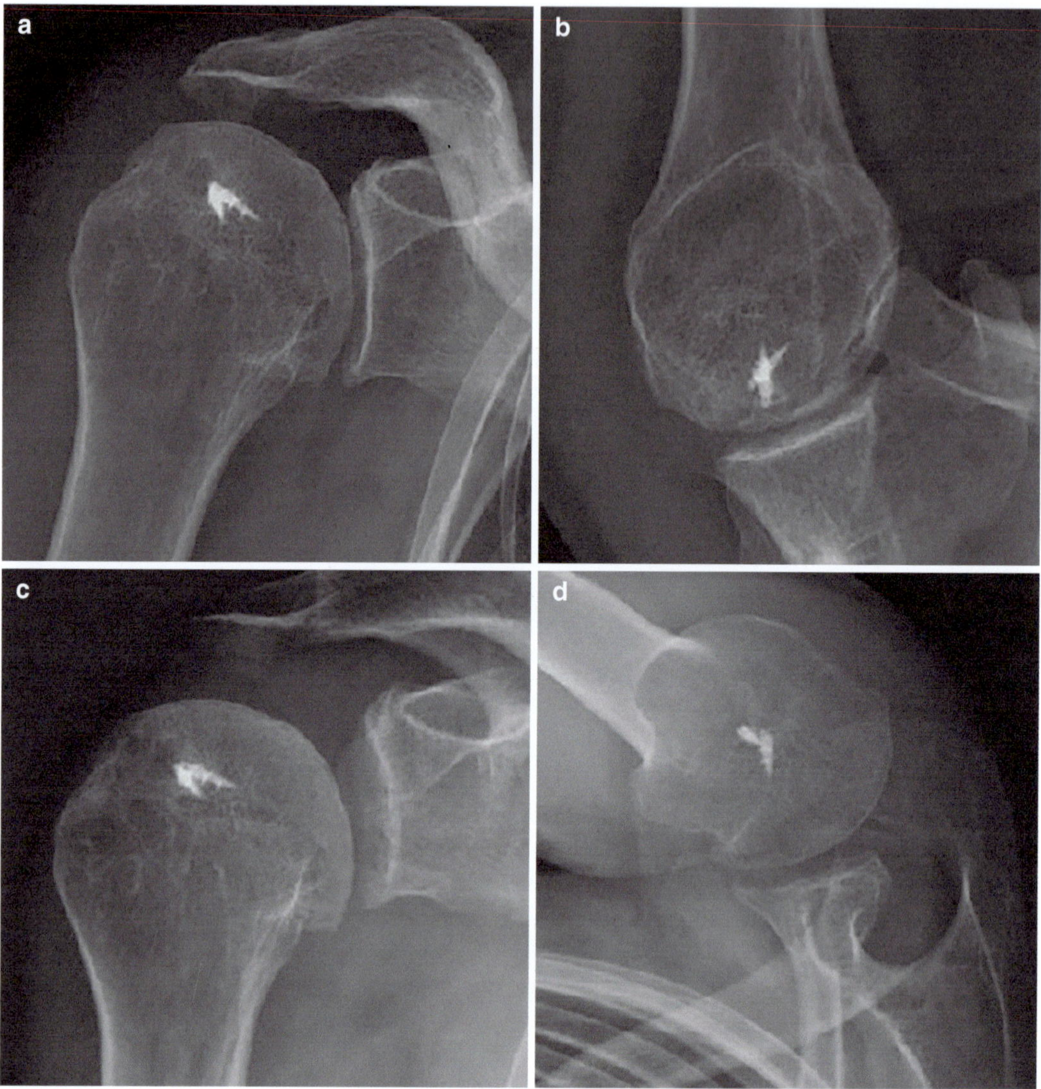

Fig. 13.9 Glenohumeral arthritis in young patients (48-year-old). (**a**, **b**) Preop AP and axial XR. (**b**) Preop axial view. (**c**, **d**) Post-op XR AP and axial view. We observe the increased joint space in a patient who underwent arthroscopic biologic glenoid resurfacing

Hemiarthroplasty with Biological Interposition

Hemiarthroplasty with biological interposition is another option to treat young patients with shoulder arthritis. Different autografts or allografts have been used to interpose between the glenoid and the humeral hemiarthroplasty. The goal of this procedure is to avoid glenoid complication specially polyethylene-related problems (wear or loosening) while creating a smooth surface on the glenoid to decrease the coefficient of friction and preserve glenoid bone stock. Wirth [25] reported a series of 24 patients with lateral meniscal allograft resurfacing with hemiarthroplasty. At a mean follow-up of 3 years, he reported good results but had concern regarding durability of the graft with progressive decreasing glenohumeral joint space. Burkhead et al. [26] reported 36 patients who underwent soft tissue resurfacing of the glenoid with hemiarthroplasty. At a mean of 7 years, results were excellent in 18 shoulders, satisfactory in 13, and unsatisfactory in 5. Other series demonstrate high failure rates of 44–77% with this operation [27, 28]. Therefore, the role of hemiarthroplasty with biologic resurfacing remains controversial.

13.7 Postoperative Protocol

We indicate sling at neutral rotation for 6 weeks. Passive range of motion at 90 degrees of anterior flexion, 70–90 degrees of abduction, and 30 degrees of external rotation begins at the first month. Internal rotation begun at 2 months after surgery. Active assisted exercises begin at 6 weeks, and strengthening starting with isometric exercises for the rotator cuff and periscapular musculature begins at 8 weeks. Full strengthening with weight progression begins at 16 weeks. Sports gesture training in athletes begins at 6 months with sports return or recreational activities according to progression at 6–9 months after surgery.

13.8 Potential Complications

Persistent chronic shoulder pain is the most frequent complication after arthroscopic glenoid resurfacing that prevents patients to return to normal activities. Perhaps persistent chronic pain means progression of osteoarthritis or glenohumeral chondrolysis. Arthrofibrosis or adhesive capsulitis, infection, and complex regional pain syndrome are rare, with a very low percentage of cases.

13.9 Discussion

Arthritic changes in the young patient may affect the surgeon's treatment algorithm and the patient's prognosis. Arthroscopic management of shoulder osteoarthritis in young patients has been shown to provide short- to midterm pain relief. Loss of the normal gliding surface and increased friction may play a role in rapid progression of disease. The CAM procedure [18, 19] associated with arthroscopic glenoid resurfacing [3, 20–22] attempts to improve the mechanical symptoms and normal gliding surface to decrease friction and slow down the degenerative process. However, the mechanism of pain relief following debridement is unknown. It has been hypothesized that the removal of debris, which can cause synovitis, as well as the dilution of degenerative enzymes, may contribute to the improvement found after surgery. In addition, the removal of mechanical factors such as chondral flaps, loose bodies, and osteophytes may improve joint function. Arthroscopic glenoid resurfacing has been performed as an alternative to total shoulder or hemiarthroplasty replacement in the young patient. The purpose of this procedure is to avoid concerns of arthroplasty longevity while preserving the joint. This biological procedure resurfaces the shoulder without the use of metal implants. The choice of the fascia lata autograft and its pluripotent cell construct will be hopefully transformed over time into a fibrous tissue covering of the glenoid. Chondrocyte ingrowth/metaplasia could be considered as another theoretical advantage of glenoid resurfacing [21]. The fascia lata autograft has not been associated with allergic-type reactions or high complication rate when used. Savoie et al. [20] reported a series of 23 patients (mean age, 32 years) who underwent arthroscopic biologic resurfacing with the Restore Patch (Depuy, Warsaw, IN). Of these patients, 15 (75%) were satisfied with their surgery at a midterm 6-year follow-up, with significant improvement of pain and function. Five patients (15%) had required humeral arthroplasty at the final follow-up. Midterm results of AGR with acellular human dermal graft have also been described for glenohumeral arthritis in 32 patients, with successful outcome in 23 (72%) patients and failure in 9 (28%). An absolute increase in the range of motion was not statistically significant, although a significant increase in overall Constant and Murley shoulder score was demonstrated ($P \setminus 0.0001$) [21]. Hartzler et al. [22] published a case series of 43 patients with a medium follow-up of 53 months (48–72) and average age of 57 years old (55–59) who underwent AGR; all patients had osteoarthritis grade 2 or 3 according to the Samilson and Prieto classification, with significant improvement in outcome measures of pain and function at final follow-up and without intraoperative or postoperative complications. In ten shoulders 23% revision to a prosthetic arthroplasty was performed at a mean of 45 months (range, 9–71 months) after the index operation. Hemiarthroplasty was performed in three shoulders, TSA in four, and reverse total shoulder arthroplasty in three patients. They concluded that AGR with dermal allograft is a safe option for joint preservation in selected patients, provides pain relief, and has an acceptable rate of revision to prosthetic arthroplasty at short- to midterm follow-up. Increased age and lower preoperative ASES score were risk factors for failure of AGR [3, 22]. Arthroscopic joint preserving treatments have the advantage of delaying arthroplasty in this younger population while maintaining the patient's natural anatomy and do not appear to compromise later arthroplasty [29, 30]. Short- to midterm studies show good outcomes with low conversion rate to arthroplasty (23% (Hartzler et al.) [3, 22], 25% (Savoie et al.) [20], and 28% (De Beer et al.) [21]). Overall, the data demonstrated improved outcomes for patient undergoing a soft tissue resurfacing. The CAM procedure and the interposition of a soft tissue (autograft or allograft) with AGR are demanding procedures that should be reserved for experienced arthroscopists. If arthroscopic glenoid resurfacing fails to relieve the patient's symptoms, the procedure does not jeopardize any further surgical treatment. Soft tissue resurfacing procedures offer an option that allows the arthritic glenoid to be addressed while removing the risk of glenoid component loosening or failure in total shoulder arthroplasty. With proper patient selection and a good surgical technique, AGR is a reliable operation to relive pain and improve function. The CAM procedure with AGR is sometimes viewed as a bridge to a shoulder arthroplasty until arthroplasty is considered more appropriate. The use of biologic glenoid resurfacing with or without humeral head replacement remains controversial. Therefore, at this time we recommend caution in the use of such

techniques until further clinical studies provide stronger levels of evidence for clinical effectiveness.

In conclusion, arthroscopic management of shoulder arthritis is a useful treatment in young or active patients for whom it is advisable to delay shoulder arthroplasty. The optimal approach to surgical management remains controversial. Limited procedures such as AGR may be considered to preserve the joint. Although arthroscopic glenoid resurfacing does not prevent osteoarthritic progression, it may provide a temporizing option to avoid prosthetic replacement and allow earlier return to recreational activities and physically demanding occupations in young patients. We consider AGR to be an excellent and safe option for selected patients with glenohumeral arthritis as an alternative or interim procedure to arthroplasty in young patient population. Symptomatic glenohumeral arthritis in young patients continues to be a challenging problem to effectively manage. Further prospective studies and a longer follow-up are necessary to establish long-term outcomes and better define the role of this procedure.

13.10 Summary and Key Points

- Management of the young patient with arthritis requires an individualized approach.
- AGR provides temporary pain relief and functional improvement.
- AGR does not prevent osteoarthritic progression.
- Midterm studies show good outcomes with low conversion rate to arthroplasty.
- This procedure is useful in young who need to avoid prosthetic replacement.

References

1. Denard PJ, Wirth MA, Orfaly RM. Current concepts: review management of glenohumeral arthritis in the young adult. J Bone Joint Surg Am. 2011;93(9):885–92. https://doi.org/10.2106/JBJS.J.00960.
2. Saltzman BM, Mercer DM, Warme WJ, Bertelsen AL, Matsen FA 3rd. Comparison of patients undergoing

primary shoulder arthroplasty before and after the age of fifty. J Bone Joint Surg Am. 2010;92:42–7. https://doi.org/10.2106/JBJS.I.00071.

3. Burkhart SS, Brady PC, Denard PJ, Adams CR, Hartzler RU. The Cowboy's conundrum: complex and advanced cases in shoulder arthroscopy. Philadelphia: Wolters Kluwer; 2017. p. 343.

4. Solomon DJ, Navaie M, Stedje-Larsen ET, Smith JC, Provencher MT. Glenohumeral chondrolysis after arthroscopy: a systematic review of potential contributors and causal pathways. Arthroscopy. 2009;25(11):1329–42. https://doi.org/10.2106/JBJS.I.00071.

5. Saltzman BM, Leroux TS, Verma NN, Romeo AA. Glenohumeral osteoarthritis in the young patient. J Am Acad Orthrop Surg. 2018;26:e361–70. https://doi.org/10.5435/JAAOS-D-16-00657.

6. Chong PY, Srikumaran U, Kuye IO, Warner JJP. Glenohumeral arthritis in the young patient. J Shoulder Elbow Surg. 2011;20:S30–40. https://doi.org/10.1016/j.jse.2010.11.014.

7. Bailie D, Ellenbecker T. Severe chondrolysis after shoulder arthroscopy: a case series. J Shoulder Elbow Surg. 2009;18(5):742–7. https://doi.org/10.1016/j.jse.2008.10.017. Epub 2009 Jan 30.

8. Buscayret F, Edwards T, Szabo I, Adeleine P, Coudane II, Walch G. Glenohumeral arthrosis in anterior instability before and after surgical treatment: incidence and contributing factors. Am J Sports Med. 2004;32:1165–72. https://doi.org/10.1177/0363546503262686.

9. Cameron M, Kocher M, Briggs K, Horan M, Hawkins R. The prevalence of glenohumeral osteoarthrosis in unstable shoulders. Am J Sports Med. 2003;31:53–5. https://doi.org/10.1177/03635465030310012001.

10. Parsons IM, Buoncristiani AM, Donion S, Campbell B, Smith KL, Matsen FA. The effect of total shoulder arthroplasty on self-assessed deficits in shoulder function in patients with capsulorrhaphy arthropathy. J Shoulder Elbow Surg. 2007;16(3 suppl):S19–26. https://doi.org/10.1016/j.jse.2006.03.001.

11. Matsen FA 3rd, Rockwood CA, Wirth MA, Lippitt SB. Glenohumeral arthritis and its management. In: Rockwood CA, Matsen 3rd FA, editors. The shoulder. 2nd ed. Philadelphia: W.B. Saunders Company; 1998. p. 840–964.

12. Cameron BD, Iannotti JP. Alternatives to total shoulder arthroplasty. In: Warner JJP, Iannotti JP, Flatow EL, editors. Complex and revision problems in shoulder surgery. 2nd ed. Philadelphia: Lippincott Williams & Wilkins; 2005. p. 445–58.

13. Wallace A. Management of glenohumeral osteoarthritis in the young adult. Shoulder Elbow. 2010;2:1–8. https://doi.org/10.1111/j.1758-5740.2009.00045.x.

14. Reineck JR, Krishnan SG, Burkhead WZ. Early glenohumeral arthritis in the competing athlete. Clin Sports Med. 2008;27:803–19. https://doi.org/10.1016/j.csm.2008.07.004.

15. Gold GE, Reeder SB, Beaulieu CF. Advanced MR imaging of the shoulder: dedicated cartilage techniques. Magn Reson Imaging Clin N Am. 2004;12:143–59. https://doi.org/10.1016/j.mric.2004.01.007.

16. Hayes ML, Collins MS, Morgan JA, Wenger DE, Dahm DL. Efficacy of diagnostic magnetic resonance imaging for articular cartilage lesions of the glenohumeral joint in patients with instability. Skeletal Radiol. 2010;39:1199–204. https://doi.org/10.1007/s00256-010-0922-4.

17. Samilson RL, Prieto V. Dislocation arthropathy of the shoulder. J Bone Joint Surg. 1983;65:1456–60. PMID: 6833319.

18. Millett PJ, Gaskill TR. Arthroscopic management of glenohumeral arthrosis: humeral osteoplasty, capsular release, and arthroscopic axillary nerve release as a joint-preserving approach. Arthroscopy. 2011;27:1296–303. https://doi.org/10.1016/j.arthro.2011.03.089.

19. Millett PJ, Horan MP, Pennock AT, Rios D. Comprehensive arthroscopic management (CAM) procedure: clinical results of a joint-preserving arthroscopic treatment for young, active patients with advanced shoulder osteoarthritis. Arthroscopy. 2013;29:440–8. https://doi.org/10.1016/j.arthro.2012.10.028.

20. Savoie FH 3rd, Brislin KJ, Argo D. Arthroscopic glenoid resurfacing as a surgical treatment for glenohumeral arthritis in the young patient: midterm results. Arthroscopy. 2009;25:864–71. https://doi.org/10.1016/j.arthro.2009.02.018.

21. De Beer JF, Bhatia DN, van Rooyen KS, Du Toit DF. Arthroscopic debridement and biological resurfacing of the glenoid in glenohumeral arthritis. Knee Surg Sports Traumatol Arthrosc. 2010;18:1767–73. https://doi.org/10.1007/s00167-010-1155-8.

22. Hartzler RU, Melapi S, de Beer JF, Burkhart SS. Arthroscopic joint preservation in severe glenohumeral arthritis using interpositional human dermal allograft. Arthroscopy. 2017;33(11):1920–5. https://doi.org/10.1016/j.arthro.2017.04.005. Epub 2017 Jun 28

23. Derwin KA, Aurora A, Iannotti JP. Allograft fascia lata as an augmentation device for musculoskeletal repairs. Conference paper. Cleveland Clinic, Cleveland OH. Google–Article; 2008.

24. Saltzman MD, Chamberlain AM, Mercer DM, Warme WJ, Bertelsen AL, Matsen FA 3rd. Shoulder hemiarthroplasty with concentric glenoid reaming in patients 55 years old or less. J Shoulder Elbow Surg. 2011;20:609–15.

25. Wirth MA. Humeral head arthroplasty and meniscal allograft resurfacing of the glenoid. J Bone Joint Surg. 2009;91:1109–19. https://doi.org/10.2106/JBJS.H.00677.

26. Burkhead WZ Jr, Krishnan SG, Lin KC. Biologic resurfacing of the arthritic glenohumeral joint: historical review and current applications. J Shoulder Elbow Surg. 2007;16:S248–53. https://doi.org/10.1016/j.jse.2007.03.006.

27. Strauss EJ, Verma NN, Salata MJ, McGill KC, Klifto C, Nicholson GP, et al. The high failure rate of bio-

logic resurfacing of the glenoid in young patients with glenohumeral arthritis. J Shoulder Elbow Surg. 2014;23:409–19. https://doi.org/10.1016/j.jse.2013.06.001.

28. Namdari S, Alosh H, Baldwin K, Glaser D, Kelly JD. Biological glenoid resurfacing for glenohumeral osteoarthritis: a systematic review. J Shoulder Elbow Surg. 2011;20:1184–90. https://doi.org/10.1016/j.jse.2011.04.031.

29. Schiffman CJ, Whitson AJ, Chawla SS, Matsen FA 3rd, Hsu JE. Arthroscopic management of glenohumeral arthritis in the young patient does not negatively impact the outcome of subsequent anatomic shoulder arthroplasty. Int Orthop. 2021;45(8):2071–9. https://doi.org/10.1007/s00264-021-05133-y. Epub 2021 Jul 13. PMID: 34255098.

30. Schiffman CJ, Hannay WM, Whitson AJ, Neradilek MB, Matsen FA 3rd, Hsu JE. Impact of previous non-arthroplasty surgery on clinical outcomes after primary anatomic shoulder arthroplasty. J Shoulder Elbow Surg. 2020;29(10):2056–64. https://doi.org/10.1016/j.jse.2020.01.088. Epub 2020 Apr 22. PMID: 32331844.

Humeral Stem Length in Glenohumeral Arthroplasty: Long-Stem, Short-Stem, or Stemless

Stephen C. Weber, Prashant Meshram, and Edward G. McFarland

14.1 History of Stem Length in Glenohumeral Arthroplasty

Glenohumeral arthroplasty has been performed since the 1800s, with the first reported implant ascribed to the French surgeon Jules Emile Péan in 1893 [1]. The era of modern shoulder replacement began with the pioneering work of Dr. Charles Neer, who originally suggested humeral hemiarthroplasty for the management of acute fractures [2]. Neer subsequently expanded this indication, ultimately including total shoulder replacement for a variety of diagnoses [3]. In his 1982 paper [3], Neer describes the rationale behind his initial choice of dimensions for his humeral components. Although a standard 150 mm stem was used in almost all cases, two cases with epiphyseal dysplasia multiplex were treated with a short 63 mm stemmed device (Fig. 14.1). These short-stem devices were marketed prior to the 1976 Medical Device Amendments passed to ensure safety and effectiveness of medical devices, including diagnostic products, and so are "pre-amendment" devices (https://www.fda.gov/about-fda/fda-history/milestones-us-food-and-drug-law), allowing later short-stem devices to be cleared by their respective manufacturers via the 510(k) pathway without clinical data requirements. The choice of 150 mm standard stem length by Dr. Neer appears to have been relatively arbitrary, but it seems that a stem length comparable to the length of stems used in early, successful hip arthroplasty was chosen.

Neer's choice of stem length and prosthesis geometry proved to be the archetype of subsequent anatomic shoulder prosthesis design. While a variety of unsolved problems exist in the realm of shoulder arthroplasty, standard length humeral stems have shown high rates of success and survivorship [4] quoted as 1.4% at a mean follow-up of 9 years (minimum 5-year follow-up) [5]. Another study showed an isolated humeral loosening that occurred in 0.3% of the shoulders reviewed after 20 years' experience at a single institution [6]. This rate is so low that early loosening of an uncemented humeral stem has been felt to be invariably a sign of infection [7]. While humeral revision for aseptic loosening remains rare, the loss of bone stock associated with humeral revision for other causes remained a concern [8].

Given the high rate of success of Neer's original choice of stem length, changing stem length without substantial supportive data can be questioned. The first significant change in humeral stem length came with the advent of resurfacing arthroplasty. Copeland noted that stemmed

S. C. Weber (✉) · P. Meshram · E. G. McFarland
Division of Shoulder Surgery, The Department of Orthopedic Surgery, The Johns Hopkins University, Baltimore, MD, USA
e-mail: emcfarl1@jhmi.edu

© ISAKOS 2023
A. D. Mazzocca et al. (eds.), *Shoulder Arthritis across the Life Span*,
https://doi.org/10.1007/978-3-031-33298-2_14

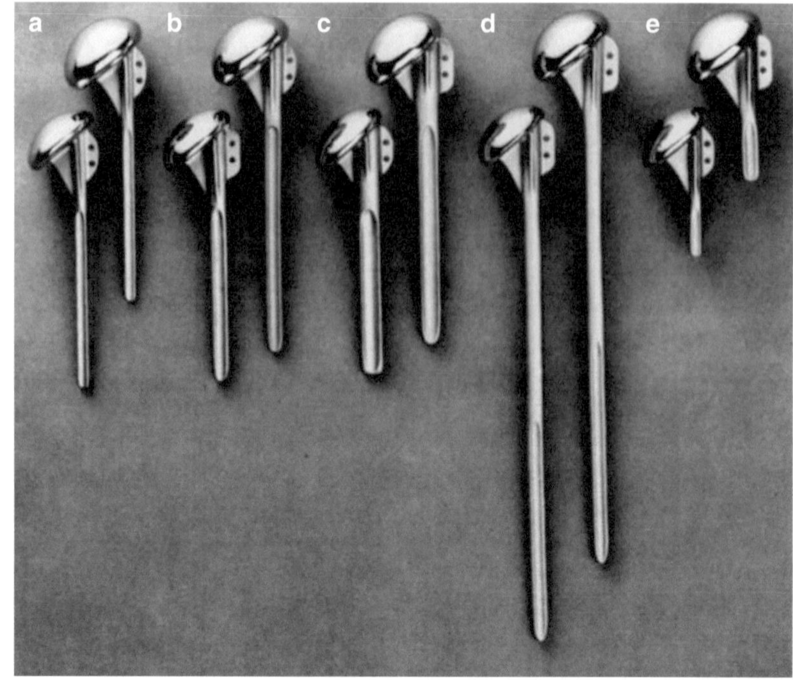

Fig. 14.1 Illustration of the original humeral stems proposed by Neer for total shoulder replacement. This illustration shows the first shorter stem shoulder arthroplasty. (Reproduced with permission from Neer, C.S., 2nd, K.C. Watson, and F.J. Stanton, Recent experience in total shoulder replacement. J Bone Joint Surg Am, 1982. 64(3): p. 319–37)

implants, while important in fracture care, may not be necessary when performing shoulder arthroplasty for osteoarthritis. In 1986, he began implanting humeral head surface replacements in patients with shoulder osteoarthritis, and by 1993, he had altered his design to include hydroxyapatite coating on the humeral component. He reported results in terms of function and survivorship that were comparable to those of a stemmed implant [9]. Glenoid replacement with resurfacing devices proved challenging, however, and complications with glenoid erosion and rotator cuff failure perhaps secondary to overstuffing the joint have caused many surgeons to abandon this approach [10]. To gain better surgical access to the glenoid, stemless arthroplasty was proposed. Introduced in 2004, the Total Evolution Shoulder System (TESS; Biomet; Warsaw, Indiana) gained widespread use in Europe [11]. The first US FDA-cleared stemless device was the Simpliciti stemless device (TORNIER Simpliciti, Wright Medical Group; Memphis, Tennessee; K143552; https://www.accessdata. fda.gov/scripts/cdrh/cfdocs/cfpmn/pmn. cfm?ID=K143552). Other stemless devices followed suit, and a variety of shorter-stem and stemless devices are now available in the United States. Although stemless reverse arthroplasty is widely used in Europe [12], there are no currently cleared stemless reverse devices in the United States. Unlike stemless devices, short-stem reverse devices are available in a reverse configuration in the United States. These shorter-stem and stemless devices have generally shown equivalent revision rates and clinical outcomes to traditional stemmed devices in short- and mid-term follow-up [12–15].

Even with limited comparative data, stemless arthroplasty is set to surpass standard stemmed arthroplasty in Europe by 2024 [16, 17]. This is despite the fact that under most hospital reimbursement systems, these implants are substantially more expensive than traditional stemmed devices. It is interesting to review the purported advantages of shorter-stem lengths based on the more recent published data, to determine how many of these claims have been supported by the subsequent literature.

Purported Advantages of Shorter-Stem Humeral Components

- Easier humeral fixation in cases with metaphyseal deformity
- Better positioning in anatomic reconstruction
- Faster surgery
- Less blood loss
- Increased bone stock preservation
- Fewer postoperative complications
- Fewer interoperative fractures
- Less stress resorption

14.2 Cases with Metaphyseal Deformity

This remains one of the best indications for shorter-stem and stemless humeral components and was Neer's original indication for these devices [3]. Patients with marked deformity due to congenital bone disorders or trauma can require an osteotomy to place a standard length stem. Humeral osteotomy can be technically challenging, and at least one study showed that this negatively affected the final outcome of the procedure [18]. Short-stem and stemless implants allow reasonable glenoid exposure and can permit humeral replacement without osteotomy in these cases [19, 20]. Data regarding these advantages are limited to case reports [19].

14.3 Better Positioning in Anatomic Reconstruction

The unique anatomy of the proximal humerus is known to make precise reconstruction of the humerus difficult with a standard stemmed prosthesis. The humeral head's center of rotation is offset from the humeral shaft medial 5 mm to 11 mm and posterior 1 mm to 5 mm. Humeral head inclination is variable at 40–45° and the head height or thickness is 15–20 mm from the anatomic neck axis. Native version is an average of 18–25° retroverted, although this can range from 5° of anteversion to 60° of retroversion [21]. Variable neck angle standard prostheses and offset humeral heads have improved the anatomic

results to a degree [22]. Short-stem and especially stemless devices theoretically allow better duplication of the normal anatomy, as the position of the humeral head is not constrained by the stem. Although desirable, clinical data to support the relationship between anatomic reconstruction and clinical outcomes are lacking, and the pathologic anatomy of the severely arthritic shoulder with its associated soft tissue contractures may make restoration to its pre-arthritic bony anatomy undesirable.

14.4 Faster Surgery

Berth and Pap in a comparative study of stemless and traditional stemmed devices showed a significant decrease in operative time [23]. In revision surgery, Tracy et al. [24] showed that primary short-stem and stemless devices can be revised significantly more quickly than standard stem devices, with stemless on average 40 min faster and 25 min for short stems than traditional length devices. These differences may be clinically significant as well. These differences become especially relevant as many as 30% of stemmed platform systems cannot be converted without removing the initial stem [25] negating the advantages of the platform system. The ease of revision with shorter stems seems likely. This becomes more important in the revision with unexpected positive intraoperative cultures, where shorter stems allow removal of all components, effecting a single-stage revision in this setting.

14.5 Less Blood Loss

While widely touted as an advantage of shorter-stem implants, comparative studies remain few. Most comparative studies [15, 26–29] do not address this issue. Berth and Pap in one of the few comparative studies did show significantly less blood loss with a stemless device [23]. Tracy et al. showed that while conversion of short-stem and stemless implants to RTSA had significantly less blood loss, transfusion rates were low in both groups and not significantly different [24], raising questions about how clinically significant this difference is despite the statistical significance cited.

14.6 Increased Bone Stock Preservation

It seems obvious that shorter-stem and stemless components would preserve humeral bone. Preservation of bone stock remains a cogent argument for shorter stems. Data to support improved survivorship upon revision of shorter-stem devices over traditional stems is lacking. Other options exist with standard stems. Boorman et al. describe a conservative broaching and impaction grafting technique for standard stem humeral component placement and fixation in shoulder arthroplasty which they call "the procrustean method" [30]. This group continues to report excellent results with this technique, citing preservation of bone stock using a standard stem length [31].

14.7 Fewer Interoperative Fractures

A reduced rate of intraoperative humeral fractures has been cited as an advantage of stemless and short-stem devices. However, data to support this remains scarce. Berth and Pap in their comparative study showed equivalent rates of intraoperative fracture (2%) [23]. Erickson et al. in their comparative study showed identical low rates of intraoperative fracture (0.3 versus 0.4%) comparing standard stem to a short-stem prosthesis [29]. Huguet et al. actually showed a 7% rate of intraoperative fractures with a stemless device, which they attributed to implantation technique. This requires immediate revision to a standard stem in four of five cases [32]. Tracy et al. in their retrospective review of short-stem and stemless revision surgery showed significantly less interoperative fractures with revision of stemless devices (3.6%) but short-stem and standard stem devices showed similar rates of fracture (23.4% and 24%, respectively). While periprosthetic fractures around short-stem and stemless prostheses will often occur in the metaphyseal portion of the humerus, and so may be more likely to heal than diaphyseal fractures around standard stem devices, there is little data to support this contention.

14.8 Less Stress Resorption/Stress Shielding

Stress shielding and bone resorption have been reported as a significant issue in standard length shoulder arthroplasty, secondary to bypassing the metaphysis with diaphyseal fixation [33]. While metaphyseal fixation has been proposed to eliminate this, more recent studies have shown that this can still be a problem, especially with short-stem devices. Habermeyer et al. noted minimal radiolucent lines using a short-stem device [34]. These authors however noted an area of lower-density cancellous bone in the proximal humerus was observed in 41.3% of the patients, which did not seem to affect clinical outcome. Giordano et al. actually showed more stress shielding with a short-stem than a standard stem device [35]. Raiss et al. showed that only 49% of anatomic short stem and 65% of reverse short stem had no evidence for radiographic changes of stress shielding or loosening [36]. These authors noted that radiographic changes were increased in cases where high filling ratios of the device to the humeral canal were noted. Other authors have noted similar findings [37]. While lower filling ratios diminished the stress shielding, this also increases the risk of valgus positioning [38]. The clinical implications of lucencies around the humeral stem remain unclear [39].

Problems Unique to Shorter Stems

(a) While better restoration of anatomy is proposed as an advantage of shorter-stem prostheses, the reverse may in fact be true. Abdic et al. noted that one-fourth of short-stem prostheses were malaligned, usually placed in valgus [38]. Varus positioning in short stem was described by Casagrande et al. as well [40]. Cox et al. noted similar issues with stemless shoulders, with 22% of implants placed in varus [41], with Kadum et al. reporting a similar high rate of malalignment [42]. Overstuffing of the joint with stemless devices, potentially leading to increased rates of stiffness and rotator cuff failure, has also been described. Grubhofer et al. showed that 66% of stemless prostheses failed to restore anatomy to within 3 mm [43]. Eighty-eight percent of these failures were caused by overstuffing, usually due to poor humeral osteotomy placement. This problem is similar to published results with resurfacing [44]. Other authors, however, have shown better alignment with short-stem than standard stem devices [8]. While the constraint on positioning imposed by a standard stem can be a disadvantage, it appears that the occasional shoulder surgeon may in fact be less likely to reproduce the native anatomy with shorter-stem and stemless devices. Lazarus et al. stated "Stemmed humeral components may help correct an imperfect humeral osteotomy because the intramedullary canal can be used to guide implant placement" [45].

(b) Loosening. Not all shorter-stem and stemless outcomes have been satisfactory in regard to early loosening. Casagrande et al. noted a 71% incidence of radiolucent lines in early follow-up of the TORNIER AEQUALIS ASCEND FLEX (Wright Medical, Escondido, California), with 10.1% judged to be loose and 12% requiring a revision [40]. Zmistowski et al. raised similar issues with the grit-blasted Univers Apex (short stem) (Arthrex, Naples, Florida) [46]. In this study, 23 (12.5%) patients presented with a painful shoulder and radiographic concern for potential humeral loosening at a mean follow-up of 1.5 years (range: 1.5 months to 3.4 years). Thirteen (7.1%) of these reviewed by Zmistowski et al. required long-stem revision shoulder arthroplasty where a loose stem was confirmed in all cases. Converting the grit-

blasted design to proximal porous coating seems to have improved these results. Morwood et al. reported improved results with the AEQUALIS ASCEND FLEX device (Wright Medical, Escondido, California) altered to have proximal porous coating instead of grit blasting, with only 7 of 34 showing radiolucencies [47]. This problem is not limited to short-stem prostheses. While Kostretzis et al. showed a loosening rate for stemless of 3.8% [37], other surgeons have reported short-term loosening rates of as high as 5.2% [48]. Subsistence of shorter stems has also been reported. Tross et al. reported an 11% subsistence rate with a short-stem device [49]. Similar results have been reported by Van de Kleut et al. using radiostereometric analysis software [50] noting that "increased early humeral stem migration may be negatively associated with clinical outcomes." Subsistence may be an issue for those patients with weight-bearing shoulders. These studies confirm that generalizing component attributes that have been effective in traditional length stems to these shorter stems may not be universally successful. Recent review of the Australian Joint Replacement Registry (AJRR) has not shown shorter stems to be outliers in terms of mid-term loosening [51]. This suggests that registry data to date has not identified any problems with early failure of shorter-stem devices.

(c) Inadequate bone quality. Many patients will have insufficient metaphyseal bone to allow for metaphyseal fixation. This requires an assessment at the time of surgery to determine if the bone quality is adequate. Churchill et al. described this as a "thumb test" where the adequacy of bone was assessed by the ability to indent the humeral osteotomy site with a thumb [13]. This subjective assessment can be challenging. Published case reports of this problem are lacking, but the 2017 UK recall of the Biomet Nano reverse stemless suggests that the failure to adequately assess bone quality at surgery is not trivial (https://www.gov.uk/

drug-device-alerts/shoulder-system-comprehensive-nano-humeral-components-increased-risk-of-revision-when-used-in-reverse-configuration). In revision settings there is rarely sufficient bone stock to allow the use of shorter-stem components [45] and traditional length stems will be required.

(d) Lesser tuberosity osteotomy. Subscapularis failure after anatomic shoulder arthroplasty has been a significant concern. Lesser tuberosity osteotomy has been proposed as a means to mitigate this problem, but compromise of metaphyseal fixation of shorter-stem devices with lesser tuberosity osteotomy has been raised as a concern [52]. Morwood [53] and others [52] in their reviews have shown reasonable outcomes with lesser tuberosity osteotomy with stemless designs, but clearly osteotomies involving a substantial part of the lesser tuberosity raise concerns for subsequent implant fixation.

14.9 Summary

While short-stem and stemless implants are being used with increasing frequency over traditional length stemmed implants, few of the theoretical advantages of these implants have been substantiated in the literature. Preservation of bone stock for subsequent revision remains the most widespread reason cited for the use of shorter-stem device, but data to support improved survivorship upon revision of shorter-stem devices is not currently available [8]. Level one evidence comparing these newer implants to traditional length stemmed implants is lacking, and these newer implants represent some distinct disadvantages over traditional length stemmed devices, including potential for implant malpositioning, problems with subscapularis reattachment, and precocious loosening if requirements for optimal proximal bone quality are not adhered to. These disadvantages and the increased cost of these implants should be born in mind when selecting the appropriate length of humeral stem in revision surgery.

References

1. Flatow EL, Harrison AK. A history of reverse total shoulder arthroplasty. Clin Orthop Relat Res. 2011;469(9):2432–9.
2. Neer CS 2nd, Brown TH, McLaughlin HL. Fracture of the neck of the humerus with dislocation of the head fragment. Am J Surg. 1953;85(3):252–8.
3. Neer CS 2nd, Watson KC, Stanton FJ. Recent experience in total shoulder replacement. J Bone Joint Surg Am. 1982;64(3):319–37.
4. Verborgt O, El-Abiad R, Gazielly DF. Long-term results of uncemented humeral components in shoulder arthroplasty. J Shoulder Elbow Surg. 2007;16(3 Suppl):S13–8.
5. Matsen FA 3rd, Iannotti JP, Rockwood CA Jr. Humeral fixation by press-fitting of a tapered metaphyseal stem: a prospective radiographic study. J Bone Joint Surg Am. 2003;85(2):304–8.
6. Cil A, et al. Survivorship of the humeral component in shoulder arthroplasty. J Shoulder Elbow Surg. 2010;19(1):143–50.
7. Paxton ES, Green A, Krueger VS. Periprosthetic infections of the shoulder: diagnosis and management. J Am Acad Orthop Surg. 2019;27(21):e935–44.
8. Erickson BJ, et al. Initial and 1-year radiographic comparison of reverse total shoulder arthroplasty with a short versus standard length stem. J Am Acad Orthop Surg. 2022;30:e968.
9. Copeland S. The continuing development of shoulder replacement: "reaching the surface". J Bone Joint Surg Am. 2006;88(4):900–5.
10. Soudy K, et al. Results and limitations of humeral head resurfacing: 105 cases at a mean follow-up of 5 years. Orthop Traumatol Surg Res. 2017;103(3):415–20.
11. Hawi N, et al. Anatomic stemless shoulder arthroplasty and related outcomes: a systematic review. BMC Musculoskelet Disord. 2016;17(1):376.
12. Ajibade DA, et al. Stemless reverse total shoulder arthroplasty: a systematic review. J Shoulder Elbow Surg. 2022;31(5):1083–95.
13. Churchill RS, et al. Clinical and radiographic outcomes of the Simpliciti canal-sparing shoulder arthroplasty system: a prospective two-year multicenter study. J Bone Joint Surg Am. 2016;98(7):552–60.
14. Erickson BJ, et al. Current state of short-stem implants in total shoulder arthroplasty: a systematic review of the literature. JSES Int. 2020;4(1):114–9.
15. Uschok S, et al. Is the stemless humeral head replacement clinically and radiographically a secure equivalent to standard stem humeral head replacement in the long-term follow-up? A prospective randomized trial. J Shoulder Elbow Surg. 2017;26(2):225–32.
16. Willems JIP, Hoffmann J, Sierevelt IN, Van den Bekerom MPJ, Alta TDW, van Noort A. Results of stemless shoulder arthroplasty: a systematic review and meta-analysis. EFORT Open Rev. 2021;6(1):35–49.

17. Sorokina Y, Spicer J. Will stemless implants dominate the shoulder arthroplasty market? In MedDevice Online.
18. Boileau P, et al. Shoulder arthroplasty for the treatment of the sequelae of fractures of the proximal humerus. J Shoulder Elbow Surg. 2001;10(4):299–308.
19. Holmes N, Virani S, Relwani J. Use of reverse stemless shoulder arthroplasty in a patient with multiple hereditary exostosis. J Clin Orthop Trauma. 2020;11(Suppl 5):S752–5.
20. Ballas R, Teissier P, Teissier J. Stemless shoulder prosthesis for treatment of proximal humeral malunion does not require tuberosity osteotomy. Int Orthop. 2016;40(7):1473–9.
21. Iannotti JP, et al. The normal glenohumeral relationships. An anatomical study of one hundred and forty shoulders. J Bone Joint Surg Am. 1992;74(4):491–500.
22. Pearl ML. Proximal humeral anatomy in shoulder arthroplasty: implications for prosthetic design and surgical technique. J Shoulder Elbow Surg. 2005;14(1 Suppl S):99s–104s.
23. Berth A, Pap G. Stemless shoulder prosthesis versus conventional anatomic shoulder prosthesis in patients with osteoarthritis: a comparison of the functional outcome after a minimum of two years follow-up. J Orthop Traumatol. 2013;14(1):31–7.
24. Tracy ST, et al. Revision to reverse total shoulder arthroplasty: do short stem and stemless implants reduce the operative burden compared to convertible stems? vol. 31. Semin Arthroplasty; 2021. p. 248.
25. Wieser K, et al. Conversion of stemmed hemi- or total to reverse total shoulder arthroplasty: advantages of a modular stem design. Clin Orthop Relat Res. 2015;473(2):651–60.
26. Razmjou H, et al. Impact of prosthetic design on clinical and radiologic outcomes of total shoulder arthroplasty: a prospective study. J Shoulder Elbow Surg. 2013;22:206.
27. Maier MW, et al. Are there differences between stemless and conventional stemmed shoulder prostheses in the treatment of glenohumeral osteoarthritis? BMC Musculoskelet Disord. 2015;16:275.
28. Spranz DM, et al. Functional midterm follow-up comparison of stemless total shoulder prostheses versus conventional stemmed anatomic shoulder prostheses using a 3D-motion-analysis. BMC Musculoskelet Disord. 2017;18(1):478.
29. Erickson BJ, et al. A 135° short inlay humeral stem leads to comparable radiographic and clinical outcomes compared to a standard-length stem for reverse shoulder arthroplasty, vol. 6. JSES Int; 2022. p. 802.
30. Boorman RS, et al. A conservative broaching and impaction grafting technique for humeral component placement and fixation in shoulder arthroplasty: the procrustean method. Tech Shoulder Elbow Surg. 2001;2:166–75.
31. Hacker SA, et al. Impaction grafting improves the fit of uncemented humeral arthroplasty. J Shoulder Elbow Surg. 2003;12(5):431–5.
32. Huguet D, et al. Results of a new stemless shoulder prosthesis: radiologic proof of maintained fixation and stability after a minimum of three years' follow-up. J Shoulder Elbow Surg. 2010;19(6):847–52.
33. Nagels J, Stokdijk M, Rozing PM. Stress shielding and bone resorption in shoulder arthroplasty. J Shoulder Elbow Surg. 2003;12(1):35–9.
34. Habermeyer P, et al. Midterm results of stemless shoulder arthroplasty: a prospective study. J Shoulder Elbow Surg. 2015;24(9):1463–72.
35. Giordano MC, et al. Comparative study of 145° onlay curved stem versus 155° inlay straight stem reverse shoulder arthroplasty: clinical and radiographic results with a minimum 2-year follow-up. J Shoulder Elbow Surg. 2022;31:2089.
36. Raiss P, et al. Radiographic changes around humeral components in shoulder arthroplasty. J Bone Joint Surg Am. 2014;96(7):e54.
37. Kostretzis L, et al. Stemless reverse total shoulder arthroplasty: a systematic review of contemporary literature. Musculoskelet Surg. 2021;105(3):209–24.
38. Abdic S, et al. Short stem humeral components in reverse shoulder arthroplasty: stem alignment influences the neck-shaft angle. Arch Orthop Trauma Surg. 2021;141(2):183–8.
39. Hawi N, et al. Nine-year outcome after anatomic stemless shoulder prosthesis: clinical and radiologic results. J Shoulder Elbow Surg. 2017;26:1609.
40. Casagrande DJ, et al. Radiographic evaluation of short-stem press-fit total shoulder arthroplasty: short-term follow-up. J Shoulder Elbow Surg. 2016;25(7):1163–9.
41. Cox RM, et al. Radiographic humeral head restoration after total shoulder arthroplasty: does the stem make a difference? J Shoulder Elbow Surg. 2021;30(1):51–6.
42. Kadum B, et al. Clinical and radiological outcome of the Total Evolutive Shoulder System (TESS(R)) reverse shoulder arthroplasty: a prospective comparative non-randomised study. Int Orthop. 2014;38(5):1001–6.
43. Grubhofer F, et al. Does computerized CT-based 3D planning of the humeral head cut help to restore the anatomy of the proximal humerus after stemless total shoulder arthroplasty? J Shoulder Elbow Surg. 2021;30(6):e309–16.
44. Geervliet PC, et al. Overstuffing in resurfacing hemiarthroplasty is a potential risk for failure. J Orthop Surg Res. 2019;14(1):474.
45. Lazarus MD, et al. Stemless prosthesis for total shoulder arthroplasty. J Am Acad Orthop Surg. 2017;25(12):e291–300.
46. Zmistowski B, et al. Symptomatic aseptic loosening of a short humeral stem following anatomic total shoulder arthroplasty. J Shoulder Elbow Surg. 2021;30:2738.
47. Morwood MP, Johnston PS, Garrigues GE. Proximal ingrowth coating decreases risk of loosening following uncemented shoulder arthroplasty using mini-stem humeral components and lesser tuberosity osteotomy. J Shoulder Elbow Surg. 2017;26(7):1246–52.

48. Liu EY, et al. Stemless reverse total shoulder arthroplasty: a systematic review of short- and mid-term results. Shoulder Elbow. 2021;13(5):482–91.
49. Tross AK, et al. Subsidence of uncemented short stems in reverse shoulder arthroplasty-a multicenter study. J Clin Med. 2020;9(10):3362.
50. Van de Kleut ML, et al. Are short press-fit stems comparable to standard length cemented stems in reverse shoulder arthroplasty? A prospective randomized clinical trial. J Shoulder Elbow Surg. 2021;31:580.
51. Australian Orthopaedic Association. Hip, knee and shoulder arthroplasty annual report. Australian Orthopaedic Association, National Joint Replacement Registry; 2016.
52. Aibinder WR, et al. Subscapularis management in stemless total shoulder arthroplasty: tenotomy versus peel versus lesser tuberosity osteotomy. J Shoulder Elbow Surg. 2019;28(10):1942–7.
53. Morwood MP, Johnston PS, Garrigues GE. Proximal ingrowth coating decreases risk of loosening following uncemented shoulder arthroplasty using mini-stem humeral components and lesser tuberosity osteotomy. J Shoulder Elbow Surg. 2017;26:1246.

Total Shoulder Arthroplasty in the Young, Athletic Patient

Alexander J. Johnson, Benjamin R. Wharton, and Eric C. McCarty

15.1 Introduction

Glenohumeral (GH) arthritis can be a debilitating, progressive disorder characterized by pain, stiffness, and loss of function. As pain and stiffness progress, it may become difficult or impossible for patients to continue recreational activities diminishing their quality of life [1–3]. Though more common in older populations, young, athletic patients may participate in activities or have medical comorbidities predisposing them to certain forms of early GH arthritis including post-traumatic arthritis after fracture or shoulder instability, avascular necrosis (AVN), post-arthroscopic or pain pump-related chondrolysis, and inflammatory joint disease [4–11]. Treatment in this age group is particularly challenging due to high baseline demands and less predictable outcomes with arthroplasty [12–14]. Exhausting nonoperative treatment modalities [15–19] is prudent, but arthroplasty remains a sensible option for surgeons and patients to consider when they can no longer easily complete activities of daily living (ADLs) or recreational activities [20–27]. As the indications for shoulder arthroplasty across different age groups con-tinue to evolve, it is essential for surgeons to develop a complete understanding of the current literature to optimize patient care in a challenging situation.

15.2 Types of Glenohumeral Arthritis in Young, Athletic Patients

Glenohumeral arthritis is most common in older patients, but it can occur at any age. There are multiple causes of GH arthritis that all may eventually require treatment with arthroplasty. Primary osteoarthritis (OA) is a common, though incompletely understood, cause of shoulder dysfunction that is diagnosed through a combination of clinical and radiographic findings [28]. Despite well-described X-ray changes, surgeons should understand that severity of symptoms may not correlate with severity of radiographic findings and patient-specific treatment is essential in young patients [5, 28–31]. Several studies have identified patient factors that do place them at elevated risk for early arthritis including body mass index (BMI), hypertension, highly demanding recurrent shoulder motion, genetics, occupation, and previous injury that may help explain the rare process in young patients [32, 33].

Shoulder instability, treated operatively or nonoperatively, is a significant risk factor for developing GH arthritis with reported incidence of 22.7% in patients with history of anterior insta-

A. J. Johnson · B. R. Wharton (✉) · E. C. McCarty
Department of Orthopedics, University of Colorado, Boulder, CO, USA
e-mail: alexander.johnson@sluhn.org;
benjamin.wharton@cuanschutz.edu;
eric.mccarty@cuanschutz.edu

© ISAKOS 2023
A. D. Mazzocca et al. (eds.), *Shoulder Arthritis across the Life Span*,
https://doi.org/10.1007/978-3-031-33298-2_15

bility [11, 34–36]. Older age at time of instability, recurrent instability, high-energy sports participation, and a history of alcohol abuse likely place patients at a higher risk [6]. Certain historic procedures have been linked to unacceptably high rates of early arthritis in a process that has been termed capsulorrhaphy arthropathy [5, 37–40]. The Latarjet procedure is another nonanatomic stabilizing procedure with high reported rates of arthritic changes in long-term follow-up. However, more recent reports have shown that most patients with arthritis after Latarjet procedure have mild disease and progression to moderate or severe disease is rare [41–45]. Surgeons who plan to perform arthroplasty procedures on patients who had previous shoulder stabilization surgery should plan for a technically demanding procedure, particularly in the presence of retained hardware or bony deformity [46].

Another possible destructive process disproportionately affecting the glenohumeral joint of young healthy patients is glenohumeral chondrolysis [5, 9, 47, 48]. Although rare, this disorder most commonly occurs after shoulder arthroscopy. Several possible causes have been investigated, but the best evidence suggests that use of post-arthroscopic, intra-articular infusion of local anesthetic is the most likely culprit. [49–53] Patients experiencing pain and dysfunction related to chondrolysis will most likely present with a history of previous arthroscopic surgery, and imaging studies will show diffuse degenerative changes and cartilage loss in the absence of osteophyte formation [5, 54].

Patients with rheumatoid arthritis (RA) commonly have shoulder involvement, often with debilitating symptoms [55]. The age at which patients present with advanced shoulder disease and undergo arthroplasty is variable across the literature, but it is clear that some patients in their fourth or fifth decade of life do undergo this procedure [56, 57]. Though disease-modifying agents have improved medical treatment of the disease, patients in this group often have extensive soft tissue involvement and may present with glenoid or humeral bone defects [5, 58]. Several studies have shown less favorable results with use of anatomic total shoulder arthroplasty (aTSA) implants, while a number of studies report improved short- and mid-term outcomes with rTSA implants. However, these results are heterogenous and several recent studies maintain that aTSA is an acceptable option in patients with RA [55, 56, 58–63]. Several authors have noted increased risk of glenoid bone defects in patient with RA, emphasizing the need for careful preoperative evaluation and planning [59].

AVN of the humeral head is another challenging pathologic process that may cause debilitating pain and loss of function in young, active patients. There are many possible root causes of the disorder [5, 64, 65]. Regardless of the cause, AVN is characterized by loss of blood flow to the humeral head leading to collapse of the articular surface leading to GH joint destruction with progressive pain and loss of function [66]. There are a number of joint-preserving surgical options that may be considered during the early stages of the disease highlighting the importance of early detection [67–69]. However, joint preservation is often not an option in advanced disease and arthroplasty may need to be considered. Literature regarding the optimal arthroplasty option in this population continues to evolve, but hemiarthroplasty, aTSA, and rTSA have a role in certain patients [70–73].

15.3 Non-arthroplasty Treatment Options

The primary treatment goals for young, athletic patients with glenohumeral arthritis are symptom relief and restoration of shoulder function and mobility. According to the 2008 study by McCarty et al. [74], the most common reason that young athletes pursued treatment was to attempt to return to their previous level of sporting activity. Though this goal is reasonable, the natural history of GH arthritis tells us that the disease is likely to progress and no treatment modality has proven to reliably alter this course [75, 76]. Understanding the progressive nature of the disease emphasizes the need to appropriately counsel patients and manage expectations throughout the treatment process. Due to inferior outcomes with arthroplasty in young patients, surgeons should strive to exhaust all evidence-based nonoperative and joint-preserving measures prior to consideration of arthroplasty. Further nonarthroplasty options are discussed in the other chapters in this text.

15.4 Glenohumeral Arthroplasty

Patients who have persistent pain and dysfunction limiting their ability to maintain an active lifestyle despite extensive attempts at nonoperative treatment may be indicated for shoulder arthroplasty. Several arthroplasty options are available, and thorough understanding of the risks, benefits, and expected outcomes of each procedure in this patient population is essential for surgeons. Every attempt should be made to appropriately educate patients during the counseling process, thereby empowering them to participate in shared decision-making. Over the last decade, there has been a large shift in the utilization of and indications for hemiarthroplasty, aTSA, and rTSA, particularly in young patients [77–80]. Indications may continue to evolve as implant innovations and additional data emerge, but each of these procedures may be appropriately indicated in young, athletic patients. A summary of key outcome studies can be found in Table 15.1.

Table 15.1 Summary of key arthroplasty outcomes in young, athletic patients

Arthroplasty outcomes in young, athletic patients					
	N	Avg. age	Age range	Avg. follow-up	Key findings
Hemiarthroplasty					
Bartelt et al. [81]	66	49	21–55	7.0 years	Pain score, ROM, and implant survival favor aTSA over hemiarthroplasty in patients <55 years
Garcia et al. [82]	80	66	42.7–87.7	5.13 years	aTSA leads to higher rates of return to sport, less pain, higher satisfaction compared to hemiarthroplasty
aTSA					
Roberson et al. [80]	154	45.6	16–64	9.17 years	aTSA in patients <65 leads to low revision rates and high implant survivorship despite high rates of periprosthetic lucency. PROs show significant increases from baseline but remain inferior to overall aTSA population
Brochin et al. [83]	34	54.4	35.5–59.8	16.1 years	aTSA significantly increased active motion, pain scores, SST, and ASES scores. There was aseptic glenoid loosening rate of 17.6, and implant survival rate of 97.1% at 10 years, 85.4% at 15 years, and 80.1% at 20 years
rTSA					
Chelli et al. [84]	417	56	21–65	4.17 years	rTSA for rotator cuff deficiency or failed arthroplasty in patients <65 years lead to improvements in function and ASES score. Complication rate (17%) and revision rate (7%) are comparable to older patient cohorts
Monir et al. [85]	52	58	53–63	6.3 years	rTSA in patients <65 years lead to improvements in active motion, SST, Constant score, ASES score, UCLA score, and pain scores above MCID. Complication rate was 7.7% and revision rate was 5.8%
Goldenberg et al. [86]	286	58.4	48.9–60.4	4.7 years	rTSA in patients <65 lead to significant improvements in active motion and all reported PROs with 18.6% complication rate and implant survival of 99% at 2 years, 91–98% at 5 years, and 88% at 10 years
Vancolen et al. [87]	245	57	39–65	4.17 years	rTSA resulted in improvements in motion, pain, and all reported outcomes measures with an 18% pooled complication rate in patients <65 years
Hanisch et al. [88]	566	67.8	Not specified	7.75 years	rTSA resulted in statistically significant difference in WOOS when comparing patients <65 and >65, but this was not clinically relevant. There was no increased risk of complication or revision in younger patients

Before undergoing a more nuanced discussion of arthroplasty options in this population, it is important to understand that evidence indicates that younger patients do have improved pain and function after shoulder arthroplasty, but they also tend to be less satisfied than older patients after the same surgeries [89]. This is a key point to consider when counseling patients and indicating them for surgery. The Patient Acceptable Symptom State (PASS) score was recently developed to define when patients feel well after surgery, as opposed to simply better. One study of 301 patients undergoing aTSA showed that patients who failed to achieve the PASS threshold were younger and persistent pain was the most common reason for failure to reach the threshold [12]. Other studies have shown similar low patient satisfaction despite improvements in pain and function from baseline after arthroplasty. In a systematic review from 2017, revision rates were low, implant survivorship was high, and patient-reported outcomes (PROs) improved from baseline but were significantly lower than those of the overall TSA population [80]. Not only can this understanding help guide counseling discussions with patients, but it again highlights the difficult nature of this pathology and the importance of exhausting non-arthroplasty options prior to proceeding with definitive surgery. Many patients may benefit from the understanding that they can expect improvements in pain and function but that they should not expect to have a normal shoulder after shoulder arthroplasty.

15.4.1 Total Shoulder Arthroplasty Vs. Hemiarthroplasty

Historically, concerns over glenoid component loosening, as well as desire to maintain normal anatomy, have led to frequent utilization of hemiarthroplasty implants in young, athletic patients [90]. As new literature provides insight into the mostly inferior outcomes of hemiarthroplasty when compared to aTSA, hemiarthroplasty is becoming less common [91]. Nonetheless, hemiarthroplasty has been shown to provide improvements in pain and function in long-term studies and is still commonly performed in this demographic [90, 92].

Bartelt et al. [81] demonstrated improved pain relief, range of motion, and implant survival with TSA when compared to hemiarthroplasty in patients younger than 55 years old [93]. A meta-analysis by Bryant et al. [94] and a multicenter study by Edwards et al. [95] confirmed superiority of aTSA in nearly all outcome measures. Another study showed that rate of return to sports was significantly better after aTSA, while hemiarthroplasty patients had significantly more pain with less satisfaction [82]. Studies focusing on AVN show similarly favorable outcomes of hemiarthroplasty and aTSA, but it is less clear which implant provides superior outcomes [65, 67, 96].

From a financial standpoint, aTSA is the more cost-effective treatment with the greatest utility to the patient at a lower overall cost to the payer [97, 98]. Finally, another systematic review comparing individuals who underwent either aTSA or hemiarthroplasty for glenohumeral arthritis at the 2-year follow-up demonstrated far better pain scores and forward elevation improvements in TSA [94].

15.4.2 Anatomic Total Shoulder Arthroplasty

Though recent literature supports the use of aTSA in young patients with appropriate indications, there are additional considerations specific to this population that are important to understand. Roberson et al. conducted a systematic review in 2017 including six studies [47, 57, 81, 99–101] evaluating the outcomes of aTSA in patients under the age of 65. The overall complication rate in these studies was 9.4%. Results showed that 54% of patients developed some degree of glenoid lucency, but the revision rate was 17.4% at an average of 9.4 years. The PROs did improve significantly from baseline but were inferior to those in the overall aTSA population. Another study reported outcomes of aTSA in patients with an average age of 54 and average follow-up of 16 years [83]. Range of motion, pain scores, and patient-reported outcomes were all significantly improved from preoperative values. 17.6% of cases were complicated by aseptic glenoid loosening, but implant survival was 80.1% at 20 years.

As surgeons seek ways to improve outcomes in younger patients undergoing aTSA, the glenoid has often been the focus of ongoing attempts at innovation. The most common reason for failure in aTSA is failure of the glenoid component [102, 103]. This is often attributed to the "rocking horse" phenomenon in which repetitive edge loading of the glenoid component causes wear and loosening over time [104]. To combat this mechanism of failure, inlay glenoid components have become increasingly employed after mechanical testing supported its utilization [105, 106]. Subsequent clinical studies show acceptable outcomes with these implants at early follow-up. In 1 study of 27 patients with an average age of 52.1 and minimum of 2-year follow-up, the use of an inlay glenoid component leads to improved outcomes, high rate of return to activity, no reoperations, and no evidence of glenoid loosening [102]. Several other studies have reported similar positive results. [102, 107, 108] Longer-term outcome studies with comparison to traditional glenoid components are necessary, but early results indicate that inlay glenoid components are worthy of additional study and may be an attractive option for young, active patients in the future.

As one example of a young, athletic patient who had successful outcome after aTSA, Fig. 15.1 shows the pre- and postoperative imaging of a 41-year-old male weight lifter and CrossFit enthusiast presenting with left shoulder pain and limited function. After several years of nonoperative treatment with NSAIDs, injections, and physical therapy, he opted to proceed with aTSA. Preoperatively he rated his pain as 8/10 and his Single Assessment Numeric Evaluation (SANE) score was 30. Postoperatively he returned to lighter weight lifting, but never felt compelled to return CrossFit. At 18-month follow-up, he reported daily average pain of 0/10 with worst episodes of 2/10, a SANE score of 95, and excellent satisfaction with the procedure.

15.4.3 Reverse Total Shoulder Arthroplasty

Initially designed for the treatment of rotator cuff arthropathy, indications for rTSA over the last decade have expanded substantially to include massive, irreparable rotator cuff tears, OA with excessive posterior glenoid wear, glenoid bone loss, and revision after failed aTSA [24, 109–113]. Despite excellent outcomes in older patients, surgeons have remained hesitant to perform the procedure in younger, athletic patients due to concerns over implant longevity and outcomes in high-demand individuals [89, 93, 114–117]. This concern is not without merit and the topic of rTSA in young patient remains controversial.

Discussing the prolonged recovery course and limitations may help manage postoperative expectations. Specifically, patients who underwent rTSA were less likely to exhibit a substantial clinical benefit and less likely to exceed the PASS threshold compared to aTSA [118]. In terms of function deficits after rTSA, internal rotation is less likely to return to an acceptable level after surgery [119]. Another recent study showed that young age was not correlated with worse outcomes after rTSA, but higher function prior to surgery did lead to significantly lower satisfaction [13].

Although the data on rTSA in young, athletic patients is lacking, there are several recent systematic reviews showing that relatively younger patients can have acceptable outcomes. One study showed the complication, reoperation, and revision rates were 17%, 12%, and 7%, respectively, in a group of patients under 65 [84]. Similar results were reported by Monir et al. in 2019 [85]. Millet and colleagues completed a systematic review of patients under the age of 65 undergoing rTSA with an average follow-up of 4.7 years showing similar outcomes, complications, reoperations, and revision compared to older populations [86]. Similar results were reported in studies by Vancolen et al. [87] and by Hanisch et al [88].

Until additional data emerges regarding rTSA in young, athletic patients, the option should only

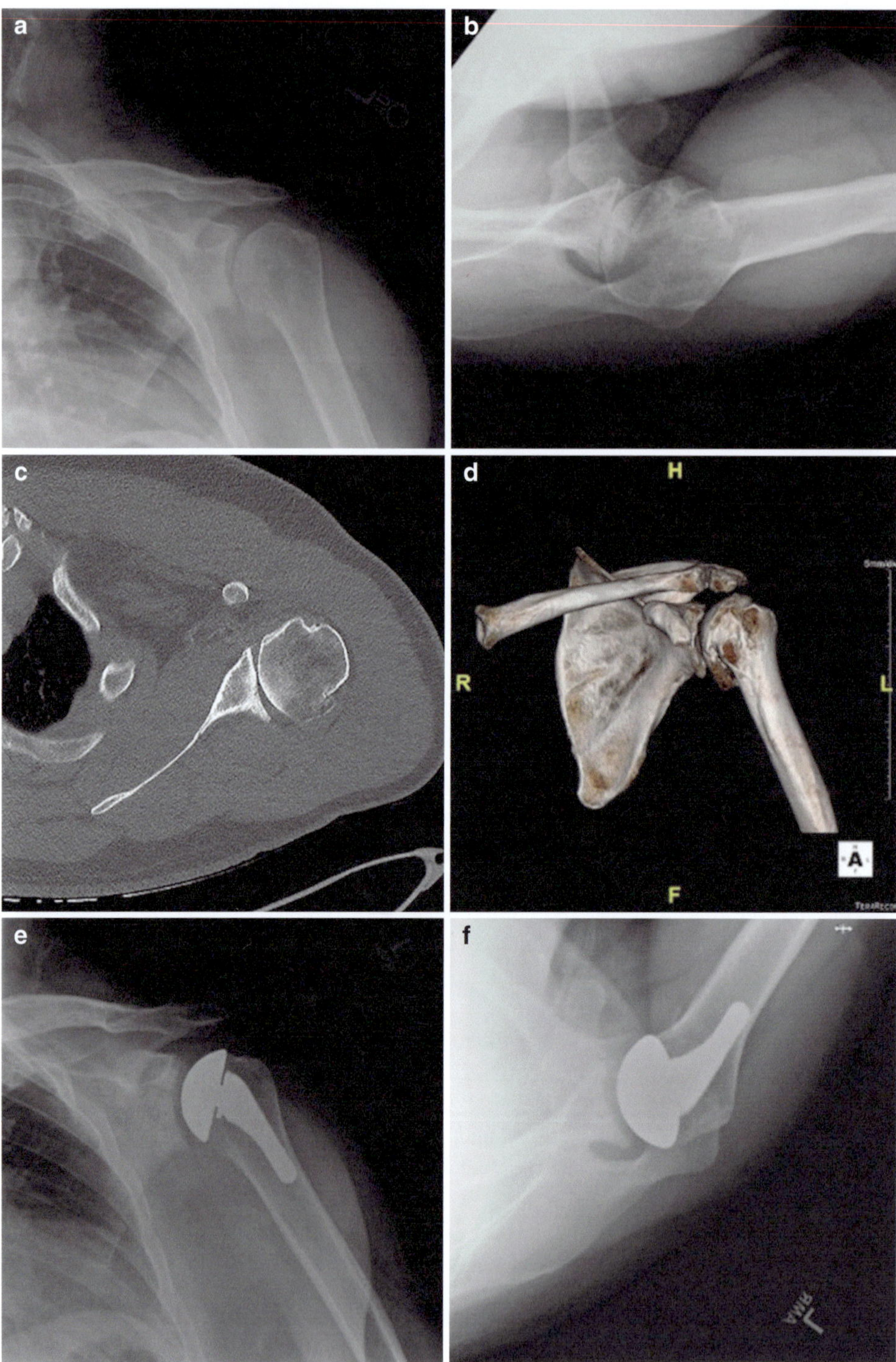

Fig. 15.1 Anatomic total shoulder arthroplasty (aTSA) in a young, athletic patient. Preoperative images of a 41-year-old male weight lifter including (**a**) Grashey view, (**b**) axillary view, (**c**) computed tomography axial view, and (**d**) preoperative 3-D reconstruction demonstrating advanced glenohumeral osteoarthritis with a Walch B2 glenoid but without excessive glenoid retroversion, bone loss, or posterior subluxation of the humeral head. The patient underwent anatomic total shoulder arthroplasty demonstrated by postoperative (**e**) Grashey and (**f**) axillary views

be considered in these patients when specific contraindications to aTSA exist and only after extensive counseling [114].

15.5 Postoperative Rehabilitation

Literature focusing on physical therapy and rehabilitation protocols following shoulder arthroplasty is surprisingly limited, let alone in younger populations. Patients have been shown to have positive perceptions of their experience with physical therapy after shoulder surgery in general [120]. However, the current body of evidence is insufficient to provide a definitive recommendation for physical therapy after shoulder arthroplasty [121, 122]. Interestingly, there is data available in the hip arthroplasty literature showing that patients do not see significant benefit from formal physical therapy after total hip arthroplasty [123]. Nevertheless, there are available guidelines and publications that provide recommendations for physical therapy after shoulder arthroplasty [121, 124–127]. Despite the lack of definitive evidence in this area, the senior author does routinely prescribe formal physical therapy to patients after shoulder arthroplasty to assist in gaining motion and strength.

15.6 Return to Sport Following Arthroplasty

Evidence regarding return to sport after shoulder arthroplasty continues to grow but remains limited for most athletic activities, especially in young patients. Patient-specific goals must be understood and discussed to provide realistic expectations and timeline for returning to activity. Regardless of what they hope to get back to, it is important that the reintegration process occurs gradually through appropriate return to play progression. Though many studies have defined high rates of return to sport after shoulder arthroplasty, the age of patients in the studies is heterogenous, rarely focusing on young patients [128, 129]. Unsurprisingly, several studies have shown patients of all ages are less likely to return to high-demand sports. [74, 130–134] Results of one study did show that patients of all ages participating in sports involving the upper extremities had similar function with less evidence of radiolucency at 5 years [103].

Another study did specifically examine return to sport after aTSA in patients 55 and younger [135]. Results showed 96.4% of patients returned to sports at an average of 6.7 months without any patients requiring glenoid revision at an average of 61 months. Interestingly, 83.8% of patients returned to upper extremity sports. Longer-term, larger studies are required, but these early results are promising.

15.7 Conclusion

Young, athletic patients with GH arthritis continue to be a challenge for orthopedic surgeons to treat. Certain patient characteristics may place these patients at higher risk of GH arthritis. The progressive nature of this disorder often leads to pain and unacceptable loss of function causing patients to seek treatment. There are many nonoperative options in these situations that are unlikely to alter progression of disease but may allow patients to delay shoulder arthroplasty procedures. Patients who are unable to continue functioning at a high level, and who have maximized relief with nonoperative options, can expect reliable improvement in pain and function with shoulder arthroplasty. More active patients are at risk for lower overall satisfaction after these procedures, but appropriate indications and extensive counseling prior to surgery may help improve outcomes. Over the last decade, aTSA has proven to be superior to hemiarthroplasty in terms of outcomes and revision rates, even in young patients. When there are specific contraindications to aTSA, rTSA has been shown to have acceptable outcomes in young patients despite early concerns for loss of function and poor implant survival. Implant innovation and additional research with longer follow-up focusing on young, athletic patients will allow surgeons to continue to solidify indications and improve outcomes in the future.

References

1. Matsen FA III, Ziegler DW, DeBartolo SE. Patient self-assessment of health status and function in glenohumeral degenerative joint disease. J Shoulder Elbow Surg. 1995;4:345–51.
2. Saltzman BM, Leroux TS, Verma NN, Romeo AA. Glenohumeral osteoarthritis in the young patient. J Am Acad Orthop Surg. 2018;26(17):e361–70.
3. Khazzam M, Gee AO, Pearl M. Management of glenohumeral joint osteoarthritis. J Am Acad Orthop Surg. 2020;28(19):781–9.
4. Laidlaw MS, Mahon HS, Werner BC. Etiology of shoulder arthritis in young patients. Clin Sports Med. 2018;37(4):505–15.
5. Brunelli J, Bravman JT, Caperton K, McCarty EC. Glenohumeral arthritis in the athlete. In: Miller MD, Thompson SR, editors. DeLee, Drez, and Miller's orthopaedic sports medicine principles and practice. Philadelphia: Elsevier; 2020.
6. Hovelius L, Saeboe M. Neer Award 2008: arthropathy after primary anterior shoulder dislocation—223 shoulders prospectively followed up for twenty-five years. J Shoulder Elbow Surg. 2009;18(3):339–47.
7. McNickle AG, L'Heureux DR, Provencher MT, Romeo AA, Cole BJ. Postsurgical glenohumeral arthritis in young adults. Am J Sports Med. 2009;37(9):1784–91.
8. Carbone A, Rodeo S. Review of current understanding of post-traumatic osteoarthritis resulting from sports injuries. J Orthop Res. 2017;35(3):397–405.
9. Hansen BP, Beck CL, Beck EP, Townsley RW. Postarthroscopic glenohumeral chondrolysis. Am J Sports Med. 2007;35(10):1628–34.
10. Herve A, Chelli M, Boileau P, et al. Clinical and radiological results of hemiarthroplasty and Total shoulder arthroplasty for primary avascular necrosis of the humeral head in patients less than 60 years old. J Clin Med. 2021;10(14):3081.
11. Coifman I, Brunner UH, Scheibel M. Dislocation arthropathy of the shoulder. J Clin Med. 2022;11(7):2019.
12. Cole EW, Moulton SG, Werner BC, Denard PJ. Why patients fail to achieve a patient acceptable symptom state (PASS) after total shoulder arthroplasty? JSES Int. 2022;6(1):49–55.
13. Rauck RC, Ruzbarsky JJ, Swarup I, et al. Predictors of patient satisfaction after reverse shoulder arthroplasty. J Shoulder Elbow Surg. 2020;29(3):e67–74.
14. Henn RF 3rd, Ghomrawi H, Rutledge JR, Mazumdar M, Mancuso CA, Marx RG. Preoperative patient expectations of total shoulder arthroplasty. J Bone Joint Surg Am. 2011;93(22):2110–5.
15. Millett PJ, Fritz EM, Frangiamore SJ, Mannava S. Arthroscopic management of glenohumeral arthritis: a joint preservation approach. J Am Acad Orthop Surg. 2018;26(21):745–52.
16. Takamura KM, Chen JB, Petrigliano FA. Nonarthroplasty options for the athlete or active individual with shoulder osteoarthritis. Clin Sports Med. 2018;37(4):517–26.
17. Metzger CM, Farooq H, Merrell GA, et al. Efficacy of a single, image-guided corticosteroid injection for glenohumeral arthritis. J Shoulder Elbow Surg. 2021;30(5):1128–34.
18. Zhang B, Thayaparan A, Horner N, Bedi A, Alolabi B, Khan M. Outcomes of hyaluronic acid injections for glenohumeral osteoarthritis: a systematic review and meta-analysis. J Shoulder Elbow Surg. 2019;28(3):596–606.
19. Rossi LA, Piuzzi NS, Shapiro SA. Glenohumeral osteoarthritis: the role for orthobiologic therapies: platelet-rich plasma and cell therapies. JBJS Rev. 2020;8(2):e0075.
20. Lugli T. Artificial shoulder joint by Péan (1893): the facts of an exceptional intervention and the prosthetic method. Clin Orthop Relat Res. 1978(133):215–218.
21. Baulot E, Sirveaux F, Boileau P. Grammont's idea: the story of Paul Grammont's functional surgery concept and the development of the reverse principle. Clin Orthop Relat Res. 2011;469(9):2425–31.
22. Boileau P, Watkinson DJ, Hatzidakis AM, Balg F. Grammont reverse prosthesis: design, rationale, and biomechanics. J Shoulder Elbow Surg. 2005;14(1 Suppl S):147s–61s.
23. Berliner JL, Regalado-Magdos A, Ma CB, Feeley BT. Biomechanics of reverse total shoulder arthroplasty. J Shoulder Elbow Surg. 2015;24(1):150–60.
24. Frank JK, Siegert P, Plachel F, Heuberer PR, Huber S, Schanda JE. The evolution of reverse total shoulder arthroplasty-from the first steps to novel implant designs and surgical techniques. J Clin Med. 2022;11(6):1512.
25. Zilber S. Shoulder arthroplasty: historical considerations. Open Orthop J. 2017;11:1100–7.
26. Zhang B, Chen G, Fan T, Chen Z. Resurfacing hemiarthroplasty versus stemmed hemiarthroplasty for glenohumeral osteoarthritis: a meta-analysis. Arthroplasty. 2020;2(1):25.
27. Goetti P, Denard PJ, Collin P, Ibrahim M, Mazzolari A, Lädermann A. Biomechanics of anatomic and reverse shoulder arthroplasty. EFORT Open Rev. 2021;6(10):918–31.
28. Jawa A, Shields MV. The evolution of the Walch classification for primary glenohumeral arthritis. J Am Acad Orthop Surg. 2021;29(13):e635–45.
29. Joyce CD, Gutman MJ, Hill BW, et al. Radiographic severity may not be associated with pain and function in glenohumeral arthritis. Clin Orthop Relat Res. 2022;480(2):354–63.
30. Vezeridis PS, Ishmael CR, Jones KJ, Petrigliano FA. Glenohumeral dislocation arthropathy: etiology, diagnosis, and management. J Am Acad Orthop Surg. 2019;27(7):227–35.
31. Neer CS 2nd. Replacement arthroplasty for glenohumeral osteoarthritis. J Bone Joint Surg Am. 1974;56(1):1–13.

32. Plachel F, Akgun D, Imiolczyk JP, Minkus M, Moroder P. Patient-specific risk profile associated with early-onset primary osteoarthritis of the shoulder: is it really primary? Arch Orthop Trauma Surg. 2021;143:699.
33. Ibounig T, Simons T, Launonen A, Paavola M. Glenohumeral osteoarthritis: an overview of etiology and diagnostics. Scand J Surg. 2021;110(3):441–51.
34. Ogawa K, Yoshida A, Ikegami H. Osteoarthritis in shoulders with traumatic anterior instability: preoperative survey using radiography and computed tomography. J Shoulder Elbow Surg. 2006;15(1):23–9.
35. Buscayret F, Edwards TB, Szabo I, Adeleine P, Coudane H, Walch G. Glenohumeral arthrosis in anterior instability before and after surgical treatment: incidence and contributing factors. Am J Sports Med. 2004;32(5):1165–72.
36. Carpinteiro EP, Barros AA. Natural history of anterior shoulder instability. Open Orthop J. 2017;11:909–18.
37. Kiss J, Mersich I, Perlaky GY, Szollas L. The results of the Putti-Platt operation with particular reference to arthritis, pain, and limitation of external rotation. J Shoulder Elbow Surg. 1998;7(5):495–500.
38. Konig DP, Rutt J, Treml O, Kausch T, Hackenbroch MH. Osteoarthrosis following the Putti-Platt operation. Arch Orthop Trauma Surg. 1996;115(3–4):231–2.
39. van der Zwaag HM, Brand R, Obermann WR, Rozing PM. Glenohumeral osteoarthrosis after Putti-Platt repair. J Shoulder Elbow Surg. 1999;8(3):252–8.
40. Magnuson PB, Stack JK. Recurrent dislocation of the shoulder. 1943. Clin Orthop Relat Res. 1991;269:4–8.
41. Kee YM, Kim HJ, Kim JY, Rhee YG. Glenohumeral arthritis after Latarjet procedure: progression and it's clinical significance. J Orthop Sci. 2017;22(5):846–51.
42. Rollick NC, Ono Y, Kurji HM, et al. Long-term outcomes of the Bankart and Latarjet repairs: a systematic review. Open Access J Sports Med. 2017;8:97–105.
43. Mizuno N, Denard PJ, Raiss P, Melis B, Walch G. Long-term results of the Latarjet procedure for anterior instability of the shoulder. J Shoulder Elbow Surg. 2014;23(11):1691–9.
44. Menon A, Fossati C, Magnani M, Boveri S, Compagnoni R, Randelli PS. Low grade of osteoarthritis development after Latarjet procedure with a minimum 5 years of follow-up: a systematic review and pooled analysis. Knee Surg Sports Traumatol Arthrosc. 2022;30(6):2074–83.
45. Gilat R, Lavoie-Gagne O, Haunschild ED, et al. Outcomes of the Latarjet procedure with minimum 5- and 10-year follow-up: a systematic review. Shoulder Elbow. 2020;12(5):315–29.
46. Willemot LB, Elhassan BT, Sperling JW, Cofield RH, Sanchez-Sotelo J. Arthroplasty for glenohumeral arthritis in shoulders with a previous Bristow or Latarjet procedure. J Shoulder Elbow Surg. 2018;27(9):1607–13.
47. Levy JC, Virani NA, Frankle MA, Cuff D, Pupello DR, Hamelin JA. Young patients with shoulder chondrolysis following arthroscopic shoulder surgery treated with total shoulder arthroplasty. J Shoulder Elbow Surg. 2008;17(3):380–8.
48. Petty DH, Jazrawi LM, Estrada LS, Andrews JR. Glenohumeral chondrolysis after shoulder arthroscopy: case reports and review of the literature. Am J Sports Med. 2004;32(2):509–15.
49. Athwal GS, Shridharani SM, O'Driscoll SW. Osteolysis and arthropathy of the shoulder after use of bioabsorbable knotless suture anchors: a report of four cases. J Bone Joint Surg Am. 2006;88-A(8):1840–5.
50. Baumgarten KM, Helsper E. Does chondrolysis occur after corticosteroid-analgesic injections? An analysis of patients treated for adhesive capsulitis of the shoulder. J Shoulder Elbow Surg. 2016;25(6):890–7.
51. Anderson SL, Buchko JZ, Taillon MR, Ernst MA. Chondrolysis of the glenohumeral joint after infusion of bupivacaine through an intra-articular pain pump catheter: a report of 18 cases. Arthroscopy. 2010;26(4):451–61.
52. Wiater BP, Neradilek MB, Polissar NL, Matsen FA 3rd. Risk factors for chondrolysis of the glenohumeral joint: a study of three hundred and seventy-five shoulder arthroscopic procedures in the practice of an individual community surgeon. J Bone Joint Surg Am. 2011;93(7):615–25.
53. Levine WN. Commentary on an article by Brett P. Wiater, MD, et al.: "Risk factors for chondrolysis of the glenohumeral joint. A study of three hundred and seventy-five shoulder arthroscopic procedures in the practice of an individual community surgeon". J Bone Joint Surg Am. 2011;93(7):e32.
54. Scheffel PT, Clinton J, Lynch JR, Warme WJ, Bertelsen AL, Matsen FA 3rd. Glenohumeral chondrolysis: a systematic review of 100 cases from the English language literature. J Shoulder Elbow Surg. 2010;19(6):944–9.
55. Haleem A, Shanmugaraj A, Horner NS, Leroux T, Khan M, Alolabi B. Anatomic total shoulder arthroplasty in rheumatoid arthritis: a systematic review. Shoulder Elbow. 2022;14(2):142–9.
56. Barlow JD, Yuan BJ, Schleck CD, Harmsen WS, Cofield RH, Sperling JW. Shoulder arthroplasty for rheumatoid arthritis: 303 consecutive cases with minimum 5-year follow-up. J Shoulder Elbow Surg. 2014;23(6):791–9.
57. Burroughs PL, Gearen PF, Petty WR, Wright TW. Shoulder arthroplasty in the young patient. J Arthroplasty. 2003;18(6):792–8.
58. Levigne C, Chelli M, Johnston TR, et al. Reverse shoulder arthroplasty in rheumatoid arthritis: survival and outcomes. J Shoulder Elbow Surg. 2021;30(10):2312–24.

59. He Y, Xiao LB, Zhai WT, Xu YL. Reverse shoulder arthroplasty in patients with rheumatoid arthritis: early outcomes, pitfalls, and challenges. Orthop Surg. 2020;12(5):1380–7.

60. Mangold DR, Wagner ER, Cofield RH, Sanchez-Sotelo J, Sperling JW. Reverse shoulder arthroplasty for rheumatoid arthritis since the introduction of disease-modifying drugs. Int Orthop. 2019;43(11):2593–600.

61. Cho CH, Kim DH, Song KS. Reverse shoulder arthroplasty in patients with rheumatoid arthritis: a systematic review. Clin Orthop Surg. 2017;9(3):325–31.

62. Christie A, Dagfinrud H, Ringen HO, Hagen KB. Beneficial and harmful effects of shoulder arthroplasty in patients with rheumatoid arthritis: results from a Cochrane review. Rheumatology (Oxford). 2011;50(3):598–602.

63. Jordan RW, Manoharan G, Van Liefland M, et al. Reliability of stemless shoulder arthroplasty in rheumatoid arthritis: observation of early lysis around the humeral component. Musculoskelet Surg. 2021;105(2):139–48.

64. Wang KC, Kantrowitz DE, Patel AV, Parsons BO, Flatow EL, Cagle PJ. Survivorship of total shoulder arthroplasty versus hemiarthroplasty for the treatment of avascular necrosis at greater than 10-year follow-up. J Shoulder Elbow Surg. 2022;31:1782.

65. Schoch BS, Barlow JD, Schleck C, Cofield RH, Sperling JW. Shoulder arthroplasty for post-traumatic osteonecrosis of the humeral head. J Shoulder Elbow Surg. 2016;25(3):406–12.

66. Keough N, Lorke DE. The humeral head: a review of the blood supply and possible link to osteonecrosis following rotator cuff repair. J Anat. 2021;239(5):973–82.

67. Franceschi F, Franceschetti E, Paciotti M, et al. Surgical management of osteonecrosis of the humeral head: a systematic review. Knee Surg Sports Traumatol Arthrosc. 2017;25(10):3270–8.

68. Alkhateeb JM, Arafah MA, Tashkandi M, Al Qahtani SM. Surgical treatment of humeral head avascular necrosis in patients with sickle cell disease: a systematic review. JSES Int. 2021;5(3):391–7.

69. Kennon JC, Smith JP, Crosby LA. Core decompression and arthroplasty outcomes for atraumatic osteonecrosis of the humeral head. J Shoulder Elbow Surg. 2016;25(9):1442–8.

70. Tauber M, Karpik S, Matis N, Schwartz M, Resch H. Shoulder arthroplasty for traumatic avascular necrosis: predictors of outcome. Clin Orthop Relat Res. 2007;465:208–14.

71. Ristow JJ, Ellison CM, Mickschl DJ, et al. Outcomes of shoulder replacement in humeral head avascular necrosis. J Shoulder Elbow Surg. 2019;28(1):9–14.

72. Feeley BT, Fealy S, Dines DM, Warren RF, Craig EV. Hemiarthroplasty and total shoulder arthroplasty for avascular necrosis of the humeral head. J Shoulder Elbow Surg. 2008;17(5):689–94.

73. McLaughlin R, Tams C, Werthel JD, et al. Reverse shoulder arthroplasty yields similar results to anatomic total shoulder arthroplasty for the treatment of humeral head avascular necrosis. J Shoulder Elbow Surg. 2022;31(6S):S94–S102.

74. McCarty EC, Marx RG, Maerz D, Altchek D, Warren RF. Sports participation after shoulder replacement surgery. Am J Sports Med. 2008;36(8):1577–81.

75. Logli AL, Pareek A, Nguyen NTV, Sanchez-Sotelo J. Natural history of glenoid bone loss in primary glenohumeral osteoarthritis: how does bone loss progress over a decade? J Shoulder Elbow Surg. 2021;30(2):324–30.

76. Walker KE, Simcock XC, Jun BJ, Iannotti JP, Ricchetti ET. Progression of glenoid morphology in glenohumeral osteoarthritis. J Bone Joint Surg Am. 2018;100(1):49–56.

77. Kim SH, Wise BL, Zhang Y, Szabo RM. Increasing incidence of shoulder arthroplasty in the United States. J Bone Joint Surg Am. 2011;93(24):2249–54.

78. Brolin TJ, Thakar OV, Abboud JA. Outcomes after shoulder replacement surgery in the young patient: how do they do and how long can we expect them to last? Clin Sports Med. 2018;37(4):593–607.

79. Bixby EC, Boddapati V, Anderson MJJ, Mueller JD, Jobin CM, Levine WN. Trends in total shoulder arthroplasty from 2005 to 2018: lower complications rates and shorter lengths of stay despite patients with more comorbidities. JSES Int. 2020;4(3):657–61.

80. Roberson TA, Bentley JC, Griscom JT, et al. Outcomes of total shoulder arthroplasty in patients younger than 65 years: a systematic review. J Shoulder Elbow Surg. 2017;26(7):1298–306.

81. Bartelt R, Sperling JW, Schleck CD, Cofield RH. Shoulder arthroplasty in patients aged fifty-five years or younger with osteoarthritis. J Shoulder Elbow Surg. 2011;20(1):123–30.

82. Garcia GH, Liu JN, Mahony GT, et al. Hemiarthroplasty versus total shoulder arthroplasty for shoulder osteoarthritis: a matched comparison of return to sports. Am J Sports Med. 2016;44(6):1417–22.

83. Brochin RL, Zastrow RK, Patel AV, et al. Long-term clinical and radiographic outcomes of total shoulder arthroplasty in patients under age 60 years. J Shoulder Elbow Surg. 2022;31(6S):S63–70.

84. Chelli M, Lo Cunsolo L, Gauci MO, et al. Reverse shoulder arthroplasty in patients aged 65 years or younger: a systematic review of the literature. JSES Open Access. 2019;3(3):162–7.

85. Monir JG, Abeyewardene D, King JJ, Wright TW, Schoch BS. Reverse shoulder arthroplasty in patients younger than 65 years, minimum 5-year follow-up. J Shoulder Elbow Surg. 2020;29(6):e215–21.

86. Goldenberg BT, Samuelsen BT, Spratt JD, Dornan GJ, Millett PJ. Complications and implant survivorship following primary reverse total shoulder arthroplasty in patients younger than 65 years: a systematic review. J Shoulder Elbow Surg. 2020;29(8):1703–11.

87. Vancolen SY, Elsawi R, Horner NS, Leroux T, Alolabi B, Khan M. Reverse total shoulder arthroplasty in the younger patient (</=65 years): a systematic review. J Shoulder Elbow Surg. 2020;29(1):202–9.

88. Hanisch K, Holte MB, Hvass I, Wedderkopp N. Clinically relevant results of reverse total shoulder arthroplasty for patients younger than 65 years compared to the older patients. Arthroplasty. 2021;3(1):30.

89. Muh SJ, Streit JJ, Wanner JP, et al. Early follow-up of reverse total shoulder arthroplasty in patients sixty years of age or younger. J Bone Joint Surg Am. 2013;95(20):1877–83.

90. Christensen J, Brockmeier S. Total shoulder arthroplasty in the athlete and active individual. Clin Sports Med. 2018;37(4):549–58.

91. Best MJ, Aziz KT, Wilckens JH, McFarland EG, Srikumaran U. Increasing incidence of primary reverse and anatomic total shoulder arthroplasty in the United States. J Shoulder Elbow Surg. 2021;30(5):1159–66.

92. Sperling JW, Cofield RH, Rowland CM. Neer hemiarthroplasty and Neer total shoulder arthroplasty in patients fifty years old or less. Long-term results. J Bone Joint Surg Am. 1998;80(4):464–73.

93. Barlow JD, Abboud J. Surgical options for the young patient with glenohumeral arthritis. Int J Shoulder Surg. 2016;10(1):28–36.

94. Bryant D, Litchfield R, Sandow M, Gartsman GM, Guyatt G, Kirkley A. A comparison of pain, strength, range of motion, and functional outcomes after hemiarthroplasty and total shoulder arthroplasty in patients with osteoarthritis of the shoulder. A systematic review and meta-analysis. J Bone Joint Surg Am. 2005;87(9):1947–56.

95. Edwards TB, Kadakia NR, Boulahia A, et al. A comparison of hemiarthroplasty and total shoulder arthroplasty in the treatment of primary glenohumeral osteoarthritis: results of a multicenter study. J Shoulder Elbow Surg. 2003;12(3):207–13.

96. Schoch BS, Barlow JD, Schleck C, Cofield RH, Sperling JW. Shoulder arthroplasty for atraumatic osteonecrosis of the humeral head. J Shoulder Elbow Surg. 2016;25(2):238–45.

97. Mather RC, Watters TS, Orlando LA, Bolognesi MP, Moorman CT. Cost effectiveness analysis of hemiarthroplasty and total shoulder arthroplasty. J Shoulder Elbow Surg. 2010;19(3):325–34.

98. Bhat SB, Lazarus M, Getz C, Williams GR Jr, Namdari S. Economic decision model suggests total shoulder arthroplasty is superior to hemiarthroplasty in young patients with end-stage shoulder arthritis. Clin Orthop Relat Res. 2016;474(11):2482–92.

99. Schoch B, Schleck C, Cofield RH, Sperling JW. Shoulder arthroplasty in patients younger than 50 years: minimum 20-year follow-up. J Shoulder Elbow Surg. 2015;24(5):705–10.

100. Raiss P, Aldinger PR, Kasten P, Rickert M, Loew M. Total shoulder replacement in young and middle-aged patients with glenohumeral osteoarthritis. J Bone Joint Surg Br. 2008;90(6):764–9.

101. Denard PJ, Raiss P, Sowa B, Walch G. Mid- to long-term follow-up of total shoulder arthroplasty using a keeled glenoid in young adults with primary glenohumeral arthritis. J Shoulder Elbow Surg. 2013;22(7):894–900.

102. Cvetanovich GL, Naylor AJ, O'Brien MC, Waterman BR, Garcia GH, Nicholson GP. Anatomic total shoulder arthroplasty with an inlay glenoid component: clinical outcomes and return to activity. J Shoulder Elbow Surg. 2020;29(6):1188–96.

103. Endell D, Audige L, Grob A, et al. Impact of sports activity on medium-term clinical and radiological outcome after reverse shoulder arthroplasty in cuff deficient arthropathy; an institutional register-based analysis. J Clin Med. 2021;10(4):828.

104. Anglin C, Wyss UP, Pichora DR. Mechanical testing of shoulder prostheses and recommendations for glenoid design. J Shoulder Elbow Surg. 2000;9:323–231.

105. Gunther SB, Lynch TL, O'Farrell D, Calyore C, Rodenhouse A. Finite element analysis and physiologic testing of a novel, inset glenoid fixation technique. J Shoulder Elbow Surg. 2012;21(6):795–803.

106. Gagliano JR, Helms SM, Colbath GP, Przestrzelski BT, Hawkins RJ, DesJardins JD. A comparison of onlay versus inlay glenoid component loosening in total shoulder arthroplasty. J Shoulder Elbow Surg. 2017;26(7):1113–20.

107. Uribe JW, Zvijac JE, Porter DA, Saxena A, Vargas LA. Inlay total shoulder arthroplasty for primary glenohumeral arthritis. JSES Int. 2021;5(6):1014–20.

108. Ross M, Glasson JM, Alexander J, et al. Medium to long-term results of a recessed glenoid for glenoid resurfacing in total shoulder arthroplasty. Shoulder Elbow. 2020;12(1 Suppl):31–9.

109. Walker M, Brooks J, Willis M, Frankle M. How reverse shoulder arthroplasty works. Clin Orthop Relat Res. 2011;469(9):2440–51.

110. Wall B, Nové-Josserand L, O'Connor DP, Edwards TB, Walch G. Reverse total shoulder arthroplasty: a review of results according to etiology. J Bone Joint Surg Am. 2007;89(7):1476–85.

111. Kim H, Kim CH, Kim M, et al. Is reverse total shoulder arthroplasty (rTSA) more advantageous than anatomic TSA (aTSA) for osteoarthritis with intact cuff tendon? A systematic review and meta-analysis. J Orthop Traumatol. 2022;23(1):3.

112. Drake GN, O'Connor DP, Edwards TB. Indications for reverse total shoulder arthroplasty in rotator cuff disease. Clin Orthop Relat Res. 2010;468(6):1526–33.

113. Erickson BJ, Bohl DD, Cole BJ, et al. Reverse total shoulder arthroplasty: indications and techniques across the world. Am J Orthop (Belle Mead NJ). 2018;47(9).

114. Kozak T, Bauer S, Walch G, Al-Karawi S, Blakeney W. An update on reverse total shoulder arthroplasty:

current indications, new designs, same old problems. EFORT Open Rev. 2021;6(3):189–201.

115. Guery JFL, Sirveaux F, Oudet D, Mole D, Walch G. Reverse total shoulder arthroplasty: survivorship analysis of eighty replacements followed for five to ten years. J Bone Joint Surg Am. 2006;88:1742–7.

116. Schoch BS, King JJ, Zuckerman J, Wright TW, Roche C, Flurin PH. Anatomic versus reverse shoulder arthroplasty: a mid-term follow-up comparison. Shoulder Elbow. 2021;13(5):518–26.

117. Wright MA, Keener JD, Chamberlain AM. Comparison of clinical outcomes after anatomic total shoulder arthroplasty and reverse shoulder arthroplasty in patients 70 years and older with glenohumeral osteoarthritis and an intact rotator cuff. J Am Acad Orthop Surg. 2020;28(5):e222–9.

118. Drager J, Polce EM, Fu M, et al. Patients undergoing anatomic total shoulder arthroplasty achieve clinically significant outcomes faster than those undergoing reverse shoulder arthroplasty. J Shoulder Elbow Surg. 2021;30(11):2523–32.

119. Kim MS, Jeong HY, Kim JD, Ro KH, Rhee SM, Rhee YG. Difficulty in performing activities of daily living associated with internal rotation after reverse total shoulder arthroplasty. J Shoulder Elbow Surg. 2020;29(1):86–94.

120. Sabesan VJ, Dawoud M, Stephens BJ, Busheme CE, Lavin AC. Patients' perception of physical therapy after shoulder surgery. JSES Int. 2022;6(2):292–6.

121. Kirsch JM, Namdari S. Rehabilitation after anatomic and reverse total shoulder arthroplasty: a critical analysis review. JBJS Rev. 2020;8(2):e0129.

122. Mulieri PJ, Holcomb JO, Dunning P, et al. Is a formal physical therapy program necessary after total shoulder arthroplasty for osteoarthritis? J Shoulder Elbow Surg. 2010;19(4):570–9.

123. Austin MS, Urbani BT, Fleischman AN, et al. Formal physical therapy after total hip arthroplasty is not required: a randomized controlled trial. J Bone Joint Surg Am. 2017;99(8):648–55.

124. Edwards PK, Ebert JR, Joss B, Ackland T, Wang A. A randomised trial comparing two rehabilitation approaches following reverse total shoulder arthroplasty. Shoulder Elbow. 2021;13(5):557–72.

125. Kennedy JS, Garrigues GE, Pozzi F, et al. The American Society of Shoulder and Elbow Therapists' consensus statement on rehabilitation for anatomic total shoulder arthroplasty. J Shoulder Elbow Surg. 2020;29(10):2149–62.

126. Edwards PK, Ebert JR, Littlewood C, Ackland T, Wang A. Effectiveness of formal physical therapy following total shoulder arthroplasty: a systematic review. Shoulder Elbow. 2020;12(2):136–43.

127. Hagen MS, Allahabadi S, Zhang AL, Feeley BT, Grace T, Ma CB. A randomized single-blinded trial of early rehabilitation versus immobilization after reverse total shoulder arthroplasty. J Shoulder Elbow Surg. 2020;29(3):442–50.

128. Wang J, Popchak A, Giugale J, Irrgang J, Lin A. Sports participation is an appropriate expectation for recreational athletes undergoing shoulder arthroplasty. Orthop J Sports Med. 2018;6(10):2325967118800666.

129. Johnson DJ, Johnson CC, Gulotta LV. Return to play after shoulder replacement surgery: what is realistic and what does the evidence tell us. Clin Sports Med. 2018;37(4):585–92.

130. Tangtiphaiboontana J, Mara KC, Jensen AR, Camp CL, Morrey ME, Sanchez-Sotelo J. Return to sports after primary reverse shoulder arthroplasty: outcomes at mean 4-year follow-up. Orthop J Sports Med. 2021;9(6):23259671211012393.

131. Dukan R, Rouillon O, Masmejean EH. Can you maintain a competitive golf swing after total shoulder arthroplasty? Eur J Orthop Surg Traumatol. 2022;33:795.

132. Robinson PG, Williamson TR, Creighton AP, et al. Rate and timing of return to golf after hip, knee, or shoulder arthroplasty: a systematic review and meta-analysis. Am J Sports Med. 2023;51(6):1644–51.

133. Schumann K, Flury MP, Schwyzer HK, Simmen BR, Drerup S, Goldhahn J. Sports activity after anatomical total shoulder arthroplasty. Am J Sports Med. 2010;38(10):2097–105.

134. Tramer JS, Klag EA, Kuhlmann NA, Sheena GJ, Muh SJ. Return to golf following reverse total shoulder arthroplasty. Arch Bone Joint Surg. 2021;9(3):306–11.

135. Garcia GH, Liu JN, Sinatro A, et al. High satisfaction and return to sports after total shoulder arthroplasty in patients aged 55 years and younger. Am J Sports Med. 2017;45(7):1664–9.

Part IV

Joint Replacement: Open Treatment in Middle-Aged

Long-term Outcomes of Anatomical Total Shoulder Replacement at 10 Years: Analysis of the Australian Joint Replacement Registry

16

Kristine Italia, Freek Hollman, Mohammad Jomaa, Roberto Pareyon, Richard Page, Kenneth Cutbush, Dylan Harries, and Ashish Gupta

16.1 Introduction

Glenohumeral arthritis is a debilitating condition causing unrelenting pain and loss of motion. This is associated with significant dysfunction affecting the activities of daily living. Total shoulder replacement (TSR) is the treatment of choice for end-stage shoulder arthritis. This has produced good to excellent outcomes [1–3]. However, this is also associated with complications such as loosening, instability, rotator cuff insufficiency, and infection [2]. Because of these, many surgeons can be reluctant in performing TSR in the younger age groups. Several studies have reported good outcomes after TSR in the young [4–8]. Despite this, higher revision rates have been associated with TSR in this age group. This can be attributed to the higher demands for the shoulder as well as longer life expectancy [4]. This chapter will analyze the published long-term data on total shoulder replacement from the Australian Orthopaedic National Joint Replacement Registry (AOANJRR).

K. Italia · F. Hollman · M. Jomaa · R. Pareyon
K. Cutbush
Queensland Unit for Advanced Shoulder Research (QUASR), Brisbane, QLD, Australia
e-mail: ken@kennethcutbush.com

R. Page · D. Harries
Australian Orthopaedic Association National Joint Replacement Registry (AOANJRR),
Adelaide, South Australia

South Australian Health and Medical Research Institute (SAHMRI), Adelaide, South Australia
e-mail: richardpage@geelongortho.com.au;
Dylan.Harries@csiro.au

A. Gupta (✉)
Queensland Unit for Advanced Shoulder Research (QUASR), Brisbane, QLD, Australia

Queensland Orthopaedic Clinic, Greenslopes Private Hospital, Brisbane, QLD, Australia
e-mail: ashish@qoc.com.au

16.2 Shoulder Replacement in the AOANJRR

The AOANJRR 2021 Annual Report includes information on 67,614 primary and revision shoulder replacement surgeries performed from 16 April 2004 to 31 December 2020 [9]. This number has increased by 188.5% since 2008. This is further evidenced by an increase in the proportion of TSR from 57.6% in 2008 to 88.4% in 2020. This is in turn accompanied by a steady decline in partial shoulder replacements (from 32.6% in 2008 to 10.9% in 2020) (Fig. 16.1) [10]. The same trend is observed in the United States [3].

© ISAKOS 2023
A. D. Mazzocca et al. (eds.), *Shoulder Arthritis across the Life Span*,
https://doi.org/10.1007/978-3-031-33298-2_16

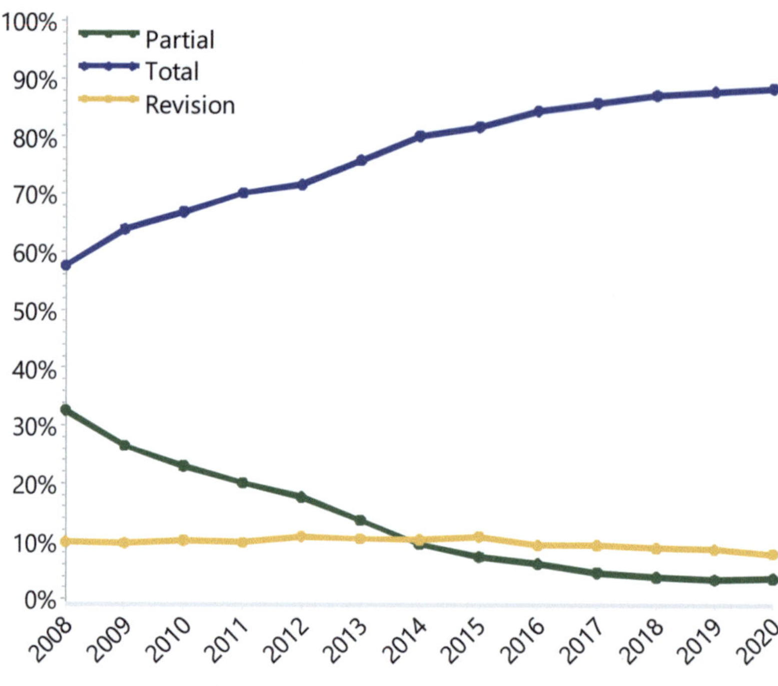

Fig. 16.1 Proportion of shoulder replacements (AOANJRR 2021, Fig. S1). (This graph is reprinted with permission from *Fig. S1 Proportion of Shoulder Replacements*, page 272 of Hip, Knee & Shoulder Arthroplasty Annual Report 2021 by the Australian Orthopaedic Association National Joint Replacement Registry (AOANJRR). 2021, Adelaide: AOA. © 2021 AOANJRR)

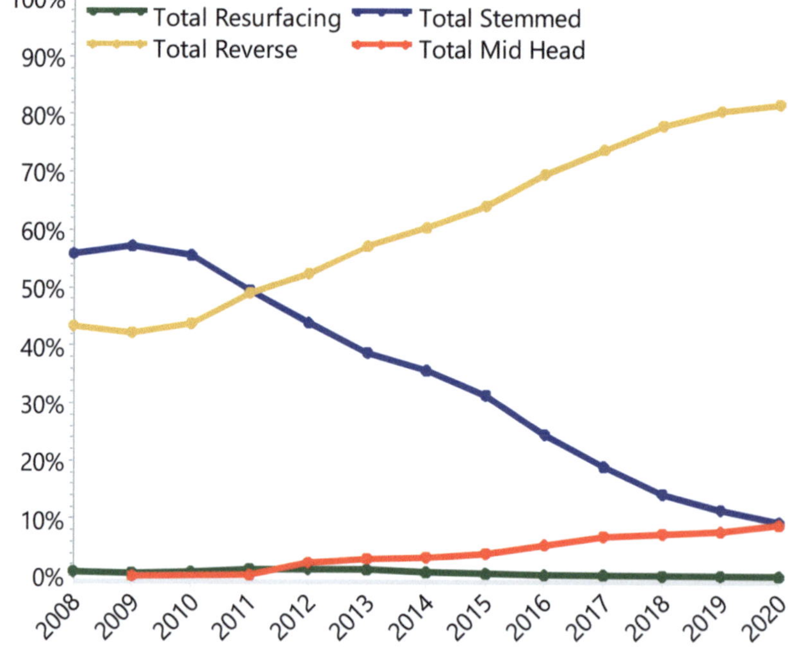

Fig. 16.2 Primary total shoulder replacement by class (AOANJRR 2021, Fig ST1). (This graph is reprinted with permission from *Figure ST1 Primary Total Shoulder Replacement by Class*, page 281 of Hip, Knee & Shoulder Arthroplasty Annual Report 2021 by the Australian Orthopaedic Association National Joint Replacement Registry (AOANJRR). 2021, Adelaide: AOA. © 2021 AOANJRR)

There were 53,815 primary TSR included in the Registry up to 2020 [9]. The most commonly performed is total reverse comprising 66.9% of all TSR. Total stemmed comprised 27.6% and were most commonly performed for osteoarthritis (94.2%). Total resurfacing and total midhead are performed much less frequently (Fig. 16.2).

The data from the AOANJRR 2021 Annual Report that will be presented in this chapter only involves procedures using prostheses that have been available and used in 2020, which are described as modern prostheses. This change was made in the Registry to ensure that it reflects the use of contemporary prostheses [9].

16.3   Arthroplasty Revision Rate

Based on the AOANJRR 2021 Annual Report, the proportion of revision procedures for all shoulder replacements has decreased to 7.9%, equating to 224 less revisions compared its peak in 2012 at 10.9% [9]. The revision burden in 2020 is the lowest since the shoulder registry's full national dataset in 2008 [9]. Focusing on TSR, total stemmed replacement has the highest cumulative percent revision among all classes (Table 16.1). It is widely acknowledged the confounding effect of the increased rate of revision of primary anatomic TSR with metal backed glenoids in this data set [9]. The most common reason for revision after this procedure is rotator cuff insufficiency (33.8%). Other reasons for revision include instability/dislocation (26.9%) and loosening (15.6%).

Table 16.1   Cumulative percent revision of primary total shoulder replacement by class (AOANJRR 2021, Table ST6)

Shoulder class	*N* revised	*N* total	1 year	3 years	5 years	7 years	9 years	10 years
Total stemmed	640	8324	3.0 (2.6, 3.4)	5.9 (5.4, 6.5)	7.4 (6.8, 8.0)	8.8 (8.1, 9.6)	10.8 (9.9, 11.8)	12.0 (10.9, 13.1)
Total reverse	1238	34,017	2.4 (2.2, 2.6)	3.6 (3.4, 3.9)	4.3 (4.1, 4.6)	4.9 (4.6, 5.2)	5.8 (5.4, 6.3)	6.2 (5.7, 6.8)
Total midhead	64	2406	1.6 (1.2, 2.3)	3.6 (2.8, 4.7)	4.5 (3.4, 5.9)	4.5 (3.4, 5.9)		
Total	**1942**	**44,747**						

Note: Restricted to modern prostheses

This table is reprinted with permission from *Table ST6 Primary Total Shoulder Replacement by Class*, page 283 of Hip, Knee & Shoulder Arthroplasty Annual Report 2021 by the Australian Orthopaedic Association National Joint Replacement Registry (AOANJRR). 2021, Adelaide: AOA. © 2021 AOANJRR

16.4　Factors Affecting Survivorship of TSR

The primary aim of the AOANJRR is as a quality to improve patient outcomes of shoulder arthroplasty. Consequently, it aims to identify important factors contributing to the risk of revision surgery. Key factors affecting survivorship are emphasized, including patient characteristics, prosthesis used, and fixation techniques. The registry also identifies specific prosthesis with higher-than-expected revision rates.

16.4.1　Patient Characteristics

Patient factors that were accounted for in the AOANJRR included age, gender, American Society of Anaesthesiologists—Physical Status Classification (ASA), body mass index (BMI), and glenoid morphology. More recently patient reported outcomes (PROMs) and expectations (PREMs) are collected preoperatively and at 6 months.

16.4.1.1　Age

Anatomic TSR (i.e., total stemmed, total midhead, total resurfacing) is usually performed in younger patients compared to those who undergo total reverse. In the AOANJRR 2021 Annual Report, patients aged 65–74 years account for the largest proportion of anatomic TSR procedures (Table 16.2) [9]. In comparison, almost 50% of the total reverse patients are 75 years and older. This can be attributed to the tendency to perform total reverse for older patients given that this age group would have high chance of having age-related rotator cuff dysfunction. As seen in the Registry, more total reverse shoulder replacements are being performed for patients 75 years and older with osteoarthritis than anatomic TSR (7497 vs 1972) (Table 16.3). Total reverse is preferred in this age group as poor rotator cuff tendon quality has been shown to result in poorer outcomes after anatomic TSR [11]. It can be noted in the registry that total stemmed shoulder arthroplasty has the highest cumulative percent revision at 7 years if performed for cuff tear arthropathy (Table 16.4).

Total stemmed replacement used for osteoarthritis had a revision rate that generally decreases as age increases (Table 16.4). At 10 years, the highest cumulative percent revision is noted in patients 55–64 years old (16.5%), whereas patients 75 years and older have the lowest cumulative percent revision (8.1%). It has been observed that younger patients are likely to have more severe and complex disease, which necessitates earlier shoulder arthroplasty [12]. The higher revision rate in younger patients can be attributed to increased demand in the presence of more severe disease, consequently placing more mechanical stress on the rotator cuff and the implants [13]. This is associated with an increased wear rate leading to earlier implant loosening and revision [14].

Table 16.2 Primary total shoulder replacement by class and age (all diagnoses) (AOANJRR 2021, Table ST4)

Shoulder class	<55		55–64		65–74		≥75		Total	
	N	%	N	%	N	%	N	%	N	%
Total resurfacing	33	14.0	77	32.8	106	45.1	19	8.1	235	100.0
Total stemmed	824	5.5	3461	23.3	6596	44.4	3991	26.8	14,872	100.0
Total reverse	558	1.6	3638	10.1	13,911	38.7	17,873	49.7	35,980	100.0
Total midhead	245	9.0	748	27.4	1221	44.8	514	18.8	2728	100.0
Total	**1660**	**3.1**	**7924**	**14.7**	**21,834**	**40.6**	**22,397**	**41.6**	**53,815**	**100.0**

This table is reprinted with permission from *Table ST4 Primary Total Shoulder Replacement by Class and Age*, page 282 of Hip, Knee & Shoulder Arthroplasty Annual Report 2021 by the Australian Orthopaedic Association National Joint Replacement Registry (AOANJRR). 2021, Adelaide: AOA. © 2021 AOANJRR

Table 16.3 Cumulative percent revision of primary shoulder replacement by type of primary and age (primary diagnosis OA) (AOANJRR 2021, Table ST27 and Table ST49)

Type of primary	Age	*N* revised	*N* total	1 year	3 years	5 years	7 years	9 years	10 years
Total stemmed	<55	42	438	3.1 (1.8, 5.4)	7.1 (4.9, 10.2)	10.2 (7.4, 14.1)	12.2 (8.8, 16.8)	13.9 (10.0, 19.1)	13.9 (10.0, 19.1)
	55–64	179	1915	3.2 (2.5, 4.1)	6.7 (5.6, 8.0)	8.2 (6.9, 9.7)	10.6 (9.0, 12.6)	14.0 (11.8, 16.7)	16.5 (13.8, 19.7)
	65–74	248	3525	2.9 (2.4, 3.5)	5.6 (4.8, 6.4)	6.8 (6.0, 7.8)	8.0 (7.0, 9.1)	10.3 (8.9, 11.9)	11.0 (9.5, 12.8)
	≥75	122	1972	2.5 (1.9, 3.3)	5.0 (4.1, 6.1)	6.2 (5.1, 7.4)	7.2 (6.0, 8.7)	7.9 (6.5, 9.5)	8.1 (6.7, 9.8)
Total reverse	<55	9	185	3.5 (1.6, 7.7)	5.4 (2.7, 10.7)	5.4 (2.7, 10.7)			
	55–64	85	1419	3.7 (2.8, 4.9)	5.9 (4.7, 7.5)	6.7 (5.3, 8.3)	7.5 (5.8, 9.7)	10.3 (7.2, 14.6)	10.3 (7.2, 14.6)
	65–74	200	5825	2.0 (1.7, 2.4)	3.4 (2.9, 3.9)	4.0 (3.5, 4.7)	5.1 (4.3, 6.0)	6.0 (4.9, 7.3)	6.3 (5.1, 7.7)
	≥75	194	7497	1.8 (1.5, 2.1)	2.5 (2.1, 2.9)	2.9 (2.5, 3.4)	3.5 (2.9, 4.1)	4.1 (3.4, 5.0)	4.6 (3.7, 5.8)
Total		**1079**	**22,776**						

Note: Restricted to modern prostheses
This table is reprinted with permission from *Table ST27 Cumulative Percent Revision of Primary Total Stemmed Shoulder Replacement by Age (Primary Diagnosis OA)*, page 296, and *Table ST49 Cumulative Percent Revision of Primary Total Reverse Shoulder Replacement by Age (Primary Diagnosis OA)*, page 321 of Hip, Knee & Shoulder Arthroplasty Annual Report 2021 by the Australian Orthopaedic Association National Joint Replacement Registry (AOANJRR). 2021, Adelaide: AOA. © 2021 AOANJRR

Table 16.4 Cumulative percent revision of primary total stemmed shoulder replacement by primary diagnosis (AOANJRR 2021, Table ST24)

Primary diagnosis	*N* revised	*N* total	1 year	3 years	5 years	7 years	9 years	10 years
Osteoarthritis	591	7850	2.9 (2.5, 3.3)	5.8 (5.3, 6.4)	7.2 (6.6, 7.8)	8.6 (7.9, 9.4)	10.7 (9.8, 11.7)	11.7 (10.7, 12.9)
Osteonecrosis	13	150	4.3 (1.9, 9.3)	7.6 (4.1, 13.7)	11.4 (6.7, 19.3)			
Rheumatoid arthritis	8	116	0.9 (0.1, 6.3)	3.0 (1.0, 9.0)	4.3 (1.6, 11.1)	6.0 (2.5, 14.2)		
Fracture	10	72	7.2 (3.1, 16.5)	14.9 (8.3, 26.0)	14.9 (8.3, 26.0)	14.9 (8.3, 26.0)	14.9 (8.3, 26.0)	14.9 (8.3, 26.0)
Rotator cuff arthropathy	9	57	7.4 (2.8, 18.4)	14.1 (7.0, 27.6)	17.3 (8.9, 32.2)	17.3 (8.9, 32.2)		
Other inflammatory arthritis	4	45	4.7 (1.2, 17.3)	4.7 (1.2, 17.3)	7.7 (2.5, 22.3)	7.7 (2.5, 22.3)	16.1 (5.2, 43.7)	16.1 (5.2, 43.7)
Other (3)	5	34	6.3 (1.6, 23.0)	15.1 (5.8, 36.0)	21.1 (9.0, 45.0)			
Total	**640**	**8324**						

This table is reprinted with permission from *Table ST24 Cumulative Percent Revision of Primary Total Stemmed Shoulder Replacement by Primary Diagnosis*, page 293 of Hip, Knee & Shoulder Arthroplasty Annual Report 2021 by the Australian Orthopaedic Association National Joint Replacement Registry (AOANJRR). 2021, Adelaide: AOA. © 2021 AOANJRR

16.4.1.2 Gender

Gender was not a significant factor in the survivorship of total stemmed prosthesis for osteoarthritis. The revision rate is slightly higher for males than females at 10 years postoperatively (12% versus 11.6%) but the difference was not significant [9]. However, AOANJRR studies of shorter time frame with more specific data sets have shown gender differences in revision outcome [15].

16.4.1.3 Comorbidity

ASA scores and BMI reflect patient comorbidities. The majority of the total stemmed replacements performed for osteoarthritis comprised patients with ASA 2 or 3 (92%) and in pre-obese or obese class 1 (63%) [9].

The highest cumulative percent revision was observed in patients with ASA 2 (7.3% at 5 years) and in patients who are obese class 1 (7.9% at 5 years). However, analysis has shown that there was no significant difference in the revision rates among different ASA scores and BMI categories over the entire follow-up period [9]. Therefore, both ASA score and BMI are not considered risk factors for revision after stemmed ATSA for osteoarthritis.

The reasons for revision of total stemmed replacements were different for each class. Rotator cuff insufficiency is the most common reason for revision in ASA 2 and 3, pre-obese, and obese patients. On the other hand, instability or dislocation was the main reason for revision in ASA 1 patients and patients with normal BMI [9].

At less than 1 year postoperatively, increased instability and dislocations were observed in the pre-obese and obese patients, especially in obese class 3 [9]. This may indicate that increased BMI is a risk factor for instability during the early postoperative period. This is similar to the findings of a meta-analysis of 15 studies involving 152,306 patients wherein obesity was linked to increased risk of dislocation from 90 days to 1 year postoperatively [16]. The authors have noted that patients with BMI of 30 kg/m^2 or greater had increased odds of dislocation compared with those with BMI less than 30 kg/m^2. Similarly, Werner et al. also reported obesity as risk factor for early revision [17]. After analysis of data from 221,381 patients who underwent shoulder arthroplasty, they have reported that obesity and morbid obesity are associated with dislocation as a cause for revision in 1 year regardless of the type of arthroplasty. This is in contrast with the findings of the study by Kusin et al. involving 9382 patients, wherein no linear association was noted between BMI and risk of dislocation of TSR. It was even noted that overweight patients (BMI 25–29.9) experienced the lowest dislocation rate while underweight patients (BMI <18.5) experienced the highest dislocation rate in the first 30 days after surgery [18].

Despite this association of higher BMI and instability during the early postoperative period, it does not seem to have a linear relationship with the revision rate as increasing BMI was not associated with poorer survivorship. This is similar to the revision rates across the range of ASA scores.

16.4.1.4 Glenoid Morphology

The majority of patients who underwent primary stemmed TSA for osteoarthritis had glenoid morphology of A1 (35.7%), followed by A2 (24%). There was a higher cumulative percent revision associated with A2 morphology at 3 years postoperatively (6.2%) and lowest rate with B2 glenoids (3.4%) (Table 16.5) [9]. This is contrast to earlier studies showing poorer outcomes of anatomic TSA when performed in patients with B2 glenoid [19, 20]. This is due to the increased risk of recurrent instability and early glenoid loosening associated with the posterior humeral head subluxation and glenoid retroversion [19–21].

Despite this, the Registry has shown that glenoid morphology does not significantly affect survivorship of stemmed TSA over the 3-year period. This is similar to several studies on TSAs and glenoid morphology showing no association between preoperative glenoid wear and humeral head decentering with the outcomes [19, 22, 23]. This may be because of the improved surgical techniques and availability of implants to effectively correct preoperative glenoid deformity and/or humeral head decentering [22, 23].

Table 16.5 Cumulative percent revision of primary total stemmed shoulder replacement by glenoid morphology (primary diagnosis OA) (AOANJRR 2021, Table ST31)

Glenoid morphology	N revised	N total	1 year	2 years	3 years
A1	26	794	2.3 (1.4, 3.7)	3.5 (2.3, 5.2)	4.9 (3.2, 7.4)
A2	22	534	2.3 (1.3, 4.2)	5.1 (3.3, 7.8)	6.2 (4.0, 9.5)
B1	14	478	2.4 (1.3, 4.4)	3.3 (1.9, 5.6)	4.0 (2.3, 6.9)
B2	6	350	0.7 (0.2, 2.7)	1.7 (0.6, 4.7)	3.4 (1.4, 7.8)
C	4	65	5.1 (1.7, 15.1)	5.1 (1.7, 15.1)	5.1 (1.7, 15.1)
Total	**72**	**2221**			

Note: Restricted to modern prostheses

Excludes 3 procedures where a glenoid morphology of B3 was recorded

This table is reprinted with permission from *Table ST31 Cumulative Percent Revision of Primary Total Stemmed Shoulder Replacement by Glenoid Morphology (Primary Diagnosis OA)*, page 302 of Hip, Knee & Shoulder Arthroplasty Annual Report 2021 by the Australian Orthopaedic Association National Joint Replacement Registry (AOANJRR). 2021, Adelaide: AOA. © 2021 AOANJRR

16.4.2 Prosthesis Characteristics

16.4.2.1 Glenoid Component

The most common cause of revision in conventional anatomic TSR is loosening of the glenoid component [24]. This is associated with the "rocking horse" phenomenon where there is eccentric loading of the component causing compression on one side and distraction on the other side [25, 26]. This produces micromotion leading to increased wear and subsequent failure [24, 26]. Moreover, radiolucent lines (RLLs) have also been linked to component loosening. These are radiolucencies noted at the bone-cement interface when cemented all-polyethylene glenoid prostheses are used [27]. RLLs can be observed as early as the immediate postoperative radiograph and in as much as 96% of cases [27, 28]. However, this does not account for the influence of polyethylene type, with a significant reduction in anatomic TSR revision when XLPE (cross-linked polyethylene) is used in the glenoid component [29, 30].

Registry data indicate 40.9% of revisions after primary total resurfacing shoulder replacement and 12.5% of primary total midhead replacements were due to loosening [9]. For total stemmed, loosening comes in third as the reason for revision (15.6%). The most common reason for revision is rotator cuff insufficiency (33.8%) [9]. This has been greatly associated with the "rocking horse" phenomenon as well. Deficiency of the superior rotator cuff interferes with the ability to contain the humeral head within the center of the glenoid component causing superior migration of the humeral head. This promotes higher force and compression on the superior aspect of the glenoid, producing the "rocking horse" phenomenon [25, 31].

Glenoid Component Design

Because of this phenomenon, several strategies have been developed in order to address this and other causes of glenoid failure. These include modifying the glenoid design. The metal-backed glenoid (MBG) prostheses were introduced in an attempt to improve implant longevity. These are uncemented implants that have a porous or similar coated component on the glenoid bone-prosthesis contact surface that is designed to induce bony ingrowth [32]. MBGs can be nonmodular or modular wherein the metal glenoid component can be retained and polyethylene insert can be replaced with a glenosphere.

The Registry has collected data on total stemmed replacements with three glenoid types: modular MBG, nonmodular MBG, and all-polyethylene. Cemented all-polyethylene glenoids are the most common type used in Australia (61%, vs modular MBG 27%, vs nonmodular MBG 12%) [9]. Although it has been theorized that MBG is an ideal component as it should

Table 16.6 Cumulative percent revision of primary total stemmed shoulder replacement by glenoid type (primary diagnosis OA) (AOANJRR 2021, ST33)

Glenoid type	N revised	N total	1 year	3 years	5 years	7 years	9 years	10 years
Modular metal backed	334	2121	6.0 (5.0, 7.1)	11.2 (9.9, 12.7)	13.7 (12.2, 15.3)	15.9 (14.2, 17.7)	19.2 (17.1, 21.5)	21.3 (19.0, 23.9)
All-polyethylene	198	4817	1.5 (1.2, 1.9)	3.2 (2.7, 3.8)	4.1 (3.5, 4.8)	5.1 (4.4, 6.0)	6.5 (5.5, 7.7)	6.9 (5.9, 8.2)
Nonmodular metal backed	59	912	3.0 (2.0, 4.3)	5.7 (4.3, 7.5)	6.1 (4.7, 8.0)	7.2 (5.5, 9.4)	8.5 (6.4, 11.3)	8.5 (6.4, 11.3)
Total	**591**	**7850**						

This table is reprinted with permission from *Table ST33 Cumulative Percent Revision of Primary Total Stemmed Shoulder Replacement by Glenoid Type (Primary Diagnosis OA)*, page 305 of Hip, Knee & Shoulder Arthroplasty Annual Report 2021 by the Australian Orthopaedic Association National Joint Replacement Registry (AOANJRR). 2021, Adelaide: AOA. © 2021 AOANJRR

afford stable fixation in the long term because of progressive bone ingrowth [33] and equal stress distribution at the bone interface, the AOANJRR has shown otherwise [24]. It has been noted that MBGs have higher revision rate than all-polyethylene glenoid components over the entire study period (Table 16.6). This is also increased when modular MBG is used (21.3% at 10 years) [9]. These findings are consistent with the existing literature comparing MBGs and all-polyethylene glenoids [34, 35].

Cementless MBGs are being revised for rotator cuff insufficiency, instability and/or dislocation, implant breakage and/or dissociation, infection, and loosening [24]. These complications can be attributed to its design. The initial design requires a thin polyethylene liner to avoid overstuffing of the joint since MBG tends to be thicker [32, 34, 36]. The thin liner makes it more prone to breakage and increased wear [32]. When the liner fails, metal-on-metal contact between the humeral head and the glenoid component occurs causing rapid metallosis, subsequently requiring revision surgery [37]. On the other hand, if a thicker liner is used, overstuffing of the joint results. This often leads to joint instability and rotator cuff insufficiency [31].

To be able to address these problems, some design modifications were made by using trabecular metal (TM) glenoids or altering the central peg [37]. TM glenoids have monoblock design made up of layers of titanium mesh welded together to form four porous pegs (first-generation TM glenoid) or porous tantalum keel (second-generation TM glenoid) covering the backside of the polyethylene implant [37, 38]. On the other hand, the second-generation SMR has a curved back and less conforming shape, stiff and thick metal back to decrease the stress in the polyethylene component and minimize wear, and initial fixation through two screws and one hollow central peg [37, 38]. These modern MBG designs have been shown by Kim et al. to have promising results that are comparable to or even better than cemented all-polyethylene glenoids [32]. When compared to the conventional MBGs, these modern MBG designs produced significantly lower loosening and failure rates [38]. However, this has not been supported by national level Registry data, with revision rates still higher than cemented all-polyethylene glenoids [9].

Two modern MBGs (SMR L2 and TM glenoid) were included in the Registry data until 31 December 2019 (2020 report data) [39]. Among all the glenoid prostheses included in the registry, SMR L2 had the highest revision rate throughout the entire follow-up period. It had a 9.7% cumulative percent revision at the first postoperative year. At 7 years, the revision rate was 34%, significantly higher than what is anticipated. This is in contrast to the systematic review of Kim et al. [32] Because of this observation in the registry, the SMR L2 prosthesis was eventually withdrawn from the market.

Glenoid Component Polyethylene: Non-cross-Linked Polyethylene (XLPE) Versus XLPE

Polyethylene used in glenoid components can either be cross-linked polyethylene (XLPE) or non-XLPE. The most common type used nationally is non-XLPE, which is available across a wider number of prostheses. The Registry shows that XLPE has a significantly lower cumulative percent revision at 10 years compared to the non-XLPE type (4.9% vs 13.1%) for all glenoid types (Table 16.7) [30]. The same has been noted when XLPE all-polyethylene is compared to non-XLPE all-polyethylene glenoids at 10 years (4.6% vs 7.8%) (Table 16.8). This may be attributed to less wear and particle generation, which decreases the risk of osteolysis and subsequent loosening and failure, as observed in hip and knee arthroplasties [40]. However, the early revisions noted may be due to other prosthesis and patient-related factors before lysis and loosening come into play.

Glenoid Component Shape: Keeled Versus Pegged All-Polyethylene

The first-generation TSRs had keeled glenoid components [37]. Because of the possibility of earlier failure due to prosthesis movement and higher risk of revision surgery after TSR especially in the younger patients, current practice has moved to preserving the bone stock on the glenoid side. Pegged design for the glenoid was introduced in order to reduce the resection of subchondral bone and to utilize stronger peripheral bone for fixation [26, 37, 41]. In addition, because of the variable number and length of pegs, it has been shown that the pegged design can withstand high shear and rotational forces resulting to decreased rate of loosening [42]. Earlier studies have shown that the keeled design

Table 16.7 Cumulative percent revision of primary total stemmed shoulder replacement using "all types" of glenoids by polyethylene type (primary diagnosis OA) (AOANJRR 2021, Table ST35)

Polyethylene type	N revised	N total	1 year	3 years	5 years	7 years	9 years	10 years
Non-XLPE	537	6076	3.4 (2.9, 3.9)	6.6 (5.9, 7.3)	8.1 (7.3, 8.9)	9.7 (8.8, 10.6)	11.9 (10.9, 13.1)	13.1 (11.9, 14.4)
XLPE	53	1754	1.1 (0.7, 1.8)	2.9 (2.1, 3.9)	3.7 (2.8, 4.9)	4.0 (3.0, 5.4)	4.9 (3.4, 6.9)	4.9 (3.4, 6.9)
Total	**590**	**7830**						

Note: Restricted to modern prostheses

This table is reprinted with permission from *Table ST35 Cumulative Percent Revision of Primary Total Stemmed Shoulder Replacement Using All Types of Glenoids by Polyethylene Type (Primary Diagnosis OA)*, page 307 of Hip, Knee & Shoulder Arthroplasty Annual Report 2021 by the Australian Orthopaedic Association National Joint Replacement Registry (AOANJRR). 2021, Adelaide: AOA. © 2021 AOANJRR

Table 16.8 Cumulative percent revision of primary total stemmed shoulder replacement using "all-polyethylene" glenoids by polyethylene type (primary diagnosis OA) (AOANJRR 2021, Table ST36)

Polyethylene type	N revised	N total	1 year	3 years	5 years	7 years	9 years	10 years
Non-XLPE	150	3073	1.7 (1.3, 2.3)	3.5 (2.9, 4.3)	4.5 (3.8, 5.4)	5.7 (4.8, 6.9)	7.3 (6.1, 8.8)	7.8 (6.5, 9.5)
XLPE	48	1742	1.0 (0.6, 1.6)	2.7 (1.9, 3.6)	3.4 (2.5, 4.6)	3.7 (2.7, 5.0)	4.6 (3.2, 6.6)	4.6 (3.2, 6.6)
Total	**198**	**4815**						

Note: Restricted to modern prostheses

This table is reprinted with permission from *Table ST36 Cumulative Percent Revision of Primary Total Stemmed Shoulder Replacement using All-polyethylene Glenoids by Polyethylene Type (Primary Diagnosis OA)*, page 308 of Hip, Knee & Shoulder Arthroplasty Annual Report 2021 by the Australian Orthopaedic Association National Joint Replacement Registry (AOANJRR). 2021, Adelaide: AOA. © 2021 AOANJRR leads to higher rates of postoperative RLLs and loosening resulting to higher revision rates than the pegged glenoid component [37, 42, 43].

The majority of cemented all-polyethylene glenoid components used in Australia have been pegged (92%). Although there was a trend of higher cumulative percent revision for keeled glenoid components, the Registry has shown that there was no significant difference in the revision rates between the two types (5.2% for pegged at 7 years, 4.6% for keeled) (Table 16.9) [9]. This is similar to several studies showing no difference in the rates of loosening and revision between the keeled and pegged designs [44–46]. This has been attributed to modern and better cementing techniques, [44, 47] as well as contemporary highly cross-linked polyethylene [30]. Also, some studies have shown that the presence of greater RLLs attributed to keeled glenoid components does not necessarily correlate with greater failure and revision rates [45].

Fixation Technique: Cementless Versus Cemented Versus Hybrid

The Registry has compared the outcomes of four different fixation techniques. Hybrid TSR fixation with cemented glenoid is the most common fixation technique (59.6%). After analysis, the Registry has shown that cementless components have the highest revision rate at 10 years postoperatively (18.2%) (Table 16.10) [9, 24]. On the other hand, hybrid fixation with cemented glenoid component has the lowest failure rate from 1 to 10 years postoperatively (6.8% at 10 years).

Table 16.9 Cumulative percent revision of all-polyethylene cemented primary total stemmed shoulder replacement by glenoid design (primary diagnosis OA) (AOANJRR 2021, Table ST34)

Glenoid design	N revised	N total	1 year	3 years	5 years	7 years	9 years	10 years
Keeled cemented	12	382	0.3 (0.0, 2.0)	2.6 (1.3, 5.1)	3.0 (1.6, 5.7)	4.6 (2.4, 8.7)	6.1 (3.1, 11.7)	
Pegged cemented	186	4428	1.6 (1.2, 2.0)	3.3 (2.7, 3.9)	4.2 (3.6, 5.0)	5.2 (4.4, 6.1)	6.6 (5.5, 7.8)	7.0 (5.9, 8.3)
Total	**198**	**4810**						

Note: Restricted to modern prostheses

This table is reprinted with permission from *Table ST34 Cumulative Percent Revision of All-Polyethylene Cemented Primary Total Stemmed Shoulder Replacement by Glenoid Design (Primary Diagnosis OA)*, page 306 of Hip, Knee & Shoulder Arthroplasty Annual Report 2021 by the Australian Orthopaedic Association National Joint Replacement Registry (AOANJRR). 2021, Adelaide: AOA. © 2021 AOANJRR

Table 16.10 Cumulative percent revision of primary total stemmed shoulder replacement by fixation (primary diagnosis OA) (AOANJRR 2021, Table ST32)

Fixation	N revised	N total	1 year	3 years	5 years	7 years	9 years	10 years
Cemented	24	393	1.9 (0.9, 3.9)	3.8 (2.2, 6.5)	4.3 (2.6, 7.3)	7.1 (4.3, 11.4)	8.0 (4.9, 12.8)	10.1 (6.3, 16.0)
Cementless	371	2730	5.2 (4.4, 6.1)	9.7 (8.7, 11.0)	11.5 (10.4, 12.9)	13.5 (12.2, 15.0)	16.4 (14.7, 18.3)	18.2 (16.2, 20.4)
Hybrid (glenoid cemented)	189	4675	1.5 (1.2, 1.9)	3.4 (2.9, 4.0)	4.3 (3.7, 5.1)	5.1 (4.4, 6.0)	6.6 (5.6, 7.8)	6.8 (5.7, 8.0)
Hybrid (glenoid cementless)	7	52	5.8 (1.9, 16.9)	7.9 (3.0, 19.7)	15.6 (7.7, 30.4)	15.6 (7.7, 30.4)	15.6 (7.7, 30.4)	
Total	**591**	**7850**						

Note: Restricted to modern prostheses

This table is reprinted with permission from *Table ST32 Cumulative Percent Revision of Primary Total Stemmed Shoulder Replacement by Fixation (Primary Diagnosis OA)*, page 304 of Hip, Knee & Shoulder Arthroplasty Annual Report 2021 by the Australian Orthopaedic Association National Joint Replacement Registry (AOANJRR). 2021, Adelaide: AOA. © 2021 AOANJRR

It can be noted also that at all time points, the cumulative percent revision is higher when the glenoid component is not cemented. This can then indicate that the revision rate is increased if the glenoid component is cementless. This is similar to the results of the New Zealand Joint Registry, which showed five times higher revision rate when the glenoid component is uncemented [35].

Page et al. [24] in 2018 has reported that cementless glenoid components for the primary surgery had higher proportion of procedures being revised for rotator cuff insufficiency (28.2%), instability and/or dislocation (24.3%), implant breakage of glenoid insert (12.9%) and/or dissociation (5.5%), and infection (4.1%). On the other hand, cemented glenoids were being revised primarily because of loosening (34.1%) [24]. Rotator cuff insufficiency and instability/dislocation presented earlier postoperatively in cementless components, whereas loosening gradually increases over time in both cementless and cemented glenoids [24].

16.4.2.2 Humeral Component

Humeral component failure can also be a reason for revision following TSR. The common humeral-sided complications include loosening, possible intraoperative fracture of the humerus during insertion, dislocation, calcar osteolysis, and infection [48]. These complications arise as a consequence of the humeral head size, stem length, or fixation technique.

Humeral Head Size

Head size has been noted to be a factor in total stemmed shoulder replacement. The Registry has shown that TSR survivorship improves with increasing head size, with >50 mm having the lowest cumulative percent revision at 10 years (9.5%) and <44 mm having the highest (14.6%) (Table 16.11) [9]. There are likely patient factors not measured that may contribute to this.

Despite the Registry showing better outcome with increasing head size, accurate humeral head size selection is key for good outcome after TSA. Increasing the humeral head thickness more than the native anatomic humeral head can result in overstuffing of the joint leading and over-tensioning of the soft tissues and significant decrease in range of motion [49, 50]. On the other hand, decreasing the size can lead to greater tuberosity impingement and point loading on the glenoid [49]. Restoration of the premorbid anatomy is ideal; hence, the resected humeral head can guide the surgeon on the correct humeral head diameter and thickness [51]. However, soft tissue status must be taken into consideration as well to afford proper tensioning and humeral bone loss can make accurate restoration difficult [49, 51].

Table 16.11 Cumulative percent revision of primary total stemmed shoulder replacement by humeral head size (primary diagnosis OA) (AOANJRR 2021, Table ST38)

Humeral head size	N revised	N total	1 year	3 years	5 years	7 years	9 years	10 years
<44 mm	97	1014	3.7 (2.7, 5.1)	8.6 (6.9, 10.6)	10.1 (8.2, 12.4)	11.5 (9.3, 14.2)	14.6 (11.5, 18.4)	14.6 (11.5, 18.4)
44–50 mm	380	4845	2.8 (2.4, 3.3)	5.9 (5.2, 6.6)	7.3 (6.5, 8.1)	8.9 (7.9, 9.9)	11.0 (9.8, 12.3)	12.0 (10.7, 13.5)
>50 mm	114	1990	2.6 (2.0, 3.4)	4.2 (3.4, 5.2)	5.4 (4.4, 6.6)	6.6 (5.3, 8.0)	8.0 (6.5, 9.9)	9.5 (7.6, 11.8)
Total	**591**	**7849**						

Note: Restricted to modern prostheses
Excludes 1 procedures with unknown head size
This table is reprinted with permission from *Table ST38 Cumulative Percent Revision of Primary Total Stemmed Shoulder Replacement by Humeral Head Size*, page 309 of Hip, Knee & Shoulder Arthroplasty Annual Report 2021 by the Australian Orthopaedic Association National Replacement Registry (AOANJRR). 2021, Adelaide: AOA. © 2021 AOANJRR

The cause of early failure across all head sizes is instability/dislocation. Starting from the second year postoperatively, rotator cuff insufficiency becomes the main reason for revision for heads 50 mm or smaller. Loosening, on the other hand, is noted to be more apparent in heads >50 mm with increasing incidence starting at year 8 after the primary surgery and becomes the main reason for revision for these sizes at 12 years postoperatively.

16.5 Summary

Anatomic TSR is a reliable operation with excellent long-term outcomes. It can be a challenging procedure especially in large males with significant glenoid deformity. Despite its nuances, anatomic TSR has gone through various modifications in the last decade. Each design modification is showing improved trends for lower revision, with a cemented, XLPE all-polyethylene glenoid having the lowest cumulative revision rate in the AOANJRR. However, this cannot be accounted for in isolation. Despite the dominance of reverse shoulder replacement in current arthroplasty landscape, anatomic TSR is good operation with dependable outcomes and high satisfaction for the suitable patient.

Acknowledgement The authors would like to thank the Australian Orthopaedic Association National Joint Registry and its staff for its help with the data for this manuscript and acknowledge all Australian surgeons who contribute data to the Registry.

References

1. Craig RS, Goodier H, Singh JA, Hopewell S, Rees JL. Shoulder replacement surgery for osteoarthritis and rotator cuff tear arthropathy. Cochrane Database Syst Rev [Internet]. 2020;(4):1–114. http://doi.wiley.com/10.1002/14651858.CD012879.pub2.
2. Jensen AR, Tangtiphaiboontana J, Marigi E, Mallett KE, Sperling JW, Sanchez-Sotelo J. Anatomic total shoulder arthroplasty for primary glenohumeral osteoarthritis is associated with excellent outcomes and low revision rates in the elderly. J Shoulder Elbow Surg [Internet]. 2021;30(7):S131–S139. https://doi.org/10.1016/j.jse.2020.11.030.
3. American Academy of Orthopaedic Surgeons. Shoulder & Elbow Registry (SER): 2020 annual report. Rosemont; 2021.
4. Raiss P, Aldinger PR, Kasten P, Rickert M, Loew M. Total shoulder replacement in young and middle-aged patients with glenohumeral osteoarthritis. J Bone Joint Surg Br [Internet]. 2008;90-B(6):764–9. https://online.boneandjoint.org.uk/doi/10.1302/0301-620X.90B6.20387.
5. Gauci MO, Bonnevialle N, Moineau G, Baba M, Walch G, Boileau P. Anatomical total shoulder arthroplasty in young patients with osteoarthritis. Bone Joint J [Internet]. 2018;100-B(4):485–92. https://online.boneandjoint.org.uk/doi/10.1302/0301-620X.100B4.BJJ-2017-0495.R2.
6. Fonte H, Amorim-Barbosa T, Diniz S, Barros L, Ramos J, Claro R. Shoulder arthroplasty options for glenohumeral osteoarthritis in young and active patients (<60 years old): a systematic review. J Shoulder Elb Arthroplast. 2022;6:247154922210870.
7. Roberson TA, Bentley JC, Griscom JT, Kissenberth MJ, Tolan SJ, Hawkins RJ, et al. Outcomes of total shoulder arthroplasty in patients younger than 65 years: a systematic review. J Shoulder Elbow Surg. 2017;26(7):1298–306.
8. McBride AP, Ross M, Duke P, Hoy G, Page R, Dyer C, et al. Shoulder joint arthroplasty in young patients: analysis of 8742 patients from the Australian Orthopaedic Association National Joint Replacement Registry. Shoulder Elbow. 2021:175857322110587.
9. Australian Orthopaedic Association. Australian Orthopaedic Association National Joint Replacement Registry (AOANJRR). Hip, knee & shoulder arthroplasty: 2021 annual report [Internet]. Adelaide; 2021. p. 1–432. https://aoanjrr.sahmri.com/annual-reports-2021.
10. Australian Orthopaedic Association. Demographics and outcomes of shoulder arthroplasty: supplementary report. 2012. p. 35–47.
11. Wright MA, Keener JD, Chamberlain AM. Comparison of clinical outcomes after anatomic total shoulder arthroplasty and reverse shoulder arthroplasty in patients 70 years and older with glenohumeral osteoarthritis and an intact rotator cuff. J Am Acad Orthop Surg [Internet]. 2020;28(5):e222–9. http://journals.lww.com/10.5435/JAAOS-D-19-00166.
12. Saltzman MD, Mercer DM, Warme WJ, Bertelsen AL, Matsen FA. Comparison of patients undergoing primary shoulder arthroplasty before and after the age of fifty. J Bone Joint Surg Am. 2010;92(1):42–7.
13. Brewley EE, Christmas KN, Gorman RA, Downes KL, Mighell MA, Frankle MA. Defining the younger patient: age as a predictive factor for outcomes in shoulder arthroplasty. J Shoulder Elbow Surg. 2020;29(7):S1–8.
14. Sowa B, Bochenek M, Bülhoff M, Zeifang F, Loew M, Bruckner T, et al. The medium- and long-term outcome of total shoulder arthroplasty for primary glenohumeral osteoarthritis in middle-aged patients. Bone Joint J [Internet]. 2017;99-B(7):939–43.

https://online.boneandjoint.org.uk/doi/10.1302/0301-620X.99B7.BJJ-2016-1365.R1.

15. Gill DRJ, Page RS, Graves SE, Rainbird S, Hatton A. A comparison of revision rates for osteoarthritis of primary reverse total shoulder arthroplasty to primary anatomic shoulder arthroplasty with a cemented all-polyethylene glenoid: analysis from the Australian Orthopaedic Association National Joint Replacement Registry. Clin Orthop Relat Res [Internet]. 2021;479(10):2216–24. https://journals.lww.com/10.1097/CORR.0000000000001869.

16. Theodoulou A, Krishnan J, Aromataris E. Risk of poor outcomes in patients who are obese following total shoulder arthroplasty and reverse total shoulder arthroplasty: a systematic review and meta-analysis. J Shoulder Elbow Surg [Internet]. 2019;28(11):e359–e376. https://doi.org/10.1016/j.jse.2019.06.017.

17. Werner BC, Burrus MT, Begho I, Gwathmey FW, Brockmeier SF. Early revision within 1 year after shoulder arthroplasty: patient factors and etiology. J Shoulder Elbow Surg [Internet]. 2015;24(12):e323–30. https://doi.org/10.1016/j.jse.2015.05.035.

18. Kusin DJ, Ungar JA, Samson KK, Teusink MJ. Body mass index as a risk factor for dislocation of total shoulder arthroplasty in the first 30 days. JSES Open Access [Internet]. 2019;3(3):179–182. https://doi.org/10.1016/j.jses.2019.07.001.

19. Petri M, Euler SA, Dornan GJ, Greenspoon JA, Horan MP, Katthagen JC, et al. Predictors for satisfaction after anatomic total shoulder arthroplasty for idiopathic glenohumeral osteoarthritis. Arch Orthop Trauma Surg [Internet]. 2016;136(6):755–62. http://link.springer.com/10.1007/s00402-016-2452-6.

20. Walch G, Moraga C, Young A, Castellanos-Rosas J. Results of anatomic nonconstrained prosthesis in primary osteoarthritis with biconcave glenoid. J Shoulder Elbow Surg. 2012;21(11):1526–33.

21. Gates S, Sager B, Khazzam M. Preoperative glenoid considerations for shoulder arthroplasty: a review. EFORT Open Rev [Internet]. 2020;5(3):126–37. https://eor.bioscientifica.com/view/journals/eor/5/3/2058-5241.5.190011.xml

22. Matsen FA, Russ SM, Vu PT, Hsu JE, Lucas RM, Comstock BA. What factors are predictive of patient-reported outcomes? A prospective study of 337 shoulder arthroplasties. Clin Orthop Relat Res [Internet]. 2016;474(11):2496–2510. https://journals.lww.com/00003086-201611000-00026.

23. Altintas B, Horan MP, Dornan GJ, Pogorzelski J, Godin JA, Millett PJ. The recovery curve of anatomic total shoulder arthroplasty for primary glenohumeral osteoarthritis: midterm results at a minimum of 5 years. JSES Int [Internet]. 2022 [cited 2022 Oct 23];6(4):587–95. https://linkinghub.elsevier.com/retrieve/pii/S2666638322001049.

24. Page RS, Pai V, Eng K, Bain G, Graves S, Lorimer M. Cementless versus cemented glenoid components in conventional total shoulder joint arthroplasty: analysis from the Australian Orthopaedic Association National Joint Replacement Registry. J Shoulder

25. Franklin JL, Barrett WP, Jackins SE, Matsen FA. Glenoid loosening in total shoulder arthroplasty. J Arthroplasty. 1988;3(1):39–46.

26. Trivedi NN, Shimberg JL, Sivasundaram L, Mengers S, Salata MJ, Voos JE, et al. Advances in glenoid design in anatomic total shoulder arthroplasty. J Bone Joint Surg. 2020;102(20):1825–35.

27. Lazarus MD, Jensen KL, Southworth C, Matsen FA. The radiographic evaluation of keeled and pegged glenoid component insertion. J Bone Joint Surg Am. 2002;84(7):1174–82.

28. Grob A, Freislederer F, Marzel A, Audigé L, Schwyzer HK, Scheibel M. Glenoid component loosening in anatomic total shoulder arthroplasty: association between radiological predictors and clinical parameters—an observational study. J Clin Med. 2021;10(2):234.

29. Sandow M, Page R, Hatton A, Peng Y. Total shoulder replacement stems in osteoarthritis—short, long or reverse? An analysis of the impact of cross-linked polyethylene. J Shoulder Elbow Surg [Internet]. 2022;31:2249. https://doi.org/10.1016/j.jse.2022.04.015.

30. Page RS, Alder-Price AC, Rainbird S, Graves SE, de Steiger RN, Peng Y, et al. Reduced revision rates in total shoulder arthroplasty with crosslinked polyethylene: results from the Australian Orthopaedic Association National Joint Replacement Registry. Clin Orthop Relat Res [Internet]. 2022;10(1907). https://journals.lww.com/10.1097/CORR.0000000000002293.

31. Thomas R, Richardson M, Patel M, Page R, Sangeux M, Ackland DC. Rotator cuff contact pressures at the tendon-implant interface after anatomic total shoulder arthroplasty using a metal-backed glenoid component. J Shoulder Elbow Surg [Internet]. 2018;27(11):2085–92. https://doi.org/10.1016/j.jse.2018.04.017.

32. Kim DM, Aldeghaither M, Alabdullatif F, Shin MJ, Kholinne E, Kim H, et al. Loosening and revision rates after total shoulder arthroplasty: a systematic review of cemented all-polyethylene glenoid and three modern designs of metal-backed glenoid. BMC Musculoskelet Disord. 2020;21(1):114.

33. Page RS, Pai V, Eng K, Bain G, Graves S, Lorimer M. Cementless versus cemented glenoid components in conventional total shoulder joint arthroplasty: analysis from the Australian Orthopaedic Association National Joint Replacement Registry. J Shoulder Elbow Surg. 2018;27(10):1859–65.

34. Papadonikolakis A, Matsen FA. Metal-backed glenoid components have a higher rate of failure and fail by different modes in comparison with all-polyethylene components. J Bone Joint Surg. 2014;96(12):1041–7.

35. Sharplin PK, Frampton CMA, Hirner M. Cemented vs. uncemented glenoid fixation in total shoulder arthroplasty for osteoarthritis: a New Zealand Joint Registry study. J Shoulder Elbow Surg. 2020;29(10):2097–103.

36. Boileau P, Avidor C, Krishnan SG, Walch G, Kempf JF, Molé D. Cemented polyethylene versus uncemented metal-backed glenoid components in total shoulder arthroplasty: a prospective, double-blind, randomized study. J Shoulder Elbow Surg. 2002;11(4):351–9.

37. Castagna A, Garofalo R. Journey of the glenoid in anatomic total shoulder replacement. Shoulder Elbow. 2019;11(2):140–8.

38. Kim DM, Alabdullatif F, Aldeghaither M, Shin MJ, Kim H, Park D, et al. Do modern designs of metal-backed glenoid components show improved clinical results in total shoulder arthroplasty? A systematic review of the literature. Orthop J Sports Med. 2020;8(9):1–12.

39. Australian Orthopaedic Association. Australian Orthopaedic Association National Joint Replacement Registry (AOANJRR). Hip, knee & shoulder arthroplasty: 2020 annual report. Adelaide; 2020. p. 1–474.

40. Carpenter SR, Urits I, Murthi AM. Porous metals and alternate bearing surfaces in shoulder arthroplasty. Curr Rev Musculoskelet Med [Internet]. 2016;9(1):59–66. http://link.springer.com/10.1007/s12178-016-9319-x.

41. Voss A, Beitzel K, Obopilwe E, Buchmann S, Apostolakos J, Di Venere J, et al. No correlation between radiolucency and biomechanical stability of keeled and pegged glenoid components. BMC Musculoskelet Disord. 2017;18(1):213.

42. Welsher A, Gohal C, Madden K, Miller B, Bedi A, Alolabi B, et al. A comparison of pegged vs. keeled glenoid components regarding functional and radiographic outcomes in anatomic total shoulder arthroplasty: a systematic review and meta-analysis. JSES Open Access. 2019;3(3):136–144.e1.

43. Vavken P, Sadoghi P, von Keudell A, Rosso C, Valderrabano V, Müller AM. Rates of radiolucency and loosening after total shoulder arthroplasty with pegged or keeled glenoid components. J Bone Joint Surg Am. 2013;95(3):215–21.

44. Kilian CM, Press CM, Smith KM, O'Connor DP, Morris BJ, Elkousy HA, et al. Radiographic and clinical comparison of pegged and keeled glenoid components using modern cementing techniques: midterm results of a prospective randomized study. J Shoulder Elbow Surg. 2017;26(12):2078–85.

45. Khazzam M, Argo M, Landrum M, Box H. Comparison of pegged and keeled glenoid components for total shoulder arthroplasty. J Shoulder Elb Arthroplast. 2017;1:247154921770532.

46. Moulton SG, Cole EW, Gobezie R, Romeo AA, Lederman E, Denard PJ. Minimum 5-year outcomes of pegged versus keeled all-polyethylene glenoids. JSES Open Access [Internet]. 2019;3(4):292–295. https://doi.org/10.1016/j.jses.2019.09.006.

47. Edwards TB, Labriola JE, Stanley RJ, O'Connor DP, Elkousy HA, Gartsman GM. Radiographic comparison of pegged and keeled glenoid components using modern cementing techniques: a prospective randomized study. J Shoulder Elbow Surg. 2010;19(2):251–7.

48. Erickson BJ, Chalmers PN, Denard PJ, Gobezie R, Romeo AA, Lederman ES. Current state of short-stem implants in total shoulder arthroplasty: a systematic review of the literature. JSES Int [Internet]. 2020;4(1):114–9. https://doi.org/10.1016/j.jses.2019.10.112.

49. Matache BA, Lapner P. Anatomic shoulder arthroplasty: technical considerations. Open Orthop J [Internet]. 2017;11(1):1115–1125. https://openorthopaedicsjournal.com/VOLUME/11/PAGE/1115/.

50. Monir JG, Hao KA, Abeyewardene D, O'Keefe KJ, King JJ, Wright TW, et al. Extra-short humeral heads reduce glenohumeral joint overstuffing compared with short heads in anatomic total shoulder arthroplasty. JSES Int. 2022;6(2):209–15.

51. Sanchez-Sotelo J. Current concepts in humeral component design for anatomic and reverse shoulder arthroplasty. J Clin Med. 2021;10(21):5151.

Long-Term RSA Surgical Outcomes

17

Denny Tjiauw Tjoen Lie, Sheng Xu,
and Gerald Joseph Zeng

17.1 Introduction

Reverse shoulder arthroplasty (RSA) has come a long way since the introduction of the first model implant by Paul Grammont in 1985 [1] to the current Delta III reverse prosthesis in 1991 [2]. However, compared to other prosthesis such as total knee and total hip, the reverse shoulder prosthesis only obtained FDA approval in the USA in November 2003, thus limiting the amount of high-quality long-term outcome studies available in the English literature.

17.2 Chapter Overview

This chapter will provide a brief overview of the long-term outcomes of RSA, how outcomes are defined, what outcomes are commonly measured for RSA, and the newer definitions of outcomes. Indications for surgery and surgical approaches could affect long-term outcomes. These will also be discussed, as would some literature on implant survivorship and revision surgery.

17.3 Definition of Study Duration

In current literature, authors usually define their study duration (long-, mid-, or short-term) arbitrarily with a wide range of variation. In a recent systematic review by Ahmad et al., the mean follow-up of papers published in the six highest ranked orthopedic journals was studied, and it was concluded that the mean follow-up of a short-term, mid-term, and long-term study was 2.5 years, 5 years, and 12.5 years respectively [3].

17.4 Exploring Different Categories of Outcomes

17.4.1 Patient Reported Outcome Measures

There exist various ways of defining outcomes. Historically, outcomes were defined based on success or failure of surgery. These gradually evolved into assessment of patient reported outcome measures (PROMs). Absolute improvement in PROMs validate interventions for specific conditions and guide informed clinical decision-

D. T. T. Lie (✉)
Duke-National University of Singapore Medical School, Singapore, Singapore

Department of Orthopaedic Surgery, Singapore General Hospital, Singapore, Singapore
e-mail: denny.lie.t.t@singhealth.com.sg

S. Xu · G. J. Zeng
Department of Orthopaedic Surgery, Singapore General Hospital, Singapore, Singapore
e-mail: sheng.xu@mohh.com.sg;
gerald.zeng@mohh.com.sg

© ISAKOS 2023
A. D. Mazzocca et al. (eds.), *Shoulder Arthritis across the Life Span*,
https://doi.org/10.1007/978-3-031-33298-2_17

making as well as provision of patient-centered care [4]. They allow patients to make decisions about their own care based on evidence-based information and gave them quality assurance regarding their surgery [5]. The most utilized PROM in the literature measuring outcome after RSA is the Constant-Murley score (CMS). CMS is a 100-point scale divided into four subscales: pain, activities of daily living, strength, and range of motion, with a higher score signifying better quality of function. Improvement in CMS after RSA is well documented, with short- and medium-term score more than doubling in most literature [6–10], and this does not appear to be influenced by patient demographics such as age or gender [11]. In longer-term follow-up, the improvement in CMS is still significant; however, similar to ROM, many authors have reported a decrease in CMS from medium- to long-term follow-up. Bacle et al. [12] noted that CMS improved from 23 to 63 at mid-term follow-up; however this declined to 55 at 150 months. Favard et al. [13] also noted that CMS increased from 23.9 to 61.5 at 5 years; however there is a drop to 56.76 at 9 years. In the study by Guery et al. [7], 88% of patient had a CMS of more than 30 at 72 months follow-up; however this decreased to only 58% at 120 months. This decrease in CMS could be due to the decreased in ROM with time as previously described, which makes up 40 points in the 100-point scale. Along with PROMs, researchers also often assess for statistical significance in improvement of PROMs with p-value being the most common statistical tool used [14] (Table 17.1).

17.4.2 Evolving Concept of Outcomes (MCID, PASS)

However, in recent years, there has been a shift and new concepts of how outcomes are perceived have evolved. With more outcome scores being developed, there is high variability between each scoring system, which posed challenges in instituting practical guidelines in man-

Table 17.1 Long-term outcomes after reverse shoulder arthroplasty

Author	Year	Journal	Number of patients	Patient reported outcome measures
Bacle et al. [12]	2017	JBJS	84 patients, 87 prostheses	CMS improvement from 23 to 63 at mid-term but declined to 55 at 150 months (long term)
Guery et al. [7]	2006	JBJS	77 patients, 80 prostheses	Decline in number of patients with CMS > 30, from 88 to 58% as patients progressed from mid-term to long-term follow-up
Favard et al. [13]	2011	CORR	506 patients, 527 prostheses	CMS increase from 23.9 to 61.5 at 5 years, but dropped to 56.76 at 9 years

agement. Statistically significant improvements in scores were usually expected after undergoing RSA, but they may not necessarily translate into fulfillment of the patients' satisfaction and expectation.

The concept of threshold scores such as minimal clinically important difference (MCID) and patient acceptable symptomatic state (PASS) have been developed as newer methods for quantifying value in shoulder arthroplasty. MCID is defined as "the smallest difference in score in the domain of interest which patients perceive as beneficial and which would mandate, in the absence of troublesome side effects and excessive cost, a change in patient's management." by Jaeschke et al. [15] In evaluating 466 cases of either anatomy TSA or reverse TSA, Simovitch et al. [16] identified the anchor-based MCID results for various outcome measures, including CMS (5.7 ± 1.9). This meant that an improvement in CMS of 5.7 points was the minimum improvement necessary for patients to achieve a

Table 17.2 Recent concepts in defining outcomes

Concept	Definition	Study
Minimal clinically important difference (MCID)	Smallest difference in score perceived as beneficial and affecting patient's management	**Simovitch et al.** [16]: MCID of CMS (5.7 ± 1.9) Interpretation: Improvement in CMS of 5.7 points was the minimum improvement necessary for patients to achieve a result they believe is clinically meaningful, and was attained by more than 80% of patients
Patient acceptable symptomatic state (PASS)	Absolute threshold, beyond which patients consider themselves well and satisfied with treatment	**Chamberlain et al.** [17]: Visual Analog Scale (VAS) pain score, the Simple Shoulder Test (SST), and American Shoulder and Elbow Surgeons (ASES) score of 1.5, 8.4, and 76 considered acceptable symptomatic states

result they believe is clinically meaningful and was attained by more than 80% of patients. PASS is defined as the highest level of symptom beyond which a patient would consider himself to be well. Chamberlain et al. [17] performed a study on PASS in 2017 and found that patients treated with shoulder arthroplasty consider Visual Analog Scale (VAS) pain score, the Simple Shoulder Test (SST), and American Shoulder and Elbow Surgeons (ASES) score of 1.5, 8.4, and 76 to be acceptable symptomatic states. Similar studies on PASS, but for different PROMs, can be derived from existing literature, to evaluate efficacy of intervention (Table 17.2).

17.4.3 Range of Movement

One significant benefit of RSA is the improvement in range of motion (ROM) postoperatively [1, 2, 7, 10–13, 18], specifically active forward flexion. In short- and medium-term follow-up studies, most patients achieved significant improving in forward flexion. At a mean follow-up of 29.9 months of 240 prosthesis in 232 patients, Wall et al. [10] found that the mean forward flexion improved from 86° to 137°. At 48 months follow-up, Stechel et al. [9] found that forward flexion improved from 47° to 105°. The longest follow-up study by Bacle et al. [12] of 87 prostheses in 84 patients with a mean follow-up of 150 months showed that forward flexion improved from 81° to 131°. Improvement in external rotation after RSA is more varied in the literature, with Stechel et al. and Favard et al. [13] reporting an increase in active external rotation at short- and median-term follow-up, but this was not seen in the long-term follow-up studies reported by Bacle et al. [12] One significant contributor to postoperative external rotation is the state of the teres minor. Boileau et al. [6] reported that in patients with <50% fatty infiltration of teres minor, mean active external rotation was 15° compared to 0° in those with >50% fatty infiltration. Interestingly, Bacle et al. [12] also reported that although significant improvement in forward flexion was achieved at a mean follow-up of 150 months, there was a significant decrease from median-term follow-up. Favard et al. [13] also noted a time-dependent reduction in ROM in their group of patients from 5 to 9 years postoperatively. This gradual reduction in ROM could be a result of impairment of active deltoid power. In RSA, the lowered and medialized center of rotation lead to a non-physiological contraction-stretching cycle of the deltoid, and an aging muscle tissue could hinder its adaptation to repetitive contraction-stretching movements and decrease its motor performance [1, 2, 12]. Therefore, patients can expect a significant improvement in ROM (forward flexion) even 10 years after RSA; however, this will tend to decrease over time. In the same study by Simovitch et al. [16], improvement in active forward flexion of 12° ± 4° and active external rotation of 3° ± 2° constituted attainment of MCID (Table 17.3).

Table 17.3 Change in range of movement after reverse shoulder arthroplasty

Author	Year	Journal	Number of patients	Change in range of movement
Wall et al. [10]	2007	BJJ	232 patients, 240 prostheses	Mean forward flexion improved from 86° to 137 at 30 months
Stechel et al. [9]	2010	Acta Ortho	59 patients, 68 prostheses	Forward flexion improved from 47° to 105 at 48 months
Bacle et al. [12]	2017	JBJS	84 patients, 87 prostheses	Forward flexion improved from 81° to 131° at 150 months, but time-dependent reduction in ROM after
Favard et al. [13]	2011	CORR	506 patients, 527 prostheses	Forward flexion increased from 69 to 129 at 5 years, but time dependent reduction in ROM after

17.5 Indications for RSA as Predictors of Outcome

One significant influencer of long-term outcome after RSA is the indication for surgery. RSA for massive cuff tear with or without glenohumeral arthropathy and primary osteoarthritis appears to confer the best outcome [10, 12] and RSA for rheumatoid arthritis, fractures, and revision surgery having poorer outcome [6, 7, 9]. It is also a good option for patients with severe glenoid bone loss, such as from tumors [19]. Bacle et al. [12] found the highest absolute CMS in patients who underwent RSA for cuff arthropathy and primary osteoarthritis (63 ± 13 points and 62 ± 8 points, respectively), compared to those where RSA were performed for revision or posttraumatic arthritis (CMS of 45 points for both). Wall et al. [10] found that patients with posttraumatic arthritis or revision arthroplasty had worse preoperative Constant scores and worse active elevation compared to those with massive cuff tear with or without arthropathy and primary osteoarthritis,

leading them to conclude that, although patients with posttraumatic arthritis and revision arthroplasty had improvement of similar magnitudes in terms of shoulder motion and function, they did not achieve the same overall level of performance compared with the other patients.

17.6 Relative Indications for RSA Leads to Poorer Outcomes

Contraindications to RSA include known damage to the axillary nerve, a non-functional deltoid muscle, glenoid vault deficiency precluding baseplate fixation, ongoing infection, as well as neuropathic joints [20]. Lädermann et al. [21] studied 49 patients with impaired deltoid function who underwent RSA and found that while postoperative complication rate was significant at 18% (including two episodes of dislocation), preoperative deltoid impairment, in certain circumstances, was not an absolute contraindication to RSA, and majority of patients managed to do well postoperatively. Additionally, RSA should be performed with caution in patients with systemic inflammatory conditions, such as rheumatoid arthritis. In the study by Rittmeister et al. [22] of eight prosthesis in seven patients with rheumatoid arthritis, even though all patients experienced a significant improvement in function and CMS, complications occurred in six shoulders, with one septic loosening, two aseptic loosening, and three failed acromion osteosynthesis following the transacromial approach. Other than increased risk of infection in patients with rheumatoid arthritis, patients with rheumatoid arthritis often have poor bone stock which increased their risk of implant failure. Another distinction is that in patients with rheumatoid cuff arthropathy, there is often involvement of the infraspinatus and teres muscles besides the supraspinatus, leading to impaired external rotation postoperatively which will directly affect their CMS. Boileau et al. [6] reported a high rate of complications in their group of patients who underwent RSA for revision surgery, leading to a significantly lower

Constant scores compared with those with primary cuff arthropathy. This was attributed to the possibility that previous shoulder arthroplasty permanently altered shoulder function, deltoid power, and tuberosity malunion can interfere with prosthetic positioning, causing changes in biomechanical behavior and a faster decrease in functional outcome over time. Thus, although RSA can significantly improve outcome after fracture and revision, clinicians need to be aware of the potential difference in outcome in order to manage patient expectations.

17.7 Impact of Surgical Approach on Outcomes

Several authors have also described that different surgical approach can potentially affect outcome after RSA. Grammont originally described the transacromial approach but subsequently converted to a deltopectoral approach. Another commonly described approach is the superior transdeltoid approach. In theory, the superior transdeltoid approach can potentially lead to poorer outcome if the deltoid split resulted in excessive damage to the deltoid muscle or if there is excessive stripping of the deltoid, especially from acromion. Furthermore, exposure to the inferior glenoid may not be optimal in a transdeltoid approach, posing additional challenges to placing the glenoid component in the ideal position. In a comparative study between 35 RSA implanted via the superolateral approach and 30 in the deltopectoral approach by Melis et al. [18], a higher incidence of scapular notching was noted in the superolateral approach. Similarly, Wall et al. [10] also described a case of superior cut out and loosening of the glenoid component with the superior approach. This was likely attributed to the tendency to place the baseplate with superior tilt and higher on the glenoid when RSA was implanted via the superior transdeltoid approach. In the series by Boileau et al. [6], their technique was revised from a transdeltoid to a deltopectoral approach due to concerns regarding possible damage to the deltoid muscle, critical for this prosthesis, and access to the humeral diaphysis that was necessary in revision and fracture cases. Naveed et al. [8] also described a change in their technique from the superior deltoid split to deltopectoral approach due to difficulty in achieving good exposure of the inferior glenoid to place the baseplate on the glenoid as inferiorly as possible. Although the type of approach may potentially impact ease of prosthesis implantation, there appears to be no clear evidence in their influence on outcome. In the series by Sirveaux et al. [11] where superolateral approach was performed in 58 shoulders, deltopectoral in 16, and transacromial in 3, they found no difference in CMS at a mean follow-up of 44.5 months.

17.8 Survivorship

Long-term survival rate after RSA has been reported to be up to 89% at 10 years follow-up. The longest follow-up study by Bacle et al. [12] with a mean follow-up of 150 months reported a mean implant survival of 110.3 month with 93% survival probability at 120 months. In the largest follow-up study by Favard et al. [13] of 527 prostheses in 506 patients with a mean follow-up of 115 months, the implant survival was 89% at 120 months. Sirveaux et al. [11] and Guery et al. [7] also reported implant survival of 95.1% and 91% at 97 months and 120 months, respectively.

17.9 Revision Surgery

Revision rate after RSA is still relatively high, with figures quoted up to 12% in the literature [2, 7, 9–13, 18, 23, 24]. However, numerous studies have found that the peak incidence for revision is in the short-term follow-up period, with the incidence of revision dropping drastically after that [7, 12, 13, 25]. This is likely because the most common causes of revision were infection and mechanical failure which tend to occur in the early follow-up period. In the study by Bacle et al. [12], the revision rate was up to 12% at mean follow-up of 150 months; however, eight of these revisions occurred in the first 2 years and another eight after 2 years. The most common reason for revision in their series was infection which accounted for six cases of revision surgery in the first 2 years, and in those who required revision after 2 years, the most common cause was implant loosening. Guery et al. [7], Favard et al. [13], and Melis et al. [18] also reported that infection was the most common reason for revision surgery with a peak incidence before 3 years. Frankle et al. [23] reported a revision rate of 11.7% in 60 prostheses at an average of 21.4 months. In all cases that required revision surgery, inspection of the porous surface of the glenoid baseplate revealed no evidence of osseous ingrowth, leading them to conclude that a critical time-period for RSA was the first 2 years during which, if ingrowth did not occur, mechanical failure would result from metal fatigue in the screws.

Several factors can affect the long-term survival and revision rate after RSA. Compared to the original design by Grammont which has a glenosphere with threaded locking system, the Delta III prosthesis makes use of a glenosphere with Morse taper. Various authors have reported a high incidence of unscrewing of the glenosphere from the metaglene in the original system leading to reduced long-term survivorship. Sirveaux et al. [11] reported five cases of unscrewing of the glenosphere from the metaglene, with a higher incidence in the right shoulder. Guery et al. [7] reported three incidences of glenoid unscrewing, with all three patients having received the earlier version of the prosthesis. This is likely because in the original design, active forward flexion, especially in the right shoulder, produced a ratchet-like effect leading to high rate of unscrewing. When the glenosphere became loose, revision surgery could occasionally have been avoided by tightening the glenoid component. However, if this complication was not picked up in time, unscrewing of the glenosphere led to loosening which necessitated revision surgery (Table 17.4).

Table 17.4 Revision surgery in reverse shoulder arthroplasty

Author	Year	Journal	Number of patients	Revision rate
Bacle et al. [12]	2017	JBJS	84 patients, 87 prostheses	**Revision rate 12% (16 cases)** Most common reason for revision being infection (8 cases), followed by glenoid loosening (4 cases), humeral loosening (2 cases), dislocation (1 case), and wear (1 case)
Guery et al. [7]	2006	JBJS	77 patients, 80 prostheses	**Revision rate 10%.** Revision rate highest in the first 3 years, due to infection or malposition implant. RA has high risk of infection
Favard et al. [13]	2011	CORR	506 patients, 527 prostheses	**Revision rate 5%.** 12 prostheses removed for infection in the first 3 years, substantial peak in revision before 2 years
Melis et al. [18]	2011	BJJ	119 patients, 122 prostheses	**Revision rate 7% (9 of 122 cases).** 6 for infection, 1 for glenosphere unscrewing, 2 for glenoid loosening
Frankle et al. [23]	2005	JBJS	60 patients, 60 prostheses	**Revision rate 11.7%,** with critical time period for these device being the first 2 years, because if ingrowth does not occur, mechanical failure may result from metal fatigue

17.10 Conclusion

RSA has revolutionized the treatment of cuff arthropathy, which previously did not have a suitable solution. Patient reported outcome measures and patient satisfaction rates are high even after long-term follow-up, with the majority of patients experiencing improvement in pain scores and better function. Revision rates are high in the long term, and more longer-term studies are needed to validate the long-term efficacy of RSA.

References

1. Grammont PLJP. Etude et réalisation d'une nouvelle prothèse d'épaule. Rheumatologie. 1987;39: 27–38.
2. Boileau P, Watkinson DJ, Hatzidakis AM, Balg F. Grammont reverse prosthesis: design, rationale, and biomechanics. J Shoulder Elbow Surg. 2005;14(1 Suppl S):147S–61S. https://doi.org/10.1016/j.jse.2004.10.006.
3. Ahmad SS, Hoos L, Perka C, Stöckle U, Braun KF, Konrads C. Follow-up definitions in clinical orthopaedic research: a systematic review. Bone Jt Open. 2021;2(5):344–50. https://doi.org/10.1302/2633-1462.25.BJO-2021-0007.R1.
4. Gagnier JJ. Patient reported outcomes in orthopaedics. J Orthop Res. 2017;35(10):2098–108. https://doi.org/10.1002/jor.23604.
5. Foong WS, Zeng GJ, Goh GS, Hao Y, Lie DTT, Chang PCC. Determining the minimal clinically important difference on the Oxford shoulder instability score in patients undergoing arthroscopic Bankart repair for shoulder instability. Orthop J Sports Med. 2022;10(1):23259671211060024. https://doi.org/10.1177/23259671211060023.
6. Boileau P, Watkinson D, Hatzidakis AM, Hovorka I. Neer award 2005: the Grammont reverse shoulder prosthesis: results in cuff tear arthritis, fracture sequelae, and revision arthroplasty. J Shoulder Elbow Surg. 2006;15(5):527–40. https://doi.org/10.1016/j.jse.2006.01.003.
7. Guery J, Favard L, Sirveaux F, Oudet D, Mole D, Walch G. Reverse total shoulder arthroplasty. Survivorship analysis of eighty replacements followed for five to ten years. J Bone Joint Surg Am. 2006;88(8):1742–7. https://doi.org/10.2106/JBJS.E.00851.
8. Naveed MA, Kitson J, Bunker TD. The Delta III reverse shoulder replacement for cuff tear arthropathy: a single-centre study of 50 consecutive procedures. J Bone Joint Surg Br. 2011;93(1):57–61. https://doi.org/10.1302/0301-620X.93B1.24218.
9. Stechel A, Fuhrmann U, Irlenbusch L, Rott O, Irlenbusch U. Reversed shoulder arthroplasty in cuff tear arthritis, fracture sequelae, and revision arthroplasty. Acta Orthop. 2010;81(3):367–72. https://doi.org/10.3109/17453674.2010.487242.
10. Wall B, Nové-Josserand L, O'Connor DP, Edwards TB, Walch G. Reverse total shoulder arthroplasty: a review of results according to etiology. J Bone Joint Surg Am. 2007;89(7):1476–85. https://doi.org/10.2106/JBJS.F.00666.
11. Sirveaux F, Favard L, Oudet D, Huquet D, Walch G, Molé D. Grammont inverted total shoulder arthroplasty in the treatment of glenohumeral osteoarthritis with massive rupture of the cuff. Results of a multicentre study of 80 shoulders. J Bone Joint Surg Br. 2004;86(3):388–95. https://doi.org/10.1302/0301-620x.86b3.14024.
12. Bacle G, Nové-Josserand L, Garaud P, Walch G. Long-term outcomes of reverse total shoulder arthroplasty: a follow-up of a previous study. J Bone Joint Surg Am. 2017;99(6):454–61. https://doi.org/10.2106/JBJS.16.00223.
13. Favard L, Levigne C, Nerot C, Gerber C, De Wilde L, Mole D. Reverse prostheses in arthropathies with cuff tear: are survivorship and function maintained over time? Clin Orthop Relat Res. 2011;469(9):2469–75. https://doi.org/10.1007/s11999-011-1833-y.
14. Sierevelt IN, van Oldenrijk J, Poolman RW. Is statistical significance clinically important?—A guide to judge the clinical relevance of study findings. J Long Term Eff Med Implants. 2007;17(2):173–9. https://doi.org/10.1615/jlongtermeffmedimplants.v17.i2.100.
15. Jaeschke R, Singer J, Guyatt GH. Measurement of health status. Ascertaining the minimal clinically important difference. Control Clin Trials. 1989;10(4):407–15. https://doi.org/10.1016/0197-2456(89)90005-6.
16. Simovitch R, Flurin PH, Wright T, Zuckerman JD, Roche CP. Quantifying success after total shoulder arthroplasty: the minimal clinically important difference. J Shoulder Elbow Surg. 2018;27(2):298–305. https://doi.org/10.1016/j.jse.2017.09.013.
17. Chamberlain AM, Hung M, Chen W, et al. Determining the patient acceptable symptomatic state for the ASES, SST, and VAS pain after total shoulder arthroplasty. J Shoulder Elbow Arthroplasty. 2017;1:247154921772004. https://doi.org/10.1177/2471549217720042.
18. Melis B, DeFranco M, Lädermann A, et al. An evaluation of the radiological changes around the Grammont reverse geometry shoulder arthroplasty after eight to 12 years. J Bone Joint Surg Br. 2011;93(9):1240–6. https://doi.org/10.1302/0301-620X.93B9.25926.
19. Hyun YS, Huri G, Garbis NG, McFarland EG. Uncommon indications for reverse total shoulder arthroplasty. Clin Orthop Surg. 2013;5(4):243–55. https://doi.org/10.4055/cios.2013.5.4.243.

20. Familiari F, Rojas J, Nedim Doral M, Huri G, McFarland EG. Reverse total shoulder arthroplasty. EFORT Open Rev. 2018;3(2):58–69. https://doi.org/10.1302/2058-5241.3.170044.

21. Lädermann A, Walch G, Denard PJ, et al. Reverse shoulder arthroplasty in patients with pre-operative impairment of the deltoid muscle. Bone Joint J. 2013;95-B(8):1106–13. https://doi.org/10.1302/0301-620X.95B8.31173.

22. Rittmeister M, Kerschbaumer F. Grammont reverse total shoulder arthroplasty in patients with rheumatoid arthritis and nonreconstructible rotator cuff lesions. J Shoulder Elbow Surg. 2001;10(1):17–22. https://doi.org/10.1067/mse.2001.110515.

23. Frankle M, Siegal S, Pupello D, Saleem A, Mighell M, Vasey M. The reverse shoulder prosthesis for glenohumeral arthritis associated with severe rotator cuff deficiency. A minimum two-year follow-up study of sixty patients. J Bone Joint Surg Am. 2005;87(8):1697–705. https://doi.org/10.2106/JBJS.D.02813.

24. Werner CML, Steinmann PA, Gilbart M, Gerber C. Treatment of painful pseudoparesis due to irreparable rotator cuff dysfunction with the Delta III reverse-ball-and-socket total shoulder prosthesis. J Bone Joint Surg Am. 2005;87(7):1476–86. https://doi.org/10.2106/JBJS.D.02342.

25. Baker BA. Efficacy of age-specific high-intensity stretch-shortening contractions in reversing dynapenia, sarcopenia, and loss of skeletal muscle quality. J Funct Morphol Kinesiol. 2018;3(2):36. https://doi.org/10.3390/jfmk3020036.

Strategies to Improve Function in Reverse Total Shoulder Arthroplasty (RTSA): Glenoid-Shaft Angle and Lateralization

Joseph P. DeAngelis

As discussed throughout this edition, the shoulder relies on a careful balance of stability and mobility, and while an anatomic total shoulder arthroplasty aims to reproduce normal shoulder kinematics, the reverse total shoulder arthroplasty (RTSA) is a non-anatomic procedure. It draws on a partially constrained design to empower the deltoid and the intact elements of the shoulder girdle to move the humerus around a fixed point, the glenosphere. When the treatment of rotator cuff tear arthropathy was revolutionized by Grammont's design, the mechanical effect of his design increased the deltoid's moment arm by 42% [1]. In time, modern reverse designs have maintained the essential elements of his approach to maintain the joint's stability, while simultaneously seeking a more anatomic position for the resulting shoulder joint to minimize complications and maximize range of motion (external rotation).

The normal inclination of the proximal humerus, or neck-shaft angle (NSA), is approximately 135°. However, person-to-person variability can range from 115 to 148°. When studied, approximately 22% of patients will have a NSA less than 130° or greater than 140°, so careful consideration needs to address the native anatomy and the intended surgical result [2]. The Grammont design had a fixed, 155-degree NSA

and enhanced the deltoid moment arm by moving the humerus inferior or distal [3]. This change in position made the deltoid more powerful in forward elevation and abduction, while shifting center of rotation medially [4]. Grammont achieved success in his design by moving the center of rotation (COR) medial to the interface between the baseplate and glenoid [5].

This change in the COR created a stable foundation for the reverse total shoulder by minimizing sheer and promoting the compression necessary for osteointegration. When combined with a 155-degree angle on the humeral prostheses, these technical considerations addressed the intrinsic disability of rotator cuff arthropathy as long as the glenosphere was placed inferior on the glenoid face and the humeral implant did not impinge.

However, these design choices also result in significant changes to the physiologic function of the shoulder's muscular supports. The anterior deltoid, the posterior deltoid, and the pectoralis major are more easily recruited as flexors and abductors, improving a patient's ability to lift the arm. The latissimus dorsi, teres major, and lower part of the pectoralis major have an increased ability to serve in adduction and extension. This change results in a corresponding decrease in their effect on both internal and external rotation [6, 7]. In patients with Grammont-style RSA, the anterior and posterior rotator cuff are weakened by medialization, limiting their active internal and external rotation [8, 9].

J. P. DeAngelis (✉)
Beth Israel Deaconess Medical Center/Harvard Medical Center, Boston, MA, USA
e-mail: jpdeange@bidmc.harvard.edu

© ISAKOS 2023
A. D. Mazzocca et al. (eds.), *Shoulder Arthritis across the Life Span*,
https://doi.org/10.1007/978-3-031-33298-2_18

In time, the medialization intrinsic to the traditional Grammont design was associated with high rates of scapular notching and concern for baseplate micro-motion, osteolysis, and potential glenoid loosening [10, 11]. This concern combined with the observation that more notching was associated with worse clinical outcomes [12–15]. To address the concerns associated with the traditional design, lateralized implants have been developed to improve the characteristics of the glenoid component, the humeral stem, or both [16].

Lateralized glenoid components employ modern materials to create a stable implant-bone interface with a COR that is lateral to the surface of the glenoid. This modification preserves rotational moment arms of the subscapularis and teres minor and enhances the active range of motion in the axial plane [17]. While the joint's COR needs to be more medial than the native, lateralization of the glenosphere from the glenoid enhances the compressive forces at the bone-implant interface and may overcome the shear forces that result from lateralization [18].

As a result, lateralized components have been shown to decrease the impingement between the scapular neck and the humeral prosthesis that results in notching. In a systematic review of 13 studies, the incidence of scapular notching was 5.4% in a lateralized glenoid group compared to 44.9% in a traditional group ($p < 0.001$) [19]. At the same time, patients with a lateralized prosthesis demonstrated more active external rotation ($46°$ vs. $24°$, $p < 0.001$). In contrast, clinically significant glenoid loosening was found in 1.8% of the traditional compared to 8.8% in the lateralized group ($p = 0.003$), raising questions of the sheer stress associated with lateralization. When one lateralized design was compared to a Grammont-style prosthesis, the same disparity was confirmed; glenoid loosening occurred in 5.8% of lateralized implants compared to 2.5% [20]. In the lab, lateralized implants have increased micromotion with a lateralized design, acknowledging that lateralization can be achieved through the implant's design or with bone grafting and/or bone augmentation of the glenoid [18].

With the ongoing evolution of reverse total shoulder designs, there may be a lag in the maturation of the data available regarding implant behavior. In a 2019 systematic review that included 103 studies, there was no difference in the rate of aseptic loosening for lateralized and medialized glenoids (1.84% vs. 1.15%, respectively) [21]. Correspondingly, patient outcomes were similar for the two designs in a 2018 review, despite a difference in external rotation (lateralized greater than Grammont) and a difference in scapular notching (Grammont greater than lateralized) [22].

In considering the relevant equivalence of the two designs' results, the debate remains unresolved. The Grammont design medializes the center of rotation, creating a compressive force at the implant-bone interface that may improve the glenoid fixation and implant longevity. Conversely, lateralized designs decrease the incidence of scapular notching and may improve external rotation.

Changes to the humeral component have been introduced to maximize the compression on the glenoid component while increasing the mechanical advantage of a lateralized center of rotation. While $155°$ is the most common humeral shaft angle, the horizontal cut may increase the impingement [23–26]. A reduced neck-shaft angle aims to reduce scapular notching, but it may increase the rate of dislocation [3].

In biomechanical studies, a decreased shaft angle will increase the range of motion, while decreasing the potential for contact with the inferior angle of the glenoid [27]. A recent meta-analysis of 2222 shoulders undergoing RTSA compared the rate of scapula notching and dislocation between implants with different neck-shaft angles [28]. While only 20% of the implants included had a neck-shaft angle of $135°$, scapular notching was found to be more common with a 155-degree implant (16.80%) than a 135-degree prosthesis (2.83%) ($p < 0.01$). There was no significant difference in dislocation rate between the two groups (2.33% and 1.74%, respectively). However, lateralization alone has been shown to decrease scapular notching, even with a 155-degree prosthesis, so the neck-shaft angle may not be the salient implant characteristic [29].

When the impact of neck-shaft angle on range of motion was examined, a similar meta-analysis revealed that a 135-degree prosthesis achieved greater external rotation ($33°$) than the 155-degree alternative (25°) ($p < 0.01$) [30]. In this way, modification to the humeral designs that lower the neck-shaft angle may reduce scapula notching and increase external rotation. How this adjustment should be combined with the lateralization of the glenoid component and the risk of loosening warrants further investigation, particularly if the risk of scapula fracture is included in the broader analysis of a patient's expected clinical result (Figs. 18.1 and 18.2; Table 18.1).

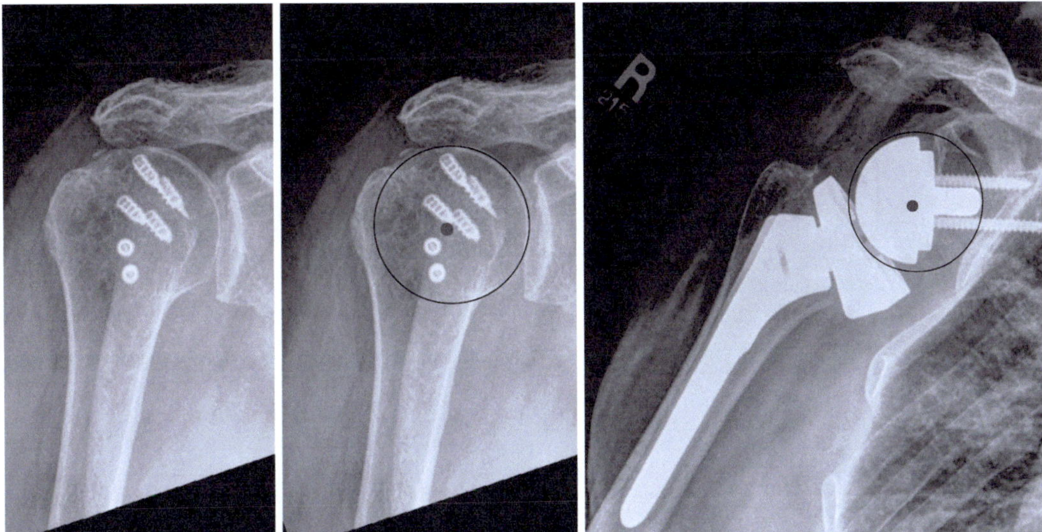

Fig. 18.1 Grammont-style prosthesis. Left—AP radiograph of a right shoulder in a patient with rotator cuff arthropathy. Center—The center of rotation relative lies in the center of the humeral head. Right—After a Grammont-style reverse total shoulder, the center of rotation is offset medially and distally

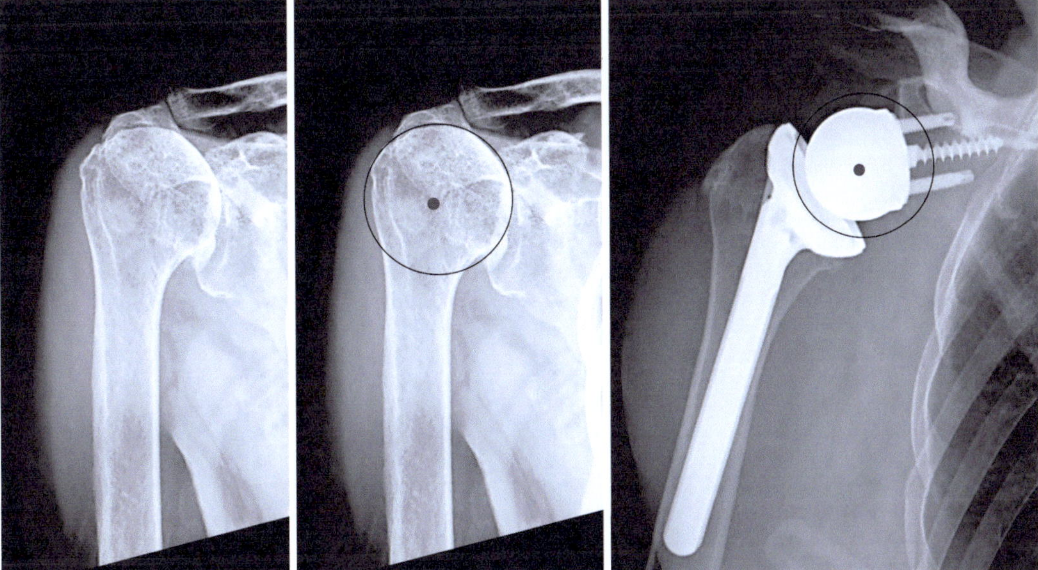

Fig. 18.2 Lateralized prosthesis. Left—AP radiograph of a right shoulder in a patient with rotator cuff arthropathy. Center—The center of rotation relative lies in the center of the humeral head. Right—After a lateralized reverse total shoulder, the center of rotation is moved laterally

Table 18.1 Methods for affecting lateralization in a reverse total shoulder arthroplasty

Glenoid	
Frankle-style glenosphere	Non-hemispherical design moves the center of rotation lateral
Bone grafting/bone augmentation of glenoid	Increased bone stock places the baseplate more lateral
Augmented-metal baseplates	Metal augment lateralizes the position of the baseplate
Lateralized baseplate	Thickness of the baseplate increases the lateral offset
Humerus	
Decreased neck-shaft angle	Moves the humeral shaft lateral rather than distal
Humeral tray/adaptor	Increases the offset of the humeral component
Humeral stem design	Curved and onlay stems

References

1. Kontaxis A, Johnson GR. The biomechanics of reverse anatomy shoulder replacement: a modelling study. Clin Biomech (Bristol, Avon). 2009;24:254–60.
2. Jeong J, Bryan J, Iannotti JP. Effect of a variable prosthetic neck-shaft angle and the surgical technique on replication of normal humeral anatomy. J Bone Joint Surg Am. 2009;91-A:1932–41.
3. Boileau P, Watkinson DJ, Hatzidakis AM, Balg F. Grammont reverse prosthesis: design, rationale, and biomechanics. J Shoulder Elbow Surg. 2005;14:147S–61S.
4. Schwartz DG, Kang SH, Lynch TS, et al. The anterior deltoid's importance in reverse shoulder arthroplasty: a cadaveric biomechanical study. J Shoulder Elbow Surg. 2013;22:357–64.
5. Grammont PM, Baulot E. Delta shoulder prosthesis for rotator cuff rupture. Orthopedics. 1993;16:65–8.
6. Ackland DC, Richardson M, Pandy MG. Axial rotation moment arms of the shoulder musculature after reverse total shoulder arthroplasty. J Bone Joint Surg Am. 2012;94-A:1886–95.
7. Ackland DC, Roshan-Zamir S, Richardson M, Pandy MG. Moment arms of the shoulder musculature after reverse total shoulder arthroplasty. J Bone Joint Surg Am. 2010;92-A:1221–30.
8. Herrmann S, König C, Heller M, Perka C, Greiner S. Reverse shoulder arthroplasty leads to significant biomechanical changes in the remaining rotator cuff. J Orthop Surg Res. 2011;6:42.
9. Simovitch RW, Helmy N, Zumstein MA, Gerber C. Impact of fatty infiltration of the teres minor muscle on the outcome of reverse total shoulder arthroplasty. J Bone Joint Surg Am. 2007;89-A:934–9.
10. Werner CML, Steinmann PA, Gilbart M, Gerber C. Treatment of painful pseudoparesis due to irreparable rotator cuff dysfunction with the Delta III reverse-ball-and-socket total shoulder prosthesis. J Bone Joint Surg Am. 2005;87:1476–86.
11. Roche CP, Stroud NJ, Martin BL, et al. The impact of scapular notching on reverse shoulder glenoid fixation. J Shoulder Elbow Surg. 2013;22:963–70.
12. Mollon B, Mahure SA, Roche CP, Zuckerman JD. Impact of scapular notching on clinical outcomes after reverse total shoulder arthroplasty: an analysis of 476 shoulders. J Shoulder Elbow Surg. 2017;26:1253–61.
13. Wellmann M, Struck M, Pastor MF, Gettmann A, Windhagen H, Smith T. Short and midterm results of reverse shoulder arthroplasty according to the preoperative etiology. Arch Orthop Trauma Surg. 2013;133:463–71.
14. Simovitch RW, Zumstein MA, Lohri E, Helmy N, Gerber C. Predictors of scapular notching in patients managed with the Delta III reverse total shoulder replacement. J Bone Joint Surg Am. 2007;89:588–600.
15. Sirveaux F, Favard L, Oudet D, Huquet D, Walch G, Molé D. Grammont inverted total shoulder arthroplasty in the treatment of glenohumeral osteoarthritis with massive rupture of the cuff: results of a multicentre study of 80 shoulders. J Bone Joint Surg Br. 2004;86:388–95.
16. Werthel J-D, Walch G, Vegehan E, Deransart P, Sanchez-Sotelo J, Valenti P. Lateralization in reverse shoulder arthroplasty: a descriptive analysis of different implants in current practice. Int Orthop. 2019;43:2349–60.
17. Greiner S, Schmidt C, König C, Perka C, Herrmann S. Lateralized reverse shoulder arthroplasty maintains rotational function of the remaining rotator cuff. Clin Orthop Relat Res. 2013;471:940–6.
18. Harman M, Frankle M, Vasey M, Banks S. Initial glenoid component fixation in 'reverse' total shoulder arthroplasty: a biomechanical evaluation. J Shoulder Elbow Surg. 2005;14:162S–7S.
19. Lawrence C, Williams GR, Namdari S. Influence of glenosphere design on outcomes and complications of reverse arthroplasty: a systematic review. Clin Orthop Surg. 2016;8:288–97.
20. Zumstein MA, Pinedo M, Old J, Boileau P. Problems, complications, reoperations, and revisions in reverse total shoulder arthroplasty: a systematic review. J Shoulder Elbow Surg. 2011;20:146–57.
21. Rojas J, Choi K, Joseph J, Srikumaran U, McFarland EG. Aseptic glenoid baseplate loosening after reverse total shoulder arthroplasty: a systematic review and meta-analysis. JBJS Rev. 2019;7:e7.
22. Helmkamp JK, Bullock GS, Amilo NR, et al. The clinical and radiographic impact of center of rotation lateralization in reverse shoulder arthroplasty: a systematic review. J Shoulder Elbow Surg. 2018;27:2099–107.
23. Wall B, Nové-Josserand L, O'Connor DP, Edwards TB, Walch G. Reverse total shoulder arthroplasty: a

review of results according to etiology. J Bone Joint Surg Am. 2007;89:1476–85.

24. De Biase CF, Delcogliano M, Borroni M, Castagna A. Reverse total shoulder arthroplasty: radiological and clinical result using an eccentric glenosphere. Musculoskelet Surg. 2012;96:S27–34.

25. Sayana MK, Kakarala G, Bandi S, Wynn-Jones C. Medium term results of reverse total shoulder replacement in patients with rotator cuff arthropathy. Ir J Med Sci. 2009;178:147–50.

26. Young AA, Smith MM, Bacle G, Moraga C, Walch G. Early results of reverse shoulder arthroplasty in patients with rheumatoid arthritis. J Bone Joint Surg Am. 2011;93:1915–23.

27. Oh JH, Shin S-J, McGarry MH, Scott JH, Heckmann N, Lee TQ. Biomechanical effects of humeral neck-shaft angle and subscapularis integrity in reverse total shoulder arthroplasty. J Shoulder Elbow Surg. 2014;23:1091–8.

28. Erickson BJ, Frank RM, Harris JD, Mall N, Romeo AA. The influence of humeral head inclination in reverse total shoulder arthroplasty: a systematic review. J Shoulder Elbow Surg. 2015;24:988–93.

29. Boileau P, Moineau G, Roussanne Y, O'Shea K. Bony increased-offset reversed shoulder arthroplasty: minimizing scapular impingement while maximizing glenoid fixation. Clin Orthop Relat Res. 2011;469:2558–67.

30. Erickson BJ, Harris JD, Romeo AA. The effect of humeral inclination on range of motion in reverse total shoulder arthroplasty: a systematic review. Am J Orthop (Belle Mead NJ). 2016;45:E174–9.

Periprosthetic Humerus Fractures After Shoulder Arthroplasty

Casey L. Wright, Maria A. Theodore, Richard Smith, and Evan A. O'Donnell

Periprosthetic humerus fractures adjacent to shoulder arthroplasty pose a challenging problem for orthopaedic surgeons and patients alike. Recent decades have seen a substantial increase in the prevalence of shoulder arthroplasty, which increased by approximately 730% between 1995 and 2017 [1]. In 2017, approximately 2% of the population over the age of 80 was living with a shoulder arthroplasty. As the prevalence of shoulder arthroplasty increases, so too does the population at risk of periprosthetic complications. Although overall complication rates may be downtrending with improvements in surgical technique and implant design [2, 3], estimates of the complication rates of anatomic and reverse total shoulder arthroplasty are variable and may be as high as 25% [3–6]. Complications include instability, periprosthetic fracture, infection, implant loosening, neurologic injury, acromial or scapular spine fracture, hematoma, deltoid injury, rotator cuff injury, and venous thromboembolism. Periprosthetic humerus fractures account for approximately 20% of all complications, with the majority of fractures occurring intraopera-

tively [3, 7]. Fractures are significantly more likely to occur in cases of reverse (OR 4.01) [3, 8] and revision arthroplasty (RR 2.8) [9, 10]; the prevalence of both of which can be expected to increase in coming years.

While humeral shaft fractures in the absence of an implant demonstrate reliable healing, periprosthetic fractures are associated with greater rates of nonunion [11, 12]. The presence of a prosthesis may disrupt endosteal blood supply, cause persistent distraction at the fracture site, and alter the mechanical environment at the fracture by altering glenohumeral joint motion [11, 13]. Patient factors predisposing to fracture, such as medical comorbidities in the aging population, rheumatoid arthritis, and osteopenia, may also hinder healing [13]. Further complicating shared decision-making among patients and surgeons is the relative lack of evidence-based guidance on management of periprosthetic humerus fractures, with most recommendations limited to expert opinion and small case series [12].

19.1 Classification Schemes

Several classification schemes for periprosthetic humerus fractures have been proposed, primarily based on fracture location. Successive classification systems have attempted to improve the utility of fracture classification in guiding management by incorporating factors such as

C. L. Wright · R. Smith · E. A. O'Donnell (✉)
Department of Orthopaedic Surgery, Massachusetts General Hospital, Boston, MA, USA
e-mail: clwright@partners.org; rsmith21@partners.org; eodonnell4@partners.org

M. A. Theodore
Harvard College, Cambridge, MA, USA
e-mail: mtheodore@college.harvard.edu

© ISAKOS 2023
A. D. Mazzocca et al. (eds.), *Shoulder Arthritis across the Life Span*,
https://doi.org/10.1007/978-3-031-33298-2_19

fracture pattern, available bone stock, and implant loosening. Only the most recent classification schemes, which were developed after the widespread adoption of reverse, short-stem, and stemless implants, consider implant design.

One of the most widely accepted periprosthetic humerus fracture classification schemes was proposed by Wright and Cofield in 1995, which utilized the tip of the implant as a reference point (Fig. 19.1) [14]. Wright and Cofield Type A and B fractures both originate at the tip of the stem, with Type A fractures demonstrating proximal extension greater than one-third the length of the stem, Type B fractures extending proximally to a lesser extent, and Type C fractures located entirely distal to the stem.

In 1998, Campbell et al. classified fractures based on the *anatomic* location of the fracture [15]. Fractures are classified based on their location within the greater and/or lesser tuberosities (region 1), metaphysis (region 2), proximal diaphysis (region 3), or mid- to distal humeral diaphysis (region 4).

Similar to the original Wright and Cofield classification, Worland et al. proposed a classification scheme centered around the location of the fracture relative to the stem, with a subclassification based on fracture pattern and stability of the implant [16]. In the Worland classification, Type A fractures involve the tuberosities, Type B occur at the level of the stem, and Type C occur distal to the implant. Type B fractures are further subdivided into spiral fractures (Type B1), oblique fractures near the stem tip (Type B2), and fractures associated with an unstable implant (Type B3). Such subclassification is designed to reduce the ambiguity in treatment of Type B fractures, as Type B2 can typically be treated nonoperatively and Type B3 fractures should be managed surgically.

In 2008, Groh et al. developed a classification scheme for both intra- and postoperative fractures, utilizing the stem as a reference point, which could guide management [17]. Type I fractures exist entirely proximal to the stem tip and are amenable to cerclage if occurring intraoperatively. Type II fractures, which extend distal to the stem tip, and Type III fractures, occurring entirely distal to the stem, are amenable to cerclage and conversion to a long-stem prosthesis when occurring intraoperatively. When occurring postoperatively, Type III fractures involving a stable implant are amenable to a trial of nonoperative management.

The above classification schemes have demonstrated only moderate inter-observer agreement, with Fleiss' kappa values between 0.483 (Groh classification) and 0.583 (Wright and Cofield classification) for fracture classification and in guiding management [18]. Fractures of the humeral diaphysis at or proximal to the stem tip, including Wright and Cofield Type A, Campbell Region 3, Worland Type B, and Groh Type II fractures, present a significant challenge to surgeons evidenced by variability in preferred management. The variability could result from degree of fracture displacement, implant instability, and/or remaining bone stock, which are not well-accounted for in the available classification schemes, as well as surgeon preference.

Recently, Kirchoff et al. proposed a more comprehensive classification system and treatment algorithm inclusive of some of these factors

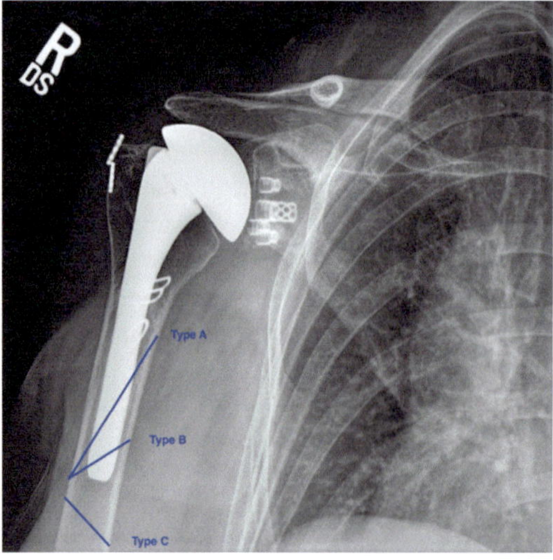

Fig. 19.1 AP X-ray of the right shoulder with an anatomic total shoulder replacement. Lines demonstrate the Wright and Cofield fracture classification. Type A fractures originate at the stem tip and extend proximally greater than one-third the length of the stem. Type B fractures originate at the stem tip and extend proximally to a lesser extent. Type C fractures occur distal to the stem tip

[19]. The system takes into consideration the type of prosthesis (anatomic, stemless, reverse), anatomic fracture location (acromion, glenoid, humerus), location of the fracture in relation to the implant, presence of a glenoid prosthesis, integrity of the rotator cuff, and implant stability. In a subsequent retrospective validation study, they found high inter-rater reliability between two board-certified trauma surgeons (Cohen's kappa of 0.94) with the sole discrepancy resulting from disagreement classifying a stem as loose or stable [20]. Eighty-four percent of the fractures were treated in accordance with the proposed treatment algorithm and 94% of these cases (15 of 16) had a good outcome. Conversely, in all three cases in which the surgeon deviated from the proposed treatment, the patient experienced a poor outcome.

To date, however, no classification scheme has been universally adopted. The lack of a standardized classification system hinders both the creation of larger data repositories on periprosthetic humerus fractures and the development of management guidelines.

19.2 Risk Factors

Proximal humerus periprosthetic fractures are best considered in two broad groups, intra- and postoperative, each of which has its own risk factor profile, management options, and clinical outcomes.

Intraoperative periprosthetic humerus fractures largely occur during implant removal in revision cases (up to 81%), during reaming and broaching (up to 31%), during trialing or implant insertion (up to 19%), or due to excessive torque or retraction (up to 13–15%) [10, 15, 21, 22]. Risk factors include both modifiable and non-modifiable patient factors, including female sex (RR 3.3 [9]–4.19 [23]), post-traumatic arthritis (RR 1.9 [9]–2.55 [23]) [15, 21], instability (RR 2.65 [10]), osteoporosis [14, 15, 23, 24], and rheumatoid arthritis [13, 14, 25–27]; implant factors, such as the use of press-fit stems (RR 2.9 [9]) or prior hemiarthroplasties in revision cases (OR 2.34 [10]); and surgical factors, such as revision cases (RR 2.8 [9]). Revision cases pose a particular challenge due to the scar tissue encountered during the approach, the need to remove the previous implant, and stress shielding of the greater tuberosity in uncemented and diaphyseal-fitting stems [15, 22]. Excessive scar tissue may necessitate increased torque to obtain adequate exposure, whereas stress shielding predisposes the tuberosities to fracture.

A comprehensive understanding of a patient's risk factors for periprosthetic fracture is imperative to pre-operative planning and informed consent discussions. In high-risk patients, the possible need for intraoperative fixation or conversion to reverse total shoulder arthroplasty should be discussed preoperatively. Surgeons may also ensure additional equipment, such as cerclage wires, plates, screws, long-stem implants, reverse components, and cement, are available.

Several mitigation techniques exist to reduce the risk of intraoperative fracture and start with patient positioning. The patient should be positioned to allow for full extension and adduction of the humerus, which allows for adequate humeral canal preparation without levering of the distal humerus. Surgeons should ensure adequate capsular release, especially in cases of severe osteoarthritis, significant medial glenoid wear, and revision cases with soft tissue contracture, to allow for adequate exposure without excessive torque on the humerus. The humerus is at particular risk of fracture due to torque and excessive external rotation during initial dislocation and glenoid preparation. Appreciating pre-existing humeral deformity in the case of post-traumatic arthritis or revision surgery is important to ensure a correct entry point and trajectory for reaming, avoiding perforation. Intraoperative fluoroscopy may be useful to plan and confirm the appropriate positioning of reamer, broaches, or implants. Overzealous reaming and endosteal notching predispose to both intra- and postoperative fractures by creating a stress riser at the tip of the implant stem. Hand reaming is particularly useful in mitigating this risk, especially in osteoporotic bone in which it allows for compression of cancellous bone. Finally, appropriate preoperative templating may mitigate the risk of fracture associated with underreaming and placement of an oversized prosthesis. Intraoperative radiographs taken prior to leaving the OR are useful in identifying unrecognized fractures or risk factors for postoperative periprosthetic fracture.

In revision cases, implant removal and disruption of the bone-implant or cement-implant interface may result in significant bone loss and is typically associated with fractures involving the greater tuberosity. The greater tuberosity is at particular risk with metaphyseal-filling ingrowth stems or cemented stems with proximal fins, which result in significant proximal bone loss during removal. Preventative measures include utilization of implant-specific removal devices and decreasing the force necessary to remove the implant by performing a corticotomy [22].

Some surgeons utilize prophylactic placement of heavy, nonabsorbable sutures or cerclage wires around the tuberosities or metaphysis. This may be especially useful in patients at high risk of fracture during stem removal, reaming, or insertion, including those with a thin greater tuberosity.

The vast majority of postoperative fractures occur after a fall [13, 14, 16, 23] or through an area of cortical weakening due to a stress riser or prosthetic loosening [14, 23]. Risk factors for postoperative fractures include osteonecrosis and increased Charlson medical comorbidity index [28]. Generally, postoperative fractures occur at the tip of the stem or cement mantle. However, with short-stem or canal-sparing implants, fractures may involve the tuberosities and proximal humeral shafts.

19.3 Patient Evaluation

Evaluation of patients with periprosthetic humeral fractures involves a thorough history, physical examination, and radiographic evaluation. A thorough history should elicit the mechanism of injury, risk factors for periprosthetic fracture as detailed above, and review of prior operative reports. Review of operative reports should note the preoperative diagnosis and implants used. Notes should also be made of any prior complications and revision surgeries. During the physical examination, it is imperative

to note neurovascular status particularly of the axillary and radial nerves, as well as distal perfusion, as revision shoulder arthroplasty and open reduction and internal fixation (ORIF) of periprosthetic fractures are higher risk operations for neurovascular complication.

X-rays of the shoulder (AP, true AP (Grashey), scapular Y, and axillary views) and full-length humerus (AP and lateral) should be assessed for previous implant, implant loosening, stress shielding, available bone stock, fracture pattern, and any pre-existing humeral deformity. Metal suppression CT is useful for assessing remaining bone stock, implant stability, fracture pattern, glenoid version, and rotator cuff integrity [29]. Axial imaging also aids the surgeon in planning the feasibility and trajectory of possible "skive" screws, or bicortical non-locking screws angled to skirt around the implant, in cases of planned ORIF.

19.4 Management and Outcomes

Management of periprosthetic humeral fractures is dependent on several factors including timing of fracture (intraoperative vs postoperative); implant type and stability; fracture location and morphology; and patient factors, such as bone quality, rotator cuff integrity, and medical comorbidities. Treatment options vary and include nonoperative treatment, open reduction, and internal fixation and revision arthroplasty. The goals of fracture management are pain relief, early range of motion, preservation of shoulder function, and promotion of fracture union while maintaining implant stability.

19.5 Intraoperative Fractures

Management of intraoperative fractures is highly dependent on fracture location. Metaphyseal, calcar, and proximal humeral diaphyseal fractures are generally amenable to bypassing the fracture by two [23] to three [15] cortical diameters with either a standard-length or long-stem prosthesis, with supplemental cerclage, tape/suture, and plate and screw fixation as needed. Tuberosity fractures may be managed with transosseous suture fixation to secure the rotator cuff attachments, with or without screw augmentation. If unable to attain stable fixation, conversion to a fracture or revision stem may improve stability by improving proximal ingrowth and providing more options for fixation through the stem. In cases in which there is persistent inability to attain stable fixation, conversion to a reverse arthroplasty may be necessary.

Intraoperative shaft fractures can similarly be managed with conversion to a longer-stemmed prosthesis, bypassing the fracture site by at least two cortical diameters. Placement of cement in the distal canal to engage the tip of the prosthesis may improve stability. When a fracture is sustained prior to cementation, it is imperative to prevent cement from escaping through the fracture site, which can impede healing and result in nerve injury. If a fracture occurs after cementation and the stem is determined to be stable, plate fixation may avoid the risk of fracture propagation and increased morbidity associated with stem removal [11]. If unable to bypass the fracture site by a sufficient length or in the setting of severe osteopenia, additional fracture fixation with cerclage cables, suture fixation, plate and screw fixation, and/or strut allograft is advisable. Supplementary fixation allows for earlier range of motion and higher union rates [11, 15].

In their report of intraoperative fractures, Athwal and colleagues noted all fractures demonstrated radiographic healing at a mean of 17 weeks postoperatively (range, 6–56 weeks) [9]. Non-displaced greater tuberosity fractures healed at a mean of 6.5 weeks, whereas displaced tuberosity fractures healed at a mean of 13.5 weeks. Humeral shaft fractures healed at a mean of 22.5 weeks.

19.6 Postoperative Fractures

19.6.1 Nonoperative Management

Many surgeons advocate for a trial of nonoperative management for postoperative shaft fractures in acceptable alignment without evidence of implant loosening [17, 23, 25, 30]. Acceptable alignment is generally defined as less than 20 degrees of flexion/extension, 15–20 degrees of rotation and 30 degrees of varus/valgus deformity [11, 31, 32]. Long oblique and spiral fractures are most amenable to nonoperative treatment [14], unless overlapping a significant portion of the stem compromising implant stability. Nonoperative management generally involves immobilization with a shoulder immobilizer, cast, or Sarmiento brace, depending on the fracture location.

Although many authors advocate for a trial of nonoperative management, it is important to understand the low success and high complication rates associated with nonoperative treatment (Table 19.1) [13–17, 23, 25, 33–36]. A recent systematic review of management of periprosthetic humerus fractures found a 50% failure rate of nonoperative treatment [12]. Of the 32 patients identified in their study who were treated entirely nonoperatively, 10 (31%) developed complications including malunion/nonunion, radial nerve palsy, shoulder stiffness, and skin necrosis from the orthosis.

19.6.2 Open Reduction and Internal Fixation

Indications for fracture fixation include failure of nonoperative management for a humeral shaft fracture surrounding a stable implant and tuberosity fracture near a hemiarthroplasty or anatomic total shoulder arthroplasty [37]. Failure of nonoperative treatment can be assumed when there is failure to maintain adequate reduction or there is nonunion of an unstable fracture after at least 3 months of attempted nonoperative management [11, 23]. Transverse and short oblique fractures are more likely to fail nonoperative management [14]. Tuberosity fractures can be repaired via transosseous sutures, tape, cerclage, or conversion to reverse total shoulder arthroplasty. Fixation of periprosthetic shaft fractures around a well-fixed implant can be achieved with either a plate, strut allograft, or both. The plate may be secured around the stem with either cerclage wires, short unicortical locking screws, or bicortical "skive" screws. To avoid the creation of

Table 19.1 Outcomes of periprosthetic humerus fractures managed conservatively

Study	No. of fractures managed non-operatively	No. of fractures that healed with non-operative management	Mean time to radiographic healing	Complications (%)	Complications
Boyd (1992) [13]	7	1 (14.3%)	3 months	1 (100%)	Union with pain
Krakauer (1994) [25]	11	6 (54.5%)	11–13 weeks[a]	None reported	Not specified
Wright (1995) [14]	8	4 (50%)	5.3 months	1 (12.5%)	Persistent pain
Campbell (1998) [15]	5	5 (100%)	3.1 months	2 (40%)	Frozen shoulder, skin slough and cellulitis
Worland (1999) [16]	2	1 (50%)	3 months	1 (100%)	Death
Kumar (2004) [23]	11	6 (54.5%)	180 days	None reported	None reported
Groh (2008) [17]	4	4 (100%)	11 weeks[b]	None reported	None reported
Wolf (2012) [33]	2	0 (0%)	N/A	1 (100%)	Nonunion, persistent pain
García-Fernández (2015) [34]	1	1 (100%)	18 weeks	None reported	None reported
Ascione (2018) [35]	5	5 (100%)	Not specified	None reported	None reported
Ragusa (2020) [36]	5	4 (80%)	4.4 months	3 (60%)	Acromial stress fracture, second fracture, hypertrophic nonuinon

[a] Range, mean value not provided
[b] Inclusive of all fractures, treated operatively and non-operatively

a stress riser, the plate should overlap the prosthesis by at least two cortical diameters. Locking plates, which may be particularly useful in osteopenic bone, have the benefit of increased bone-implant stability and screw pull out [11]. Contraindications to operative management include medical comorbidities precluding general anesthesia and active infection.

Operative management with internal fixation has demonstrated good outcomes with respect to healing among appropriately selected patient cohorts. In 2022, Mourkus and colleagues published a systematic review of clinical outcomes following periprosthetic humerus fractures [12]. The review included 99 patients who underwent open reduction and internal fixation, in which union was achieved in 93.07% (95% CI 87.15–97.45) without further intervention. Eighty-four of these patients underwent fixation acutely, whereas 15 had previously failed a trial of nonoperative management. The overwhelming majority (95%) involved a well-fixed prosthesis and fracture healing, which was reported for 75.7% of the patients, occurred at a mean of 5.5 months (range, 2–10). Of those studies which reported patient satisfaction scores, 72% of patients reported being satisfied with their outcome. Complications included hardware irritation, transient nerve palsies, deep infection, fracture extension, or failure of fixation and nonunion.

Despite reliable radiographic healing, functional deficits may persist. Among five patients treated with open reduction and internal fixation using a locking plate, Kurowicki et al. noted a mean time to radiographic union of 19 weeks (range, 9–53 weeks) with only one patient reporting a VAS pain score above 0 (average 0.5) [38]. However, functionally limiting range of motion deficits were not uncommon. The average active shoulder flexion was 86° (range, 60–130°), abduction 70° (range, 50–90°), and external rotation 18° (range, −10 to 60°). The mean ASES total score was 75 (range, 62–100) while the mean ASES Function score was 28 (range, 15–50).

The largest case series to date, published by Andersen et al., included 17 fractures treated with ORIF occurring after anatomic (nine) or reverse (eight) shoulder arthroplasties [39]. Eight of the fractures were augmented with strut allograft. All fractures demonstrated radiographic healing at a mean 6.8 months postoperatively (range, 3.25–12 months). Mean ASES scores at time of final follow-up was 45.1 (95% CI: 26.8–63.5). Five of six patients in whom pre-fracture ASES scores were available returned to their pre-fracture score. Seven of the 17 fractures experienced complications, four of which required subsequent re-operation. These included a remote broken anatomic humeral stem due to recurrent trauma, failure of glenosphere baseplate fixation and the humeral socket, distal plate fixation failure, and distal fracture-line extension. The latter two occurred in shortly postoperatively and required extension of fixation with an additional locking plate. Radial nerve palsies occurred in three additional cases and were managed nonoperatively.

19.6.3 Revision Arthroplasty

Revision arthroplasty is indicated in fractures involving a loose implant or those in which surrounding bone stock is insufficient for fracture fixation. Implant loosening can be assessed by changes in implant positioning on serial radiographs or when radiolucency is noted in at least three of eight humeral zones [40, 41]. Traumatic loosening can occur when a fracture line extends along a significant portion of the implant, destabilizing it [11]. Revision arthroplasty typically involves conversion to a long-stemmed implant that bypasses the fracture by at least two to three cortical diameters. The long-stem implant can be either press fit or cemented, dependent on the implant chosen and available bone stock [11, 14, 16, 23]. Implant revision is often accompanied by additional fixation, usually with a strut allograft and cerclage or a plate and screws. Osteolysis and loss of available bone stock may complicate management of periprosthetic humeral fractures and may necessitate component-allograft composites or humeral endoprostheses.

Andersen and colleagues reported on 19 periprosthetic fractures involving 9 reverse and 10 anatomic implants treated with revision arthroplasty [39]. All stems were loose at the time of surgery. Fourteen were treated with a long-stem prosthesis, whereas five were treated with a short stem supplemented by ORIF. They noted an average time to radiographic union of 7.7 months (range, 3.5–13.5 months). Allograft augmentation was utilized in 17 of the cases and 18 went on to union. Pre-fracture ASES scores were available for five of the patients (32.0 (95% CI: 14.0–50.0), with all post-fracture ASES scores exceeding pre-injury scores (54.4 (95% CI: 44.6–64.2). Complications occurred in seven cases, three of which required reoperation. These included subsequent periprosthetic fracture, nonunion following multiple surgeries, and dissociation of the humeral socket-stem Morse taper. Complications treated nonoperatively included a transient radial nerve palsy, loosening of the stem, postoperative hematoma, and dislocation.

19.7 Conclusion

Periprosthetic humeral fractures are increasing in their incidence and represent a challenging clinical problem. A thorough preoperative evaluation including previous operative notes with implant specifics, radiographs, and axial imaging are necessary. Classification systems remain cumbersome and complex. Nonoperative management can be considered, though with high rates of nonunion and malunion. Surgical interventions include ORIF and revision shoulder arthroplasty and should be tailored to patient and fracture morphology.

References

1. Farley KX, Wilson JM, Kumar A, Gottschalk MB, Daly C, Sanchez-Sotelo J, et al. Prevalence of shoulder arthroplasty in the United States and the increasing burden of revision shoulder arthroplasty. JBJS Open Access [Internet]. 2021 [cited 2022 Jun 4];6(3). https://doi.org/10.2106/JBJS.OA.20.00156.

2. Bohsali KI, Wirth MA, Rockwood CA. Complications of total shoulder arthroplasty. J Bone Joint Surg Am. 2006;88(10):2279–92.

3. Bohsali KI, Bois AJ, Wirth MA. Complications of shoulder arthroplasty. J Bone Joint Surg Am. 2017;99(3):256–69.

4. Kristensen MR, Rasmussen JV, Elmengaard B, Jensen SL, Olsen BS, Brorson S. High risk for revision after shoulder arthroplasty for failed osteosynthesis of proximal humeral fractures. Acta Orthop. 2018;89(3):345–50.

5. Ascione F, Domos P, Guarrella V, Chelli M, Boileau P, Walch G. Long-term humeral complications after Grammont-style reverse shoulder arthroplasty. 2018 [cited 2022 May 21]; 27(6):1065–1071. https://doi.org/10.1016/j.jse.2017.11.028.

6. Saltzman BM, Chalmers PN, Gupta AK, Romeo AA, Nicholson GP. Complication rates comparing primary with revision reverse total shoulder arthroplasty. J Shoulder Elbow Surg. 2014;23(11):1647–54.

7. Gombera MM, Laughlin MS, Vidal EA, Brown BS, Morris BJ, Bradley Edwards T, et al. The impact of fellowship type on trends and complications following total shoulder arthroplasty for osteoarthrosis by recently trained board-eligible orthopedic surgeons. J Shoulder Elbow Surg [Internet]. 2020 [cited 2022 Jun 4];29(7):e279–ee86. https://doi.org/10.1016/j.jse.2019.11.023.

8. Ross BJ, Wu VJ, McCluskey LC, O'Brien MJ, Sherman WJ, Savoie FH. Postoperative complication rates following total shoulder arthroplasty (TSA) vs. reverse shoulder arthroplasty (RSA): a nationwide analysis. Semin Arthroplasty. 2020;30(2):83–8.

9. Athwal GS, Sperling JW, Rispoli DM, Cofield RH. Periprosthetic humeral fractures during shoulder arthroplasty. J Bone Joint Surg Am. 2009;91(3):594–603.

10. Wagner ER, Houdek MT, Elhassan BT, Sanchez-Sotelo J, Cofield RH, Sperling JW. What are risk factors for intraoperative humerus fractures during revision reverse shoulder arthroplasty and do they influence outcomes? Clin Orthop Relat Res. 2015;473(10):3228–34.

11. Steinmann SP, Cheung E. Treatment of periprosthetic humerus fractures associated with shoulder arthroplasty. J Am Acad Orthop Surg. 2008;16(4):199–207.

12. Mourkus H, Phillips NJ, Rangan A, Peach CA. Management of periprosthetic fractures of the humerus: a systematic review. Bone Joint J. 2022;104-B(4):416–23.

13. Boyd AD, Thornhill TS, Barnes CL. Fractures adjacent to humeral prostheses. J Bone Joint Surg Am. 1992;74(10):1498–504.

14. Wright TW, Cofield RH. Humeral fractures after shoulder arthroplasty. J Bone Joint Surg Am. 1995;77(9):1340–6.

15. Campbell JT, Moore RS, Iannotti JP, Norris TR, Williams GR. Periprosthetic humeral fractures: mechanisms of fracture and treatment options. J Shoulder Elbow Surg. 1998;7(4):406–13.

16. Worland RL, Kim DY, Arredondo J. Periprosthetic humeral fractures: management and classification. J Shoulder Elbow Surg. 1999;8(6):590–4.

17. Groh GI, Heckman MM, Wirth MA, Curtis RJ, Rockwood CA, Antonio S. Treatment of fractures adjacent to humeral prostheses. J Shoulder Elbow Surg. 2008;17(1):85–9.

18. Kuhn MZ, King JJ, Wright TW, Farmer KW, Levy JC, Hao KA, et al. Periprosthetic humerus fractures after shoulder arthroplasty: an evaluation of available classification systems. J Shoulder Elbow Surg [Internet]. 2022 [cited 2022 Jun 4]; S1058-2746(22)00439-6. https://doi.org/10.1016/j.jse.2022.05.011. Epub ahead of print. https://pubmed.ncbi.nlm.nih.gov/35562034/

19. Kirchhoff C, Kirchhoff S, Biberthaler P. Classification of periprosthetic shoulder fractures. Unfallchirurg. 2016;119(4):264–72.

20. Kirchhoff C, Beirer M, Brunner U, Buchholz A, Biberthaler P, Crönlein M. Validation of a new classification for periprosthetic shoulder fractures. Int Orthop. 2018;42(6):1371–7.

21. Williams GR, Iannotti JP. Management of periprosthetic fractures: the shoulder. J Arthroplasty. 2002;17(4):14–6.

22. Fram B, Elder A, Namdari S. Periprosthetic humeral fractures in shoulder arthroplasty. JBJS Rev [Internet]. 2019 [cited 2022 Jun 6];7(11):e6. https://doi.org/10.2106/JBJS.RVW.19.00017.

23. Kumar S, Sperling JW, Haidukewych GH, Cofield RH. Periprosthetic humeral fractures after shoulder arthroplasty. J Bone Joint Surg Am. 2004;86(4):680–9.

24. Bonutti PM, Hawkins RJ. Fracture of the humeral shaft associated with total replacement arthroplasty of the shoulder: a case report. J Bone Joint Surg Am. 1992;74(4):617–8.

25. Krakauer JD, Cofield RH. Periprosthetic fractures in total shoulder replacement. Oper Tech Orthop. 1994;4(4):243–52.

26. Brenner BC, Ferlic DC, Clayton ML, Dennis DA. Survivorship of unconstrained total shoulder arthroplasty. J Bone Joint Surg Am. 1989;71(9):1289–96.

27. Barrett WP, Franklin JL, Jackins SE, Wyss CR, Matsen FA 3rd. Total shoulder arthroplasty. J Bone Joint Surg Am. 1987;69(6):865–72.

28. Singh JA, Sperling J, Schleck C, Harmsen W, Cofield R. Periprosthetic fractures associated with primary total shoulder arthroplasty and primary humeral head replacement: a thirty-three-year study. J Bone Joint Surg Am. 2012;94(19):1777–85.

29. Buck FM, Jost B, Hodler J. Shoulder arthroplasty. Eur Radiol. 2008;18(12):2937–48.
30. Updegrove GF, Mourad W, Abboud JA. Humeral shaft fractures. J Shoulder Elbow Surg. 2018;27:87–97.
31. Klenerman L. Fractures of the shaft of the humerus. Bone Joint J. 1966;48(1):105–11.
32. Shields E, Sundem L, Childs S, Maceroli M, Humphrey C, Ketz JP, et al. The impact of residual angulation on patient reported functional outcome scores after non-operative treatment for humeral shaft fractures. Injury. 2016;47(4):914–8.
33. Wolf H, Pajenda G, Sarahrudi K. Analysis of factors predicting success and failure of treatment after type B periprosthetic humeral fractures: a case series study. Eur J Trauma Emerg Surg. 2012;38(2):177–83.
34. García-Fernández C, Lópiz-Morales Y, Rodríguez A, López-Durán L, Martínez FM. Periprosthetic humeral fractures associated with reverse total shoulder arthroplasty: incidence and management. Int Orthop. 2015;39(10):1965–9.
35. Ascione F, Domos P, Guarrella V, Chelli M, Boileau P, Walch G. Long-term humeral complications after Grammont-style reverse shoulder arthroplasty. J Shoulder Elbow Surg. 2018;27(6):1065–71.
36. Ragusa PS, Vadhera A, Jang JM, Ali I, McFarland EG, Srikumaran U. Nonoperative treatment of periprosthetic humeral shaft fractures after reverse total shoulder arthroplasty. Orthopedics [Internet]. 2020 Sep [cited on 2022 Sep 6];43(6):E553–60. https://doi.org/10.3928/01477447-20200910-06.
37. Sanchez-Sotelo J, Athwal GS. Periprosthetic postoperative humeral fractures after shoulder arthroplasty. J Am Acad Orthop Surg [Internet]. 2022 (cited on 2022 Sep 6). https://doi.org/10.5435/JAAOS-D-21-01001. Epub ahead of print.
38. Kurowicki J, Momoh E, Levy JC. Treatment of periprosthetic humerus fractures with open reduction and internal fixation. J Orthop Trauma [Internet]. 2016 Nov [cited 2022 Jun 4];30(11):e369–ee74. https://doi.org/10.1097/BOT.0000000000000646.
39. Andersen JR, Williams CD, Cain R, Mighell M, Frankle M. Surgically treated humeral shaft fractures following shoulder arthroplasty. J Bone Joint Surg Am. 2013;95(1):9–18.
40. Sanchez-Sotelo J, Wright TW, O'Driscoll SW, Cofield RH, Rowland CM. Radiographic assessment of uncemented humeral components in total shoulder arthroplasty. J Arthroplasty. 2001;16(2):180–7.
41. Sperling JW, Cofield RH, O'Driscoll SW, Torchia ME, Rowland CM. Radiographic assessment of ingrowth total shoulder arthroplasty. J Shoulder Elbow Surg. 2000;9(6):507–13.

Ignacio Pasqualini, Javier Ardebol,
Jeffrey L. Horinek, Cameron J. Phillips,
and Patrick J. Denard

20.1 Introduction

Subscapularis healing plays a critical role in postoperative outcomes for patients undergoing total shoulder arthroplasty (TSA) [1]. Subscapularis failure after TSA has been linked to decreased function, instability, and early implant failure [1–4]. Therefore, much attention has been placed on subscapularis management during TSA.

While subscapularis-sparing approaches are an option, the subscapularis is most commonly taken down during TSA to access the glenohumeral joint and optimize component position. Options for subscapularis taken down include tenotomy, peel, and lesser tuberosity osteotomy [5–9]. Several anatomic, biomechanical, and clinical studies have compared the advantages and disadvantages of these techniques [7, 8, 10, 11]. However, controversy continues regarding which is the best technique for addressing the subscapularis. One issue is that a variety of repair techniques exist which often cloud comparative analysis of takedown techniques.

To optimize results after TSA, it is important for surgeons to be knowledgeable and comfortable with subscapularis management. This chapter aims to provide an overview of subscapularis anatomy, approach, repair techniques, and clinical outcomes in the setting of TSA.

20.2 Subscapularis Anatomy

The subscapularis is the largest rotator cuff muscle, originating from the subscapular fossa and extending laterally to its insertion on the lesser tuberosity of the humerus [12]. The insertion is fully tendinous superiorly and more muscular at the inferior extent. Innervation is supplied from the upper and lower subscapular nerves [12]. The subscapularis muscle internally rotates and helps to adduct the humerus. Most importantly, because it is the only anterior rotator cuff muscle, it plays a critical role in dynamic glenohumeral stability. Notably, the subscapularis delivers half of the overall rotator cuff force, making it the strongest of the complex [13, 14].

20.3 Surgical Techniques

20.3.1 Subscapularis Tenotomy

20.3.1.1 Approach

Subscapularis tenotomy is performed with a vertical incision within the tendon approximately 1 cm medial to the subscapularis insertion, leaving a cuff of the tendon on the lesser tuberosity to

I. Pasqualini · J. Ardebol · J. L. Horinek ·
C. J. Phillips · P. J. Denard (✉)
Oregon Shoulder Institute, Medford, OR, USA

© ISAKOS 2023
A. D. Mazzocca et al. (eds.), *Shoulder Arthritis across the Life Span*,
https://doi.org/10.1007/978-3-031-33298-2_20

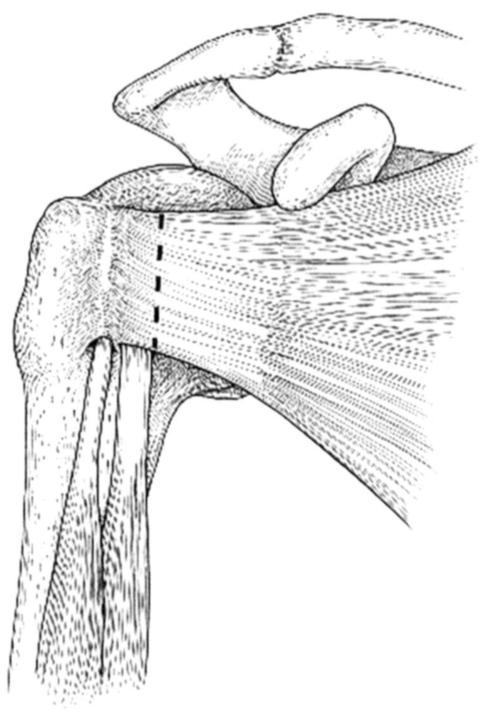

Fig. 20.1 Subscapularis tenotomy. (Reproduced with permission from Defranco MJ, Higgins LD, Warner JJP (2010) Subscapularis management in open shoulder surgery. J Am Acad Orthop Surg 18:707–717)

facilitate repair after the prosthesis is implanted [5, 6, 13]. Traction sutures are used to tag and mobilize the tendon (Fig. 20.1).

20.3.1.2 Repair
Side-to-side repair is usually achieved by using high-strength, absorbable, or nonabsorbable sutures in a configuration based on the surgeon's preference (Fig. 20.1). Double-row anchor-based repairs have also been described [15]. Additionally, the tendon-to-tendon repair can be augmented by using a transosseous technique through bone tunnels with nonabsorbable sutures [16].

20.3.2 Subscapularis Peel

20.3.2.1 Approach
With a peel approach, the tendon is completely released from the lesser tuberosity using a scalpel

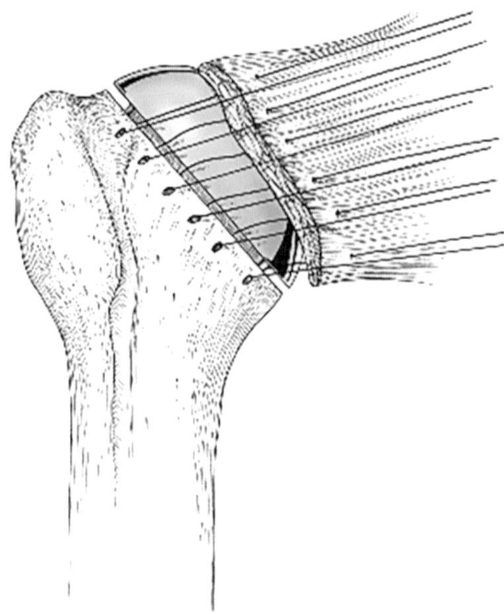

Fig. 20.2 A transosseous repair of subscapularis peel. (Reproduced with permission from Defranco MJ, Higgins LD, Warner JJP (2010) Subscapularis management in open shoulder surgery. J Am Acad Orthop Surg 18:707–717)

or electrocautery [5, 6, 13]. This is done from lateral to medial with increasing external rotation of the arm. Traction sutures may be used in the same manner as mentioned above. It is important to maintain the fully intact tendon during release.

20.3.2.2 Repair
Tendon footprint repair can be accomplished transosseously by creating bone tunnels or by passing sutures through drill holes and around a stem implant (Fig. 20.2) [17, 18]. The use of a backpack technique and knotless, anchor-based double row repairs have been described [15]. In cases of poor bone quality, the sutures can also be tied over a mini plate on the lateral side of the greater tuberosity [19].

20.3.3 Lesser Tuberosity Osteotomy

20.3.3.1 Approach
LTO maintains a portion of the subscapularis insertion to lesser tuberosity with the theoretical

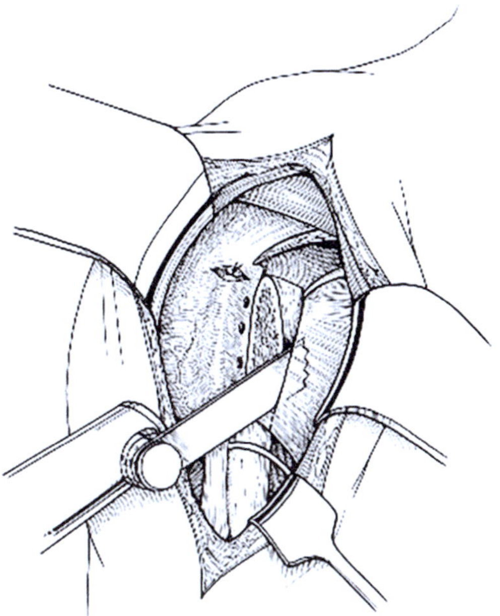

Fig. 20.3 Lesser tuberosity osteotomy. (Reproduced with permission from Defranco MJ, Higgins LD, Warner JJP (2010) Subscapularis management in open shoulder surgery. J Am Acad Orthop Surg 18:707–717)

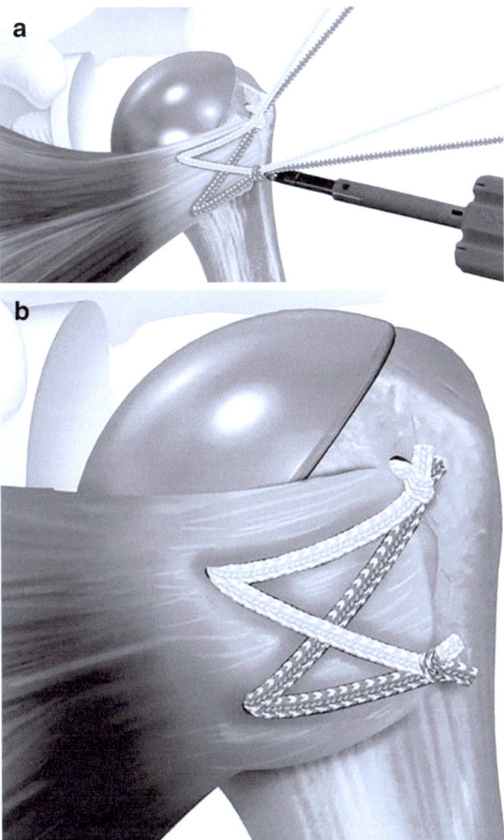

Fig. 20.4 (**a**) The suture limbs are tensioned after passing through the half-racking suture. (**b**) Final repair. (Reproduced with permission from Denard PJ, Noyes MP, Lädermann A. A Tensionable Method for Subscapularis Repair after Shoulder Arthroplasty. JSES Open Access. 2018 Dec;2(4):205–210. https://doi.org/10.1016/j.jses.2018.08.003)

advantage of bone-to-bone healing rather than tendon-to-bone healing [13]. It also allows for easier postoperative surveillance via radiography. Several LTO techniques have been described [20–23]. Generally, an osteotomy is created by sagittal saw or osteotome to obtain 0.5–1 cm or 50% of the depth of the lesser tuberosity (Fig. 20.3).

20.3.3.2 Repair
LTO repair is achieved by creating drill holes about the bicipital groove and medial to the LTO where sutures can be passed around the stem or through the stem. Different suturing methods have also been described, including backpack, single-row, and dual-row [7]. Sutures are preferably tied with the arm positioned at 30 degrees of external rotation. Moreover, a tensioning device can help generate additional compression to the construct [24] (Fig. 20.4).

20.3.4 Subscapularis-Sparing

Another technique to gain access to the glenohumeral joint without violating the subscapularis is a subscapularis sparing approach [25]. Theoretical advantages of this technique include the lack of need to achieve tendon and accelerated postoperative rehabilitation. Despite the term "sparing", this technique varies with regard to the amount of tissue that is actually removed, with reports suggesting that 30–50% of either the superior or inferior portion of the insertion may be taken down [26]. Although the technique is appealing, it has yet to gain widespread adoption due to the technical difficulty and high rate of postoperative components [6].

20.4 Biomechanical Outcomes

20.4.1 Subscapularis Approach

Several biomechanical studies have compared subscapularis management techniques. Generally, LTO technique has showed the best results or at least similar to other techniques. Van den Berghe [27] evaluated the performance of each traditional technique under fatigue, concluding that bone-to-bone repair provided the best combination of strength and restoration of subscapularis length. Ponce et al. [21] found that LTO repairs exhibited superior load to failure and decreased cyclic displacement compared to SubscapularisP and SubscapularisT. LTO has also shown biomechanical superiorities when only compared to SubscapularisT [20, 28]. Two systematic reviews supported these findings, concluding that the LTO technique provides the strongest fixation of all techniques [7, 29]. However, other authors have found no differences between techniques. Van Thiel et al. [10] and Virk et al. [30] found similar cyclic elongation, failure testing for maximum load, mode of failure, and stiffness in the three techniques. Similarly, Giuseffi et al. [31] showed no differences in load to failure when tenotomy was compared to LTO. Lederman et al. [32] compared SubscapularisP with LTO repairs finding no biomechanical differences in cadaveric shoulders with short-stemmed humeral prosthesis. Similarly, Buraimoh et al. [33] reported no significant differences regarding repair gapping, fatigue failure, and load to failure in peel compared to LTO.

20.4.2 Repair Techniques

Tenotomy appears to benefit from augmenting the traditional side-to-side repair. Ahmad et al. [34] demonstrated superior fixation strength in tenotomy augmented with transosseous sutures in comparison to side-to-side sutures alone. In stemless prostheses, Werner et al. [15] demonstrated that a double-row anchor-based repair had a higher load-to-failure than a traditional tenotomy repair. Additionally, Werner et al. [35] evaluated two SubscapularisP repair techniques (backpack versus knotless double-row), which showed similar biomechanical properties in stemless shoulder arthroplasty. LTO has been repaired using several techniques [7]. Krishnan et al. [20] found single row and double row LTO repairs to be stronger than tenotomy repairs. Moreover, Heckman et al. [36] reported less cyclic displacement in LTO repaired with a double row repair compared to a backpack technique. In contrast, other authors have found that compression and tension repairs are the best methods for LTO repair [7, 37]. Passing the sutures around the stem during LTO repair provides significant biomechanical benefits [7]. The biomechanical properties of this technique are equivalent to those of a stem-based repair using a peel approach [32]. Lastly, Denard et al. [24] compared a traditional LTO repair to a suture tape repair with a prefashioned racking hitch that can be tensioned, finding significantly higher load to failure outcomes with the latter.

20.5 Healed Vs Not Healed

Tenotomy has historically been used to mobilize the subscapularis; however, previous reports of poor healing have increased awareness of the procedure [38]. This has led to the popularity of peel and LTO techniques in recent years [39]. However, the latter is not without challenges, including technical difficulties, risk of humeral fractures during surgery, and risk for nonunion, especially in stemless and short-stem prostheses [39].

LTO has generally been associated with higher healing rates than tenotomy. Buckley et al. [40] described normal ultrasound subscapularis in 100% of LTOs compared to 88% of tenotomies. As well, Levine et al. [41] found that 93% of the

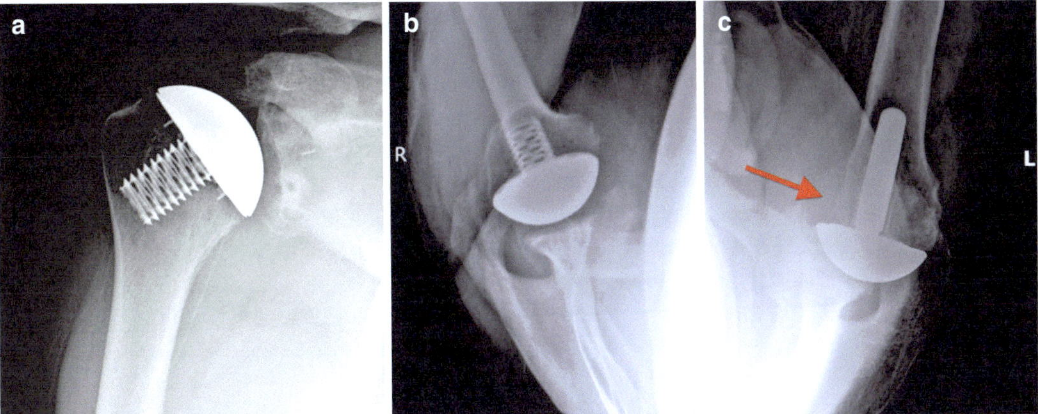

Fig. 20.5 Anteroposterior (**a**) and axillary radiographs of left shoulder demonstrate a healed (**b**) and non-healed (**c**) lesser tuberosity osteotomy following a total shoulder arthroplasty

LTOs healed compared to 86.7% of the SubscapularisTs. In contrast, LTO and peel techniques showed consistently high healing rates. Lapner et al. [42] examined healing rates through computed tomography reporting 100% in peel vs 95% in LTO (*p-value*= 0.493). Interestingly, few studies compared the healing rates of peel and tenotomy, with Lapner et al. [43] finding no difference between the two (71% vs 72%, respectively). Overall, systematic reviews have favored LTOs over other approaches. Choate et al. [8] described LTO as having the best healing rate (93.1%), followed by subscapularis peel (84.1%), and finally mid substance tenotomy (75.7%). Del Core et al. [11] also concluded that LTO had significantly higher ultrasound healing rates than the other techniques (Fig. 20.5).

20.6 Clinical Outcomes

Clinical outcomes are usually assessed with patient-reported outcomes, range of motion, and subscapularis strength testing. Each technique has proven to be effective in improving clinical outcomes [20, 44–46]. However, when these techniques are compared, results are often mixed.

In a randomized controlled trial, Lapner et al. [43] compared tenotomy to peel, finding no significant differences in internal rotation strength or WOOS and ASES scores. However, when tenotomy was compared to LTO, the results are diverse. Budge et al. [47], Levine et al. [41], and O'Brien et al. [48] showed no superiority of tenotomy in clinical outcomes compared to LTO. However, Scalise et al. [38] concluded that LTO was associated with better functional scores. In contrast, most studies comparing LTO and peels showed significant clinical improvements regardless of the treatment method [19, 39]. However, it was suggested by Shafritz et al. [49] that LTO had 4.5 times greater chances of achieving a normal postoperative lift-off test than peel.

The heterogeneity of individual studies makes it difficult to draw conclusions based on clinical outcomes. However, some authors tried to analyze these results in a more comprehensive manner. In a systematic review by Louie et al. [50], LTO vs tenotomy were compared. The authors found no differences in functional outcomes, but tenotomy was associated with a greater increase in forward elevation. In 2017, Choate et al. [8] performed another systematic review in which 14 studies were included comparing outcomes among the three techniques. The investigators found that LTO had more consistently normal belly press and lift-off test results compared to tenotomy. This difference was also reflected in the Constant and Western Ontario Osteoarthritis of the Shoulder Index (WOOS) outcome scores. Interestingly, they reported better American Shoulder and Elbow Surgeon (ASES) scores in tenotomy compared to peel and LTO. Moreover, strength and range of motion were similar between techniques. In a similar but more recent systematic review, Del Core et al. [11] analyzed these techniques through eight studies reporting no differences in the range of motion except for internal rotation, which was significantly higher in peel when compared to tenotomy. LTO was associated with significantly more negative belly press tests compared to the other techniques. Finally, all techniques showed good ASES scores and low complication rates with no significant differences.

20.7 Subscapularis Failure

Even with high strength repairs and high healing rates, subscapularis failures may still occur [51]. This can adversely affect patient function and well-being [4]. However, given the multiple subscapularis approaches, fixation techniques, imaging evaluation, and variable clinical signs, it is difficult to determine failure rates.

In a study by Armstrong et al. [52], 13% of subscapularis failed; however, the majority of patients remained asymptomatic. On the contrary, Miller et al. [4], reported pain, loss of range of motion, and instability in their patients with subscapularis tears. As well, Ives et al. [53] reported that 50% of their symptomatic patients had a subscapularis tear. Furthermore, Moeckel et al. [2] reported anterior instability in ten patients, of which 70% had a ruptured subscapularis tendon. Therefore, subscapularis failure should be evaluated on an individual basis and highly suspected in symptomatic patients.

In the event of subscapularis failure after TSA, patients may require revision surgery. Treatment options vary depending on age, activity level, comorbidities, timing and mechanism of failure, and functional expectations [54]. These include conservative treatment, soft-tissue repair, tendon or graft augmentation, and reverse shoulder arthroplasty. Nevertheless, subsequent reoperations are not uncommon, demonstrating the importance of a proper primary repair [55, 56].

20.8 Conclusion

Overall, all techniques improve outcomes after TSA. When approaches are compared, results may be heterogeneous, but they appear to slightly favor LTO. However, the authors believe surgeons can confidently perform any of the techniques provided if they perform them well and understand the pitfalls to avoid.

References

1. Terrier A, Larrea X, Malfroy Camine V, Pioletti DP, Farron A. Importance of the subscapularis muscle after total shoulder arthroplasty. Clin Biomech. 2013;28:146–50.
2. Moeckel BH, Altchek DW, Warren RF, Wickiewicz TL, Dines DM. Instability of the shoulder after arthroplasty. J Bone Joint Surg Am. 1993;75:492–7.
3. Miller BS, Joseph TA, Noonan TJ, Horan MP, Hawkins RJ. Rupture of the subscapularis tendon after shoulder arthroplasty: diagnosis, treatment, and outcome. J Shoulder Elbow Surg. 2005;14:492–6.
4. Miller SL, Hazrati Y, Klepps S, Chiang A, Flatow EL. Loss of subscapularis function after total shoulder replacement: a seldom recognized problem. J Shoulder Elbow Surg. 2003;12:29–34.
5. Dunn R, Joyce CD, Bravman JT. Comparison of subscapularis management and repair techniques. J Shoulder Elb Arthroplast. 2019;3:2471549219848152.
6. Shields E, Ho A, Wiater JM. Management of the subscapularis tendon during total shoulder arthroplasty. J Shoulder Elbow Surg. 2017;26:723–31.
7. Schrock JB, Kraeutler MJ, Crellin CT, McCarty EC, Bravman JT. How should I fixate the subscapularis in total shoulder arthroplasty? A systematic review of pertinent subscapularis repair biomechanics. Shoulder Elbow. 2017;9:153–9.
8. Choate WS, Kwapisz A, Momaya AM, Hawkins RJ, Tokish JM. Outcomes for subscapularis management techniques in shoulder arthroplasty: a systematic review. J Shoulder Elbow Surg. 2018;27:363–70.
9. Sacevich N, Athwal GS, Lapner P. Subscapularis management in total shoulder arthroplasty. J Hand Surg Am. 2015;40:1009–11.
10. Van Thiel GS, Wang VM, Wang F-C, Nho SJ, Piasecki DP, Bach BR Jr, Romeo AA. Biomechanical similarities among subscapularis repairs after shoulder arthroplasty. J Shoulder Elbow Surg. 2010;19:657–63.
11. Del Core MA, Cutler HS, Ahn J, Khazzam M. Systematic review and network meta-analysis of subscapularis management techniques in anatomic total shoulder arthroplasty. J Shoulder Elbow Surg. 2021;30:1714–24.

12. Miller MD, Sekiya JK. Shoulder anatomy and biomechanics. In: Core knowledge in orthopaedics: sports medicine. 2006. p. 239–251.
13. Defranco MJ, Higgins LD, Warner JJP. Subscapularis management in open shoulder surgery. J Am Acad Orthop Surg. 2010;18:707–17.
14. Keating JF, Waterworth P, Shaw-Dunn J, Crossan J. The relative strengths of the rotator cuff muscles. A cadaver study. J Bone Joint Surg Br. 1993;75-B:137–40.
15. Werner BC, McClish SJ, Mealey NC, Wijdicks C, Thompson T, Higgins LD. A biomechanical comparison of subscapularis tenotomy repair techniques for stemless shoulder arthroplasty. J Shoulder Elbow Surg. 2021;31:711. https://doi.org/10.1016/j.jse.2021.10.017.
16. Liem D, Kleeschulte K, Dedy N, Schulte TL, Steinbeck J, Marquardt B. Subscapularis function after transosseous repair in shoulder arthroplasty: transosseous subscapularis repair in shoulder arthroplasty. J Shoulder Elbow Surg. 2012;21:1322–7.
17. Denard PJ, Lederman E, Gobezie R, Hanypsiak BT. Stem-based repair of the subscapularis in total shoulder arthroplasty. Am J Orthop. 2016;45:228–30.
18. Clyde CT, Throckmorton TW, Duquin TR. Subscapularis peel in anatomic total shoulder arthroplasty. J Shoulder Elb Arthroplast. 2018;2:247154921881340.
19. Lapner PLC, Sabri E, Rakhra K, Bell K, Athwal GS. Comparison of lesser tuberosity osteotomy to subscapularis peel in shoulder arthroplasty: a randomized controlled trial. J Bone Joint Surg Am. 2012;94:2239–46.
20. Krishnan SG, Stewart DG, Reineck JR, Lin KC, Buzzell JE, Burkhead WZ. Subscapularis repair after shoulder arthroplasty: biomechanical and clinical validation of a novel technique. J Shoulder Elbow Surg. 2009;18:184–92; discussion 197–8.
21. Ponce BA, Ahluwalia RS, Mazzocca AD, Gobezie RG, Warner JJP, Millett PJ. Biomechanical and clinical evaluation of a novel lesser tuberosity repair technique in total shoulder arthroplasty. J Bone Joint Surg Am. 2005;87(Suppl 2):1–8.
22. Knudsen ML, Levine WN. The lesser tuberosity osteotomy exposure for total shoulder arthroplasty. JBJS Essent Surg Tech. 2021;11:e19.00031. https://doi.org/10.2106/JBJS.ST.19.00031.
23. Gerber C, Pennington SD, Yian EH, Pfirrmann CAW, Werner CML, Zumstein MA. Lesser tuberosity osteotomy for total shoulder arthroplasty. Surgical technique. J Bone Joint Surg Am. 2006;88 Suppl 1(Pt 2):170–7.
24. Denard PJ, Noyes MP, Lädermann A. A tensionable method for subscapularis repair after shoulder arthroplasty. JSES Open Access. 2018;2:205–10.
25. Lafosse L, Schnaser E, Haag M, Gobezie R. Primary total shoulder arthroplasty performed entirely thru the rotator interval: technique and minimum two-year outcomes. J Shoulder Elbow Surg. 2009;18:864–73.
26. Simovitch R, Fullick R, Zuckerman JD. Use of the subscapularis preserving technique in anatomic total shoulder arthroplasty. Bull Hosp Jt Dis. 2013;71(Suppl 2):94–100.
27. Van den Berghe GR, Nguyen B, Patil S, D'Lima DD, Mahar A, Pedowitz R, Hoenecke HR. A biomechanical evaluation of three surgical techniques for subscapularis repair. J Shoulder Elbow Surg. 2008;17:156–61.
28. Fishman MP, Budge MD, Moravek JE Jr, Mayer M, Kurdziel MD, Baker KC, Wiater JM. Biomechanical testing of small versus large lesser tuberosity osteotomies: effect on gap formation and ultimate failure load. J Shoulder Elbow Surg. 2014;23:470–6.
29. Schrock JB, Kraeutler MJ, Houck DA, Provenzano GG, McCarty EC, Bravman JT. Lesser tuberosity osteotomy and subscapularis tenotomy repair techniques during total shoulder arthroplasty: a meta-analysis of cadaveric studies. Clin Biomech. 2016;40:33–6.
30. Virk MS, Aiyash SS, Frank RM, Mellano CS, Shewman EF, Wang VM, Romeo AA. Biomechanical comparison of subscapularis peel and lesser tuberosity osteotomy for double-row subscapularis repair technique in a cadaveric arthroplasty model. J Orthop Surg Res. 2019;14:391.
31. Giuseffi SA, Wongtriratanachai P, Omae H, Cil A, Zobitz ME, An K-N, Sperling JW, Steinmann SP. Biomechanical comparison of lesser tuberosity osteotomy versus subscapularis tenotomy in total shoulder arthroplasty. J Shoulder Elbow Surg. 2012;21:1087–95.
32. Lederman E, Streit J, Idoine J, Shishani Y, Gobezie R. Biomechanical study of a subscapularis repair technique for total shoulder arthroplasty. Orthopedics. 2016;39:e937–43.
33. Buraimoh MA, Okoroha KR, Oravec DJ, Peltz CD, Yeni YN, Muh SJ. A biomechanical comparison of subscapularis repair techniques in total shoulder arthroplasty: lesser tuberosity osteotomy versus subscapularis peel. JSES Open Access. 2018;2:8–12.
34. Ahmad CS, Wing D, Gardner TR, Levine WN, Bigliani LU. Biomechanical evaluation of subscapularis repair used during shoulder arthroplasty. J Shoulder Elbow Surg. 2007;16:S59–64.
35. Werner BC, Griffin JW, Thompson T, Lendhey M, Higgins LD, Denard PJ. Biomechanical evaluation of 2 techniques of repair after subscapularis peel for stemless shoulder arthroplasty. J Shoulder Elbow Surg. 2021;30:2240–6.
36. Heckman DS, Hoover SA, Weinhold PS, Spang JT, Creighton RA. Repair of lesser tuberosity osteotomy for shoulder arthroplasty: biomechanical evaluation of the backpack and dual row techniques. J Shoulder Elbow Surg. 2011;20:491–6.
37. Schmidt CC, Jarrett CD, Brown BT, DeGravelle M Jr, Sawardeker P, Weir DM, Latona CR, Miller MC. Effect of lesser tuberosity osteotomy size and repair construct during total shoulder arthroplasty. J Shoulder Elbow Surg. 2014;23:117–27.

38. Scalise JJ, Ciccone J, Iannotti JP. Clinical, radiographic, and ultrasonographic comparison of subscapularis tenotomy and lesser tuberosity osteotomy for total shoulder arthroplasty. J Bone Joint Surg Am. 2010;92:1627–34.

39. Aibinder WR, Bicknell RT, Bartsch S, Scheibel M, Athwal GS. Subscapularis management in stemless total shoulder arthroplasty: tenotomy versus peel versus lesser tuberosity osteotomy. J Shoulder Elbow Surg. 2019;28:1942–7.

40. Buckley T, Miller R, Nicandri G, Lewis R, Voloshin I. Analysis of subscapularis integrity and function after lesser tuberosity osteotomy versus subscapularis tenotomy in total shoulder arthroplasty using ultrasound and validated clinical outcome measures. J Shoulder Elbow Surg. 2014;23:1309–17.

41. Levine WN, Munoz J, Hsu S, Byram IR, Bigliani LU, Ahmad CS, Kongmalai P, Shillingford JN. Subscapularis tenotomy versus lesser tuberosity osteotomy during total shoulder arthroplasty for primary osteoarthritis: a prospective, randomized controlled trial. J Shoulder Elbow Surg. 2019;28:407–14.

42. Lapner PLC, Sabri E, Rakhra K, Bell K, Athwal GS. Healing rates and subscapularis fatty infiltration after lesser tuberosity osteotomy versus subscapularis peel for exposure during shoulder arthroplasty. J Shoulder Elbow Surg. 2013;22:396–402.

43. Lapner P, Pollock JW, Zhang T, Ruggiero S, Momoli F, Sheikh A, Athwal GS. A randomized controlled trial comparing subscapularis tenotomy with peel in anatomic shoulder arthroplasty. J Shoulder Elbow Surg. 2020;29:225–34.

44. Caplan JL, Whitfield B, Neviaser RJ. Subscapularis function after primary tendon to tendon repair in patients after replacement arthroplasty of the shoulder. J Shoulder Elbow Surg. 2009;18:193–6; discussion 197–8.

45. Baumgarten KM, Osborn R, Schweinle WE Jr, Zens MJ. The influence of anatomic total shoulder arthroplasty using a subscapularis tenotomy on shoulder strength. J Shoulder Elbow Surg. 2018;27:82–9.

46. Gobezie R, Denard PJ, Shishani Y, Romeo AA, Lederman E. Healing and functional outcome of a subscapularis peel repair with a stem-based repair after total shoulder arthroplasty. J Shoulder Elbow Surg. 2017;26:1603–8.

47. Budge MD, Nolan EM, Michael Wiater J. Lesser tuberosity osteotomy versus subscapularis Tenotomy: technique and rationale. Oper Tech Orthop. 2011;21:39–43.

48. O'Brien PM, Kazanjian JE, Kelly JD 2nd, Hobgood ER. Subscapularis function after total shoulder arthroplasty using lesser tuberosity osteotomy or tenotomy. J Am Acad Orthop Surg Glob Res Rev. 2020;4:e2000032.

49. Shafritz AB, Fitzgerald MG, Beynnon BD, DeSarno MJ. Lift-off test results after lesser tuberosity osteotomy versus subscapularis peel in primary total shoulder arthroplasty. J Am Acad Orthop Surg. 2017;25:304–13.

50. Louie PK, Levy DM, Bach BR Jr, Nicholson GP, Romeo AA. Subscapularis tenotomy versus lesser tuberosity osteotomy for total shoulder arthroplasty: a systematic review. Am J Orthop. 2017;46:E131–8.

51. Shi LL, Jiang JJ, Ek ET, Higgins LD. Failure of the lesser tuberosity osteotomy after total shoulder arthroplasty. J Shoulder Elbow Surg. 2015;24:203–9.

52. Armstrong A, Lashgari C, Teefey S, Menendez J, Yamaguchi K, Galatz LM. Ultrasound evaluation and clinical correlation of subscapularis repair after total shoulder arthroplasty. J Shoulder Elbow Surg. 2006;15:541–8.

53. Ives EP, Nazarian LN, Parker L, Garrigues GE, Williams GR. Subscapularis tendon tears: a common sonographic finding in symptomatic postarthroplasty shoulders. J Clin Ultrasound. 2013;41:129–33.

54. Entezari V, Henry T, Zmistowski B, Sheth M, Nicholson T, Namdari S. Clinically significant subscapularis failure after anatomic shoulder arthroplasty: is it worth repairing? J Shoulder Elbow Surg. 2020;29:1831–5.

55. Lopez CD, Maier SP, Bloom ZJ, Shiu BB, Petkovic D, Jobin CM. Outcomes of lesser tuberosity osteotomy in revision anatomic shoulder arthroplasty. J Shoulder Elbow Surg. 2018;27:e219–24.

56. Elhassan B, Ozbaydar M, Massimini D, Diller D, Higgins L, Warner JJP. Transfer of pectoralis major for the treatment of irreparable tears of subscapularis: does it work? J Bone Joint Surg Br. 2008;90:1059–65.

Total Shoulder Arthroplasty in Patients with Rotator Cuff Tear

21

S. Cerciello, G. Ciolli, Dario Candura, K. Corona, F. Mocini, and L. Proietti

21.1 Introduction

Anatomic shoulder arthroplasty (hemiarthroplasty or total) (ASR) aims at replacing the degenerated joint surfaces while preserving its biomechanics thanks to the intact cuff function. Rotator cuff tears (RCT) may be encountered in the setting of a shoulder replacement or may develop after such a procedure. Cuff tears and previous cuff repair surgeries on the index shoulder may influence the outcomes of shoulder replacement and therefore must carefully evaluated.

Similarly late cuff tears after shoulder arthroplasty may severely affect functional outcomes of especially when anatomic implants are considered. The aim of the present study was to analyze the available literature to point out whether previous cuff tears may influence the outcomes of shoulder replacements (either anatomic or reverse). Similarly, the role of late cuff tears after shoulder replacements was investigated.

21.2 Epidemiology of Cuff Tears in Patients with Osteoarthritis

Cuff tears alter normal shoulder function and should be therefore carefully evaluated while planning an anatomic replacement. The analysis of the literature shows that cuff tears are uncommon in patients with osteoarthritis (OA) (Table 21.1); Edwards et al. in a series of 555 osteoarthritic shoulders found a RCT in 42 (7.6%) patients [1]. Similarly, Norris and Iannotti identified 16 full-thickness supraspinatus (SS) tears in 176 shoulders (9.1%) with primary OA,

S. Cerciello
Catholic University of the Sacred Heart, Rome, Italy

Casa di Cura Villa Betania, Rome, Italy

G. Ciolli · D. Candura (✉)
Catholic University of the Sacred Heart, Rome, Italy

K. Corona
Department of Medicine and Health Sciences, "Vincenzo Tiberio", Rome, Italy
e-mail: Katia.corona@unimol.it

F. Mocini
Casa di Cura Villa Betania, Rome, Italy

L. Proietti
Casa di Cura Villa Betania, Rome, Italy

San Pietro Hospital, Rome, Italy

Table 21.1 Prevalence of cuff tears in patients undergoing total shoulder arthroplasty

	Initial cohort	Cuff tears	%
Edwards (2002)	555	83	14.9
Norris (2002)	176	16	9.1
Sperling (2004)	114	15	13.1
Haines (2006)	124	29	23.4
Fouria (2010)	50	5	10
Simone (2014)	932	45	4.8
Levy (2016)	1259	110	8.7
Overall	3210	303	12

© ISAKOS 2023

A. D. Mazzocca et al. (eds.), *Shoulder Arthritis across the Life Span*,
https://doi.org/10.1007/978-3-031-33298-2_21

which were treated by shoulder replacement [2]. Foruria et al. reported on 50 TSRs in patients with OA aged ≥80 years and identified five rotator cuff tears (10%) [3]. Haines et al. reported on 124 TSRs performed for both primary and secondary OA and identified that cuff tears were not always small. A small tear was present in ten shoulders (8.1%) and a large tear in 19 (15.3%) [4]. Therefore, rotator cuff tears in association with OA are relatively uncommon and are often confined to the supraspinatus tendon. Levy et al. in a systematic review on 15 studies reported 110 cases of concomitant cuff tears among the study population (1259 TSA) [5].

21.3 Analysis of the Literature of Total Shoulder Arthroplasty and Concomitant Cuff Repair

Three studies analyzed the outcomes of TSA and concomitant cuff repair (Tables 21.2 and 21.3). Edwards et al. reviewed 555 shoulders in 514 patients who had an arthroplasty for the treatment of primary glenohumeral osteoarthritis [6]. Forty-one shoulders had a partial-thickness tear of the supraspinatus, and 42 had a full-thickness tear. Ninety shoulders had moderate (stage 2) fatty degeneration of the infraspinatus (IS), and 19 had severe (stage 3 or 4) degeneration. Eighty-four shoulders had moderate fatty degeneration of the subscapularis (SSc), and 15 had severe degeneration. At an average FU of 43 months, patients with healthy cuff showed an average Constant score of 95.3 those with partial supraspinatus tear 94.5 and those with complete supraspinatus tear 93.7. When analyzing IS fatty degeneration, the average Constant score was 97.1, 89, and 78.2 if the atrophy was stage 0–1, stage 2, and stage 3, respectively. When analyzing SSc fatty degeneration, the average Constant score was 96.4, 91.3, and 76 if the atrophy was stage 0–1, stage 2, and stage 3, respectively. The authors concluded that minimally retracted or non-retracted rotator SS tears did not affect most shoulder-specific outcome parameters in shoulder arthroplasty performed for the treatment of primary osteoarthritis. Conversely, fatty degeneration of the infraspinatus and subscapularis muscles adversely influenced many of these parameters.

Norris et al. reviewed their series of 176 TSA and hemiarthroplasty (HA) at a minimum FU of 2 years [2]. Sixteen patients showed a cuff tear. Tears greater than 1 cm were found in 8 patients, but all were confined to the supraspinatus tendon (<3 cm). Of the 16 with rotator cuff tears, 10 underwent hemiarthroplasty and 6 underwent total shoulder arthroplasty. Of the 8 with tears greater than 1 cm, 7 underwent hemiarthroplasty and 1 total shoulder arthroplasty. The rotator cuff was reparable in all shoulders. Intraoperative complications occurred in 5.4% of cases, and postoperative complications occurred in 7.8%. The presence of a reparable supraspinatus rotator cuff tear did not affect pain scores, SST scores, or ASES scores. There were no differences in outcome if the patient underwent total shoulder arthroplasty or hemiarthroplasty in those with a reparable rotator cuff tear.

Simone et al. reviewed 33 patients undergoing TSA and concomitant cuff repair at an average FU of 4.7 years [7]. Tears were classified into

Table 21.2 Demographics of patients undergoing total shoulder arthroplasty and concomitant cuff tear

	Implant design	Cuff tears	Overall series	Age SG/overall	Male/female	FU (months)
Edwards (2002)	TSA	83	446	65.1/67.1	85.5% 72%	47.4/42.3
Edwards (2002)	TSA	109 (fatty deg. SS)	422	65.1/66.9	74.7% 73.1%	42.5/43.3
Edwards (2002)	TSA	99 (fatty deg. SSc)	431	65.1/67.2	78.9% 72.5%	44.2/43.1
Norris (2002)	TSA/HA	16	176	na	38/62	24
Simone (2014)	TSA	33	932	na/73	63.6/36.4	55

Table 21.3 Outcomes and complications of patients undergoing total shoulder arthroplasty and concomitant cuff tear

	Outcome	Primary outcome cuff tears	Primary outcome overall series	Complications overall series (%)	Conclusion
Edwards (2002) Cuff tears	Constant	94.1	95.3	16	No difference
Edwards (2002) IS fatty deg	Constant	83.6	97.1	16	Inferior outcomes
Edwards (2002) SSc fatty deg	Constant	83.6	96.4	16	Inferior outcomes
Norris (2002)	ASES	na	na	13.2	No difference
Simone (2014)	Forward elevation	139°	na	15	No difference for small tears

small (10), medium (14), large (9), or massive (0). The mean forward elevation improved from 99° (60°–170°) to 139° (15°–180°) ($p = <0.0001$). This improvement was greater in those with a small tear ($p = 0.03$). In four patients, with one large and three medium-sized tears, active elevation was <90°, and all had clinical or radiographic evidence of instability, three in an anterosuperior and one in a superior direction. Radiographic evidence of instability developed in six patients with medium or large tears. Complications were reported in 5 patients (15%), all with medium or large tears. The authors concluded that TSA in association with cuff repair yielded good results at mid-term FU in case of small tears and relatively young patients. RSA should be considered for older, less active patients with larger tears.

The analysis of the three studies confirms that small tears of the supraspinatus especially in younger patients can be repaired at the time of TSA with clinical outcomes comparable to TSAs in intact cuff. Larger tears and older patients may have better results with RSA.

21.4 Treatment Options of the Failed Rotator Cuff Repair

Rotator cuff repair (RCR) is a common procedure with increasing numbers each year, as more active patients suffer from symptomatic rotator cuff tears [8]. Despite the evolution of repair techniques and the development of instrumentation and suture anchors, the rate of unhealed or recurrent rotator cuff tears remains relatively high (in many studies >20%) [9]. Failure after rotator cuff surgery in patients with concomitant arthritis or not represents a difficult and challenging problem. Patients may complain of persistent pain and/or pseudo-paralysis of the shoulder with impairment in activities of daily living [10]. Re-repairing the rotator cuff may not be technically feasible and even contraindicated because of rotator cuff tendon loss, muscle fatty infiltration, and/or proximal migration of the humeral head under the acromial arch [11]. Furthermore, palliative surgery, like cuff debridement and/or biceps tenotomy or tenodesis, may also have failed to relieve pain and restore shoulder function [12]. Tendon transfers can be an option for young and demanding patients but require extensive rehabilitation with somewhat unpredictable results and may not be as successful in older patients or those with arthritis [13]. Historically, non-constrained hemiarthroplasty was proposed with the hope that this would provide pain relief [14]. However functional results were unpredictable and generally poor in terms of elevation above the horizontal level. Moreover, deterioration of the functional results after hemiarthroplasty in cuff deficient patients was commonly observed at medium- or long-term follow-up because of glenoid and/or acromial erosion and wear. Conversely RSA proposed by Grammont et al. in the 1980s [15] has proven to restore elevation above the horizontal level in patients with cuff tear arthropathy.

21.5 Analysis of the Literature of Total Shoulder Arthroplasty in Prior Cuff Repair

Three studies reported the outcomes of anatomic replacements after cuff repair surgery (Tables 21.4 and 21.5) [16–18]. Schoch et al. compared the outcomes of 30 patients with TSA after healed cuff repair with 90 patients with TSA and intact cuff [16]. At an average FU of 43 months, the ASES score was 77.1 and 82.7, respectively. Corresponding complication rate was 33% and 14%. Interestingly the rate of cuff failure after TSA was 13% in the post cuff repair group and 1% in the primary TSA group. The authors concluded that although functional improvements appear similar, gains in forward elevation and overhead strength were less compared with patients without prior surgery but did not reach statistical significance. Schiffman et al. performed a retrospective review of 345 anatomic shoulder arthroplasties; of these patients, 72 underwent previous non-arthroplasty surgery (13 cuff repair) [18]. At 2 years FU, the mean SANE score was 74 and 86, respectively ($P < 0.001$). The rate of manipulation under anesthesia and open revision was 17% in the study group and 1% in the control group. Therefore, the authors concluded that previous surgery is associated with inferior clinical outcomes and higher revision rates in patients undergoing index TSA. Erickson et al. reported on 14 patients with prior RCR who underwent TSA [17]. ASES scores significantly improved from 42.9 to 78.5 at 2 years and to 86.6 at 5 years. When compared with 42 matched control patients who underwent TSA with no history of RCR, similar outcomes were observed at 2 years (78.5 vs 85.3; $P = 0.19$) and 5 years (86.6 vs 90.9; $P = 0.72$). The authors concluded that no difference in clinical outcomes at 2 or 5 years after TSA was found between patients with and without a history of prior ipsilateral RCR.

Of the three studies, one showed similar outcomes, one inferior, and one slightly inferior although not significant. When dealing with patients with prior cuff repair and candi-

Table 21.4 Demographics of patients undergoing total shoulder arthroplasty after prior cuff repair

	Implant design	Previous surgery	Control group	Age SG/CG	Male/female	FU (months)
Erickson (2020)	TSA	14	42	65.1/65.4	9/5 27/15	24
Schiffmann (2020)	TSA	72 (13 cuff repair)	221	59/68	106/115 42/30	24
Schoch (2020)	TSA	30	90	64/64	20/10 61/29	43

Table 21.5 Outcomes and complications of patients undergoing total shoulder arthroplasty after prior cuff repair

	Outcome	Primary outcome cuff repair	Primary outcome control group	p value	Complications cuff repair (%)	Complications control group (%)	Conclusion
Erickson (2020)	ASES	78.5	85.3	0.19	na	na	No difference
Schiffmann (2020)	SANE	74 (all previous surgeries)	86	<0.001	(9 + 8) MUA + open revision	(0 + 1) MUA + open revision	Inferior outcomes
Schoch (2020)	ASES	*77.1*	82.7	0.26	10 (33%)	12 (14%)	Slightly inferior

date to TSA, it is important to consider that the repaired cuff has usually lower tissue quality than intact cuff.

21.6 Cuff Tears After Total Shoulder Arthroplasty

Although relatively uncommon, rotator cuff tears after TSA are one of the most common late complications. They are primarily due to overstuffing the joint, tendon insufficiency after multiple open surgeries, or secondary to fatty infiltration or aggressive passive external rotation rehabilitation. When the subscapularis tendon is involved, and the tissue is of sufficient quality and amenable to repair, this represents an effective option. Pectoralis major tendon transfer can be considered in the setting of an irreparable subscapularis tear. This is a salvage procedure and is contraindicated when the humeral head is no longer centered into the glenoid fossa or it is statically subluxated anteriorly. Furthermore, the success of a pectoralis major tendon transfer appears also to be dependent on the quality of the existing subscapularis muscle. Patients with chronic fatty infiltrated subscapularis tears should be addressed with caution as pectoralis major tendon transfer does not provide an acceptable outcome in these patients [19]. Disruption of the subscapularis and supraspinatus results in the so-called rotator interval lesion and is exemplified by anterior and superior escape on radiographs. The integrity of the rotator cuff is critical for physiologic total shoulder arthroplasty function. A recent biomechanics study showed that in case of anatomic replacement, the maximum deltoid forces were increased by 36% under the subscapularis deficiency and by 53% under the supraspinatus, infraspinatus, subscapularis, and teres minor deficiencies [20]. The maximum glenohumeral contact forces were decreased by 11.3% in case

of supraspinatus and infraspinatus deficiencies but increased by 24.8% in case of subscapularis deficiency. The results suggested that the changes in the biomechanics of the GH joint induced by rotator cuff deficiencies after ATSA increase the deltoid muscle energy expenditure and joint instability, which result in postoperative less satisfactory clinical outcomes. The changes in rotator cuff muscle forces deserve more attention for understanding the evolution of rotator cuff tear after TSA. (Tables 21.6 and 21.7).

Gonzales et al. in a systematic review of the complications after TSA/HA reported 110 secondary cuff tears (2.7%) among the cohort of 4010 anatomic replacements [21]. The diagnosis was made most often clinically or radiographically through superior migration of the humeral head component. Reoperation for most of these cases involved more conservative procedures: acromioplasty, cuff repair, or even a muscle transfer or flap. Certain teams proposed conversion to HHA with a large humeral head. Others preferred performing glenohumeral arthrodesis or resection arthroplasty. Yet, only revision to a reverse TSA has produced satisfactory results [22].

Bohsali et al. in a review of the literature evaluated 33 studies on unconstrained total shoulder arthroplasty (in a total of 2540 shoulders) with average follow-up of 5.3 years [23]. Thirty-two patients (1.3%) showed late cuff tears.

Table 21.6 Prevalence of cuff tears after total shoulder arthroplasty

	Initial cohort	Cuff tears	%
Chin (2006)	431	17	3.9
Bohsali (2006)	2540	32	1.3
Gonzales (2011)	4010	110	2.7
Young (2012)	518	87	16.8
Levy (2016)	1259	na	14.3
Overall	8758	246	7.8

Table 21.7 Demographic of patients with rotator cuff tear after total shoulder arthroplasty

	Implant design	Overall	Cuff tears	Age	Male/female	FU (months)
Hattrupp (2006)	TSA	No	20	65.9	na	109
Young (2012)	TSA	518	87	68.2	39.3%	103.6

21.7 Epidemiology of Cuff Tears After Total Shoulder Arthroplasty

Cofield and Edgerton at the beginning of the 1990s reported an incidence of secondary cuff tears after TSA varying from 2.2 to 2.7% [24]. Chin et al. reported rotator cuff tears to be the most encountered complication following TSA, particularly late [25]. Young et al. reported a much higher 16.8% incidence of rotator cuff dysfunction following TSA, with "dysfunction" defined as >25% superior migration of the humeral component on a true anterior–posterior radiograph of the glenohumeral joint [26]. Post-TSA rotator cuff tearing or dysfunction is associated with proximal migration of the humeral component, which can accelerate polyethylene wear and loosening of the glenoid component through the rocking-horse phenomenon [27]. In an early meta-analysis at short average follow-up, Wirth and Rockwood reported rotator cuff tearing in 2% [28]. Bohsali et al. in a review of the literature evaluated 33 studies on unconstrained total shoulder arthroplasty (2540 shoulders) at an average FU of 5.3 years reported an incidence of rotator cuff tears of 1.3% TSA (32 shoulders) [23]. The subscapularis accounted for slightly more than 50% of these tears. Levy et al. in a more recent systematic review on 15 studies (1259 TSA) reported 11.3% ± 7.9 of superior cuff tears and 3.0% ± 13.6 of subscapularis cuff tears at an average FU 6.8 ± 3.2 years [5]. The authors pointed out that the diagnosis of secondary cuff tear after TSA may be not easy and should rely on X-rays (superior or anterior migration of the humeral head) rather than on clinical evaluation. They found that nearly 30% of shoulders demonstrated radiographic superior migration and 12% showed anterior migration of the humeral head at a final FU (Table 21.8).

Table 21.8 Outcomes and complications of patients with rotator cuff tear after total shoulder arthroplasty

	Outcome	Overall	Cuff tears	p value	Complications SG (%)	Complications CG (%)	Conclusion
Hattrupp (2006)	AAE	No	85°	No	77.7	No	Poor outcomes
Young (2012)	Constant	93.8	79.2	<0.001	na	na	Inferior outcomes

21.8 Analysis of the Literature of Cuff Tears After Total Shoulder Arthroplasty

Hattrupp et al. reviewed the database of the Mayo Clinic to evaluate the outcomes of patients who had a subsequent operation for cuff repair with or without component revision after TSA [29]. At the end, 20 shoulders were reviewed at an average FU of 109 months. The tear involved the subscapularis in 7 shoulders, the supraspinatus in 15, and the infraspinatus in 8. Average delay from TSA to cuff repair was 23 months. The diagnosis of secondary cuff tear was based on clinical findings and antero-superior migration of the humeral head. Active forward flexion decreased from 109° before TSA to 85° after the diagnosis of cuff tear. Other than cuff failure, 14 complications were observed. The authors concluded that the results of cuff repair in patients with late cuff tears after TSA are poor.

Young et al. reviewed 518 TSAs for primary osteoarthritis at an average FU of 103.6 months [26]. The diagnosis of secondary rotator cuff dysfunction was made when moderate or severe superior subluxation of the prosthetic humeral head was present on radiographs. The rate of secondary rotator cuff dysfunction was 16.8%. A partial or complete tear of the supraspinatus tendon at the time of surgery was not statistically associated with secondary rotator cuff dysfunction ($p = 0.16$). Survivorship free of secondary cuff dysfunction was 100% at 5 years, 84% at 10 years, and 45% at 15 years. Duration of follow-up ($p < 0.0001$), implantation of the glenoid implant with superior tilt ($p < 0.001$), and fatty infiltration of the infraspinatus muscle ($p < 0.05$) were risk factors for the development of secondary cuff dysfunction. Patients with secondary rotator cuff dysfunction had significantly worse clinical outcomes (Constant score, subjective assessment, and range of motion; $p < 0.0001$) and radiographic results (radiolucent line score, radiographic loosening, glenoid component migration; $p < 0.0001$). Although the rates of revision were not significantly different, an important finding in our study was that secondary rotator cuff dysfunction was associated with less satisfactory clinical outcomes. The authors concluded that duration of follow-up was the most significant factor associated with the development of secondary rotator cuff dysfunction, which helps to explain the variable results reported in the literature for proximal humeral migration following TSA.

21.9 Conclusions

Cuff tears may be encountered before TSA/HA and as well may develop after such operations. They influence the biomechanics of the shoulder, and therefore they must be carefully evaluated when planning these operations. Partial tears or small tears of the superior cuff may be forgiving especially in young patients and therefore do not represent a contraindication to anatomic replacement. They can be repaired or left alone at the time of replacement since no statistically significant difference is reported with respect of this choice. Similarly, the impact of previous cuff repairs before anatomic replacement is controversial. Some studies reported inferior results when compared to primary replacements while other showed similar outcomes.

Late cuff tears after anatomic replacements are uncommon even if they represent one of the most common complications. The diagnosis may be not easy especially if it only relies on clinical findings. X-rays signs of superior and anterior migration are reliable aspects of late cuff dysfunction. This occurrence is detrimental since it leads to deterioration of the clinical results and to accelerated polyethylene wear because of the altered biomechanics.

References

1. Edwards TB, Boulahia A, Kempf JF, Boileau P, Nèmoz C, Walch G. The influence of rotator cuff disease on the results of shoulder arthroplasty for primary osteoarthritis: results of a multicenter study. J Bone Jt Surg. 2002;84-A:2240–8.
2. Norris TR, Iannotti JP. Functional outcome after shoulder arthroplasty for primary osteoarthritis: a multicenter study. J Shoulder Elb Surg. 2002;11:130–5.
3. Fouria AM, Sperling JW, Ankem HK, Oh LS, Cofield RH. Total shoulder replacement for osteoarthritis in patients 80 years of age and older. J Bone Jt Surg (Br). 2010;92-B:970–4.
4. Haines JF, Trail IA, Nuttall D, Birch A, Barrow A. The results of arthroplasty in osteoarthritis of the shoulder. J Bone Jt Surg (Br). 2006;88-B:496–501.
5. Levy JC, Everding NG, Gil CC Jr, Stephens S, Giveans MR. Speed of recovery after shoulder arthroplasty: a comparison of reverse and anatomic total shoulder arthroplasty. J Shoulder Elb Surg. 2014;23(12):1872–81.
6. Edwards TB, Boulahia A, Kempf JF, Boileau P, Némoz C, Walch G. The influence of rotator cuff disease on the results of shoulder arthroplasty for primary osteoarthritis: results of a multicenter study. J Bone Jt Surg Am. 2002;84-A:2240–8.
7. Simone JP, Streubel PH, Sperling JW, Schleck CD, Cofield RH, Athwal GS. Anatomical total shoulder replacement with rotator cuff repair for osteoarthritis of the shoulder. Bone Jt J. 2014;96-B(2):224–8. https://doi.org/10.1302/0301-620X.96B.32890.
8. Paloneva J, Lepola V, Aarimaa V, Joukainen A, Ylinen J, Mattila VM. Increasing incidence of rotator cuff repairs—a nationwide registry study in Finland. BMC Musculoskelet Disord. 2015;16:189.
9. Galanopoulos I, Aslanidis I, Karliaftis K, Papadopoulos D, Ashwood N. The impact of re-tear on the clinical outcome after rotator cuff repair using open or arthroscopic techniques—a systematic review. Open Orthop J. 2017;11:95–107. https://doi.org/10.2174/1874325001711010095.
10. Neviaser RJ. Evaluation and management of failed rotator cuff repairs. Orthop Clin N Am. 1997;28(2):215–24. https://doi.org/10.1016/s0030-5898(05)70281-9.
11. DeButtet A, Bouchon Y, Capon D, Delfosse J. Grammont shoulder arthroplasty for osteoarthritis with massive rotator cuff tears: report of 71 cases. J Shoulder Elb Surg. 1997;6:19.
12. Walch G, Edwards TB, Boulahia A, Nove-Josserand L, Neyton L, Szabo I. Arthroscopic tenotomy of the long head of the biceps in the treatment of rotator cuff tears: clinical and radiographic results of 307 cases. J Shoulder Elb Surg. 2005;14:238–46.
13. Clark NJ, Elhassan BT. The role of tendon transfers for irreparable rotator cuff tears. Curr Rev Musculoskelet Med. 2018;11(1):141–9. https://doi.org/10.1007/s12178-018-9468.
14. Field LD, Dines DM, Zabinski SJ, Warren RF. Hemiarthroplasty of the shoulder for rotator cuff arthroplasty. J Shoulder Elb Surg. 1997;6:18–23.
15. Grammont P, Trouilloud P, Laffay JP, Deries X. Etude et réalisation d'une nouvelle prothése d'épaule. Rhumatologie. 1987;39:17–22.
16. Schoch BS, Tams C, Eichinger J, Wright TW, Jospeh J, King JJ, et al. Anatomic total shoulder arthroplasty after healed rotator cuff repair: a matched cohort. J Shoulder Elb Surg. 2020;29(11):2221–8. https://doi.org/10.1016/j.jse.2020.03.029.
17. Erickson BJ, Ling D, Wong A, Dines DM, Gulotta LV. Does having a rotator cuff repair before total shoulder arthroplasty influence outcomes? Orthop J Sports Med. 2020;8(8):2325967120942773. https://doi.org/10.1177/2325967120942773.
18. Schiffman CJ, Hannay WM, Whitson AJ, Neradile KMB, Matsen FA, Hsu JE. Impact of previous non-arthroplasty surgery on clinical outcomes after primary anatomic shoulder arthroplasty. J Shoulder Elb Surg. 2020;29(10):2056–64. https://doi.org/10.1016/j.jse.2020.01.088.
19. Elhassan B, Ozbaydar M, Massimini D, et al. Transfer of pectoralis major for the treatment of irreparable tears of subscapularis: does it work? J Bone Jt Surg (Br). 2008;90(8):1059–65.
20. Chen Z, Fan X, Gao Y, Zhang J, Guo L, Chen S, et al. Effect of rotator cuff deficiencies on muscle forces and glenohumeral contact force after anatomic total shoulder arthroplasty using musculoskeletal multibody dynamics simulation. Front Bioeng Biotechnol. 2021;9:691450. https://doi.org/10.3389/fbioe.2021.691450.
21. Gonzalez JF, Alami GB, Baque F, Walch G, Boileau P. Complications of unconstrained shoulder prostheses. J Shoulder Elb Surg. 2011;20(4):666–82. https://doi.org/10.1016/j.jse.2010.11.017.
22. Walch G, Boileau P, Mole D. 2000 shoulder prostheses 2–10-year follow-up. Montpellier: Sauramps Medical; 2001.
23. Bohsali KI, Wirth MA, Rockwood CA Jr. Complications of total shoulder arthroplasty. J Bone Jt Surg Am. 2006;88:2279–92.
24. Cofield RH, Edgerton BC. Total shoulder arthroplasty: complications and revision surgery. Instr Course Lect. 1990;39:449–62.
25. Chin PY, Sperling JW, Cofield RH, Schleck C. Complications of total shoulder arthroplasty: are they fewer or different? J Shoulder Elb Surg. 2006;15:19–22.
26. Young AA, Walch G, Pape G, Gohlke F, Favard L. Secondary rotator cuff dysfunction following total shoulder arthroplasty for primary glenohumeral osteoarthritis: results of a multicenter study with more than 5 years of follow-up. J Bone Jt Surg Am. 2012;94(8):685–93. https://doi.org/10.2106/JBJS.J.00727.
27. Franklin JL, Barrett WP, Jackins SE, Matsen FA 3rd. Glenoid loosening in total shoulder arthroplasty.

Association with rotator cuff deficiency. J Arthroplast. 1988;3:39–46.

28. Wirth MA, Rockwood CA Jr. Complications of total shoulder-replacement arthroplasty. J Bone Jt Surg Am. 1996;78:603–16.

29. Hattrup SJ, Cofield RH, Cha SS. Rotator cuff repair after shoulder replacement. J Shoulder Elb Surg. 2006;15(1):78–83. https://doi.org/10.1016/j.jse.2005.06.002.

Shoulder Arthroplasty and Inflammatory Arthritis

22

Daichi Morikawa, Yoshimasa Saigo, and Muneaki Ishijima

22.1 Introduction

Inflammatory arthritis encompasses several systemic diseases that cause autoimmune disorders and affect several joints. There are many variable factors for each disease regarding severity, prognosis, and treatment. Rheumatoid arthritis (RA) is one of the most common forms of inflammatory arthritis, and arthroplasty is undertaken for several joints including the shoulder in cases of severe joint destruction [1]. In this chapter, we mainly focus on RA in inflammatory arthritis, especially shoulder arthroplasty.

Recently, with the increasing use of disease-modifying antirheumatic drugs (DMARDs) and immunosuppressive medications, the occurrence of rapid joint destruction and the rate of total joint replacement (TJR) among patients with RA have significantly decreased [2, 3]. However, Mertelsmann et al. reported that the rate of TJR minimally decreased among patients with RA from 4.6 per 100,000 persons in 1991 to 4.5 per 100,000 persons in 2005 (average year's decrease: 0.01%) using administrative discharge databases [1]. Moreover, Jain et al. reported the number of cases of primary total shoulder arthroplasty (TSA) increased over time from 1992 to 2005 in patients with RA using the Nationwide Inpatient Sample database [4]. These data showed TJR including shoulder arthroplasty was still needed in patients with RA.

22.2 Perioperative Concerns in Shoulder Arthroplasty for Inflammatory Arthritis

There are several perioperative concerns in shoulder arthroplasty for patients with RA, such as surgical site infection, osteoporosis, and joint destruction.

Surgical site infection is one of the biggest concerns in shoulder arthroplasty with inflammatory arthritis. Leroux et al. reported that the rates of early surgical site infection in shoulder arthroplasty were 0.13% in RA patients and 0.09% in non-RA patients (odds ratio, 1.4; $p = 0.52$) [5]. Recently, Nezwek et al. reported that the rate of infection after reverse shoulder arthroplasty (RSA) was three times higher in patients with RA (9%) compared with patients without RA (3%) [6]. Although the early use of DMARDs and/or immunosuppressants is associated with longer time to joint replacement surgery, RA patients using these drugs have a potential risk of surgical site infection [7].

RA is associated with an increased risk of osteoporosis and fracture [8–10]. Lee et al.

D. Morikawa (✉) · Y. Saigo · M. Ishijima
Department of Orthopaedics, Juntendo University
School of Medicine, Tokyo, Japan
e-mail: dmorikaw@juntendo.ac.jp;
y.saigo.ux@juntendo.ac.jp; ishijima@juntendo.ac.jp

© ISAKOS 2023

A. D. Mazzocca et al. (eds.), *Shoulder Arthritis across the Life Span*,
https://doi.org/10.1007/978-3-031-33298-2_22

reported that the prevalence of osteoporosis in RA patients was 1.9 times higher than that in healthy subjects, and the use of glucocorticoids was a risk factor for the reduction in bone mineral density in RA patients [11]. Miller et al. reported that symptomatic acromial and scapular stress fractures after RSA were significantly more common in patients with RA (24% vs 5.2%) [12]. Thus, the surgeon should take precautions for osteoporosis in RA patients.

Joint destruction is also a perioperative concern in shoulder arthroplasty with inflammatory arthritis, especially because the glenoid bone influences the type of surgery performed [13]. Larsen's grading system is a well-established categorization scheme and assesses all limb joints for RA [14]. Levigne et al. reported the classification of a rheumatoid shoulder that had three radiological patterns defined by the morphology of the humeral head and glenoid (Fig. 22.1): Type A (ascending, 54%), Type C (centered, 20%), and Type D (destructive, 26%) [15]. They revealed that the rates of complications and repeat surgery was equivalent in all three forms of RA and that there was no correlation between the preoperative radiological pattern and the postoperative functional results after reverse shoulder arthroplasty [15]. The type of radiological pattern may influence the optimal surgical treatment, alongside the patient's age, functional demand, and rotator cuff status [13].

22.2.1 Surface Replacement

Resurfacing arthroplasty is a shoulder arthroplasty procedure for inflammatory arthritis. The objective of resurfacing arthroplasty is to correct the deformed head with minimal bone loss [13]. The advantages of resurfacing arthroplasty are short surgical times, low risk of fracture, and minimal resection. The disadvantage is difficult anatomical fitting in cases of severely deformed humeral heads. Several researchers published mid-term clinical results after resurfacing arthroplasty for RA shoulders [16–21]. Although most of the reported results of RA with resurfacing arthroplasty are good, superior migration of the humeral head was encountered in two-thirds of patients, and glenoid erosion was shown in one-third of patients [17].

22.2.2 Hemiarthroplasty

Hemiarthroplasty (HA) is another shoulder arthroplasty procedure for inflammatory arthritis. The approach for hemiarthroplasty is to replace the deformed head with or without bone loss [13]. The advantages of HA are the resulting pain relief and easier accessibility for revision. HA is preferred for patients with an intact rotator cuff and minimal glenoid bone erosion [13]. Barlow et al. reported that HA achieved pain relief and

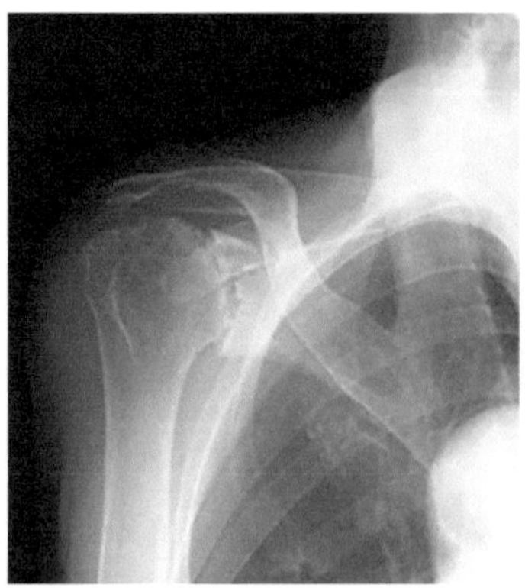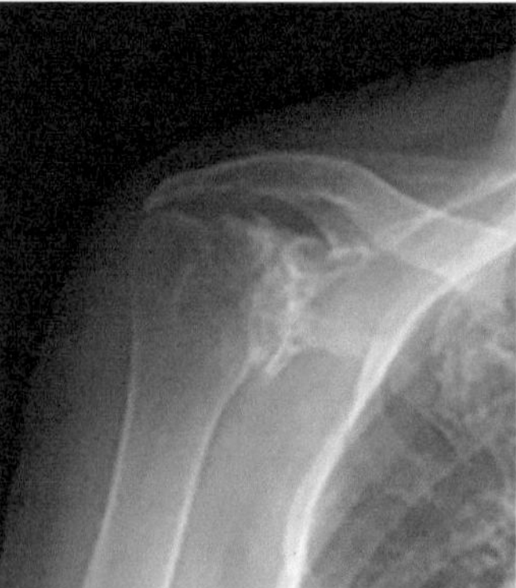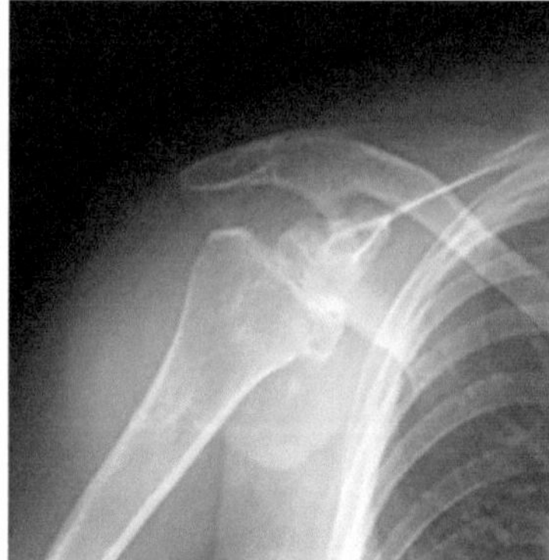

Fig. 22.1 Classification of rheumatoid shoulder according to Lévigne, with three radiological presentations: Type A (ascending), Type C (centered), and Type D (destructive)

improved motion in patients with RA as well as TSA, with a minimum 5-year follow-up period [22]. Moreover, there was significantly better pain relief and a trend toward improved motion and survivorship with TSA compared with HA in patients with an intact rotator cuff [22]. Colin et al. also confirmed these findings [23], while Trail et al. reported that medial migration was evident in 16.3% of patients at 2 years or more after HA in patients with RA [24]. Survival rates after HA for inflammatory arthritis were 80.0%, 75.8%, and 75.8% at 5, 10, and 20 years, respectively, in patients with an intact rotator cuff and 92.6% at 5, 10, and 20 years in patients without an intact rotator cuff [22].

22.2.3 Total Shoulder Arthroplasty

TSA is another shoulder arthroplasty procedure for inflammatory arthritis. The advantages of TSA are long-term pain relief and prevention of medial erosion [13, 22–25]. The average postoperative range of motion (ROM) is 66.0°–102° on forward elevation and 32°–48° on external rotation at mid- or long-term follow-up [22, 24, 26]. Barlow et al. reported that periprosthetic lucencies were 29% in the humerus and 73% in the glenoid, and survival rates after TSA for inflammatory arthritis were 96.7%, 96.7%, and 89.0% at 5, 10, and 20 years, respectively, in patients with an intact rotator cuff and 95.8%, 90.7%, and 86.0% at 5, 10, and 20 years, respectively, in patients without an intact rotator cuff [22].

22.2.4 Reverse Shoulder Arthroplasty

Reverse shoulder arthroplasty (RSA) has been widely used in patients with cuff tear arthropathy and irreparable massive rotator cuff tears.

Recently, the indications have expanded to include inflammatory arthritis, acute fractures, fracture sequelae, and revision surgery. Several studies emphasized that RSA in patients with RA had poorer clinical outcomes and higher complication and revision rates including intraoperative fractures, glenoid loosening, and infection than RSA in patients with other etiologies [27–29]. However, a recent systematic review reported that RSA in RA showed similar short- to mid-term results without higher complication rates as compared with RSA in cuff tear arthropathy [30]. Moreover, two studies showed that RSA provided excellent pain relief and function and minimal complications for patients with inflammatory arthritis [15, 31]. They also reported revision-free survivorships were 96% at 7 years and 97% at 2 and 5 years. Average postoperative ROM was 132° and 138° for forward elevation and 22° and 45° for external rotation at mid-term follow-up. They discussed their improved results were likely multifactorial, including a combination of improved surgical technique and implant design, as well as medical control of the underlying disease process. Glenoid bone grafting from the humeral head was required in 24% and 45% because of severe glenoid bone loss [15, 31]. RSA with glenoid bone grafting is one of the most challenging shoulder surgeries and depends on bone loss and the quality of the humeral head and glenoid. Recently, a patient-matched glenoid implant for severe glenoid bone deficiency was developed, and the early results of RSA were reported [32–35]. Bodendorfer et al. reported the use of a patient-matched glenoid implant for severe glenoid dysplasia of patients with RA [33]. RSA with a patient-matched glenoid implant is an option for the surgical treatment of inflammatory arthritis with severe glenoid bone loss (Fig. 22.2).

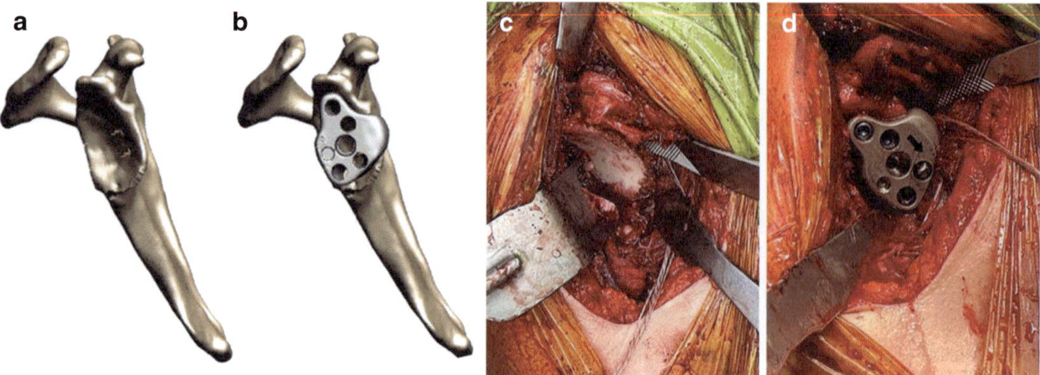

Fig. 22.2 Patient-matched glenoid implant (vault reconstruction system, Zimmer Biomet) (**a**) 3D reconstruction produced from CT scan. (**b**) Computer-aided design used to create a proposed implant. (**c**) Glenoid with severe bone loss. (**d**) Glenoid with the patient-matched implant

22.3 Conclusions

Shoulder arthroplasties remain important surgical options for inflammatory arthritis patients with shoulder pain, despite the increasing use of DMARDs and immunosuppressive medications. Optimal surgical treatment is determined according to the patient's age, functional demand, rotator cuff status, glenoid bone stock, and the advantages and disadvantages of shoulder arthroplasties.

References

1. Mertelsmann-Voss C, Lyman S, Pan TJ, Goodman SM, Figgie MP, Mandl LA. US trends in rates of arthroplasty for inflammatory arthritis including rheumatoid arthritis, juvenile idiopathic arthritis, and spondyloarthritis. Arthritis Rheumatol. 2014;66(6):1432–9.
2. Wolfe F, Zwillich SH. The long-term outcomes of rheumatoid arthritis: a 23-year prospective, longitudinal study of total joint replacement and its predictors in 1600 patients with rheumatoid arthritis. Arthritis Rheum. 1998;41(6):1072–82.
3. Jamsen E, Virta LJ, Hakala M, Kauppi MJ, Malmivaara A, Lehto MU. The decline in joint replacement surgery in rheumatoid arthritis is associated with a concomitant increase in the intensity of anti-rheumatic therapy: a nationwide register-based study from 1995 through 2010. Acta Orthop. 2013;84(4):331–7.
4. Jain A, Stein BE, Skolasky RL, Jones LC, Hungerford MW. Total joint arthroplasty in patients with rheumatoid arthritis: a United States experience from 1992 through 2005. J Arthroplast. 2012;27(6):881–8.
5. Leroux TS, Basques BA, Saltzman BM, Nicholson GP, Romeo AA, Verma NN. Shoulder arthroplasty in patients with rheumatoid arthritis: a population-based study examining utilization, adverse events, length of stay, and cost. Am J Orthop (Belle Mead NJ). 2018;47(6):46.
6. Nezwek TA, Dutcher L, Mascarenhas L, Woltemath A, Thirumavalavan J, Lund J, et al. Prior shoulder surgery and rheumatoid arthritis increase early risk of infection after primary reverse total shoulder arthroplasty. JSES Int. 2021;5(6):1062–6.
7. Moura CS, Abrahamowicz M, Beauchamp ME, Lacaille D, Wang Y, Boire G, et al. Early medication use in new-onset rheumatoid arthritis may delay joint replacement: results of a large population-based study. Arthritis Res Ther. 2015;17:197.
8. Xue AL, Wu SY, Jiang L, Feng AM, Guo HF, Zhao P. Bone fracture risk in patients with rheumatoid arthritis: a meta-analysis. Medicine (Baltimore). 2017;96(36):e6983.
9. Wright NC, Lisse JR, Walitt BT, Eaton CB, Chen Z. Women's Health Initiative I. Arthritis increases the risk for fractures—results from the Women's Health Initiative. J Rheumatol. 2011;38(8):1680–8.
10. Kim D, Cho SK, Choi CB, Jun JB, Kim TH, Lee HS, et al. Incidence and risk factors of fractures in patients with rheumatoid arthritis: an Asian prospective cohort study. Rheumatol Int. 2016;36(9):1205–14.
11. Lee SG, Park YE, Park SH, Kim TK, Choi HJ, Lee SJ, et al. Increased frequency of osteoporosis and BMD below the expected range for age among South Korean women with rheumatoid arthritis. Int J Rheum Dis. 2012;15(3):289–96.
12. Miller M, Chalmers PN, Nyfeler J, Mhyre L, Wheelwright C, Konery K, et al. Rheumatoid arthritis is associated with increased symptomatic acromial and scapular spine stress fracture after reverse total shoulder arthroplasty. JSES Int. 2021;5(2):261–5.

13. Aydin N, Aslan L, Lehtinen J, Hamuryudan V. Current surgical treatment options of rheumatoid shoulder. Curr Rheumatol Rev. 2018;14(3):200–12.

14. Larsen A, Dale K, Eek M. Radiographic evaluation of rheumatoid arthritis and related conditions by standard reference films. Acta Radiol Diagn (Stockh). 1977;18(4):481–91.

15. Levigne C, Chelli M, Johnston TR, Trojani MC, Mole D, Walch G, et al. Reverse shoulder arthroplasty in rheumatoid arthritis: survival and outcomes. J Shoulder Elb Surg. 2021;30(10):2312–24.

16. Fink B, Singer J, Lamla U, Rüther W. Surface replacement of the humeral head in rheumatoid arthritis. Arch Orthop Trauma Surg. 2004;124(6):366–73.

17. Fuerst M, Fink B, Rüther W. The DUROM cup humeral surface replacement in patients with rheumatoid arthritis. Surgical technique. J Bone Jt Surg Am. 2008;90(Suppl 2 Pt 2):287–98.

18. Rydholm U, Sjogren J. Surface replacement of the humeral head in the rheumatoid shoulder. J Shoulder Elb Surg. 1993;2(6):286–95.

19. Alund M, Hoe-Hansen C, Tillander B, Heden BA, Norlin R. Outcome after cup hemiarthroplasty in the rheumatoid shoulder: a retrospective evaluation of 39 patients followed for 2–6 years. Acta Orthop Scand. 2000;71(2):180–4.

20. Levy O, Copeland SA. Cementless surface replacement arthroplasty of the shoulder. 5- to 10-year results with the Copeland mark-2 prosthesis. J Bone Jt Surg Br. 2001;83(2):213–21.

21. Thomas SR, Wilson AJ, Chambler A, Harding I, Thomas M. Outcome of Copcland surface replacement shoulder arthroplasty. J Shoulder Elb Surg. 2005;14(5):485–91.

22. Barlow JD, Yuan BJ, Schleck CD, Harmsen WS, Cofield RH, Sperling JW. Shoulder arthroplasty for rheumatoid arthritis: 303 consecutive cases with minimum 5-year follow-up. J Shoulder Elb Surg. 2014;23(6):791–9.

23. Collins DN, Harryman DT 2nd, Wirth MA. Shoulder arthroplasty for the treatment of inflammatory arthritis. J Bone Jt Surg Am. 2004;86(11):2489–96.

24. Trail IA, Nuttall D. The results of shoulder arthroplasty in patients with rheumatoid arthritis. J Bone Jt Surg Br. 2002;84(8):1121–5.

25. Sperling JW, Cofield RH, Schleck CD, Harmsen WS. Total shoulder arthroplasty versus hemiarthroplasty for rheumatoid arthritis of the shoulder: results of 303 consecutive cases. J Shoulder Elb Surg. 2007;16(6):683–90.

26. Clement ND, Mathur K, Colling R, Stirrat AN. The metal-backed glenoid component in rheumatoid disease: 8–14-year follow-up. J Shoulder Elb Surg. 2010;19(5):749–56.

27. Favard L, Katz D, Colmar M, Benkalfate T, Thomazeau H, Emily S. Total shoulder arthroplasty—arthroplasty for glenohumeral arthropathies: results and complications after a minimum follow-up of 8 years according to the type of arthroplasty and etiology. Orthop Traumatol Surg Res. 2012;98(4 Suppl):S41–7.

28. Guery J, Favard L, Sirveaux F, Oudet D, Mole D, Walch G. Reverse total shoulder arthroplasty. Survivorship analysis of 80 replacements followed for 5–10 years. J Bone Jt Surg Am. 2006;88(8):1742–7.

29. Zumstein MA, Pinedo M, Old J, Boileau P. Problems, complications, reoperations, and revisions in reverse total shoulder arthroplasty: a systematic review. J Shoulder Elb Surg. 2011;20(1):146–57.

30. Cho CH, Kim DH, Song KS. Reverse shoulder arthroplasty in patients with rheumatoid arthritis: a systematic review. Clin Orthop Surg. 2017;9(3):325–31.

31. Mangold DR, Wagner ER, Cofield RH, Sanchez-Sotelo J, Sperling JW. Reverse shoulder arthroplasty for rheumatoid arthritis since the introduction of disease-modifying drugs. Int Orthop. 2019;43(11):2593–600.

32. Rangarajan R, Blout CK, Patel VV, Bastian SA, Lee BK, Itamura JM. Early results of reverse total shoulder arthroplasty using a patient-matched glenoid implant for severe glenoid bone deficiency. J Shoulder Elb Surg. 2020;29(7S):S139–S48.

33. Bodendorfer BM, Loughran GJ, Looney AM, Velott AT, Stein JA, Lutton DM, et al. Short-term outcomes of reverse shoulder arthroplasty using a custom baseplate for severe glenoid deficiency. J Shoulder Elb Surg. 2021;30(5):1060–7.

34. Dines DM, Gulotta L, Craig EV, Dines JS. Novel solution for massive glenoid defects in shoulder arthroplasty: a patient-specific glenoid vault reconstruction system. Am J Orthop (Belle Mead NJ). 2017;46(2):104–8.

35. De Martino I, Dines DM, Warren RF, Craig EV, Gulotta LV. Patient-specific implants in severe glenoid bone loss. Am J Orthop (Belle Mead NJ). 2018;47(2):9.

Shoulder Arthroplasty and Infection

23

Vanessa Charubhumi and Andrew Jawa

23.1 Introduction

Over the past 10 years, the incidence of primary and revision shoulder arthroplasty has increased dramatically in the USA, climbing from an estimated 64,125 arthroplasties in 2012 to 108,300 primary and 10,290 revision shoulder arthroplasties in 2017 [1–3]. Additionally, growth rate projections currently outpace those of total hip and knee arthroplasties, and the increasing incidence highlights the potential increasing revision burden, including those due to infection. Periprosthetic shoulder infections after primary arthroplasties are rare with a prevalence as low as 0.7% [4] and similar rates between anatomic and reverse shoulder arthroplasties [5]. However, studies have reported infection rates after revision surgery as high as 15.4% [6].

The most common organism responsible for infection is *Cutibacterium acnes* (formerly *Propionibacterium acnes*), a lower virulence organism. This unique microbiology of the shoulder poses a diagnostic challenge to surgeons as the criteria for hip and knee periprosthetic joint infections (PJI) may not be applicable.

23.2 Clinical Presentation

The clinical presentation of shoulder PJI varies depending on timing, the virulence of the causative pathogen, and the response of the host. The presentation can be classified as acute (less than 3 months after the index procedure), subacute (between 3 and 12 months), and chronic (greater than 12 months) [7].

The typical signs of infection, such as pain, swelling, fever, erythema, and drainage, are seen in acute PJI. While acute infections can be caused by *C.* acnes, other more virulent pathogens, including *S. aureus* and *Streptococcus*, can also be found in culture isolates. Subacute and chronic infections are more commonly caused by lower virulence organisms and often lack the common clinical signs of infection [8]. When evaluating a patient with a poorly performing shoulder arthroplasty, a high index of suspicion for infection must be maintained.

V. Charubhumi (✉)
Department of Orthopaedic Surgery, New England Baptist Hospital, Boston, MA, USA

A. Jawa
Department of Orthopaedic Surgery, New England Baptist Hospital, Boston, MA, USA

Boston Sports and Shoulder Center, Waltham, MA, USA

© ISAKOS 2023
A. D. Mazzocca et al. (eds.), *Shoulder Arthritis across the Life Span*,
https://doi.org/10.1007/978-3-031-33298-2_23

23.3 Clinical Evaluation

23.3.1 Patient Evaluation

The first step should be obtaining a comprehensive clinical history and thorough physical examination of the shoulder. Risk factors for periprosthetic shoulder infections, including obesity, diabetes mellitus, radiation, lymphedema, prior non-shoulder periprosthetic joint infection, and previous surgery, especially patients who have undergone shoulder arthroscopy less than 3 months prior to their arthroplasty procedure [9], should be noted. Of these risk factors, younger age, male sex [10, 11], postoperative hematoma [12], arthroplasty after trauma [10], and previous surgery are the most significant. Richards et al. found that with every 1 year increase in age, there was a 5% reduction in infection risk [13]. Additionally, potential sources of hematogenous spread should also be identified, such as recent pneumonia, urinary tract infection, or oral abscess. Postoperative issues, such as prolonged drainage, erythema, swelling, fever, or wound dehiscence, should be elicited and could be indicative of an infection caused by a more virulent organism.

In patients with periprosthetic shoulder infections, the most common complaint is shoulder pain, followed by a draining sinus, stiffness, erythema, and effusion. Fever, night sweats, and chills are seen less commonly [14].

23.3.2 Imaging

High-quality radiographs should be obtained to rule out other causes of shoulder pain and dysfunction that can imitate or coincide with shoulder PJI. Sequential radiographs are particularly important for evaluation of implant loosening and osteolysis. Findings concerning for PJI are radiolucent lines, osteolysis, bone erosion, endosteal scalloping, new periosteal bone formation, and component migration (Fig. 23.1). Pottinger et al. [11] also reported that humeral loosening and humeral osteolysis had triple and 10 times increased risk for a positive *C. acnes* culture.

The use of advanced imaging varies from case to case. CT can be used to assess osseous structures and evaluate for glenoid component loosening, while MRI can evaluate the integrity of the rotator cuff and other soft tissue structures. Nuclear imaging is not routinely used in the evaluation of shoulder PJI. Technetium-99m three-phase bone scan is sensitive for arthroplasty failure but has limited utility in identifying etiology [16]. Indium-labeled white blood cell (WBC) studies are also poor at detecting shoulder PJI caused by low virulence organisms [17].

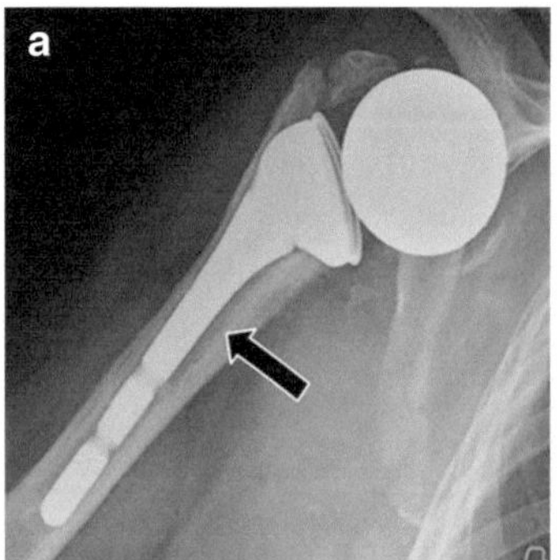
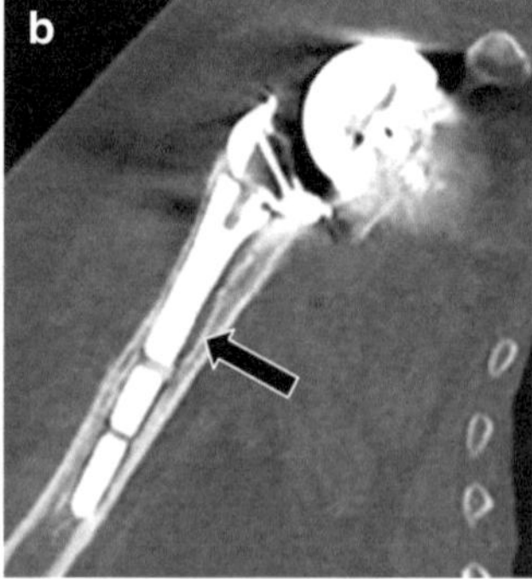
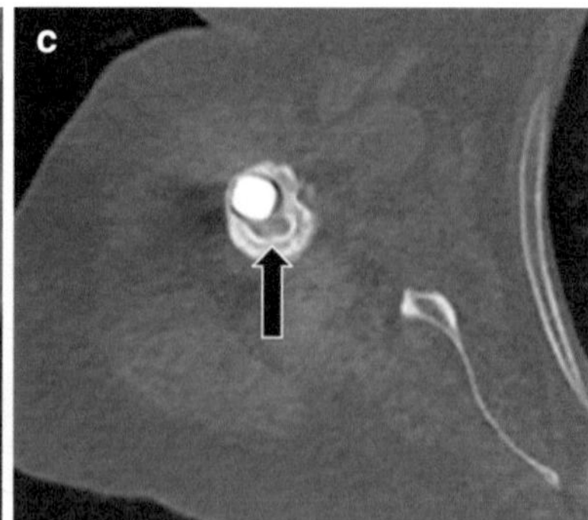

Fig. 23.1 Anteroposterior radiograph (**a**) and coronal (**b**) and axial CT (**c**) images of a 79-year-old woman with humeral component loosening manifested by an irregular radiolucent line >2 mm around the prosthetic stem (arrows) [15]

23.3.3 Serologic Tests

Serum WBC, erythrocyte sedimentation rate (ESR), and C-reactive protein (CRP) are standard serologic tests obtained in the workup for shoulder PJI. These inflammatory markers have a high specificity and positive predictive value, but lower sensitivity and negative predictive value in shoulder PJI as most infections are caused by low virulence organisms [18, 19]. These tests are often normal late after the index procedure and infection cannot be excluded based on inflammatory markers alone.

23.3.4 Arthrocentesis/Joint Aspiration

The utility of joint aspiration in the evaluation of shoulder PJI is controversial, unlike its knee and hip counterparts [20]. This is in part due to the low yield of shoulder arthrocentesis, even under image guidance, which is rarely sufficient for analysis and culture. Antibiotics should be discontinued for 2 weeks prior to aspiration in order to obtain optimal culture results. When enough synovial fluid is obtained, the cultures have a high specificity and PPV, but low sensitivity and NPV [21]. Therefore, a dry tap or negative cultures do not rule out an infection, much like normal serologic testing in shoulder PJI. Additionally, the cutoff values for synovial fluid cell count has not been determined for an infected shoulder arthroplasty. While synovial fluid with an elevated WBC and positive cultures may guide surgical treatment, the decision to perform a joint aspiration in the setting of normal serologic markers and no other risk factors is left up to the surgeon's clinical judgment.

23.3.5 Synovial Fluid Analysis

There has been increasing interest and experience with synovial fluid analysis in the diagnosis of shoulder PJI. Frangiamore et al. [22]

found that synovial interleukin (IL)-6 yielded higher sensitivity (87%) and specificity (90%) than ESR and CRP. However, Grosso et al. [23] and Villacis et al. [24] demonstrated that IL-6 has not been an effective marker in diagnosis of shoulder PJI but may have a role in confirmation. In a follow-up to his previous study, Frangiamore et al. [25] found that IL-6, tumor necrosis factor-alpha, and IL-2 in combination demonstrated superior diagnostic ability than any cytokine alone, yielding a sensitivity and specificity of 80% and 93%.

Alpha-defensin has also been studied as another infection marker. Frangiamore et al. [26] found a correlation between alpha-defensin and patients with shoulder PJI and reported a sensitivity and specificity of 63% and 95%. Subsequent studies by Bonanzinga et al. [27] and Bauer et al. [28] demonstrated that alpha-defensin has better sensitivity and specificity in patients with hip or knee PJI, when compared to those with shoulder PJI.

23.3.6 Arthroscopic Tissue Biopsy

Dilisio et al. [21] performed arthroscopic tissue biopsies in 19 patients with painful arthroplasties and demonstrated their improved utility over glenohumeral arthrocentesis in the diagnosis of shoulder PJI. Arthroscopic biopsies yielded 100% sensitivity, specificity, and positive and negative predictive values, while joint aspiration yielded 16.7% sensitivity, 100% specificity, 100% positive predictive value, and 58.3% negative predictive value. Similarly, Tashjian et al. [29] and Akgun et al. [30] also analyzed the utility of prerevision tissue biopsy and found comparable results, but not as conclusive as Dilisio's earlier study.

Arthroscopic tissue biopsy is likely most beneficial in patients with a painful arthroplasty who do not have typical signs of infection or those with supposed aseptic loosening. The culture results may allow the surgeon to determine a cause for the pain and guide treatment.

23.3.7 Intraoperative Evaluation

Wound cultures are necessary for the identification of the causative pathogen and guide antimicrobial therapy in patients with apparent shoulder PJI. In those without obvious infection, intraoperative culture is essential to establishing the diagnosis of PJI, as well as guiding treatment. These cases of failed arthroplasties with positive cultures, in which the preoperative evaluation has not definitively identified an infection, i.e., normal inflammatory markers, normal aspiration results, and normal imaging findings, have been termed unexpected positive cultures (UPCs) [7, 31].

The role of routine tissue cultures in all revisions continues to be unclear. If a positive culture results in the setting of an additional reason for failure that requires revision, such as fracture, rotator cuff failure, or component malposition, further management is controversial. It is uncertain whether a positive culture is indicative of a contaminant, an infection, or a commensal organism to deep tissue [32]. It should also be noted that several studies have found positive cultures in patients undergoing open shoulder surgery without any previous surgical history [33], as well as in those undergoing primary shoulder arthroplasty [34]. Therefore, it is left to the surgeon's discretion in obtaining routine tissue cultures during revision surgery.

23.3.8 Frozen Section Histopathology

Intraoperative samples sent for frozen section histopathology may assist in diagnosing shoulder PJI. While Mirra et al. [35] developed the criteria for PJI diagnosis in hip and knee arthroplasty as more than five neutrophils in five or more high-power microscopic fields, this does not appear to be applicable to low-virulence organisms. Patients with positive *C. acnes* cultures rarely demonstrate acute inflammation on intraoperative histology. Topolski et al. [36] found that only 8% of patients with positive intraoperative cultures demonstrated positive intraoperative histologic findings. Subsequently, Grosso et al. [37] analyzed 45 patients undergoing revision shoulder arthroplasty for which intraoperative tissue culture and frozen section histology was obtained. Using the criteria described by Mirra, the sensitivity was lower for patients with *C. acnes* infection when compared with those infected with other pathogens. They proposed a threshold of 10 or more total neutrophils in five high-power fields for the diagnosis of shoulder PJI, which yielded a 72% sensitivity and 100% specificity. It should be noted that frozen sectioning is subject to operator variability and is institution dependent.

23.3.9 Tissue Culture

Positive intraoperative tissue cultures are essential to the diagnosis and treatment of shoulder PJI. At least four samples should be obtained from tissue adjacent to the implants. Tissue cultures are preferred to swab cultures, as the latter has a lower yield, particularly for *C. acnes* which can be intracellular. Perioperative antibiotics do not need to be held until intraoperative samples have been obtained according to the hip and knee literature [38].

Cultures should be held for a minimum of 14 days [31]. Frangiamore et al. [39] classified positive *P. acnes* cultures as either "probable true positives" or "probable contaminants" (false positives) based on culture results and perioperative findings. He found that cultures that were "probable true positives" grew positive in 5 days (range, 4–6 days) and none became positive after 11 days, while cultures that were "probable contaminants" grew in 9 days (range, 6–12 days). Therefore, there is a possibility that holding cultures for up to 4 weeks, as suggested by Pottinger et al. [11], may increase the possibility of false-positive results.

Determining the significance of a positive intraoperative culture in revision shoulder arthroplasty can be challenging. Hudek et al. [32] proposed that a positive culture can be indicative of contamination, infection, or a commensal organism to deep tissue. In first-time shoulder cases, 36.4% of patients had a positive *C. acnes* culture. Several subsequent studies had similar findings. Mook et al. [33] found positive cultures in 20.5% of patients undergoing open shoulder surgery without any previous surgical history, and Wong et al. [34] identified positive cultures in 38% of patients undergoing primary shoulder arthroplasty. Tissue samples taken during revision surgery in apparently aseptic shoulders can also demonstrate significant positivity rates. McGoldrick et al. [40] performed revision shoulder arthroplasty for loosening or stiffness in patient at least 3 years after the index procedure and found that 77% of intraoperative samples were positive for *C. acnes*.

23.4 Diagnostic Criteria

The International Consensus Meeting (ICM) on Orthopedic Infections in 2018 established guidelines for the diagnosis and management of shoulder PJI [41]. Shoulder PJI was divided into four categories: definite infection, probable infection, possible infection, and unlikely infection. These are summarized in Table 23.1. A definite infection meets at least one of the following criteria: (1) presence of a sinus tract from the skin surface to the prosthesis, (2) gross intra-articular pus, or (3) two positive tissue cultures with phenotypically identical virulent organisms. A probable infection is defined as the presence of six or more minor criteria with an identified organism. A possible infection is defined as one of the following scenarios: (1) the presence of six or more minor criteria without an identified organism, (2) less than six minor criteria with a single positive culture with a virulent organism, or (3) fewer than six minor criteria with two positive cultures with a low virulence organism. An unlikely infection is defined as the presence of less than 6 minor criteria with negative cultures or one positive culture with a low virulence organism. The minor criteria are described in Table 23.2.

Table 23.1 Definition of periprosthetic shoulder infection established at the 2018 International Consensus Meeting on Orthopedic Infections [41]

Definite	Meets one of the following: • Presence of a sinus tract from the skin surface to the prosthesis • Gross intra-articular pus • Two positive tissue cultures with phenotypically identical virulent organisms
Probable	6 or greater minor criteria with an identified organism
Possible	Meets one of the following: • 6 or greater minor criteria without an identified organism • Single positive culture with a virulent organism • 2 positive cultures with a low-virulence organism
Unlikely	Meets one of the following: • Negative cultures • Single positive culture with a low-virulence organism

Table 23.2 Minor criteria for the definition of shoulder PJI

Minor criteria	Weight
Unexpected wound drainage	4
Single positive tissue culture with virulent organism	3
Single positive tissue culture with low-virulence organism	1
Second positive tissue culture (identical low-virulence organism)	3
Humeral loosening	3
Positive frozen section (5 PMNs in ≥ 5 high-power fields)	3
Positive preoperative aspirate culture (low or high virulence)	3
Elevated synovial neutrophil percentage (>80%)[a]	2
Elevated synovial WBC count (>3000 cells/μL)[a]	2
Elevated ESR (>30 mm/h)[a]	2
Elevated CRP level (>10 mg/L)[a]	2
Elevated synovial α-defensin level	2
Cloudy fluid	2

(Adapted from the 2018 International Consensus Meeting on Orthopedic Infections) [41]
PJI periprosthetic joint infection, *PMN* polymorphonuclear leukocyte, *WBC* white blood cell, *ESR* erythrocyte sedimentation rate, *CRP* C-reactive protein
[a]Beyond 6 weeks from recent surgery

23.5 Treatment

The mainstay of shoulder PJI treatment is surgery with adjuvant antimicrobial therapy. In patients who are unable to tolerate surgical intervention or when the revision surgery would incur more morbidity than the infection, chronic antibiotic suppression alone may be considered. It must be noted that failure rates approach 60–70% [14, 42].

23.5.1 Debridement with Implant Retention

Irrigation and debridement (I&D) with retention of the implants is reserved for the treatment of some case of acute shoulder PJI. According to studies by Coste et al. [42] and Rangan et al. [43], these patients are those with PJI diagnosed within 6 weeks of the index procedure or 3 weeks of symptom onset, stable implants, and identifiable pathogens of low virulence. The literature on outcomes of I&D with implant retention is limited with some studies reporting a failure rate of 50–63% [14, 42]. More recently, Dennison et al. reported 70% long-term retention rate in 10 cases of acute shoulder PJI, and these patients may require long-term antibiotic therapy [44].

23.5.2 Single-Stage Versus Two-Stage Revision

In patients with shoulder PJI greater than 4 weeks postoperatively, removal of the shoulder implants is indicated. Traditionally, the standard treatment protocol for shoulder PJI entailed of complete removal of the prosthesis, thorough I&D, and implantation of an antibiotic cement spacer, followed by a second procedure for a revision shoulder arthroplasty [45]. After the first stage, the patient is treated with IV antibiotics for at least 6 weeks, sometimes followed by a course of oral antibiotics. Prior to implantation of a new prosthesis, patients are evaluated with serial serologic testing. When there are no clinical signs of infection and inflammatory markers have normalized, a patient may be considered for re-implantation

[46]. Joint aspiration or tissue biopsy prior to second stage revision is not routinely performed. Zhang et al. [47] performed an open biopsy on 18 patients with shoulder PJI who underwent a first stage revision and completed a course of antibiotics. Persistent infection was demonstrated in 22% of all patients and 38% of patients with a *C. acnes* infection.

In some cases, an antibiotic spacer can be considered a definitive option for the treatment of shoulder PJI, if the patient is not a good surgical candidate or the patient declines additional surgery. Nelson et al. [48] reported a systematic review of 13 studies of shoulder PJI patients. Infection eradication rates were 90.3% for antibiotic spacer retention, 91.7% for single-stage revision, and 93.8% for two-stage revision. In a cohort of 19 low demand, elderly patients, Pellegrini et al. [49] found no infection recurrence after a mean follow-up of 8 years. This was followed by a retrospective case-control study of 30 patients, 19 of which underwent definitive antibiotic spacer implantation and the remaining 11 underwent a 2-stage revision. There was no infection recurrence in either group and there was no statistically significant differences in Constant or VAS scores, although range of motion was better in the patients who underwent a two-stage revision [50].

While the precedent for two-stage revision was set by knee and hip arthroplasty, there has been success with single-stage revision in the treatment of shoulder PJI. This entails removal of the components, a thorough I&D, and placement of a new prosthesis, followed by a course of antibiotics. Interest in single-stage revision has risen because it causes less insult to the soft tissue, has a shorter recovery time, and is cost effective [51]. Garrigues et al. [52] performed a systematic review of 39 articles evaluating single-stage and two-stage revision for shoulder PJI. The re-infection rate was 5.6% for single-stage and 11.4% for two-stage, and the complication rate was 12.7% for single-stage and 21.9% for two-stage. These results were statistically significant; however, the analysis did not account for selection bias. Less severe infections may have been treated preferentially with single-stage revision, whereas more severe infections may have been treated with two-stage revision. Most recently, Belay et al. [53] reported a systemic review and meta-analysis of 13 studies on single-stage and 30 studies on 2-stage revision for shoulder PJI. The re-infection rate was 6.3% for single-stage and 10.1% for 2-stage revision, but this was not statistically significant. Constant scores and range of motion were similar between the groups. Single-stage revision had a 11.4% complication rate, while two-stage revision was 22.5%. The authors concluded that one-stage revision may be as effective as two-stage revision in select patients with shoulder PJI.

23.5.3 Salvage Procedures

Resection arthroplasty is an option for low demand or elderly patients or those with recalcitrant PJI. Nelson et al. [48] reported a 93.3% rate of infection resolution. However, there are high rates of residual pain and poor function in up to 50% [54]. Additionally, resection arthroplasty may compromise potential for future prosthesis implantation due to rotator cuff atrophy and disuse osteopenia [55].

23.5.4 Unexpected Positive Cultures

There is little consensus regarding the treatment of UPCs and additional research is necessary. Hsu et al. [56] treated 55 patients undergoing a single-stage revision, in which 27 shoulders had at least 2 positive intraoperative cultures for *C. acnes* and were treated with 6 weeks of IV antibiotics, followed by at least 6 months of oral antibiotics. While the functional outcomes were comparable to the control group, this study was limited by how the control group was defined (0 or 1 UPC). Padegimas et al. [57] also analyzed patients undergoing revision shoulder arthroplasty for presumably noninfectious reasons. 28 (23.9%) of 117 individuals had at least 1 UPC. All patients received empirical oral antibiotics for 2 weeks according to the authors' revision surgery protocol. Depending on culture results,

patients received antibiotics for an additional 6 weeks. While UPC patients underwent reoperation more often than those without UPCs (20.2% versus 7.1%), this did not reach statistical significance ($p = 0.109$). These studies do not clearly demonstrate the advantage of prolonged antibiotic treatment in patient undergoing revision shoulder arthroplasty with UPCs. Additionally, greater than 80% of UPCs are low virulent organisms and due to small numbers, distinct treatment regarding UPCs with more virulent organisms is unclear [52]. The relevance of UPCs and the appropriate treatment protocol for UPCs remain to be determined.

23.5.5 Antibiotics

Antibiotic therapy should be guided by the culture results. Typically, IV antibiotics are continued for a duration of 6 weeks, followed by a period of oral antibiotics. Infectious disease specialists are commonly consulted; however, as their familiarity with *C. acnes* and other unique shoulder pathogens varies between institutions, close collaboration is necessary. As discussed above, the use of antibiotics in cases with UPCs is controversial.

23.6 Prevention

There are several measures implemented during the index shoulder arthroplasty to prevent shoulder PJI. Patients undergoing total knee and hip arthroplasty are screened for methicillin-resistant *Staphylococcus aureus* (MRSA) via nasal swab. This can also be performed for patients undergoing shoulder arthroplasty, but there is limited research verifying its efficacy. There have been several studies, however, evaluating the utility of different skin preparations. Sabetta et al. [58] found that topical benzoyl peroxide (BPO) reduced *P. acnes* on the skin but did not completely eliminate it. The skin of 50 patients undergoing arthroscopic shoulder surgery were sampled at the initiation and completion of surgery. At the beginning of surgery, 6% of cultures were positive, while 10% were positive at the end of surgery. Kolakowski et al. [59] subsequently compared BPO with chlorhexidine gluconate (CHG) in a randomized controlled trial. 80 patients were treated preoperatively with either 5% BPO or 4% CHG, and skin cultures were obtained on the day of surgery. BPO decreased the skin burden of *C. acnes* more effectively than CHG but again did not completely eliminate it. In a separate randomized controlled trial, van Diek et al. [60] compared BPO to placebo, which resulted in a 51.4% reduction in *C. acnes*.

Hydrogen peroxide has also been studied as a preoperative skin preparation. Chalmers et al. [61] compared hydrogen peroxide to placebo in a randomized controlled trial containing 124 primary shoulder arthroplasties. Cultures were taken from the skin, dermis, and joint. There were fewer patients with triple-positive cultures (0% vs. 19%, $P = 0.024$) and joint positive cultures (10% vs. 35%, $P = 0.031$) in group treated with hydrogen peroxide.

The surgical site should be prepared with an alcohol-based CHG solution, which is more effective than an iodophor and alcohol preparation or a povidone–iodine scrub and paint preparation at eliminating bacteria from the shoulder region [62]. Prophylactic antibiotics should be started within 1 h of the initiation of surgery. After draping the patient, gloves should be changed. The skin knife should also be discarded as *P. acnes* has been cultured from the subdermal layer, forceps, tip of gloves, and scalpel blades [63]. Gloves should also be changed prior to touching the implant as these can also be contaminated. 1 g of vancomycin powder may be applied to the surgical wound during closure as it can reduce surgical site infections [64] and is cost-effective [65].

23.7 Summary

PJI is a serious complication after shoulder arthroplasty, which is compounded by difficulties in diagnosis. Due to the unique milieu of the shoulder and the propensity for infection by indolent microorganisms, patients with PJI do not always present with the typical signs of infection. Additionally, serologic testing does not have the same utility as in hip and knee arthroplasty. Recent studies on IL-6 and alpha-defensin have had promising results, but the evidence support their diagnostic utility is limited.

Surgical management of shoulder PJI traditionally involves a 2-stage revision and targeted antibiotic treatment. Resection arthroplasty is typically reserved for low demand or elderly patients or those with recalcitrant PJI. Single-stage revision has demonstrated comparable rates of infection eradication with two-stage revision and has the advantages of a shorter treatment period and being more cost-effective. However, future studies should compare the functional outcomes and infection eradication rates of two surgical interventions directly.

References

1. Wagner ER, Farley KX, Higgins I, Wilson JM, Daly CA, Gottschalk MB. The incidence of shoulder arthroplasty: rise and future projections compared with hip and knee arthroplasty. J Shoulder Elb Surg. 2020;29(12):2601–9.
2. Best MJ, Aziz KT, Wilckens JH, McFarland EG, Srikumaran U. Increasing incidence of primary reverse and anatomic total shoulder arthroplasty in the United States. J Shoulder Elb Surg. 2021;30(5):1159–66.
3. Farley KX, Wilson JM, Kumar A, Gottschalk MB, Daly C, Sanchez-Sotelo J, et al. Prevalence of shoulder arthroplasty in the United States and the increasing burden of revision shoulder arthroplasty. JB JS Open Access. 2021;6(3):e20.00156.
4. Bohsali KI, Wirth MA, Rockwood CA Jr. Complications of total shoulder arthroplasty. J Bone Jt Surg Am. 2006;88(10):2279–92.
5. Florschutz AV, Lane PD, Crosby LA. Infection after primary anatomic versus primary reverse total shoulder arthroplasty. J Shoulder Elb Surg. 2015;24(8):1296–301.
6. Cofield RH, Edgerton BC. Total shoulder arthroplasty: complications and revision surgery. Instr Course Lect. 1990;39:449–62.
7. Mook WR, Garrigues GE. Diagnosis and management of periprosthetic shoulder infections. J Bone Jt Surg Am. 2014;96(11):956–65.
8. Paxton ES, Green A, Krueger VS. Periprosthetic infections of the shoulder: diagnosis and management. J Am Acad Orthop Surg. 2019;27(21): e935–e44.

9. Malik AT, Morris J, Bishop JY, Neviaser AS, Khan SN, Cvetanovich GL. Undergoing an arthroscopic procedure prior to shoulder arthroplasty is associated with greater risk of prosthetic joint infection. Arthroscopy. 2021;37(6):1748–54.e1.

10. Singh JA, Sperling JW, Schleck C, Harmsen WS, Cofield RH. Periprosthetic infections after total shoulder arthroplasty: a 33-year perspective. J Shoulder Elb Surg. 2012;21(11):1534–41.

11. Pottinger P, Butler-Wu S, Neradilek MB, Merritt A, Bertelsen A, Jette JL, et al. Prognostic factors for bacterial cultures positive for Propionibacterium acnes and other organisms in a large series of revision shoulder arthroplasties performed for stiffness, pain, or loosening. J Bone Jt Surg Am. 2012;94(22):2075–83.

12. Cheung EV, Sperling JW, Cofield RH. Infection associated with hematoma formation after shoulder arthroplasty. Clin Orthop Relat Res. 2008;466(6):1363–7.

13. Richards J, Inacio MC, Beckett M, Navarro RA, Singh A, Dillon MT, et al. Patient and procedure-specific risk factors for deep infection after primary shoulder arthroplasty. Clin Orthop Relat Res. 2014;472(9):2809–15.

14. Sperling JW, Kozak TK, Hanssen AD, Cofield RH. Infection after shoulder arthroplasty. Clin Orthop Relat Res. 2001;382:206–16.

15. Combes D, Lancigu R, Desbordes de Cepoy P, Caporilli-Razza F, Hubert L, Rony L, et al. Imaging of shoulder arthroplasties and their complications: a pictorial review. Insights Imaging. 2019;10(1):90.

16. Gyftopoulos S, Rosenberg ZS, Roberts CC, Bencardino JT, Appel M, Baccei SJ, et al. ACR appropriateness criteria imaging after shoulder arthroplasty. J Am Coll Radiol. 2016;13(11):1324–36.

17. Strickland JP, Sperling JW, Cofield RH. The results of two-stage re-implantation for infected shoulder replacement. J Bone Jt Surg Br. 2008;90(4):460–5.

18. Kheir MM, Tan TL, Shohat N, Foltz C, Parvizi J. Routine diagnostic tests for periprosthetic joint infection demonstrate a high false-negative rate and are influenced by the infecting organism. J Bone Jt Surg Am. 2018;100(23):2057–65.

19. Akgun D, Wietholter M, Siegert P, Danzinger V, Minkus M, Braun KF, et al. The role of serum C-reactive protein in the diagnosis of periprosthetic shoulder infection. Arch Orthop Trauma Surg. 2021;142(8):1715–21.

20. Della Valle C, Parvizi J, Bauer TW, DiCesare PE, Evans RP, Segreti J, et al. American Academy of Orthopaedic Surgeons clinical practice guideline on: the diagnosis of periprosthetic joint infections of the hip and knee. J Bone Jt Surg Am. 2011;93(14):1355–7.

21. Dilisio MF, Miller LR, Warner JJ, Higgins LD. Arthroscopic tissue culture for the evaluation of periprosthetic shoulder infection. J Bone Jt Surg Am. 2014;96(23):1952–8.

22. Frangiamore SJ, Saleh A, Kovac MF, Grosso MJ, Zhang X, Bauer TW, et al. Synovial fluid interleukin-6 as a predictor of periprosthetic shoulder infection. J Bone Jt Surg Am. 2015;97(1):63–70.

23. Grosso MJ, Frangiamore SJ, Saleh A, Kovac MF, Hayashi R, Ricchetti ET, et al. Poor utility of serum interleukin-6 levels to predict indolent periprosthetic shoulder infections. J Shoulder Elb Surg. 2014;23(9):1277–81.

24. Villacis D, Merriman JA, Yalamanchili R, Omid R, Itamura J, Rick Hatch GF 3rd. Serum interleukin-6 as a marker of periprosthetic shoulder infection. J Bone Jt Surg Am. 2014;96(1):41–5.

25. Frangiamore SJ, Saleh A, Grosso MJ, Farias Kovac M, Zhang X, Daly TM, et al. Neer Award 2015: Analysis of cytokine profiles in the diagnosis of periprosthetic joint infections of the shoulder. J Shoulder Elb Surg. 2017;26(2):186–96.

26. Frangiamore SJ, Saleh A, Grosso MJ, Kovac MF, Higuera CA, Iannotti JP, et al. Alpha-defensin as a predictor of periprosthetic shoulder infection. J Shoulder Elb Surg. 2015;24(7):1021–7.

27. Bonanzinga T, Zahar A, Dutsch M, Lausmann C, Kendoff D, Gehrke T. How reliable is the alpha-defensin immunoassay test for diagnosing periprosthetic joint infection? A prospective study. Clin Orthop Relat Res. 2017;475(2):408–15.

28. Bauer TW. CORR Insights®: how reliable is the alpha-defensin immunoassay test for diagnosing periprosthetic joint infection? A prospective study. Clin Orthop Relat Res. 2017;475(2):416–8.

29. Tashjian RZ, Granger EK, Zhang Y. Utility of prerevision tissue biopsy sample to predict revision shoulder arthroplasty culture results in at-risk patients. J Shoulder Elb Surg. 2017;26(2):197–203.

30. Akgun D, Maziak N, Plachel F, Minkus M, Scheibel M, Perka C, et al. Diagnostic arthroscopy for detection of periprosthetic infection in painful shoulder arthroplasty. Arthroscopy. 2019;35(9):2571–7.

31. Matsen FA 3rd, Butler-Wu S, Carofino BC, Jette JL, Bertelsen A, Bumgarner R. Origin of propionibacterium in surgical wounds and evidence-based approach for culturing propionibacterium from surgical sites. J Bone Jt Surg Am. 2013;95(23):e1811–7.

32. Hudek R, Sommer F, Kerwat M, Abdelkawi AF, Loos F, Gohlke F. Propionibacterium acnes in shoulder surgery: true infection, contamination, or commensal of the deep tissue? J Shoulder Elb Surg. 2014;23(12):1763–71.

33. Mook WR, Klement MR, Green CL, Hazen KC, Garrigues GE. The incidence of Propionibacterium acnes in open shoulder surgery: a controlled diagnostic study. J Bone Jt Surg Am. 2015;97(12):957–63.

34. Wong JC, Schoch BS, Lee BK, Sholder D, Nicholson T, Namdari S, et al. Culture positivity in primary total shoulder arthroplasty. J Shoulder Elb Surg. 2018;27(8):1422–8.

35. Mirra JM, Amstutz HC, Matos M, Gold R. The pathology of the joint tissues and its clinical relevance in prosthesis failure. Clin Orthop Relat Res. 1976;117:221–40.

36. Topolski MS, Chin PY, Sperling JW, Cofield RH. Revision shoulder arthroplasty with positive intraoperative cultures: the value of preoperative stud-

ies and intraoperative histology. J Shoulder Elb Surg. 2006;15(4):402–6.

37. Grosso MJ, Frangiamore SJ, Ricchetti ET, Bauer TW, Iannotti JP. Sensitivity of frozen section histology for identifying Propionibacterium acnes infections in revision shoulder arthroplasty. J Bone Jt Surg Am. 2014;96(6):442–7.

38. Ghanem E, Parvizi J, Clohisy J, Burnett S, Sharkey PF, Barrack R. Perioperative antibiotics should not be withheld in proven cases of periprosthetic infection. Clin Orthop Relat Res. 2007;461:44–7.

39. Frangiamore SJ, Saleh A, Grosso MJ, Alolabi B, Bauer TW, Iannotti JP, et al. Early versus late culture growth of Propionibacterium acnes in revision shoulder arthroplasty. J Bone Jt Surg Am. 2015;97(14):1149–58.

40. McGoldrick E, McElvany MD, Butler-Wu S, Pottinger PS, Matsen FA 3rd. Substantial cultures of Propionibacterium can be found in apparently aseptic shoulders revised 3 years or more after the index arthroplasty. J Shoulder Elb Surg. 2015;24(1):31–5.

41. Garrigues GE, Zmistowski B, Cooper AM, Green A, Group ICMS. Proceedings from the 2018 International Consensus Meeting on Orthopedic Infections: the definition of periprosthetic shoulder infection. J Shoulder Elb Surg. 2019;28(6S):S8–S12.

42. Coste JS, Reig S, Trojani C, Berg M, Walch G, Boileau P. The management of infection in arthroplasty of the shoulder. J Bone Jt Surg Br. 2004;86(1):65–9.

43. Rangan A, Falworth M, Watts AC, Scarborough M, Thomas M, Kulkarni R, et al. Investigation and management of periprosthetic joint infection in the shoulder and elbow: evidence and consensus based guidelines of the British Elbow and Shoulder Society. Shoulder Elb. 2018;10(1 Suppl):S5–S19.

44. Dennison T, Alentorn-Geli E, Assenmacher AT, Sperling JW, Sanchez-Sotelo J, Cofield RH. Management of acute or late hematogenous infection after shoulder arthroplasty with irrigation, debridement, and component retention. J Shoulder Elb Surg. 2017;26(1):73–8.

45. Sabesan VJ, Ho JC, Kovacevic D, Iannotti JP. Two-stage reimplantation for treating prosthetic shoulder infections. Clin Orthop Relat Res. 2011;469(9):2538–43.

46. Buchalter DB, Mahure SA, Mollon B, Yu S, Kwon YW, Zuckerman JD. Two-stage revision for infected shoulder arthroplasty. J Shoulder Elb Surg. 2017;26(6):939–47.

47. Zhang AL, Feeley BT, Schwartz BS, Chung TT, Ma CB. Management of deep postoperative shoulder infections: is there a role for open biopsy during staged treatment? J Shoulder Elb Surg. 2015;24(1):e15–20.

48. Nelson GN, Davis DE, Namdari S. Outcomes in the treatment of periprosthetic joint infection after shoulder arthroplasty: a systematic review. J Shoulder Elb Surg. 2016;25(8):1337–45.

49. Pellegrini A, Legnani C, Macchi V, Meani E. Management of periprosthetic shoulder infec-

50. Pellegrini A, Legnani C, Macchi V, Meani E. Two-stage revision shoulder prosthesis vs. permanent articulating antibiotic spacer in the treatment of periprosthetic shoulder infections. Orthop Traumatol Surg Res. 2019;105(2):237–40.

51. Weber P, Utzschneider S, Sadoghi P, Andress HJ, Jansson V, Muller PE. Management of the infected shoulder prosthesis: a retrospective analysis and review of the literature. Int Orthop. 2011;35(3):365–73.

52. Garrigues GE, Zmistowski B, Cooper AM, Green A, Group ICMS. Proceedings from the 2018 International Consensus Meeting on Orthopedic Infections: management of periprosthetic shoulder infection. J Shoulder Elb Surg. 2019;28(6S):S67–99.

53. Belay ES, Danilkowicz R, Bullock G, Wall K, Garrigues GE. Single-stage versus two-stage revision for shoulder periprosthetic joint infection: a systematic review and meta-analysis. J Shoulder Elb Surg. 2020;29(12):2476–86.

54. Sperling JW, Galatz LM, Higgins LD, Levine WN, Ramsey ML, Dunn J. Avoidance and treatment of complications in shoulder arthroplasty. Instr Course Lect. 2009;58:459–72.

55. Stine IA, Lee B, Zalavras CG, Hatch G 3rd, Itamura JM. Management of chronic shoulder infections utilizing a fixed articulating antibiotic-loaded spacer. J Shoulder Elb Surg. 2010;19(5):739–48.

56. Hsu JE, Gorbaty JD, Whitney IJ, Matsen FA 3rd. Single-stage revision is effective for failed shoulder arthroplasty with positive cultures for Propionibacterium. J Bone Jt Surg Am. 2016;98(24):2047–51.

57. Padegimas EM, Lawrence C, Narzikul AC, Zmistowski BM, Abboud JA, Williams GR, et al. Future surgery after revision shoulder arthroplasty: the impact of unexpected positive cultures. J Shoulder Elb Surg. 2017;26(6):975–81.

58. Sabetta JR, Rana VP, Vadasdi KB, Greene RT, Cunningham JG, Miller SR, et al. Efficacy of topical benzoyl peroxide on the reduction of Propionibacterium acnes during shoulder surgery. J Shoulder Elb Surg. 2015;24(7):995–1004.

59. Kolakowski L, Lai JK, Duvall GT, Jauregui JJ, Dubina AG, Jones DL, et al. Neer Award 2018: Benzoyl peroxide effectively decreases preoperative Cutibacterium acnes shoulder burden: a prospective randomized controlled trial. J Shoulder Elb Surg. 2018;27(9):1539–44.

60. van Diek FM, Pruijn N, Spijkers KM, Mulder B, Kosse NM, Dorrestijn O. The presence of Cutibacterium acnes on the skin of the shoulder after the use of benzoyl peroxide: a placebo-controlled, double-blinded, randomized trial. J Shoulder Elb Surg. 2020;29(4):768–74.

61. Chalmers PN, Beck L, Stertz I, Tashjian RZ. Hydrogen peroxide skin preparation reduces

Cutibacterium acnes in shoulder arthroplasty: a prospective, blinded, controlled trial. J Shoulder Elb Surg. 2019;28(8):1554–61.

62. Saltzman MD, Nuber GW, Gryzlo SM, Marecek GS, Koh JL. Efficacy of surgical preparation solutions in shoulder surgery. J Bone Jt Surg Am. 2009;91(8):1949–53.

63. Falconer TM, Baba M, Kruse LM, Dorrestijn O, Donaldson MJ, Smith MM, et al. Contamination of the surgical field with Propionibacterium acnes in primary shoulder arthroplasty. J Bone Jt Surg Am. 2016;98(20):1722–8.

64. Clark JJC, Abildgaard JT, Backes J, Hawkins RJ. Preventing infection in shoulder surgery. J Shoulder Elb Surg. 2018;27(7):1333–41.

65. Hatch MD, Daniels SD, Glerum KM, Higgins LD. The cost effectiveness of vancomycin for preventing infections after shoulder arthroplasty: a break-even analysis. J Shoulder Elb Surg. 2017;26(3):472–7.

Shoulder Arthroplasty and Instability

24

Denny Tjiauw Tjoen Lie, Wayne Yong Xiang Foo, and Andrew Chia Chen Chou

24.1 Introduction

Common indications for total shoulder arthroplasty (TSA) include osteoarthritis, inflammatory arthritis, failed partial joint prosthesis, and avascular necrosis of the humeral head. Performing a TSA requires an intact rotator cuff and adequate glenoid bone stock. Reverse shoulder arthroplasty (RSA) is commonly indicated for rotator cuff arthropathy, pseudoparalysis, three- or four-part fracture of the proximal humerus, or revisions of failed shoulder prosthesis caused by irreparable rotator cuff tears. RSA does not require intact rotator cuff tendons but does require an intact deltoid [1].

The incidence of shoulder arthroplasty has been increasing over the years, outpacing the rate of primary total hip arthroplasties (THA) and total knee arthroplasties (TKA). In the United States, the incidence of primary shoulder arthroplasty increased by 103.7% from 2011 to 2017 and is projected to further increase by approximately 235% from 2017 to 2025 [2]. While the incidence of hemiarthroplasty has decreased, the incidence of TSA and RSA has increased [3, 4].

The stability of the glenohumeral joint is dependent on soft tissue stabilizers, both static and dynamic. Static stabilizers include the labrum and capsuloligamentous structures. Dynamic stabilizers, most notably the rotator cuff muscles and deltoid, are responsible for the local dynamic stability of the glenohumeral joint and are crucial to the stability of shoulder arthroplasty. Activation of the rotator cuff muscles provides stability to the glenohumeral joint by compressing the humeral head against the glenoid surface for concentric rotation to take place. Known as the concavity-compression mechanism, the rotator cuff muscles are well aligned for compression of the glenohumeral joint to effectively take place at all shoulder positions [5]. The rotator cuff muscles exert in a downward and centering force, while the deltoid muscle acts superiorly on the humeral head. This allows for the rotator cuff muscles to act as a fulcrum while the deltoid acts as a lever for the arm to elevate and abduct [1].

Shoulder arthroplasty can alter the complex interplay of mechanisms that contribute to the stability of the glenohumeral joint. Rotator cuff dysfunction after TSA can result in instability due to the loss of compressive forces on the glenohumeral joint. Deltoid dysfunction due to increased deltoid activation and forces after RSA can also contribute to instability.

D. T. T. Lie (✉) · A. C. C. Chou
Duke-National University of Singapore Medical School, Singapore, Singapore

Department of Orthopaedic Surgery, Singapore General Hospital, Singapore, Singapore
e-mail: denny.lie.t.t@singhealth.com.sg;
andrew.chou@alumni.stanford.edu

W. Y. X. Foo
Duke-National University of Singapore Medical School, Singapore, Singapore

© ISAKOS 2023
A. D. Mazzocca et al. (eds.), *Shoulder Arthritis across the Life Span*,
https://doi.org/10.1007/978-3-031-33298-2_24

24.2 Incidence of Dislocation After Shoulder Arthroplasty

With the increasing rate of shoulder arthroplasties, the incidence of failure leading to revision arthroplasties will also increase. A 2017 review study revealed that the overall complication rate of TSAs and RSAs was 11%, which decreased from 14.7% in 2006 [6, 7]. The mean complication rate for RSA was 16.1%, with instability being the most common complication of RSA with a mean rate of 5.0%, ranging from 1.5 to 31% [6, 8]. Among TSAs, which had a mean complication rate of 10.3%, instability was the third most common complication, with a mean rate of 1.0% [6]. A 2021 systematic review showed that the instability rate after revision RSA was significantly greater than primary RSA (5.7% vs. 2.5%). In addition, the Grammont design for RSA had a significantly higher instability rate compared to all other designs combined (4.0% vs. 1.3%) [9].

24.3 Common Causes of Instability After Shoulder Arthroplasty

24.3.1 Total Shoulder Arthroplasty

The causes of postoperative instability after TSA are best characterized by direction, with resultant treatment aimed at correcting the underlying pathology [10].

1. *Superior instability.* Superior instability is the most common direction of instability after TSA and occurs in 3% of all patients who undergo TSA. Most commonly, instability is due to a non-functional rotator cuff and/or deficient coracoacromial arch. Other causes include a superiorly malpositioned humeral component, superiorly tilted glenoid component, or prior coracoacromial release [11]. It is crucial to recognize that the functional status of the cuff, not the presence of a tear itself, determines prosthesis stability. If the cuff itself is grossly functional despite the presence of a tear, the humeral head remains central and the presence of a tear does not lead to instability; conversely, an atrophic, poorly functioning cuff with no tear is unable to maintain the humeral head position and can still lead to instability [10, 12, 13].

2. *Anterior instability.* Anterior instability occurs in 0.9% of TSAs and is usually due to insufficiency of the subscapularis. Other potential causes include insufficient soft tissue tensioning, component malpositioning, and bony deficiency [7, 14]. Treatment generally addresses the deficient subscapularis with re-repair, tendon transfer, or lesser tuberosity osteotomy.

3. *Posterior instability.* Posterior instability occurs in 1% of patients after TSA and is often attributed to the underlying osteoarthritis, which frequently results in posterior glenoid wear, posterior bone loss, capsular laxity, and subluxation, which can sometimes be recognized intraoperatively [14, 15]. Rotator cuff dysfunction may also contribute to posterior instability. Early recognition of posterior glenoid bone loss, either preoperatively on imaging or intraoperatively, can allow for intraoperative eccentric reaming of the anterior glenoid to correct the version accordingly [16].

4. *Inferior instability.* Inferior instability is commonly seen in the context of fracture arthroplasty and is usually due to difficulty with obtaining adequate humeral length. Deltoid atony is another common contributor to instability. Preoperative templating using the contralateral humerus and intraoperative orientation with bony landmarks can be useful in establishing adequate humeral length [10].

24.3.2 Reverse Shoulder Arthroplasty

Balancing soft tissue tension appropriately is the most important factor to consider in achieving joint stability after RSA. While there are numerous causes of instability after RSA, they can be broadly categorized into the following three categories as described by Abdelfattah et al. [17]:

1. ***Loss of compression***. RSA laxity or gapping between the glenosphere and humerosocket can lead to instability and is often due to undersized implants, loss of the deltoid contour, loss of humeral height, subscapularis deficiency, acromial or scapular fracture, and deltoid dysfunction. Deltoid dysfunction is a common contributor to instability and should be worked up for a cause, which can include axillary nerve injury, cervical radiculopathy, and muscle atrophy.

2. ***Loss of containment***. Failure of the glenosphere-humerosocket articulation destabilizes the fulcrum required for arm elevation and can lead to dislocation during ranging of the shoulder. Causes can be due to (a) eccentric polyethylene wear leading to alteration of the humerosocket depth, thus resulting in dislocation, (b) mechanical failure of the humeral cup, or (c) loss of humero-glenosphere articulation due to glenosphere dissociation, humerosocket dissociation at the trunnion, and humeral stem fracture.

3. ***Impingement***. Obstruction of the glenosphere-humerosocket articulation can lead to levering out during shoulder range of motion, resulting in dislocation. This is most commonly due to soft tissue and/or bony impingement, which may be secondary to prior fracture, malunion of the tuberosities, and heterotopic ossification. Other possible causes include prosthetic malalignment and large body habitus.

24.4 Implant Factors That Affect Stability

Several implant characteristics and biomechanical principles have been studied to improve stability; these are summarized below.

Implant factor	Factors that improve stability
Glenosphere size	A larger glenosphere is known to improve abduction ROM and is more stable, requiring a larger force to dislocate the humeral cup [18]. However, Clouthier et al. showed that glenosphere size did not have any significant effect on stability [19]
Glenosphere position	Placing the glenosphere eccentrically more inferior, rather than at the center of the glenoid, prevents impingement and notch formation and improves stability by 17% [19]
Glenosphere tilt	An inferior tilt of 15° is known to reduce notch formation, which results in a larger compressive force, and thus is less likely to dislocate, compared to a neutral tilt (0°) or a superior 15° tilt [20]. The clinical significance of this factor however is less clear
Lateralized glenosphere	Lateralizing the glenosphere caused an increase in joint loading and thus, requires a larger force to cause anterior dislocation. However, it can cause an increase in torque at the implant-bone interface and may cause failure [21]. It may also cause an increased strain of the deltoids, which may predispose to acromial fractures [22]
Depth of humeral cup	A deeper humeral cup increases the socket constraint and was shown to significantly increase the forces required to dislocate the RSA, though a more constrained cup may reduce ROM and may predispose to impingement [19, 23]
Neck shaft angle	Reducing the neck-shaft angle from 155° to 135°, thus making the cup more vertical, increases adduction ROM and reduces impingement, though this factor did not affect overall stability [24]
Humeral length	A correlation was shown that loss of humeral length was associated with increased risk of dislocation, likely due to loss of soft tissue tension [25]. An increase in implant thickness was shown to increase deltoid tension and hence stability but may limit adduction. Overall, lengthening the humerus is helpful only in revision cases secondary to instability [26]
Humeral lateralization	This is known to increase soft tissue tension and may increase stability, yet did not increase deltoid forces as much as humeral lengthening [25]
Humeral version	A cadaveric study showed that humeral version did not significantly affect the dislocation forces. A humeral retroversion of 30° was able to improve external rotation. Retroversion of 0°–30° is currently recommended [26]

24.5 Clinical Assessment of Stability After Shoulder Arthroplasty

The initial evaluation of a patient presenting with instability after shoulder arthroplasty should consist of a detailed patient history and physical examination. A thorough clinical evaluation is crucial in identifying a potential cause of instability, as well as in guiding appropriate further investigations and management of the patient.

History
- Onset and duration of symptoms, exacerbating or alleviating factors, any prior history of trauma to the shoulder, and precipitating factors.
- Specific position of the arm when dislocation occurs.
- It is also paramount to rule out infection and patients should be assessed for any fever, chills, rigors, night sweats, or constitutional symptoms.
- Lastly, patients should also be asked regarding their hand dominance, occupation, hobbies, and general health, as well as their past medical history, previous operations, and any chronic medications use.

Examination
- The skin and surgical site should be carefully assessed for any signs suggestive of infection, such as erythema, edema, tenderness, sinus tracts, or discharge.
- The deltoid should be inspected, palpated, and assessed for contractility and atrophy.
- Both active and passive range of motion should be documented and compared to preoperative measurements in terms of abduction, forward flexion, extension, and external rotation. If examination shows a reduced shoulder range of motion, a possible cause should be identified, such as soft tissue contractures, mechanical block, weakness, or poor effort. The contralateral shoulder should also be assessed [27].

- A comprehensive neurological examination of the upper limbs and cervical spine should be performed, as well as the peripheral pulses.

Imaging
- **Plain radiographs**. Plain X-rays consisting of plain anteroposterior (AP), lateral, true anteroposterior (Grashey), Y-scapular, and axillary lateral views. A systematic approach to evaluating shoulder arthroplasty films can be particularly useful and the following items should be checked in the radiographs:
  1. Overall joint alignment
  2. Signs of prosthesis failure, such as component dissociation or screw breakage.
  3. Humeral component for subsidence, change in alignment, osteolysis, or radiolucent lines (RLL)
  4. Humeral diaphysis for periprosthetic fracture
  5. Humeral tuberosities for signs of fracture, bony resorption, or non-union
  6. Glenoid component for migration or RLL
  7. Implant seating
  8. Scapular notching

  For TSAs, radiolucencies around the humeral stem can be classified as per the Gruen zones as adapted to the humeral stem, with stems considered at risk if there are radiolucent lines (RLLs) of at least 2 mm in 3 or more zones. Humeral stems with circumferential RLLs and/or progressive shift in position on successive radiographs raise the suspicion of loose stems [28]. Radiolucencies on the glenoid are best visualized on the Grashey view.

  For RSAs, full length bilateral humeral radiographs with markers are useful to assess for humeral shortening as described by Ladermann et al. and excessive glenoid medialization as described by Boileau et al. [29, 30]. Excessive glenoid medialization is usually defined by a humeral axis medialized >15 mm measured from the lateral acromion. Glenosphere version is best visualized on the axillary lateral view, with an adequately positioned glenosphere sitting just flush or slightly overhanging the inferior glenoid. Inferior subluxation of the humeral implant seen on the AP view may suggest of poor soft tissue tension, while deficient tuberosities and reduced humeral length are suggestive of humeral implants placed too low [8].

- **Computed tomography (CT).** CT imaging provides greater detail for insufficiency fractures of the scapula or acromion, periprosthetic loosening, component migration, malalignment, and templating and assessing the remaining bone stock.
- **Ultrasound (US).** US is useful as an adjunct imaging for evaluation of cuff tendon integrity, muscle atrophy, and the presence of effusion or bursitis [31].

Laboratory investigations are primarily useful in ruling out prosthetic joint infection (PJI), which may cause instability. Common inflammatory markers are white blood cell count (WBC), C-reactive protein (CRP), and erythrocyte sedimentation rate (ESR). However, their clinical sensitivities are not well established for shoulder PJI, with studies showing that WBC is abnormal in 7% of patients, elevated ESR in 14%, and raised CRP in 25% of cases [32].

Nerve conduction studies (NCS) and electromyography (EMG) are generally only indicated if acute or chronic neuropathy is suspected and can provide data on both the localization and severity of the nerve injury. It is recommended to only obtain NCS/EMG studies 10–21 days after the onset of symptoms. If no significant axonal loss is noted, follow-up studies performed at least 3 months later can be useful to assess for any meaningful reinnervation [8].

24.6 Tips to Improve Stability During TSA

In managing instability after TSA, it is far easier to prevent instability from occurring in the first place. The patient is assessed preoperatively, intraoperatively, and postoperatively to address risk factors that may predispose toward instability.

1. **Preoperative.** A preoperative CT scan can be useful to assess the bone stock and glenoid version, while an MRI may be used to assess for rotator cuff tears and fatty infiltration.
2. **Intraoperative.** TSA is an anatomic joint replacement. Hence the humeral component is placed in the anatomic native version. Similarly, the height of the implant should recreate the original height of the humeral head. Leaving the implant proud may impinge on the supraspinatus tendon causing its attrition and rupture. However, allowing it to subside in the humerus will compromise the glenohumeral compression and hence predispose to instability.

   Similarly, the glenoid component is placed in its native version (for type A glenoids). For abnormal (types B and C) glenoid, eccentric drilling is recommended to prevent abnormal version, which predisposes to instability.

   After TSA, the shoulder should be assessed in multiple positions and directions to assess for any obvious instability. For example, in the presence of posterior capsular laxity, capsular imbrication sutures may be useful in stabilizing the TSA construct. It is imperative to ensure the supraspinatus tendon is intact, of adequate thickness and tension. When the tendon is thinned out and degenerate, consider augmenting the tendon with a dermal allograft patch or even converting the construct to RSA. Ensure the subscapularis tendon is repaired well.

   Intraoperative fluoroscopy may also be a useful adjunct to assess for implant positioning and to detect the presence of any potential periprosthetic fractures [10]. Matching of the natural anatomy, particularly by comparing with the contralateral limb, is integral to preventing dislocation events and restoration of the "gothic arch" in assessing the anatomic relationship of the humeral neck to the shoulder neck may be useful [33].
3. **Postoperative.** Postoperative rehabilitation should be physician directed and based on intraoperative findings. For example, if the subscapularis was found to be of poor quality

intraoperatively, a more conservative rehabilitation regime may be recommended to prevent rupture. Similarly, if posterior capsular laxity was identified, immobilization in external rotation can be considered to improve healing in the correct position [10].

24.7 Surgical Tips to Improve Stability During RSA

In the absence of the supraspinatus, maintaining stability of the shoulder joint after RSA can be challenging, even if the implant is semi-constrained. Thus, balancing the soft tissue tension is critical.

- **Surgical Approach and Exposure**

  Most surgeons are familiar with the super-olateral or deltopectoral approach. The latter takes down the subscapularis tendon and is associated with higher rates of dislocation, thus stressing the importance of the integrity of the subscapularis tendon [34]. Overall, the rates of dislocations after the deltopectoral approach, however, remain relatively low [35]. The deltopectoral approach permits a much better access to perform a complete inferior capsular release and clearance of inferior glenoid osteophytes; these, if uncleared, can cause impingement and potential dislocations. Ultimately, surgeons should adopt the surgical approach of their choice.
- **Humeral Head Osteotomy: How Much to Cut?**

  Making the humeral osteotomy too low and removing more bone may predispose to loss of deltoid tension and loss of compression, despite using a thicker insert and humeral neck. Poor tensioning is associated with increased risks of dislocation; hence it is safer to cut less initially. A good tip would be to assess the height of the humeral osteotomy. When viewed against the glenoid under normal deltoid tension, the top of humerus should be *in the middle of the glenoid* (Fig. 24.1). If the entire glenoid is easily seen, the osteotomy is too low. If the glenoid cannot be seen and

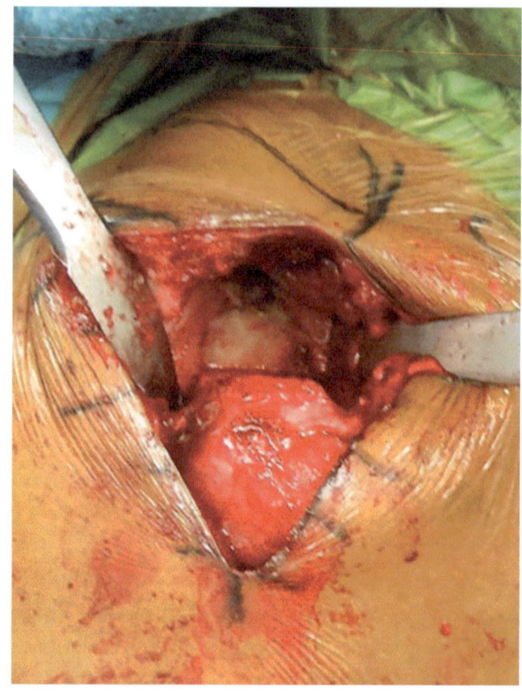

Fig. 24.1 Adequacy of the humeral osteotomy. When viewed against the glenoid, the top of the osteotomized humerus should be at the equator of the glenoid, revealing the upper half

required traction of the arm to view it, too little of the humeral head is removed and a revision osteotomy is recommended.

- **Humeral Version: Does It Matter?**

  As discussed above, humeral version of 0°–30° retroversion is recommended and is not associated with increased risks of dislocation. It is better to follow the version of the native humerus in primary cases. Surgeons should also use implants of their choice; each implant having its inherent neck-shaft angle of 135° or 155°. Other factors such as the lengthening or lateralizing of the humerus should be surgical options reserved for revision cases secondary to instability.
- **Glenosphere Position**

  It is recommended to place the glenosphere as inferior on the glenoid as possible, and even with a little inferior overhang, as long as there is sufficient bone for fixation of the inferior screw. This improves stability and prevents notching [36]. It is observed, however, that in

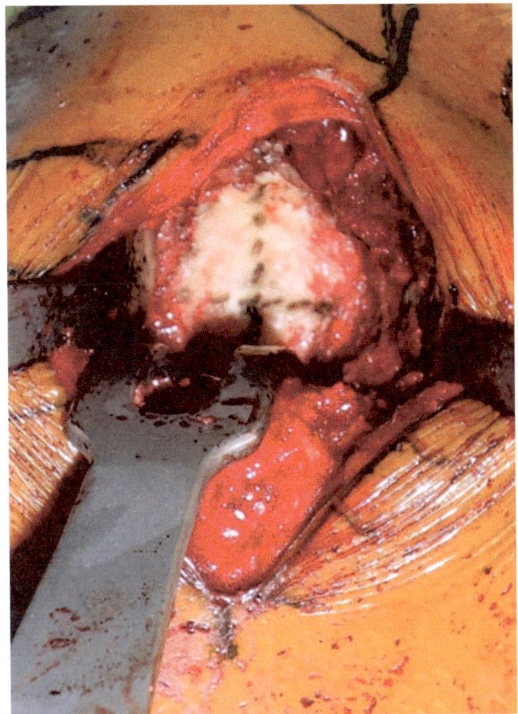

Fig. 24.2 Position of the glenosphere. The vertical axis and equator of the glenoid are clearly marked. In smaller glenoids, the glenosphere is placed in the geometric center, though positioning it inferior confers increased stability

smaller glenoids usually among Asian patients, placing the glenosphere inferior is not possible, and a central position is adequate (Fig. 24.2). Other factors like increasing glenoid size and lateralizing the glenoid remain as surgical options to be used in revision cases to improve stability.

- **Humeral Cup**

  This is a critical factor in improving stability of the RSA. Begin with the thinnest insert and perform the trial with increasing thickness of the insert. It should feel firm and should not be too easy to dislocate and reduce the humeral cup. Assess for stability (see below). If in doubt, increase the thickness of the insert or use a deep cup (increased constraint).

- **Subscapularis Repair**

  Restoring the integrity of the subscapularis is critical to maintaining stability of the RSA. There is an increased risk of dislocation

if the subscapularis is not repaired [37, 38]. Yet others have shown that repairing the subscapularis or not did not affect the complication or dislocation rates [39]. The case example below illustrated the importance of repairing the subscapularis or if not possible, to do a pectoralis major transfer to restore stability.

24.7.1 Intraoperative Assessment of Stability

Several tests have been described to assess stability during surgery [40]. These are commonly practiced:

- Bring the arm to full flexion and internal rotation, then as the arm is in neutral flexion, perform internal and external rotation. Finally bring the arm to extension and external rotation. Ensure that there is full passive ROM, with no restrictions or impingement. Assess and look out for "lifting-off" of the humeral-glenosphere articulation, especially in extremes of ROM.
- Apply a longitudinal axial traction on the arm to perform a shuck test and ensure the joint is stable while feeling the conjoint tendon remains firm.
- While performing internal–external rotation of the arm, gently apply an antero-posterior translation on the arm. The humeral cup must remain stable and not permit any translations. If in doubt, use a thicker insert of deeper cup.

24.8 Case Example

This is a clinical example of recurrent dislocation after RSA due to loss of soft tissue compression. The patient was a 77-year-old male who initially presented with right shoulder pain and weakness. X-rays showed cuff arthropathy and ultrasound confirmed massive retracted tears of the supraspinatus and infraspinatus tendons (Fig. 24.3a–d). He underwent right RSA about 6 months after initial presentation. Immediate postoperative X-rays

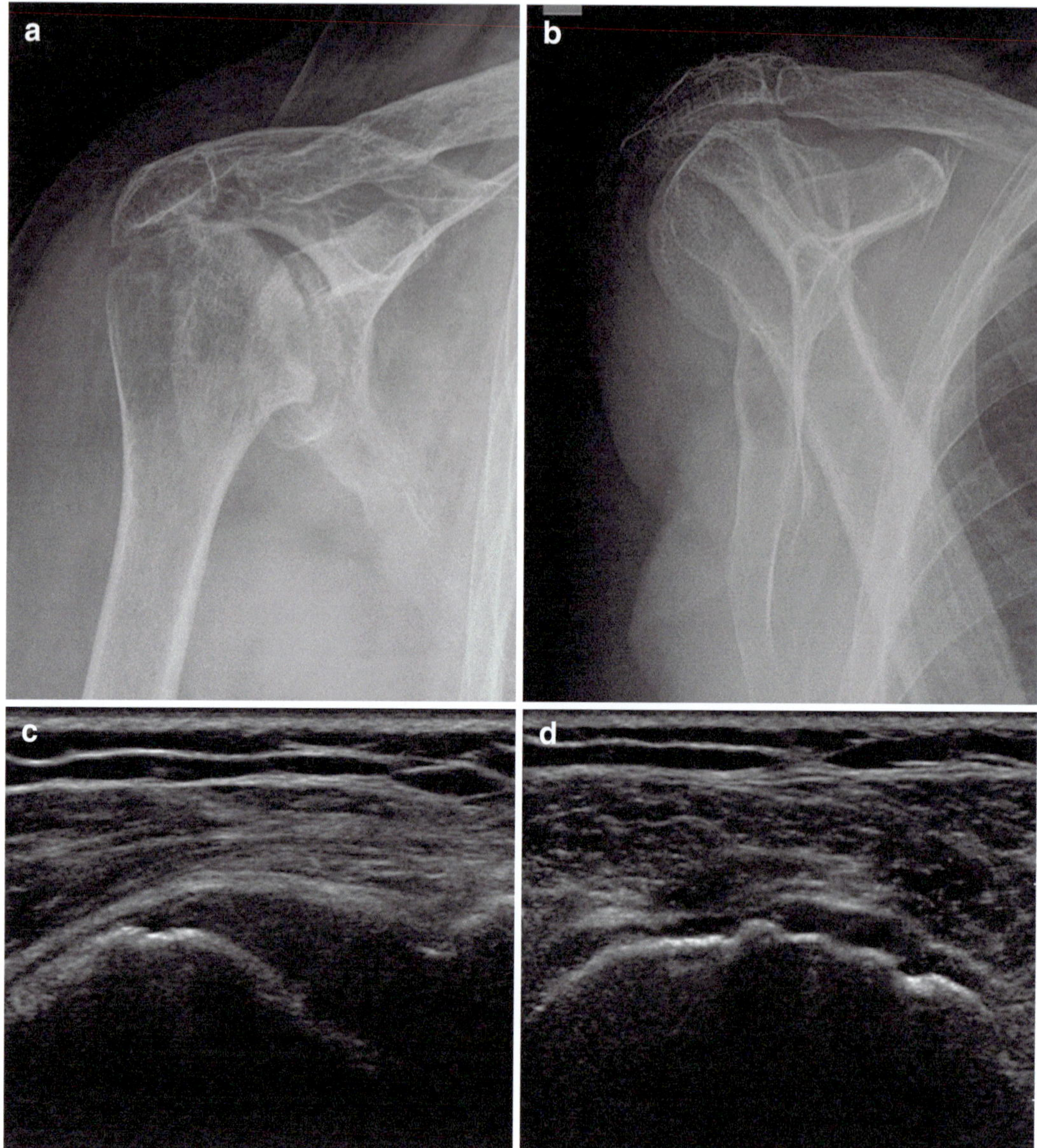

Fig. 24.3 (**a–d**) X-rays and ultrasound images of cuff arthropathy. (**a**, **b**) Shows the AP and lateral view of the right shoulder of an elderly patient with several features of cuff arthropathy: collapsed sclerotic high-riding humeral head, loss of Maloney's line, and gleno-humeral arthritis. (**c**) Shows the longitudinal and (**d**) shows the transverse sonographic views of the right supraspinatus tendon, which is torn and massively retracted

showed enlocated components (Fig. 24.4a, b) but within 1 month postoperatively, he presented with persistent pain and stiffness with no new trauma. X-rays then showed antero-superior dislocation of the humeral cup (Fig. 24.5a, b). During the open reduction performed on the same month, it was noted that the components were stable, with no overt signs of infection. After reduction the soft tissue tension felt adequate, though the subscapularis was noted as deficient.

Despite what appeared to be adequate soft tissue containment and strong deltoid muscles, the humeral cup continued to dislocate. He was then seen in our center the following month about 2 months after the index surgery and underwent open reduction. It was then noted that the del-

Fig. 24.4 (**a**, **b**)
Immediate post-op
X-rays. (**a**, **b**) Show the
AP and lateral views of
the right shoulder after a
reverse arthroplasty was
performed

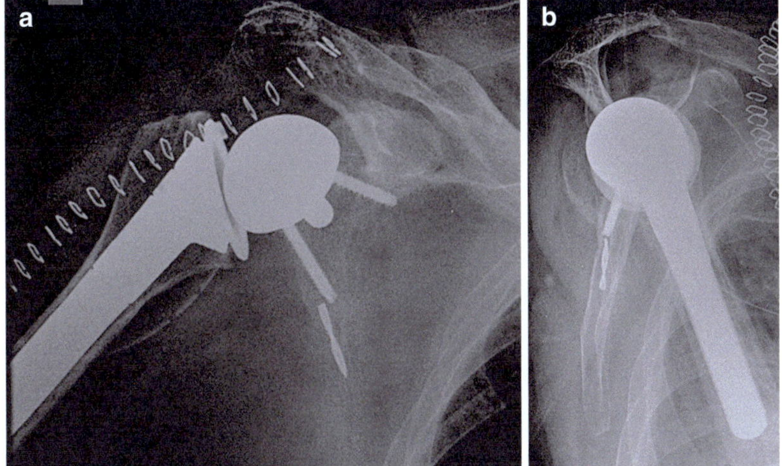

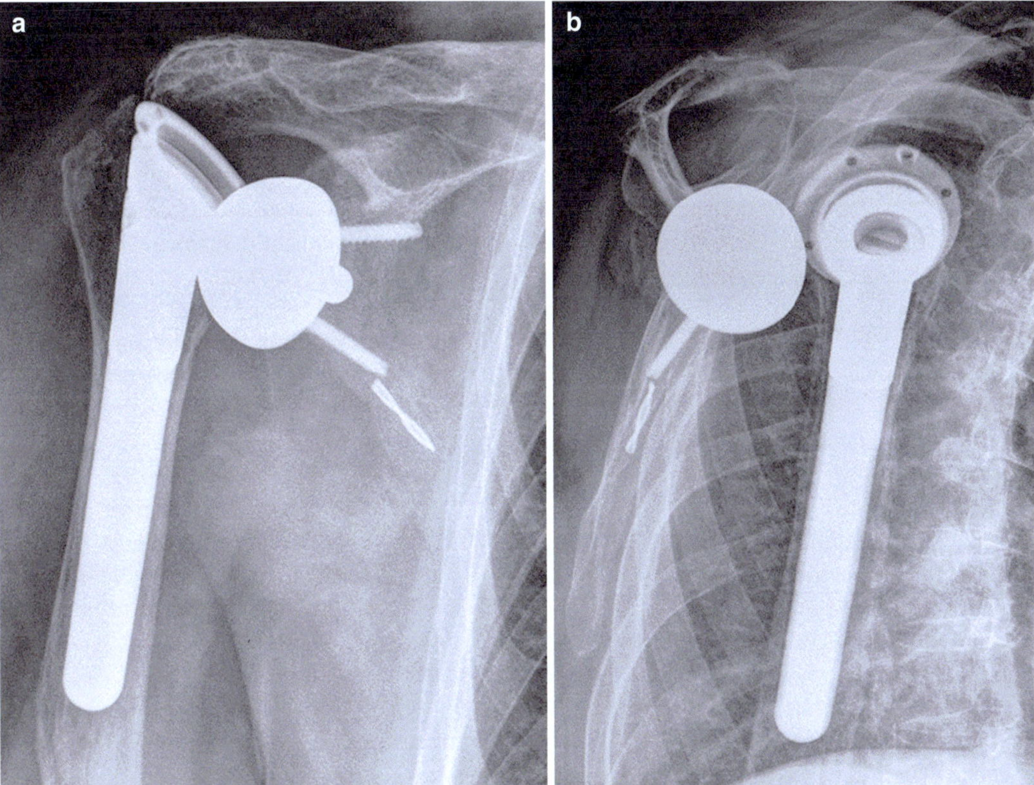

Fig. 24.5 (**a**, **b**) X-rays taken about 1 month after the index surgery. (**a**, **b**) Show the AP and lateral views of the dislocated RSA, with the humeral cup dislocating antero-superiorly

toids had atrophied slightly and that the subscapularis was deficient. Soft tissue containment and stability was achieved only after a pectoralis major transfer was performed to compensate for the deficient subscapularis tendon. The RSA remained stable with no further dislocations up to 2 years postoperatively (Fig. 24.6a, b), after which the patient was lost to follow-up.

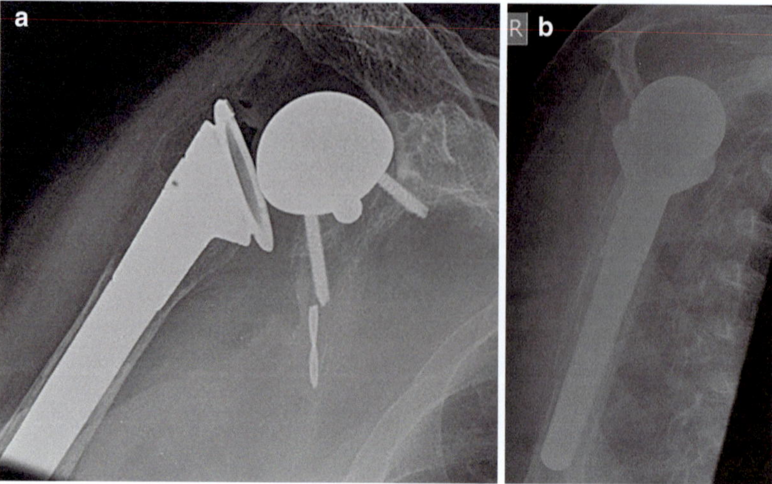

Fig. 24.6 (a, b) X-rays after revision surgery and pectoralis major transfer. After open reduction, stability and soft tissue containment was achieved after a pectoralis major transfer. (**a, b**) Show the AP and lateral views of the enlocated RSA about 9 months after the revision surgery

24.9 Algorithmic Management of Instability After RSA

There is a lack of accepted protocols to treat dislocations or instability after RSA. Chalmers et al. advocated a trial of closed reduction after which the shoulder is rested in an arm-sling for 6 weeks [34]. A technique was described by Chae et al. whereby an axial traction was applied to the arm in slight abduction as a posteriorly and inferiorly directed force was applied to the humerus [8]. Gerber et al., however, considered early dislocations to be related to surgical factors and held the opinion that closed reductions were less likely to be successful [41].

The algorithm below (Fig. 24.7) brings together the common causes and offers an approach to diagnosing the cause of the post-RSA instability and addressing the problem. The first step would be to exclude fractures of the glenoid, humeral shaft, or acromion. Acromial stress fractures can be treated by resting the arm in an abduction sling for 6 weeks [8]. A series of possible causes and cascade of steps then follow:

(a) **Joint Infections**

This is not common after shoulder arthroplasty, ranging from 1 to 3.9% [7]. The diagnosis may be evident during open reduction when inflamed synovium and purulent discharge is seen. More commonly however, it is an index of suspicion and the synovium and fluid should be sent for culture and sensitivity tests, in addition to blood tests (total white count, ESR, CRP). If infection is strongly suspected within 3 months after the index surgery, antibiotics, a thorough washout, and change of the humeral cup liner are required [7]. However, if the infection occurred more than 3 months after the index surgery, long-term antibiotic suppression is needed, in addition to a staged revision.

(b) **Impingement**

Impingement of the humeral cup with soft tissue and bony osteophytes can rarely cause the humeral cup to dislocate or limit the ROM. This uncommon cause is evident during open reduction, and the interposing soft tissues and bone debrided away to ensure full and stable ROM.

(c) **Loss of Containment**

The following two groups of mechanical causes, loss of containment or loss of compression, are more common causes of instability after shoulder arthroplasty. This concept was developed from the algorithm proposed by Boileau et al. in which he quantified the magnitude of loss of humeral length and loss of humeral lateralization [30]. A humeral shortening of less than 15 mm or humeral medialization of 15 mm is considered mild. Within this group, it is proposed

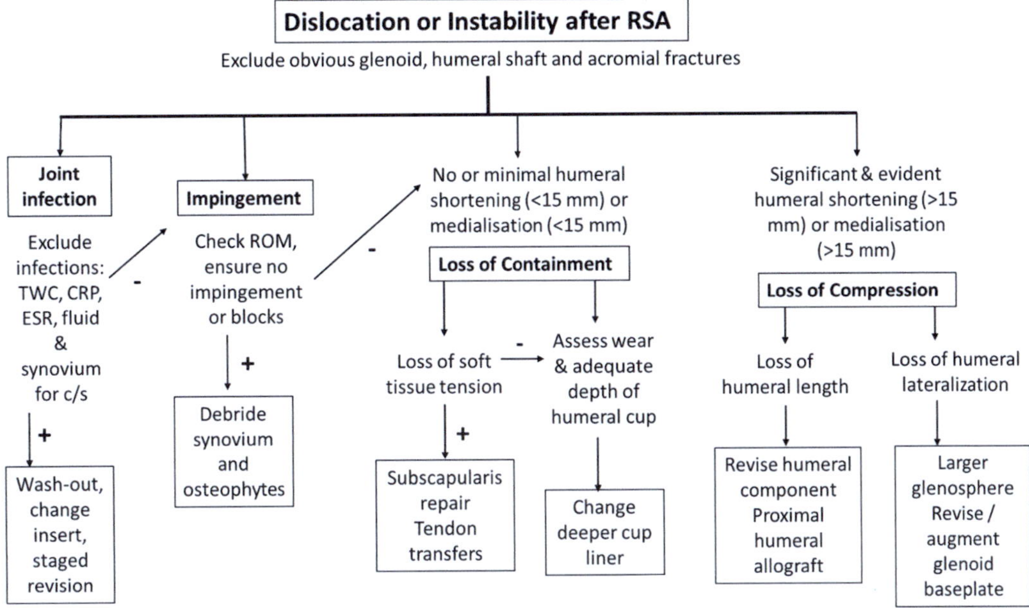

Fig. 24.7 Algorithm in managing instability after RSA

that the soft tissue tension of the remaining subscapularis and infraspinatus tendons be checked first. Inadequacy of these tendons warrant a repair or tendon transfers. The pectoralis major tendon transfer can be done to provide anterior stability when the subscapularis is irreparable, similarly the latissimus dorsi tendon transfer can be done if the infraspinatus tendon is irreparable and degenerate. If the tendons are of adequate tension however, then the humeral cup should be checked for eccentric wear that may precipitate in dislocations. Even if the wear is not evident, an option is to change the humeral cup liner to a more constrained deeper cup.

(d) **Loss of Compression**

If the humeral medialization is greater than 15 mm, lateralization can be achieved by up-sizing the glenosphere or augmenting the base of the glenosphere with bone [8]. It is uncommon to explant the well-fixed metaglene even if the implants are less than optimal [8]. Increasing the humeral length and distalizing the deltoid insertion (thus increasing deltoid tension) is more commonly done.

This can be achieved by using a thicker humeral cup insert, using a metal spacer on top of the humeral component or an allograft [42]. Distalizing and lateralizing the humerus both serve to increase the deltoid tension and thus improve stability.

24.10 In Summary

Both TSA and RSA procedures are increasing in incidence. Instability is one of the most common complications after RSA (about 5%) and third most common after TSA (1%). Of the many causes discussed earlier in this chapter, soft tissue tension stands out as being critical. The various attempts at improving implant designs to increase stability were also discussed. Rotator cuff integrity is critical in TSA; thus instability is prevented and treated by addressing rotator cuff integrity. Stability after RSA is more challenging. The semi-constrained RSA implant can be further stabilized by using a more constrained deeper humeral cup, and soft tissue tension can be improved by tendon transfers, as the case example illustrated. In uncommon cases of significant loss of tension, bony augmentation to distalize and lateralize the humerus may be required to increase deltoid tension and hence improve stability.

References

1. Lin DJ, Wong TT, Kazam JK. Shoulder arthroplasty, from indications to complications: what the radiologist needs to know. Radiographics. 2016;36:192–208. https://doi.org/10.1148/rg.2016150055.

2. Wagner ER, Farley KX, Higgins I, Wilson JM, Daly CA, Gottschalk MB. The incidence of shoulder arthroplasty: rise and future projections compared with hip and knee arthroplasty. J Shoulder Elb Surg. 2020;29:2601–9. https://doi.org/10.1016/j.jse.2020.03.049.

3. Harjula JNE, Paloneva J, Haapakoski J, Kukkonen J, Äärimaa V, Honkanen P, et al. Increasing incidence of primary shoulder arthroplasty in Finland—a nationwide registry study. BMC Musculoskelet Disord. 2018;19:245. https://doi.org/10.1186/s12891-018-2150-3.

4. Best MJ, Aziz KT, Wilckens JH, McFarland EG, Srikumaran U. Increasing incidence of primary reverse and anatomic total shoulder arthroplasty in the United States. J Shoulder Elb Surg. 2021;30:1159–66. https://doi.org/10.1016/j.jse.2020.08.010.

5. Labriola JE, Lee TQ, Debski RE, McMahon PJ. Stability and instability of the glenohumeral joint: the role of shoulder muscles. J Shoulder Elb Surg. 2005;14:S32–8. https://doi.org/10.1016/j.jse.2004.09.014.

6. Bohsali KI, Bois AJ, Wirth MA. Complications of shoulder arthroplasty. JBJS. 2017;99:256–69. https://doi.org/10.2106/JBJS.16.00935.

7. Bohsali KI, Wirth MA, Rockwood CA. Complications of total shoulder arthroplasty. J Bone Jt Surg Am. 2006;88:2279–92. https://doi.org/10.2106/JBJS.F.00125.

8. Chae J, Siljander M, Wiater JM. Instability in reverse total shoulder arthroplasty. J Am Acad Orthop Surg. 2018;26:587–96. https://doi.org/10.5435/JAAOS-D-16-00408.

9. Shah SS, Roche AM, Sullivan SW, Gaal BT, Dalton S, Sharma A, et al. The modern reverse shoulder arthroplasty and an updated systematic review for each complication: part II. JSES Int. 2021;5:121–37. https://doi.org/10.1016/j.jseint.2020.07.018.

10. Lo EY, Moen TC, Burkhead WZ. Instability failure in total shoulder arthroplasty. Semin Arthroplast JSES. 2013;24:28–32. https://doi.org/10.1053/j.sart.2013.04.005.

11. Warren RF, Coleman SH, Dines JS. Instability after arthroplasty: the shoulder. J Arthroplast. 2002;17:28–31. https://doi.org/10.1054/arth.2002.32543.

12. Iannotti JP, Norris TR. Influence of preoperative factors on outcome of shoulder arthroplasty for glenohumeral osteoarthritis. J Bone Jt Surg Am. 2003;85:251–8. https://doi.org/10.2106/00004623-200302000-00011.

13. Sperling JW, Cofield RH, Rowland CM. Minimum 15-year follow-up of Neer hemiarthroplasty and total shoulder arthroplasty in patients aged 50 years or younger. J Shoulder Elb Surg. 2004;13:604–13. https://doi.org/10.1016/S1058274604001296.

14. Moeckel BH, Altchek DW, Warren RF, Wickiewicz TL, Dines DM. Instability of the shoulder after arthroplasty. J Bone Jt Surg Am. 1993;75:492–7. https://doi.org/10.2106/00004623-199304000-00003.

15. Sanchez-Sotelo J, Sperling JW, Rowland CM, Cofield RH. Instability after shoulder arthroplasty: results of surgical treatment. J Bone Jt Surg Am. 2003;85:622–31.

16. Gerber C, Costouros JG, Sukthankar A, Fucentese SF. Static posterior humeral head subluxation and total shoulder arthroplasty. J Shoulder Elb Surg. 2009;18:505–10. https://doi.org/10.1016/j.jse.2009.03.003.

17. Abdelfattah A, Otto RJ, Simon P, Christmas KN, Tanner G, LaMartina J, et al. Classification of instability after reverse shoulder arthroplasty guides surgical management and outcomes. J Shoulder Elb Surg. 2018;27:e107–18. https://doi.org/10.1016/j.jse.2017.09.031.

18. Langohr GDG, Giles JW, Athwal GS, Johnson JA. The effect of glenosphere diameter in reverse shoulder arthroplasty on muscle force, joint load, and range of motion. J Shoulder Elb Surg. 2015;24:972–9. https://doi.org/10.1016/j.jse.2014.10.018.

19. Clouthier AL, Hetzler MA, Fedorak G, Bryant JT, Deluzio KJ, Bicknell RT. Factors affecting the stability of reverse shoulder arthroplasty: a biomechanical study. J Shoulder Elb Surg. 2013;22:439–44. https://doi.org/10.1016/j.jse.2012.05.032.

20. Gutiérrez S, Greiwe RM, Frankle MA, Siegal S, Lee WE. Biomechanical comparison of component position and hardware failure in the reverse shoulder prosthesis. J Shoulder Elb Surg. 2007;16:S9–12. https://doi.org/10.1016/j.jse.2005.11.008.

21. Ackland DC, Patel M, Knox D. Prosthesis design and placement in reverse total shoulder arthroplasty. J Orthop Surg. 2015;10:101. https://doi.org/10.1186/s13018-015-0244-2.

22. Henninger HB, Barg A, Anderson AE, Bachus KN, Burks RT, Tashjian RZ. Effect of lateral offset center of rotation in reverse total shoulder arthroplasty: a biomechanical study. J Shoulder Elb Surg. 2012;21:1128–35. https://doi.org/10.1016/j.jse.2011.07.034.

23. Gutiérrez S, Luo Z-P, Levy J, Frankle MA. Arc of motion and socket depth in reverse shoulder implants. Clin Biomech Bristol Avon. 2009;24:473–9. https://doi.org/10.1016/j.clinbiomech.2009.02.008.

24. Oh JH, Shin S-J, McGarry MH, Scott JH, Heckmann N, Lee TQ. Biomechanical effects of humeral

neck-shaft angle and subscapularis integrity in reverse total shoulder arthroplasty. J Shoulder Elb Surg. 2014;23:1091–8. https://doi.org/10.1016/j.jse.2013.11.003.

25. Giles JW, Langohr GDG, Johnson JA, Athwal GS. Implant design variations in reverse total shoulder arthroplasty influence the required deltoid force and resultant joint load. Clin Orthop. 2015;473:3615–26. https://doi.org/10.1007/s11999-015-4526-0.

26. Henninger HB, Barg A, Anderson AE, Bachus KN, Tashjian RZ, Burks RT. Effect of deltoid tension and humeral version in reverse total shoulder arthroplasty: a biomechanical study. J Shoulder Elb Surg. 2012;21:483–90. https://doi.org/10.1016/j.jse.2011.01.040.

27. Sperling JW, Kaufman KR, Schleck CD, Cofield RH. A biomechanical analysis of strength and motion following total shoulder arthroplasty. Int J Shoulder Surg. 2008;2:1–3. https://doi.org/10.4103/0973-6042.39579.

28. Sperling JW, Cofield RH, O'Driscoll SW, Torchia ME, Rowland CM. Radiographic assessment of ingrowth total shoulder arthroplasty. J Shoulder Elb Surg. 2000;9:507–13. https://doi.org/10.1067/mse.2000.109384.

29. Lädermann A, Williams MD, Melis B, Hoffmeyer P, Walch G. Objective evaluation of lengthening in reverse shoulder arthroplasty. J Shoulder Elb Surg. 2009;18:588–95. https://doi.org/10.1016/j.jse.2009.03.012.

30. Boileau P, Melis B, Duperron D, Moineau G, Rumian AP, Han Y. Revision surgery of reverse shoulder arthroplasty. J Shoulder Elb Surg. 2013;22:1359–70. https://doi.org/10.1016/j.jse.2013.02.004.

31. Sofka CM, Adler RS, Original report. Sonographic evaluation of shoulder arthroplasty. AJR Am J Roentgenol. 2003;180:1117–20. https://doi.org/10.2214/ajr.180.4.1801117.

32. Topolski MS, Chin PYK, Sperling JW, Cofield RH. Revision shoulder arthroplasty with positive intraoperative cultures: the value of preoperative studies and intraoperative histology. J Shoulder Elb Surg. 2006;15:402–6. https://doi.org/10.1016/j.jse.2005.10.001.

33. Krishnan SG, Pennington SD, Burkhead WZ, Boileau P. Shoulder arthroplasty for fracture: restoration of the "Gothic Arch". Tech Shoulder Elb Surg. 2005;6:57–66. https://doi.org/10.1097/01.bte.0000156561.97672.ea.

34. Chalmers PN, Rahman Z, Romeo AA, Nicholson GP. Early dislocation after reverse total shoulder arthroplasty. J Shoulder Elb Surg. 2014;23:737–44. https://doi.org/10.1016/j.jse.2013.08.015.

35. Wiater JM, Moravek JE, Budge MD, Koueiter DM, Marcantonio D, Wiater BP. Clinical and radiographic results of cementless reverse total shoulder arthroplasty: a comparative study with 2–5 years of follow-up. J Shoulder Elb Surg. 2014;23:1208–14. https://doi.org/10.1016/j.jse.2013.11.032.

36. De Biase CF, Delcogliano M, Borroni M, Castagna A. Reverse total shoulder arthroplasty: radiological and clinical result using an eccentric glenosphere. Musculoskelet Surg. 2012;96(Suppl 1):S27–34. https://doi.org/10.1007/s12306-012-0193-4.

37. Edwards TB, Williams MD, Labriola JE, Elkousy HA, Gartsman GM, O'Connor DP. Subscapularis insufficiency and the risk of shoulder dislocation after reverse shoulder arthroplasty. J Shoulder Elb Surg. 2009;18:892–6. https://doi.org/10.1016/j.jse.2008.12.013.

38. Bigdon SF, Bolliger L, Albers CE, Collin P, Zumstein MA. Subscapularis in reverse total shoulder arthroplasty. J Shoulder Elb Arthroplast. 2019;3:2471549219834192. https://doi.org/10.1177/2471549219834192.

39. Friedman RJ, Flurin P-H, Wright TW, Zuckerman JD, Roche CP. Comparison of reverse total shoulder arthroplasty outcomes with and without subscapularis repair. J Shoulder Elb Surg. 2017;26:662–8. https://doi.org/10.1016/j.jse.2016.09.027.

40. Javed S, Imam MA, Monga P. Intraoperative stability assessment in reverse shoulder arthroplasty. J Clin Orthop Trauma. 2019;10:617–9. https://doi.org/10.1016/j.jcot.2018.11.006.

41. Gerber C, Pennington SD, Nyffeler RW. Reverse total shoulder arthroplasty. J Am Acad Orthop Surg. 2009;17:284–95. https://doi.org/10.5435/00124635-200905000-00003.

42. Cheung E, Willis M, Walker M, Clark R, Frankle MA. Complications in reverse total shoulder arthroplasty. J Am Acad Orthop Surg. 2011;19:439–49.

Total Shoulder Arthroplasty in Middle-Aged Patients

Eoghan T. Hurley, Martin S. Davey,
Christopher Klifto, Oke Anakwenze,
Hannan Mullett, and Leo Pauzenberger

25.1 Introduction

Glenohumeral osteoarthritis is a challenging clinical problem in middle-aged and elderly patients alike. The lower the patient age, the more often the goal is to delay arthroplasty. Thus, nonoperative management is frequently the first-line treatment, which may include physiotherapy and injections. Injections most commonly consist of corticosteroid, hyaluronic acid, or platelet-rich plasma, although there is limited evidence to support their use in glenohumeral osteoarthritis. Additionally, physical therapy may be of benefit only to some patients with less advanced degeneration. However, if patients ultimately require surgical management, there exists a variety of surgical treatment options including arthroscopic management, biologic resurfacing, hemi-arthroplasty, total shoulder arthroplasty (TSA), and reverse shoulder arthroplasty (RSA). Arthroplasty of the glenohumeral joint, despite historically lacking behind hip and knee replacements in numbers and development, is now the fastest growing type of arthroplasty overall.

Due to the recent enormous progress of reverse shoulder arthroplasty and the expansion of joint and rotator cuff preserving surgeries, the relevance of anatomical shoulder replacement has been continuously subsiding for the last decade. However, the best functional outcomes are still reported after anatomic shoulder arthroplasty, which positions anatomical replacement as the most desirable treatment option in the younger and/or active patient with glenohumeral osteoarthritis. However, adequate indications and surgical technique are essential to achieve optimal outcomes. Furthermore, while TSA has been shown to provide consistently good clinical results, possibly reduced implant survival in active patients and potential revision surgeries have to be accounted for.

E. T. Hurley · O. Anakwenze
Department of Orthopaedic Surgery, Duke University,
Durham, NC, USA
e-mail: eoghan.hurley@duke.edu;
oke.anakwenze@duke.edu

M. S. Davey
Sports Surgery Clinic, Dublin, Ireland

Galway University Hospitals, Galway, Ireland
e-mail: martindavey@rcsi.ie

C. Klifto
Department of Orthopaedic Surgery, Duke University
School of Medicine, Durham, NC, USA
e-mail: christopher.klifto@duke.edu

H. Mullett
Sports Surgery Clinic, Dublin, Ireland

L. Pauzenberger (✉)
Department of Orthopaedic Surgery, Herz Jesu
Krankenhaus, Vienna, Austria
e-mail: ordination@ortho-pauzenberger.at;
leo.pauzenberger@kh-herzjesu.at

© ISAKOS 2023
A. D. Mazzocca et al. (eds.), *Shoulder Arthritis across the Life Span*,
https://doi.org/10.1007/978-3-031-33298-2_25

The purpose of this chapter is to discuss the indications, intraoperative surgical considerations, and outcomes including longevity and complications for TSA in middle-aged patients.

25.2 Indications and Contraindications

25.2.1 Indications

The predominant indication for TSA in younger patients is primary glenohumeral osteoarthritis, with high demand, and without rotator-cuff tears. However, those with rotator cuff tears, which are amenable to repair, may be considered for a TSA and can have good outcomes. Around 5% of patients undergoing TSA require repair of a torn rotator cuff, while significant improvements in range of motion and pain are possible. However, the rate of instability is increased with medium to large tears, indicating lack of rotator cuff healing in TSA. About half of patients with rotator cuff tears following TSA require revision surgery. Younger patients are potential candidates for outpatient arthroplasty as there is a move to this across healthcare systems with evidence showing it can reduce cost and improve patient outcomes. Patient selection for outpatient TSA is primarily focused on age, body mass index (BMI), absence of serious medical comorbidities, and the presence of home support, with considerable cost savings.

25.2.2 Contraindications

Complex shoulder arthritis complicated by irreparable rotator cuff tears, severe deformities, excessive glenoid retroversion, or fractures may not be suitable for TSA and thus may be better served with a primary RSA even at a younger age. There has been increasing use of RSA overall with ever-expanding indications, but especially in the middle-aged, active population due to their high demand, the rate of revisions is considerably higher. Furthermore, TSA has biomechanical limitations that negatively affect longevity if not respected. Most importantly, if adequate glenoid positioning with a final $<10°$ retroversion, $<10°$ superior inclination, contact area of $>80\%$, and $<80\%$ humeral head subluxation cannot be achieved with TSA, RSA is the more reliable choice.

25.3 Surgical Considerations

25.3.1 Glenoid

The glenoid has been the primary problem for longevity in anatomical shoulder arthroplasty, while polyethylene wear remains the main issue. All-polyethylene glenoid components have shown progressive radiolucent lines and loosening, which led to the development of metal-backed glenoid implants and hybrid variations. Continuous innovations regarding materials at the bone-implant interface and improved tribology (e.g., cross-linking polyethylene and addition of vitamin E) seem promising. The introduction of convertible baseplates allows easy revision to RSA with promising clinical results [1]. However, the available results are still not clear, which makes it difficult to define the best option for glenoid component use.

In general, there are two distinct types of glenohumeral OA: a concentric, central degeneration with a centered humeral head and a decentered form with a subluxated humerus and muscle imbalances.

These were classified by Walch et al. in Types A (concentric degeneration), B (posteriorly decentered humeral head), and C (posterior degeneration). Posterior glenoid bone defects are caused by irregular force distribution at the glenohumeral joint. Cases with OA and posterior subluxation of the humeral head have been shown to a be associated with higher complication and revision rates [2].

B2 configurated OA is not only the most common form, but it is also especially prevalent in young and/or active patients. In order to achieve good long-term outcomes, it is considered necessary to fill the posterior defect, correct the pathological glenoid version, and restore the premorbid joint line. Although there are no solid evidence-based guidelines for optimal positioning of glenoid components in TSA, a set of rules based on clinical and biomechanical observations has been postulated as guidance [3]. According to these rules, the glenoid component should be implanted in <10° retroversion and <10° superior inclination, have a contact area of >80%, and allow <80% humeral head subluxation, while avoiding anterior reaming. If these reference values cannot be achieved with anatomical components, RSA is the more reliable choice.

Surgical strategies to account for glenoid deformities include asymmetric reaming, auto- or allograft bone grafting alone or in combination with asymmetric reaming, cemented all-polyethylene or cementless metallic augmented glenoid components or their hybrid variations, and combinations of the above [4].

Due to the limited bone stock and bone quality of the glenoid vault, asymmetric reaming is reserved for only minor deformity and should be used cautiously [5–7]. The choice of auto- or allograft use for bone grafting primarily is a question of the socioeconomic, legislative, and healthcare environments in different countries [6]. The exact techniques for bone grafting depend on the type of bone defect. Contained defects can be filled with impacted cancellous bone chips. However, impaction bone grafting needs an intact vault and is therefore usually not suitable for posterior glenoid erosion. It can be combined with structural bone grafting in larger defects after restoration of containment. This can also be performed as a two-stage procedure to create a stable foundation for implant fixation in the most complex bone defects [8–14].

In cases of considerable posterior erosion or medialization of the joint line, appropriately sized structural bone grafting can be combined with long pegs or screw fixation for uncemented components or cemented all-polyethylene glenoid implants. Smaller defects in Walch type B2 or B3 deformities are more difficult to address with bone grafting, as suboptimal asymmetric force distribution potentially interferes with fixation and bone integration [15]. Filling such defects with bone cement does not provide suffi-cient long-term fixation and should thus be avoided. A better alternative could be augmented glenoid components, whereas uncemented implants seem favorable as cemented all-polyethylene versions have failed in the past. However, substantial evidence for the successful use and long-term survival of metallic augmented glenoid components is still missing.

As highlighted, optimal positioning of the glenoid can be challenging in TSA, especially in cases of severe degeneration and deformity. Preoperative planning can help to identify technical pitfalls before surgery and intraoperative guidance (e.g., patient-specific guides, classic computer navigation, or augmented reality) can help to precisely transfer the plan to the surgical environment. However, so far it could not be clarified if the extra efforts and expenses translate to improved patient outcomes, which will be needed to justify the use of all new technologies [4].

25.3.2 Humeral Head

The literature suggests long-term survival of the humeral component may be affected by type of fixation (e.g., pressfit, cemented, metaphyseal vs. diaphyseal) [16, 17]. The traditional long-stem arthroplasty design has become a reliable surgical treatment option in patients with OA of the shoulder. In younger and/or active patients, who have a high risk to face revision surgery, bone-sparing solutions are preferable to avoid humeral bone loss during long-stem removal [18].

There has been a trend toward uncemented short stems and stemless implants in primary, anatomical shoulder arthroplasty. The proposed advantages of such designs are bone stock preservation, reduced periprosthetic fractures, simpler stem positioning, reduced operating time, and easier revision surgery [19]. While short- to mid-term results are promising [20], there is still a paucity of long-term clinical data following short-stem arthroplasty. The available long-term data show good clinical results with low rates of complications [21]. However, as short-stem and stemless implants seem to provide comparable clinical outcomes and revision rates as long-stem implants, these designs seem to be preferable in middle-aged patients.

Optimal anatomical reconstruction of the humeral component is often not in the focus of surgical considerations, although it has been shown that the restoration of a native humeral morphology positively influences long-term outcomes [22]. The rate of inadequately restored humeral head morphology was recently found to be 35% despite preoperative 3D planning. The most common error on the humeral side is overstuffing of the joint, which lateralizes the center of rotation. Rather than choosing oversized components, most frequently this is caused by resecting the humeral head too far proximally [23].

Another field of potential improvements are further developments in materials. In the shoulder, currently the most controversial innovation is the introduction of humeral head components made of pyrolytic carbon for hemiarthroplasty. Pyrocarbon seems to possess better tribological characteristics against cartilage than standard metallic (i.e., CoCr) components [24]. Recent literature suggests promising results from pyrocarbon compared to metallic hemiarthroplasty, but long-term data is not yet available [25–28]. Nonetheless, pyrocarbon resurfacing is a very interesting option especially in younger and/or active patients or patients with mainly humeral degeneration.

25.3.3 Rotator Cuff Management

Rotator cuff tears remain a relevant risk following anatomical shoulder arthroplasty, accounting for 6.9–9% of all complications. The rate of rotator cuff dysfunction at midterm follow-up has been reported to be as high as 17% with all-polyethylene glenoid components [29–31].

Rotator cuff tears following TSA result in inferior clinical and radiographic outcomes. Biomechanically, the disrupted joint mechanics lead to abnormal joint loads resulting in accelerated joint wear and increased risk of dislocation, which could be detrimental for long-term implant survival.

Due to the inherent trauma of standard deltopectoral approaches, the subscapularis tendon is most at risk for failure following TSA. The subscapularis muscle is essential as part of the anterior–posterior force couple, anterior restraint, and important mover of the shoulder. Subscapularis dysfunction following TSA manifests as pain, instability, and a lack of active maximal internal rotation and is associated with poorer outcomes [32, 33]. Besides reduced shoulder function, SSC disruption leads to anterior humeral head migration and eccentric glenoid loading, which results in more stress at the glenoid interface. Therefore, SSC integrity plays a pivotal in long-term TSA survival.

Revision repair for SSC tears following TSA can be performed as a salvage option before conversion to RSA, but studies showed only moderate outcomes [34]. Ideally, the initial repair technique is secure enough to reduce the risk of postoperative tears. The main options for SSC management during TSA are subscapularis peel (peeling of the complete SSC tendon from the lesser tuberosity), tenotomy (mid substance tenotomy about 1 cm medial to the lesser tuberosity), or lesser tuberosity osteotomy (a sliver of bone of about 5 mm wide and 1 cm high is osteotomized off the lesser tuberosity at the border of the intertubercular groove) [35]. Multiple studies evaluated the different techniques but did not find relevant differences between the techniques regarding function, range of motion, SSC strength, pain, or complication rate. However, lesser tuberosity osteotomy showed superior healing and performance in SSC specific functional testing, which might make it the slightly favorable option [36–38]. Alternatively, a SSC sparing approach can be used to avoid removing the SSC altogether. However, available studies do not provide conclusive evidence for clinically relevant improvements by using a SSC sparing technique, while increasing the risk for component malpositioning, sizing issues, and residual osteophytes due to the limited exposure [39].

In close proximity, the long head of biceps tendon (LHBT) runs distally in the bicipital groove. Options to address pathologically altered LHBT are tenotomy and tenodesis.

There is broad consensus and supporting evidence that excision of the proximal part and fixing the stump to the pectoralis major insertion at the humeral head is superior and thus should be favored [39–41].

25.4 Clinical Outcomes, Complications, and Survivorship

Overall, there are excellent clinical outcomes reported following TSA in middle-aged patients. Brochin et al. performed a retrospective review of patients with TSA under 60 and found significant improvements in American Shoulder and Elbow Surgeons score (32 ± 20 to 64 ± 27, $P = 0.0008$) [42]. Simple Shoulder Test scores (3 ± 2 to 7 ± 4, $P = 0.0004$) and reduced visual analog scale pain scores (7 ± 3 to 3 ± 3, $P = 0.0001$). Furthermore, there was significant improvement in forward elevation ($119° \pm 26°$ to $146° \pm 21°$, $P = 0.0002$), external rotation ($21° \pm 25°$ to $52° \pm 15°$, $P = 0.0001$), and internal rotation (from L5 to L1, $P = 0.002$). Furthermore, Bartlet et al. found TSA resulted in significantly less pain, greater active elevation, and higher satisfaction at final follow-up compared with those who underwent hemiarthroplasty at long-term follow-up [43].

TSA has been shown to have a comparable complication rate compared to RSA and lower than hemiarthroplasty, in the treatment of arthritis in patients under 60, with Fonte et al. finding a 19.4% complication rate in their systematic review [44]. The primary concern is glenoid component loosening as this may lead to the need for an early revision. Brochin et al. found at a minimum of 10 years follow-up that 17.6% patients of patients under 60 had aseptic glenoid loosening, with 4 patients requiring conversion to an RSA and 2 undergoing arthroscopic glenoid removal, but there was an 81% survivorship rate in their series at 20 year follow-up [42]. Additionally, Bartelt et al. found a 94% survivorship rate at 10-year follow-up with TSA, which was significantly higher than those who underwent a hemiarthroplasty [43]. In contrast, Denard et al. found a 62.5% survivorship rate at 10-year follow-up in patients under 55; thus surgeons should still exercise caution when indicating younger patients for TSA [45].

25.5 Return to Play and Return to Work

Return to play is still an important consideration in this population, as high demand is a relative indication for TSA as it can allow for increased activity levels compared to RSA or hemiarthroplasty. Thus, these patients are often concerned with their ability to return to sports or other demanding activities. Several studies have examined the rates of return of to play following shoulder arthroplasty with Liu et al. finding 92.6% of those with TSA able to return compared with 74.9% following RSA and 71.1% following hemiarthroplasty [46]. The systematic review by Liu et al. also found 79.6% were able to return to sports at the same level as prior to pathological decline and surgery. Additionally, reported rates of return to golf ranged from 89 to 100% with mean time to return ranging from 5.1 to 8.4 months [47]. Furthermore, rates of return to golf following RSA and hemiarthroplasty were far lower in the literature, with 50–79% returning following RSA and 54% following hemiarthroplasty [48]. However, it remains unclear how long patients should wait before returning to activities following TSA, and further study is needed on this area to minimize complications. However, surgeons should focus on individualizing patient's timeline based on stability, strength, range of motion, and proprioception.

Return to work can be an outcome for many patients in this population, as they may have only a few years left of employment. Steinhaus et al. evaluated this in their systematic review of 7 studies and 447 patients [49]. Overall, they found the rate of return to work was 63.6% (58.8–68.2%) at a mean 2.3 months postoperatively. The rate of return to work was significantly lower for patients with heavy-intensity occupations vs.

all intensity types (61.7% vs. 67.6%). However, they found no difference among TSA, RSA, and hemiarthroplasty or among those with different indications or workman's compensation status.

25.6 Revision Options for TSA

Revision surgery for failed TSA almost exclusively means conversion to RSA, as most reasons for failure cannot be sufficiently addressed with revision TSA or component exchanges. As responsible and future-minded shoulder surgeons, it is imperative to keep possible modes of failure and ultimately revision surgeries in mind already at the time of primary arthroplasty to prevent future disaster. This is especially important in the younger and/or active patient population with a high risk of needing future surgeries in their lifetime. In general, this could mean to consider hemiarthroplasty as first-line treatment in high-demand patients, for example, using pyrocarbon humeral heads, that can be potentially converted to TSA and ultimately RSA if necessary. On the glenoid side, this could mean to consider implants that are revisable without creating massive bone loss or convertible systems that can be changed to RSA with relative ease and little trauma. The majority of modern humeral implant designs allow the conversion from anatomic humeral head components to reverse geometry. If the preferred system does not offer the option of such conversion, bone-sparing implants (i.e., short-stem or stemless options) should be considered. Nonetheless, revisions from anatomical to reverse arthroplasty often provide inferior outcomes to primary procedures, but planning ahead at primary surgery can go a long way in achieving the best results for the patients.

25.7 Summary

Glenohumeral arthritis is a challenging clinical pathology in middle-aged patients. TSA is a reliable option allowing patients to return to high-demand activities, with significant improvement in range of motion, pain, and function. Continuous innovations led to improved longevity, but TSA has inherent limitations and is thus not feasible for all patients or pathologies. As responsible shoulder surgeons, we need to keep the possibility of revision surgery in mind and choose implants and patients accordingly to avoid future problems.

References

1. Castagna A, Delcogliano M, de Caro F, Ziveri G, Borroni M, Gumina S, et al. Conversion of shoulder arthroplasty to reverse implants: clinical and radiological results using a modular system. Int Orthop. 2013;37(7):1297–305.
2. Walch G, Moraga C, Young A, Castellanos-Rosas J. Results of anatomic nonconstrained prosthesis in primary osteoarthritis with biconcave glenoid. J Shoulder Elb Surg. 2012;21(11):1526–33.
3. Walch G. Golden rules for total shoulder arthroplasty treatment. Tennessee: Wright Medical Group N.V.; 2016.
4. Grubhofer F, Wieser K. Die Bedeutung von computerunterstützter Operationstechnik und Planung der Glenoidpositionierung bei anatomischer Schultertotalprothese. The role of computerized planning and surgical technique in anatomic total shoulder arthroplasty glenoid component positioning. Obere Extremität. 2022;17:67–73.
5. Walch G, Badet R, Boulahia A, Khoury A. Morphologic study of the glenoid in primary glenohumeral osteoarthritis. J Arthroplast. 1999;14(6):756–60.
6. Albers S, Hudek R, Kircher J. How to deal with posterior glenoid erosion in anatomic total shoulder arthroplasty. Obere Extremitat. 2022;17(2):74–83.
7. Mimar R, Limb D, Hall R. Evaluation of the mechanical and architectural properties of glenoid bone. J Shoulder Elb Surg. 2008;17:336–41.
8. Gowda A, Pinkas D, Wiater JM. Treatment of glenoid bone deficiency in total shoulder arthroplasty: a critical analysis review. JBJS Rev. 2015;3(7):e2.
9. Scalise JJ, Iannotti JP. Bone grafting severe glenoid defects in revision shoulder arthroplasty. Clin Orthop Relat Res. 2008;466(1):139–45.
10. Steinmann SP, Cofield RH. Bone grafting for glenoid deficiency in total shoulder replacement. J Shoulder Elb Surg. 2000;9(5):361–7.
11. Neyton L, Walch G, Nové-Josserand L, Edwards TB. Glenoid corticocancellous bone grafting after glenoid component removal in the treatment of glenoid loosening. J Shoulder Elb Surg. 2006;15(2):173–9.
12. Bonnevialle N, Melis B, Neyton L, Favard L, Molé D, Walch G, et al. Aseptic glenoid loosening or failure in total shoulder arthroplasty: revision with glenoid reimplantation. J Shoulder Elb Surg. 2013;22(6):745–51.

13. Hill J, Norris T. Long-term results of total shoulder arthroplasty following bone-grafting of the glenoid. J Bone Jt Surg Am. 2001;83-A:877–83.

14. Gohlke F, Werner B, Wiese I. Glenoid reconstruction in revision shoulder arthroplasty. Oper Orthop Traumatol. 2019;31(2):98–114.

15. Nyffeler R, Sheikh R, Atkinson T, Jacob H, Favre P, Gerber C. Effects of glenoid component version on humeral head displacement and joint reaction forces: an experimental study. J Shoulder Elb Surg. 2006;15:625–9.

16. Tross A-K, Bülhoff M, Renkawitz T, Kretzer JP. Stem length in anatomic total shoulder arthroplasty: long stem, short stem, and stemless. Obere Extremität. 2022;17:84–91.

17. Bohsali KI, Bois AJ, Wirth MA. Complications of shoulder arthroplasty. J Bone Jt Surg Am. 2017;99(3):256–69.

18. Churchill RS, Athwal GS. Stemless shoulder arthroplasty-current results and designs. Curr Rev Musculoskelet Med. 2016;9(1):10–6.

19. Schnetzke M, Loew M, Raiss P, Walch G. Short-stem anatomical shoulder replacement—a systematic review Die Kurzschaftprothese beim anatomischen Schultergelenkersatz—eine systematische Literaturübersicht. Obere Extremität. 2019;14:139–48.

20. Schnetzke M, Rick S, Raiss P, Walch G, Loew M. Mid-term results of anatomical total shoulder arthroplasty for primary osteoarthritis using a short-stemmed cementless humeral component. Bone Jt J. 2018;100-B:603–9.

21. Magosch P, Lichtenberg S, Habermeyer H. Survival of stemless humeral head replacement in anatomic shoulder arthroplasty. A prospective study. J Shoulder Elb Surg. 2020;30(7):e343–55.

22. Flurin PH, Roche CP, Wright TW, Marczuk Y, Zuckerman JD. A comparison and correlation of clinical outcome metrics in anatomic and reverse total shoulder arthroplasty. Bull Hosp Jt Dis (2013). 2015;73(Suppl 1):S118–23.

23. Grubhofer F, Muniz Martinez AR, Haberli J, Selig ME, Ernstbrunner L, Price MD, et al. Does computerized CT-based 3D planning of the humeral head cut help to restore the anatomy of the proximal humerus after stemless total shoulder arthroplasty? J Shoulder Elb Surg. 2021;30(6):e309–e16.

24. Klawitter JJ, Patton J, More R, Peter N, Podnos E, Ross M. In vitro comparison of wear characteristics of pyrocarbon and metal on bone: shoulder hemiarthroplasty. Shoulder Elb. 2020;12(1 Suppl):11–22.

25. McBride AP, Ross M, Hoy G, Duke P, Page R, Peng Y, et al. Mid-term outcomes of pyrolytic carbon humeral resurfacing hemiarthroplasty compared with metal humeral resurfacing and metal stemmed hemiarthroplasty for osteoarthritis in young patients: analysis from the Australian Orthopaedic Association National Joint Replacement Registry. J Shoulder Elb Surg. 2022;31(4):755–62.

26. Garret J, Harly É, Le Huec J-C, Brunner UH, Rotini R, Godeneche A. Pyrolytic carbon humeral head in hemi-shoulder arthroplasty: preliminary results at 2-year follow-up. JSES Open Access. 2019;3:37–42.

27. Cointat C, Raynier JL, Vasseur H, Lareyre F, Raffort J, Gauci MO, et al. Short-term outcomes and survival of pyrocarbon hemiarthroplasty in the young arthritic shoulder. J Shoulder Elb Surg. 2022;31(1):113–22.

28. Tsitlakidis S, Doll J, Westhauser F, Wolf M, Hetto P, Maier M, et al. Promising results after hemi shoulder arthroplasty using pyrolytic carbon heads in young and middle-aged patients. Orthop Traumatol Surg Res. 2021;107:102896.

29. Jackson JD, Cil A, Smith J, Steinmann SP. Integrity and function of the subscapularis after total shoulder arthroplasty. J Shoulder Elb Surg. 2010;19(7):1085–90.

30. Bornes TD, Rollins MD, Lapner PL, Bouliane MJ. Subscapularis management in total shoulder arthroplasty: current evidence comparing peel, osteotomy, and tenotomy. J Shoulder Elb Arthroplast. 2018;2:2471549218807772.

31. Armstrong A, Lashgari C, Teefey S, Menendez J, Yamaguchi K, Galatz L. Ultrasound evaluation and clinical correlation of subscapularis repair after total shoulder arthroplasty. J Shoulder Elb Surg. 2006;15:541–8.

32. Miller B, Joseph T, Noonan T, Horan M, Hawkins R. Rupture of the subscapularis tendon after shoulder arthroplasty: diagnosis, treatment, and outcome. J Shoulder Elb Surg. 2005;14:492–6.

33. Miller S, Hazrati Y, Klepps S, Chiang A, Flatow E. Loss of subscapularis function after total shoulder replacement: a seldom recognized problem. J Shoulder Elb Surg. 2003;12:29–34.

34. Moeckel BH, Altchek DW, Warren RF, Wickiewicz TL, Dines DM. Instability of the shoulder after arthroplasty. JBJS. 1993;75(4):492–7.

35. Matache BA, Lapner PL. Anatomic shoulder arthroplasty: technical considerations. Open Orthop J. 2017;11:1115–25.

36. Choate WS, Kwapisz A, Momaya AM, Hawkins RJ, Tokish JM. Outcomes for subscapularis management techniques in shoulder arthroplasty: a systematic review. J Shoulder Elb Surg. 2018;27(2):363–70.

37. Del Core MA, Cutler HS, Ahn J, Khazzam M. Systematic review and network meta-analysis of subscapularis management techniques in anatomic total shoulder arthroplasty. J Shoulder Elb Surg. 2021;30(7):1714–24.

38. Lee S, Sardar H, Horner NS, Al Mana L, Miller BS, Khan M, et al. Subscapularis-sparing approaches in shoulder arthroplasty: a systematic review. J Orthop. 2021;24:165–72.

39. Tuckman DV, Dines DM. Long head of the biceps pathology as a cause of anterior shoulder pain after shoulder arthroplasty. J Shoulder Elb Surg. 2006;15(4):415–8.

40. Fama G, Edwards TB, Boulahia A, Kempf J-F, Boileau P, Némoz C, et al. The role of concomitant

biceps tenodesis in shoulder arthroplasty for primary osteoarthritis: results of a multicentric study. Thorofare: SLACK Incorporated; 2004. p. 401–5.

41. Simmen B, Bachmann L, Drerup S, Schwyzer H-K, Burkhart A, Flury M, et al. Usefulness of concomitant biceps tenodesis in total shoulder arthroplasty: a prospective cohort study. J Shoulder Elb Surg. 2008;17:921–4.

42. Brochin RL, Zastrow RK, Patel AV, Parsons BO, Galatz LM, Flatow EL, et al. Long-term clinical and radiographic outcomes of total shoulder arthroplasty in patients under age 60 years. J Shoulder Elb Surg. 2022;31(6, Supplement):S63–70.

43. Bartelt R, Sperling JW, Schleck CD, Cofield RH. Shoulder arthroplasty in patients aged 55 years or younger with osteoarthritis. J Shoulder Elb Surg. 2011;20(1):123–30.

44. Fonte H, Amorim-Barbosa T, Diniz S, Barros L, Ramos J, Claro R. Shoulder arthroplasty options for glenohumeral osteoarthritis in young and active patients (<60 years old): a systematic review. J Shoulder Elb Arthroplast. 2022;6:24715492221087014.

45. Denard PJ, Raiss P, Sowa B, Walch G. Mid- to long-term follow-up of total shoulder arthroplasty using a keeled glenoid in young adults with primary glenohumeral arthritis. J Shoulder Elb Surg. 2013;22(7):894–900.

46. Liu J, Steinhaus M, Garcia G, Chang B, Fields K, Dines D, et al. Return to sport after shoulder arthroplasty: a systematic review and meta-analysis. Knee Surg Sports Traumatol Arthrosc. 2017;26:1–13.

47. Salem HS, Park DH, Thon SG, Bravman JT, Seidl AJ, McCarty EC, et al. Return to golf after shoulder arthroplasty: a systematic review. Am J Sports Med. 2020;49(4):1109–15.

48. Davey MG, Davey MS, Hurley ET, Gaafar M, Pauzenberger L, Mullett H. Return to sport following reverse shoulder arthroplasty: a systematic review. J Shoulder Elb Surg. 2021;30(1):216–21.

49. Steinhaus M, Gowd A, Hurwit D, Lieber A, Liu J. Return to work after shoulder arthroplasty: a systematic review and meta-analysis. J Shoulder Elb Surg. 2019;28(5):998–1008.

Reverse Total Shoulder Arthroplasty (RTSA) in a Middle-Aged Patient

26

Joseph P. DeAngelis

Since reverse total shoulder arthroplasty was introduced, the indications have expanded beyond Grammont's original plan to address shoulder pain due to chronic rotator cuff insufficiency in the elderly. In addition to rotator cuff arthropathy, the reverse total shoulder is now being used to address proximal humerus fractures and glenoid bone loss, and, in some locales, RTSA is the preferred treatment for primary glenohumeral arthritis. Many of these additional applications are described in this volume, and these proposed benefits of the RTSA will be tested in time.

Along with these broadening indications for surgery, the role of the RTSA is being examined as a function of patient age. At present, RTSA is being performed in patients younger than those originally indicated. However, it is unclear at what age an RTSA is an appropriate intervention. Just as the indications for implant utilization have been expanded, the age of implantation has also decreased. These changes have occurred in concert with the rapid adoption of RTSA and offer some insight into the future of shoulder arthroplasty. As more RTSAs are performed, the expanding patient cohort offers us a broader and more nuanced perspective into what patients and their surgeons can expect over the life of a RTSA. Correspondingly, with each passing year, the available data have matured allowing for a closer consideration of complications and patient concerns. The resulting quality control has grown into an opportunity for improvement, and this process has fueled further innovation.

Historically, surgeons have been reluctant to perform RTSAs in younger patients due to concerns about the longevity of the implant. As with all large-joint replacements, the risk of revision increases with time. However, it is impossible to know how long a prosthesis will last at the time of its implantation, and we are unable to identify in whom a catastrophic failure will occur. Because younger patients typically have higher expectations of their artificial shoulders than older patients, and because younger patients typically have more active lifestyles, orthopaedic surgeons frequently dissuade patients from joint arthroplasty until their disease has crossed a threshold of severity [1]. While the shared decision-making aims to balance a patient's expectations and satisfaction, the process is heavily influenced by the patient's experience of their condition (the reported severity of their impairment) and their surgeon's presentation of the risk of surgical complications (implant failure) [2]. Surgeons often advise their younger patients to delay intervention in an effort to improve implant survival.

J. P. DeAngelis (✉)
Harvard Medical School, Boston, MA, USA

Beth Israel Deaconess Medical Center,
Boston, MA, USA

© ISAKOS 2023
A. D. Mazzocca et al. (eds.), *Shoulder Arthritis across the Life Span*,
https://doi.org/10.1007/978-3-031-33298-2_26

Ironically, this delay in treatment may increase the complexity of their subsequent surgery and therefore decrease the implants survival [3].

When RTSA is compared to hip and knee replacement, the relative novelty of the procedure limits our experience and therefore our long-term follow-up. In the United States, the RTSA was first approved for use in 2003, so 20-year outcomes are not known. Looking to the French experience for guidance, the original cohorts were not encouraging as the clinical outcomes of RTSA have been shown to deteriorate after 6–10 years [4, 5]. Correspondingly, when Gerber considered the effect of patient age on the outcomes after RTSA, he found that patients younger than 65 years of age demonstrated high rates of complications [6].

Unfortunately, this experience has been affirmed in other larger studies. In the Australian National Joint Registry (NJR), significantly increased revision rates were reported in younger age groups [7]. Their 2019 annual report revealed that the 7-year revision rate increased with declining age (55–64 5.7%; 65–74 3.6%; older than 75 2.7%). In a recently published series, the 10-year RTSA survival was only 81% for a Grammond-style prosthesis in a cohort with an average age of 66 years at the time of surgery [8]. This observation raises a fundamental question: How should an orthopaedic surgeon advise a middle-aged patient on the appropriateness of a RTSA?

Importantly, the trend towards higher revision rates in younger patients is not unique to RTSA. It can be seen in all types of shoulder arthroplasty. A review of 5494 consecutive shoulder arthroplasties (anatomic, reverse, and hemiarthroplasty), performed between 1970 and 2012, found a 3% decrease in the need for revision with each year of increased age [9]. When the individual subgroups were considered, the same age-based association was seen.

An argument has been made that modern implant designs will improve implant survival following RTSA. The introduction of lateralized glenoids along with changes in the humeral neck shaft angle may influence the revision rate after RTSA, but more time is needed for the data to mature. Optimistically, these improvements could benefit middle-aged patients who are considering an intervention to address their shoulder pain and function.

Recent studies have offered some hope for the survivability of RTSA. In a cohort of 20 patients with a mean age of 57 years, the reported implant survivorship was 91% at a mean follow-up of 11.7 years [10]. In a meta-analysis of patients younger than 65 undergoing RTSA with 4 years of follow-up, the survivorship was 93%, and the complication rate was 17% (4% infection, 5% instability) [11]. In 2020, a separate meta-analysis affirmed that RTSA was safe and effective in patients under 65 years of age, acknowledging that the rates of complication, reoperation, and revision to those of patients older than 65 at a mean of 4.7 years of follow-up [12]. A similar comparison was made in another meta-analysis examining RTSA in patients younger than 60 years [13]. They found similar clinical outcomes in both younger and older patients, with comparable implant survivorship. Altogether, these data are encouraging because they suggest that age alone may not be a significant risk factor for implant failure or the need for a revision.

If our long-term experience with RTSA affirms this conclusion, the middle-aged patient may be best positioned to benefit from surgery. Improved clinical outcomes and function are additive over time. Performing a RTSA in relatively younger individuals should afford them a better quality of life over a longer duration [14]. In the literature, this utility appears to be present regardless of patient's age and the surgical indication for RTSA [15, 16].

The middle-aged patient also presents a unique challenge because of their expected level of postoperative activity. In an effort to set appropriate expectations, most orthopaedic surgeons caution their patients prior to RTSA. However, there is no common consensus on what activities are safe or appropriate following RTSA. In a 2018 meta-analysis that included 621 patients, ranging in age from 22 to 92 years old, more than 60% of patients returned to sports [17]. Franceschetti et al. found the same rate of return to sports in their review of 457 RTSA patients and added that the time to return was only 5.3 months [18].

As the utilization of RTSA continues to grow, the middle-aged patient is best positioned to benefit from the knowledge gained through our collective experience. Larger clinical trials will offer insights into how the RTSA performs within specific groups of patients. The maturity of registry data should provide the long-term follow-up necessary for more detailed subgroup analysis. In combination, this information should guide the middle-aged patient for the longest potential benefit.

References

1. Husain A, Lee GC. Establishing realistic patient expectations following total knee arthroplasty. J Am Acad Orthop Surg. 2015;23(12):707–13. https://doi.org/10.5435/JAAOS-D-14-00049.
2. Slover J, Alvarado C, Nelson C. Shared decision making in total joint replacement. JBJS Rev. 2014;2(3):e1. https://doi.org/10.2106/JBJS.RVW.M.00044.
3. Boselli KJ, Ahmad CS, Levine WN. Treatment of glenohumeral arthrosis. Am J Sports Med. 2010;38(12):2558–72. https://doi.org/10.1177/0363546510369250.
4. Guery J, Favard L, Sirveaux F, Oudet D, Mole D, Walch G. Reverse total shoulder arthroplasty: survivorship analysis of 80 replacements followed for 5–10 years. J Bone Jt Surg Am. 2006;88:1742–7.
5. Favard L, Levigne C, Nerot C, Gerber C, De Wilde L, Mole D. Reverse prostheses in arthropathies with cuff tear: are survivorship and function maintained over time? Clin Orthop Relat Res. 2011;469:2469–75.
6. Ek ETH, Neukom L, Catanzaro S, Gerber C. Reverse total shoulder arthroplasty for massive irreparable rotator cuff tears in patients younger than 65 years old: results after 5–15 years. J Shoulder Elb Surg. 2013;22:1199–208.
7. Australian Orthopaedic Association National Joint Replacement Registry. Hip, knee and shoulder arthroplasty annual report 2019. Adelaide: AOA; 2019.
8. Sheth MM, Heldt BL, Spell JH, Vidal EA, Laughlin MS, Morris BJ, Elkousy HA, Edwards TB. Patient satisfaction and clinical outcomes of reverse shoulder arthroplasty: a minimum of 10 years' follow-up. J Shoulder Elb Surg. 2022;31(4):875–83. https://doi.org/10.1016/j.jse.2021.09.012.
9. Wagner ER, Houdek MT, Schleck CD, et al. The role age plays in the outcomes and complications of shoulder arthroplasty. J Shoulder Elb Surg. 2017;26:1573–80.
10. Ernstbrunner L, Suter A, Catanzaro S, Rahm S, Gerber C. Reverse total shoulder arthroplasty for massive, irreparable rotator cuff tears before the age of 60 years: long-term results. J Bone Jt Surg Am. 2017;99:1721–9.
11. Chelli M, Lo Cunsolo L, Gauci M-O, et al. Reverse shoulder arthroplasty in patients aged 65 years or younger: a systematic review of the literature. JSES Open Access. 2019;3:162–7.
12. Goldenberg BT, Samuelsen BT, Spratt JD, Dornan GJ, Millett PJ. Complications and implant survivorship following primary reverse total shoulder arthroplasty in patients younger than 65 years: a systematic review. J Shoulder Elb Surg. 2020;29:1703–11.
13. Bedeir YH, Gawish HM, Grawe BM. Outcomes of reverse total shoulder arthroplasty in patients 60 years of age or younger: a systematic review. J Hand Surg Am. 2020;45:254.e1–8.
14. Nicholson JA, Jones R, MacDonald DJ, Brown I, McBirnie J. Cost-effectiveness of the reverse total shoulder arthroplasty. Does indication affect outcome? Shoulder Elb. 2021;13(1):90–7. https://doi.org/10.1177/1758573219897860.
15. Hanisch K, Holte MB, Hvass I, Wedderkopp N. Clinically relevant results of reverse total shoulder arthroplasty for patients younger than 65 years compared to the older patients. Arthroplasty. 2021;3(1):30. https://doi.org/10.1186/s42836-021-00086-4.
16. Castricini R, Gasparini G, Di Luggo F, De Benedetto M, De Gori M, Galasso O. Health-related quality of life and functionality after reverse shoulder arthroplasty. J Shoulder Elb Surg. 2013;22(12):1639–49. https://doi.org/10.1016/j.jse.2013.01.020.
17. MacInnes SJ, Mackie KE, Titchener A, Gibbons R, Wang AW. Activity following reverse total shoulder arthroplasty: what should surgeons be advising? Shoulder Elb. 2019;11(2 Suppl):4–15. https://doi.org/10.1177/1758573218793648.
18. Franceschetti E, Giovannetti de Sanctis E, Gregori P, Palumbo A, Paciotti M, Di Giacomo G, Franceschi F. Return to sport after reverse total shoulder arthroplasty is highly frequent: a systematic review. J ISAKOS. 2021;6(6):363–6. https://doi.org/10.1136/jisakos-2020-000581.

Outcomes of Reverse Shoulder Arthroplasty Following Failed Superior Capsular Reconstruction Versus Rotator Cuff Repair

Annabelle Davey, Antonio Cusano, and Augustus D. Mazzocca

27.1 Introduction

Rotator cuff tears (RCTs) are a common injury, with a prevalence of approximately 40% in adults aged over 60 years [1]. Up to 50% of RCTs may be asymptomatic, but tears may progress in size over time and eventually become symptomatic [2]. Rotator cuff repair (RCR) is the preferred treatment option in younger patients with symptomatic full-thickness rotator cuff tears to restore function and prevent tear progression and subsequent degenerative changes [2]. However, while RCR has shown favorable outcomes in many cases, there remains a high failure rate, with nearly 40% of patients with massive RCTs suffering re-tear [3]. Additionally, many RCTs may be irreparable at the time of initial presentation and so considerable effort has been placed into developing effective treatment strategies [4]. The natural history of failed RCR or superior capsular reconstruction (SCR) results in progression of tear size, with eventual cuff tear arthropathy (CTA) due to altered biomechanics of the shoulder [5–7].

Originally described by Mihata using fascia lata autograft, the SCR has emerged as a potential surgical option for younger patients with massive irreparable tears and limited glenohumeral arthritis [8, 9]. This technique holds considerable joint-preserving potential and seeks to provide several years of pain and functionality so as to delay future arthroplasty procedures. Initial results following SCR have yielded promising outcomes, with failure rates dependent on graft choice and technique and reported up to 36% [10]. Nonetheless, the gold standard for treatment of CTA continues to be the reverse total shoulder arthroplasty (RSA), which has been shown to have excellent outcomes [11].

Outcomes of RSA following a failed SCR versus RCR are not well studied. Given the aging population and the evolving indications of RCR and SCR for massive RCTs, it is likely that there will be an increasing number of RSAs performed in patients following failed RCR or SCR. The current chapter sought to provide an overview of the existing literature regarding RSA outcomes following RCR or SCR.

A. Davey · A. Cusano (✉)
Department of Orthopaedic Surgery, University of Connecticut, Farmington, CT, USA
e-mail: adavey@uchc.edu; acusano@uchc.edu

A. D. Mazzocca
Department of Orthopedic Surgery, Massachusetts General Hospital/Harvard Medical School, Boston, MA, USA
e-mail: amazzocca@mgh.harvard.edu

© ISAKOS 2023
A. D. Mazzocca et al. (eds.), *Shoulder Arthritis across the Life Span*,
https://doi.org/10.1007/978-3-031-33298-2_27

27.2 Outcomes Following RSA

RSA has shown favorable results in the setting of rotator cuff arthropathy, with reported 10-year survival rates of 89% [12–14]. Predictive variables of poor clinical outcomes following RSA, however, are controversial. Several studies have suggested that age [15, 16], higher body mass index, gender, and prior rotator cuff repair [17–19] may be associated with worse postoperative outcomes following RSA. More recent data [20, 21] has also found that patients with an increased number of reported allergies, history of preoperative opioid use, and/or previous ipsilateral shoulder surgery were associated with worse postoperative outcomes. Further, the presence of functional somatic symptoms, or chronic physical symptoms without an identifiable organic cause, portend to worse 2-year postoperative Single Assessment Numeric Evaluation (SANE) and American Shoulder Elbow Score (ASES) scores [20, 21].

In an effort to guide patient-centered care and clinical decision-making, clinically significant outcome measures, such as the minimal clinically significant difference (MCID) and substantial clinical benefit (SCB), have been developed and studied in the context of SANE, Constant, and ASES scores in orthopedics [22–24] and shoulder arthroplasty [25]. To that end, Gowd et al. [26] retrospectively reviewed patients undergoing total shoulder arthroplasties from 2014 to 2017 and found that achievement of clinically significant outcomes in SANE correlated with achieving meaningful outcomes as per the Constant and ASES scores. Based on their results, a change in SANE score from pre- to final postoperative of 29 points constituted the MCID, a change in SANE from 50 points constituted the SCB, and a SANE ≥ 75 constituted the patient acceptable symptomatic state (PASS). Having an understanding of these clinically relevant thresholds is critical to interpreting outcomes after shoulder-directed interventions.

27.3 RSA After Failed RCR

Nearly 40% of RCRs will show evidence of re-tear on advanced imaging [3]; however, many will be asymptomatic [3]. For those patients with symptomatic re-tears following RCR with limited degenerative changes of the shoulder, an additional soft tissue procedure—such as revision RCR, SCR, or tendon transfer—may be indicated. However, in patients with advanced degenerative changes of the glenohumeral joint (Hamada class 3 or greater), RSA remains the gold standard (Fig. 27.1a–c) [11, 27]. RSA relies on deltoid function for joint stability and motion, so deltoid muscle or axillary nerve dysfunction is an absolute contraindication to RSA. There has traditionally been concern that prior open rotator cuff repair, which may require deltoid detachment for full visualization of the rotator cuff tendons, may lead to deltoid dysfunction [28]. However, there has been no reported difference in outcomes between patients who underwent prior arthroscopic versus open RCR prior to RSA [28, 29]. Similarly, RSA may also be considered in patients with failed RCR in the absence of CTA [11]. However, there are high rates of aseptic loosening and decreased implant survival in younger, higher-demand patients. As such, patient age and functional status should be taken into account when indicating patients for RSA following failed RCR.

Several studies have looked at the outcomes of RSA following failed RCR. In a retrospective multicenter study of 42 RSAs in 40 patients by Boileau et al. [29] the authors found that while RSA can improve overall functionality in cuff-deficient shoulders after failure of previous cuff surgery, results were inferior to those following primary RSA. Similarly, in their review 83 patients with previous RCR compared to 189 matched controls undergoing primary RSA, Shields et al. [19] found that while patients who had undergone prior failed RCR had improved patient reported outcome measure (PROM) scores and range of motion

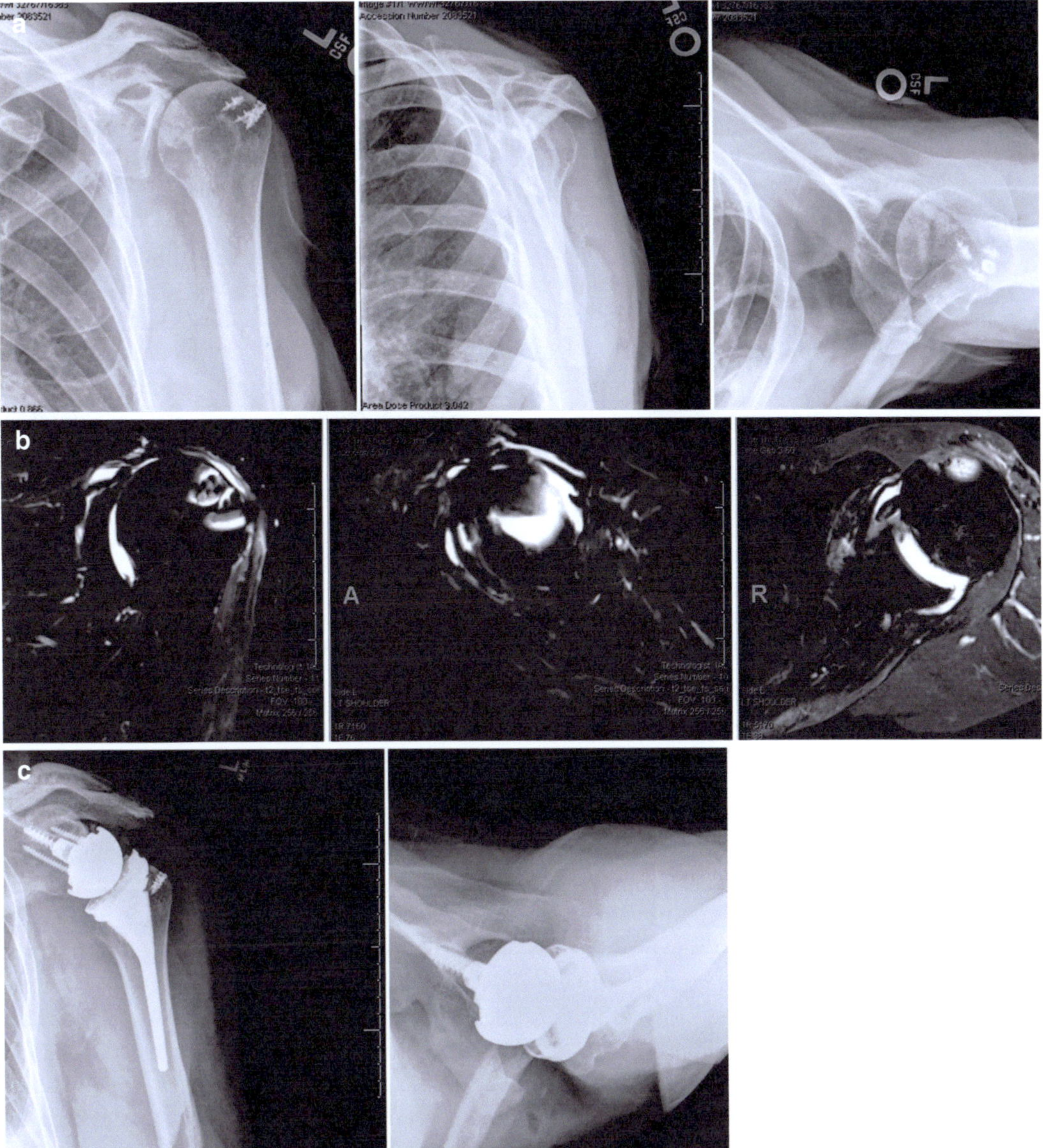

Fig. 27.1 (**a**) Three-view radiographs of the left shoulder show mild osteoarthritic glenohumeral joint changes with mild proximal humeral head migration. There are anchors within the greater tuberosity from a previous rotator cuff repair with adjacent lucencies concerning for hardware loosening. (**b**) Representative select coronal, sagittal, and axial MRI cuts show full-thickness supraspinatus and infraspinatus tears, as well as a near full-thickness tear of the subscapularis. Also visualized are fatty atrophy of the rotator cuff musculature and dislocation of the long head of the biceps tendon out of its groove with its anchor attached. (**c**) Anteroposterior and axillary images of the left shoulder status post reverse shoulder arthroplasty with intact hardware in appropriate position and no evidence of gross failure or loosening

(ROM) at 2-year follow-up, they had lower postoperative PROM scores, less improvement in PROM scores, and less improvement in range of motion compared to controls [19]. However, the differences in PROM scores between groups were less than the published minimal clinically important difference (MCID) thresholds, so the clinical significance of these findings is uncertain [19]. Sadoghi et al. evaluated 66 shoulders (66 patients) and found that RSA resulted in a significantly improved benefits in terms of less shoulder pain, greater range of motion, and greater shoulder stability, irrespective of having undergone a previous arthroscopic rotator cuff reconstruction [18]. Conversely, Marigi et al. reported similar results in a study using a large multicenter database to compare 438 RSAs in patients with prior RCR to 876 matched controls [30]. The prior RCR group had improvements in PROMs and ROM, but these improvements were less than those seen in the control group. However, there were no differences in rates of complications and reoperations [30].

Despite the inferior outcomes compared to RSA without prior RCR, the complication rate is not increased in patients undergoing RSA after prior RCR [19, 29–32]. Additionally, survival rates are comparable between groups. In a study of 22 shoulders with minimum 15-year follow-up, 13 of which had undergone at least 1 prior RCR, Gerber et al. noted improvements in PROMs that remained stable throughout the follow-up period, and an 84% survival rate without failure at 15 years with no significant association of failure and prior RCR [31]. This survival rate is comparable to reports elsewhere in the literature of RSA survival at long-term follow-up [33].

Still, while outcomes for RSA following failed RCR may be inferior to outcomes following primary RSA for massive RCTs, the outcomes are still favorable with the majority of patients with prior failed RCR experiencing improvement in pain and function of the shoulder following RSA.

27.4 The SCR: Biomechanics and Factors Associated with Its Failure

The superior shoulder capsule is a thin continuous sheet of interwoven collagen fibrils that span from the glenoid labrum out laterally to the humerus. At its insertion on the humerus, the superior capsule encompasses 30–61% of the greater tuberosity and is 4.4–9.1 mm thick [34, 35]. The superior capsule functions as a hammock that overlies the glenohumeral joint and critically prevents proximal humeral migration and contact with the acromial undersurface. Biomechanically, this band of tissue has been shown to provide passive stability to the glenohumeral joint. Ishihara et al. [36] showed that a superior capsular tear significantly increased anterior and inferior translation when compared to those shoulders with an intact capsule and that the creation of a superior capsular defect resulted in increased glenohumeral translation in all directions and increased subacromial contact pressure. A cadaveric study by Mihata et al. [37] which evaluated proximal humerus migration under various conditions found that excising the supraspinatus tendon significantly increased superior translation of the proximal humerus, which was only fully restored when the superior capsule was reconstructed with graft. As such, some have described a superior capsular defect as the "essential lesion" that may be responsible for suboptimal outcomes in patients with superior rotator cuff tears, as its presence significantly alters shoulder biomechanics [38].

While the aforementioned studies certainly support the rationale behind a superior capsular reconstruction, studies reporting on risk factors associated with its failure are limited. Graft size and failure to restore posterior continuity between the graft, residual infraspinatus tendon, and underlying shoulder capsule have been suggested to portend to worse outcomes. Another biomechanical study by Mihata et al. [39] found that an 8 mm graft compared to a 4 mm graft significantly reduced both subacromial peak contact pressure and superior translation and that the SCR normalized superior shoulder stability when the graft was attached at 10° or 30° of glenohumeral abduction. In a separate study, Mihata et al. [40] evaluated subacromial peak contact pressure, glenohumeral superior translation, glenohumeral compression force, and glenohumeral range of motion across five conditions: an intact shoulder, simulated irreparable supraspinatus tear, SCR without side-to-side suturing, SCR with posterior side-to-side suturing, and an SCR with both anterior and posterior side-to-side suturing. The authors found that an SCR with side-to-side suturing reestablished superior glenohumeral joint stability by restoring posterior continuity between the graft, residual infraspinatus tendon, and underlying shoulder capsule. Similarly, in their review of 32 patients (36 shoulders) who underwent arthroscopic SCR at a mean follow-up of 24.8 ± 6.9 months, Lee et al. [41] found that inadequate restoration of the acromiohumeral distance (1.6 ± 2.2 mm vs. 3.8 ± 2.8 mm) and poor posterior remnant tissue significantly increased graft failure risk. Further, Denard et al. [42] showed that subscapularis atrophy was lower in patients with healed graft on postoperative MRI following arthroscopic SCR with a dermal allograft. Patient factors have also been implicated in failure rates following SCR. A retrospective review by Gilat et al. [43] found that female sex and the presence of a subscapularis tear were associated with increased clinical failure after SCR. Other factors, including lower preoperative forward flexion and acromiohumeral distance and larger BMI trended toward an association with clinical, although did not reach statistical significance.

To improve failure rates, various technical modifications have been suggested. For example, Mihata's team [44] advocated for a concomitant acromioplasty done at the time of SCR in order to help decrease postoperative risk of abrasion and graft tear beneath the acromion. While such modifications have objectively led to improvements in patient outcomes, their clinical implications and relevance are not as well understood. This effort to more objectively define patient satisfaction has led to the emergence of the MCID, SCB, and PASS scores as they pertain to outcomes following SCR. To that end, a recent review by Evuarherhe et al. [45] calculated the MCID, SCB, and PASS to be 11.2, 18.02, and 68.82 for ASES; 14.5, 23.13, and 69.9 for SANE; and 3.6, 10, and 18 for Constant, respectively, as they pertain to patients who underwent SCR with an acellular dermal allograft. On the basis of these calculated values, subscapularis tearing, workers compensation status, advanced age, and female sex were associated with failure to achieve these clinically significant outcomes. Conversely, concomitant distal clavicle excision during SCR and lower preoperative ASES were prognostic for achievement of the MCID and SCB. Further understanding of these clinically significant outcomes following SCR will undoubtedly allow providers to better counsel patients prior to SCR.

27.5 RSA After Failed SCR

SCR is a relatively novel procedure that has increased in popularity over the past decade [46]. Techniques and indications for SCR continue to evolve, with outcomes varying widely with different available graft choices and patient selection. As the indications have narrowed, outcomes have improved, with clinical failure rates reported as low as 3.1 in patients without advanced degenerative glenohumeral changes (Hamada <3) (Fig. 27.2a, b) [10]. Despite these promising results, the increasing number of SCRs performed coupled with their limited survivorships will inevitably lead to a greater number of clinical failures progressing to CTA.

SCR failure can be defined as persistent or worsening pain and is often associated with graft tear [43]. Graft tear is conventionally diagnosed with MRI, although plain radiographs may show progression of CTA [42, 43]. Patients with failed SCR and progression of CTA will frequently not be candidates for other soft tissue procedures, thereby leaving RSA as the procedure of choice

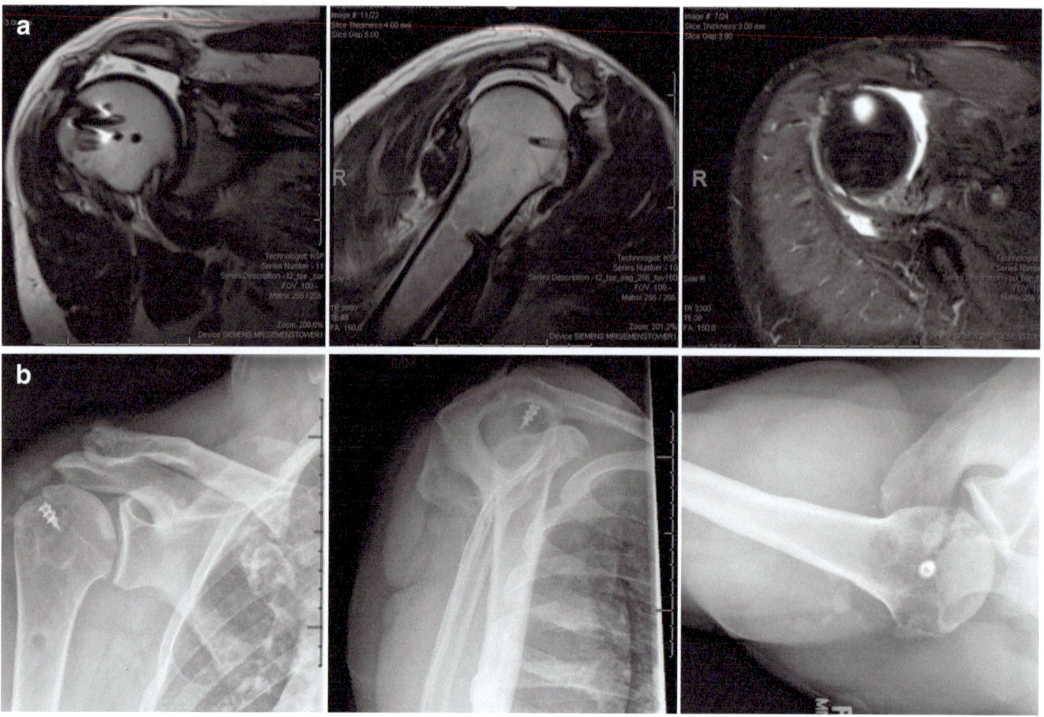

Fig. 27.2 Pre-SCR. (**a**) Representative coronal, sagittal, and axial MRI cuts demonstrate a recurrent full-thickness supraspinatus tear and near full-thickness infraspinatus tear with medial tendon retraction to the level of the glenoid, as well as mild glenohumeral joint osteoarthritis and a large joint effusion with reactive synovitis. Also appreciated are postoperative changes consistent with the patient's previous revision rotator cuff repair, subacromial decompression, and biceps tenodesis. (**b**) Three-view radiographs show a well-maintained glenohumeral joint without significant proximal humeral head migration. Previous surgical hardware is intact and without obvious signs of loosening

(Fig. 27.3a–c). This is problematic in that the SCR is most commonly indicated for younger and higher demand patients with massive RCTs who are not candidates for RSA, due to concerns with implant survivorship and high risks of aseptic loosening and failure [8]. As with all younger patients undergoing RSA, patients should be counseled preoperatively on the relatively higher risk of failure and need for future revision, as well as the need for activity modification.

Reports on outcomes of RSA following failed SCR are limited. Cusano et al. [47] was the first to directly evaluate the effects of a previously failed SCR versus RCR on functional outcomes following conversion to RSA. These authors matched 13 patients undergoing RSA after failed SCR to 32 patients undergoing RSA following failed RCR by number of procedures to the ipsilateral extremity (e.g., 1, 2, ≥3) and secondarily by age within 5 years. While both groups had significant improvements from preoperative to postoperative PROMs, there was greater improvement and decreased pain in the RCR group. There were similar rates of patients achieving the MCID and substantial clinical benefit (SCB) thresholds in both groups, but no members of the SCR group met the patient acceptable symptomatic state (PASS) threshold for the SANE score compared to 56.7% in the RCR group [47]. Similarly, Magone et al. reported on 13 patients who underwent RSA following failed SCR, with a control group of 15 patients who underwent RSA following failed RCR [48]. At a minimum 1 year follow-up, the SCR group had significantly less improvements in PROM scores and ROM compared to the RCR group. Despite the inferior outcomes in the SCR group, there was no difference in complication

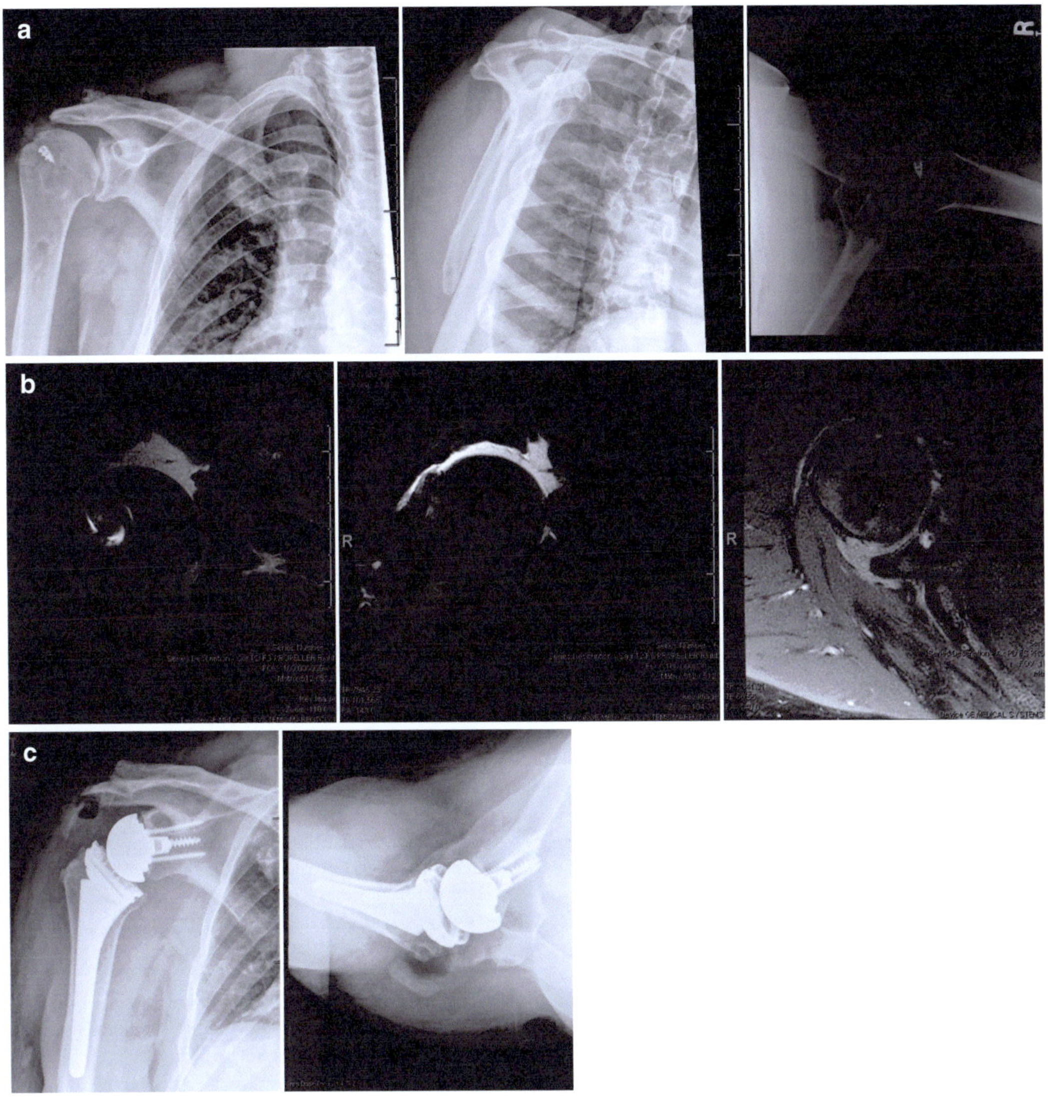

Fig. 27.3 Post- SCR. (**a**) Three-view radiographs show minimal to no significant proximal humeral head migration or degenerative glenohumeral joint disease. There is, however, evidence of heterotopic ossification around the greater tuberosity metal anchor and biceps tenodesis tunnel, with stable type 1 acromion. (**b**) MRI identifies a full-thickness complete tear of the supraspinatus and subscapularis tendons, as well as most of the infraspinatus tendon. (**c**) Radiographs status post right reverse shoulder arthroplasty with intact hardware and no evidence of gross failure or periprosthetic loosening

rates [48]. From a technical standpoint, the authors advocated that prior humeral sided anchors should be removed before reaming and broaching the humeral canal to avoid varus placement of the humeral component [48]. Additionally, the SCR graft and glenoid sided anchors should be removed prior to preparation of the glenoid to avoid interference and malposi-tioning with implantation of the glenoid compo-nent [48]. The authors found that patients undergoing conversion to RTSA from SCR had extensive subdeltoid and subacromial scarring which required more surgical dissection and may have implications on their residual postop-erative pain and poor function despite improve-ments in range of motion following RTSA.

27.6 Conclusions

RSA is an effective procedure for patients with persistent shoulder pain and dysfunction due to RCR or SCR failure. Outcomes in RSA after failed SCR are inferior to outcomes after failed RCR, and outcomes after both failed RCR and SCR are inferior to outcomes of primary RSA. However, there is no evidence of increased complication rates or decreased survivorship. Much of the current literature is limited to small case series and retrospective reviews, which introduce selection biases and potential intrinsic differences between RCR and SCR cohorts that confound analyses. Ultimately, the discrepancy in outcomes of RSA following SCR versus RCR is likely multifactorial and not entirely explained by existing data. With the advent of new graft options and refined surgical techniques, it is possible that such differences may not be appreciated moving forward.

Disclaimer Augustus D. Mazzocca receives consulting fees as well as research support from Arthrex Inc. (Naples, FL). The company had no involvement in the study design, data collection, or final manuscript.

Disclosure All other authors have nothing to disclose.

References

1. Lawrence RL, Moutzouros V, Bey MJ. Asymptomatic rotator cuff tears. JBJS Rev. 2019;7(6):e9.
2. Tashjian RZ. Epidemiology, natural history, and indications for treatment of rotator cuff tears. Clin Sports Med. 2012;31(4):589–604.
3. Shah NS, et al. Long-term outcomes of massive rotator cuff tear repair: a systematic review. HSS J. 2022;18(1):130–7.
4. Cvetanovich GL, et al. Management of the irreparable rotator cuff tear. J Am Acad Orthop Surg. 2019;27(24):909–17.
5. Ecklund KJ, et al. Rotator cuff tear arthropathy. J Am Acad Orthop Surg. 2007;15(6):340–9.
6. Fucentese SF, et al. Evolution of nonoperatively treated symptomatic isolated full-thickness supraspinatus tears. J Bone Jt Surg Am. 2012;94(9):801–8.
7. Maman E, et al. Outcome of nonoperative treatment of symptomatic rotator cuff tears monitored by magnetic resonance imaging. J Bone Jt Surg Am. 2009;91(8):1898–906.
8. Frank RM, et al. Superior capsular reconstruction: indications, techniques, and clinical outcomes. JBJS Rev. 2018;6(7):e10.
9. Mihata T, et al. Clinical results of arthroscopic superior capsule reconstruction for irreparable rotator cuff tears. Arthroscopy. 2013;29(3):459–70.
10. Catapano M, et al. Arthroscopic superior capsular reconstruction for massive, irreparable rotator cuff tears: a systematic review of modern literature. Arthroscopy. 2019;35(4):1243–53.
11. Gerber C, Pennington SD, Nyffeler RW. Reverse total shoulder arthroplasty. J Am Acad Orthop Surg. 2009;17(5):284–95.
12. Al-Hadithy N, Domos P, Sewell MD, Pandit R. Reverse shoulder arthroplasty in 41 patients with cuff tear arthropathy with a mean follow-up period of 5 years. J Shoulder Elb Surg. 2014;23(11):1662–8.
13. Favard L, Levigne C, Nerot C, Gerber C, De Wilde L, Mole D. Reverse prostheses in arthropathies with cuff tear: are survivorship and function maintained over time? Clin Orthop Relat Res. 2011;469(9):2469–75.
14. Puskas B, Kevin H, Clark R, Downes K, Virani NA, Frankle M. Isometric strength, range of motion, and impairment before and after total and reverse shoulder arthroplasty. J Shoulder Elb Surg. 2013;22:869–76.
15. Friedman R, Cheung E, Flurin P-H, Wright T, Simovitch R, Roche C. Are age and patient gender associated with different rates and magnitudes of clinical improvement after reverse shoulder arthroplasty? Clin Orthop Relat Res. 2018;476:1264–73.
16. Wong SE, et al. The effect of patient gender on outcomes after reverse total shoulder arthroplasty. J Shoulder Elb Surg. 2017;26(11):1889–96.
17. Boileau P, et al. Risk factors for recurrence of shoulder instability after arthroscopic Bankart repair. J Bone Jt Surg Am. 2006;88(8):1755–63.
18. Sadoghi P, Vavken P, Leithner A, Hochreiter J, Weber G, Pietschmann MF. Impact of previous rotator cuff repair on the outcome of reverse shoulder arthroplasty. J Shoulder Elb Surg. 2011;20:1138–46.
19. Shields EJW, et al. Previous rotator cuff repair is associated with inferior clinical outcomes after reverse total shoulder arthroplasty. Orthop J Sports Med. 2017;5(10):2325967117730311.
20. Carducci MP, Zimmer ZR, Jawa A. Predictors of unsatisfactory patient outcomes in primary reverse total shoulder arthroplasty. J Shoulder Elb Surg. 2019;28(11):2113–20.
21. Forlizzi JM, et al. Predictors of poor and excellent outcomes after reverse shoulder arthroplasty. J Shoulder Elb Surg. 2021;31(2):294–301.
22. Berliner JL, Brodke D, Chan V, SooHoo NF, Bozic KJ. John Charnley award: preoperative patient-reported outcome measures predict clinically mean-

ingful improvement in function after THA. Clin Orthop Relat Res. 2016;474:321–9.

23. Glassman SD, Copay A, Berven SH, Polly DW, Subach BR, Carreon LY. Defining substantial clinical benefit following lumbar spine arthrodesis. J Bone Jt Surg Am. 2008;90:1839–47.

24. Nwachukwu BU, et al. Preoperative short form health survey score is predictive of return to play and minimal clinically important difference at a minimum 2-year follow-up after anterior cruciate ligament reconstruction. Am J Sports Med. 2017;45(12):2784–90.

25. Gordon D, et al. Minimal clinically important difference, substantial clinical benefit, and patient acceptable symptom state of PROMIS upper extremity after total shoulder arthroplasty. JSES Int. 2021;5(5):894–9.

26. Gowd AK, et al. Single Assessment Numeric Evaluation (SANE) is a reliable metric to measure clinically significant improvements following shoulder arthroplasty. J Shoulder Elb Surg. 2019;28(11):2238–46.

27. Bacle G, et al. Long-term outcomes of reverse total shoulder arthroplasty: a follow-up of a previous study. J Bone Jt Surg Am. 2017;99(6):454–61.

28. Cho NS, Cha SW, Rhee YG. Alterations of the deltoid muscle after open versus arthroscopic rotator cuff repair. Am J Sports Med. 2015;43(12):2927–34.

29. Boileau P, et al. Reverse total shoulder arthroplasty after failed rotator cuff surgery. J Shoulder Elb Surg. 2009;18(4):600–6.

30. Marigi EM, et al. Reverse shoulder arthroplasty after prior rotator cuff repair: a matched cohort analysis. J Am Acad Orthop Surg. 2021;30(3):e395–404.

31. Gerber C, et al. Longitudinal observational study of reverse total shoulder arthroplasty for irreparable rotator cuff dysfunction: results after 15 years. J Shoulder Elb Surg. 2018;27(5):831–8.

32. Sadoghi P, et al. Impact of previous rotator cuff repair on the outcome of reverse shoulder arthroplasty. J Shoulder Elb Surg. 2011;20(7):1138–46.

33. van Ochten JHM, et al. Long-term survivorship and clinical and radiological follow-up of the primary uncemented Delta III reverse shoulder prosthesis. J Orthop. 2019;16(4):342–6.

34. Burkhart SS, et al. Arthroscopic superior capsular reconstruction for massive irreparable rotator cuff repair. Arthrosc Tech. 2016;5(6):e1407–18.

35. Nimura A, et al. The superior capsule of the shoulder joint complements the insertion of the rotator cuff. J Shoulder Elb Surg. 2012;21(7):867–72.

36. Ishihara Y, et al. Role of the superior shoulder capsule in passive stability of the glenohumeral joint. J Shoulder Elb Surg. 2014;23(5):642–8.

37. Mihata T, et al. Superior capsule reconstruction to restore superior stability in irreparable rotator cuff tears: a biomechanical cadaveric study. Am J Sports Med. 2012;40(10):2248–55.

38. Adams CR, et al. The rotator cuff and the superior capsule: why we need both. Arthroscopy. 2016;32(12):2628–37.

39. Mihata T, et al. Biomechanical effect of thickness and tension of fascia lata graft on glenohumeral stability for superior capsule reconstruction in irreparable supraspinatus tears. Arthroscopy. 2016;32(3):418–26.

40. Mihata T, et al. Biomechanical role of capsular continuity in superior capsule reconstruction for irreparable tears of the supraspinatus tendon. Am J Sports Med. 2016;44(6):1423–30.

41. Lee SJ, Min YK. Can inadequate acromiohumeral distance improvement and poor posterior remnant tissue be the predictive factors of re-tear? Preliminary outcomes of arthroscopic superior capsular reconstruction. Knee Surg Sports Traumatol Arthrosc. 2018;26(7):2205–13.

42. Denard PJ, et al. Preliminary results of arthroscopic superior capsule reconstruction with dermal allograft. Arthroscopy. 2018;34(1):93–9.

43. Gilat R, et al. Patient factors associated with clinical failure following arthroscopic superior capsular reconstruction. Arthroscopy. 2021;37(2):460–7.

44. Mihata T, et al. Biomechanical effects of acromioplasty on superior capsule reconstruction for irreparable supraspinatus tendon tears. Am J Sports Med. 2016;44(1):191–7.

45. Evuarherhe A Jr, et al. Defining clinically significant outcomes following superior capsular reconstruction with acellular dermal allograft. Arthroscopy. 2022;38(5):1444–1453.e1.

46. Tokish JM, Makovicka JL. The superior capsular reconstruction: lessons learned and future directions. J Am Acad Orthop Surg. 2020;28(13):528–37.

47. Cusano A, et al. Outcomes of reverse shoulder arthroplasty following failed superior capsular reconstruction. J Shoulder Elb Surg. 2022;31(7):1426–35.

48. Magone KM, et al. Outcomes of reverse shoulder arthroplasty following failed superior capsular reconstruction. JSES Int. 2022;6(2):216–20.

Management of Bone Deficiency in Shoulder Arthroplasty

Edoardo Giovannetti de Sanctis, Federico Bozzi, Alessio Palumbo, and Francesco Franceschi

28.1 Introduction

Complex glenoid and humeral bone deficits continue to present significant challenges in both primary and revision arthroplasty. As shoulder arthroplasty is increasingly being implanted, so does the overall number of revisions to be expected in the future. Bone deficiency results in decreased surface area and bony support for glenoid and humeral components, and it is associated with an increased risk of loosening and implant failure. Both the quantity and quality of remaining bone are important considerations to be evaluated in the management of these patients.

28.2 Humeral Bone Deficiency

Proximal humeral bone loss (PHBL) is one of the main challenging obstacles to achieving a well-fixed, stable prosthesis [1].

E. Giovannetti de Sanctis (✉) · A. Palumbo
F. Franceschi
Department of Orthopaedic and Trauma Surgery, San Pietro Fatebenefratelli Hospital, Rome, Italy

UniCamillus-Saint Camillus International University of Health Sciences, Rome, Italy
e-mail: francesco.franceschi@unicamillus.org

F. Bozzi
Department of Orthopaedic and Trauma Surgery, Fondazione Poliambulanza, Brescia, Italy

PHBL occurs in cases of periprosthetic infection, stress shielding, difficult stem extraction of a well-fixed humeral stem, aseptic loosening of previous implant, osteolysis secondary to wear debris, and following humeral resection for tumor.

It has been shown through a biomechanical analysis that a significant bone loss leads to increased bending and torsional forces on the humeral component [2]. As proximal humeral bone loss compromises proximal bony fixation, the implant relies on rotational stability only within the diaphysis.

The increased stress on the humeral implant is often further exacerbated using larger glenospheres as a way of preventing instability. The greater the contact area between the glenosphere and humeral socket, the higher the constraint then transmitted to the humeral stem [3]. This is particularly true in case of reverse shoulder arthroplasty (rTSA), where due to the specific design, substantial rotational forces are transmitted to the humeral stem.

Significant PHBL is associated to postoperative instability and an increased risk of mechanical failure with humeral stem loosening and implant derotation [4].

Severe PHBL influences also the glenohumeral soft tissue envelope: in case of greater tuberosity absence, the ROM is altered, with loss of active external rotation.

© ISAKOS 2023
A. D. Mazzocca et al. (eds.), *Shoulder Arthritis across the Life Span*,
https://doi.org/10.1007/978-3-031-33298-2_28

Achieving secure fixation and long-term stability of the stem in case of humeral bone deficiency is therefore paramount.

28.2.1 Evaluation and Classification

Anticipating humeral bone deficiency with preoperative appropriate planning enables the surgeon to achieve adequate fixation and stability.

Humeral bone loss and intramedullary diameter of the remaining bone should be evaluated with both bilateral full-length radiographs of the humeri in neutral rotation and computed tomography (CT) scans.

Radiographic signs of loosening and the length of the humeral implant in place (to provide data regarding the possible cortical window needed to remove a well-fixed stem) should be assessed.

In case of humeral component loosening or osteolysis, inflammation-related laboratory data (complete blood count, erythrocyte sedimentation rate, C-reactive protein) are needed preoperatively to exclude any periprosthetic infections.

In case of a high suspicion of infection with normal laboratory values, shoulder aspiration or biopsy should be performed before surgical planning.

Two classification systems have been proposed to assess humeral bone loss.

The first one has been proposed by Boileau et al. dividing PHBL in 4 types [4].

- **A**: bone loss of the epiphysis (≤ 2 cm)
- **B**: bone loss of the metaphysis (≤ 4)
- **C**: bone loss extending into the humeral diaphysis proximally to the deltoid insertion (≤ 8)
- **D**: bone loss extending below the deltoid insertion (≥ 8)

Chalmers et al. developed the Proximal Humeral Arthroplasty Revision Osseous inSufficiency (PHAROS) system, divided in three types, further subdivided in six subtypes [5].

1. Type 1: epiphyseal bone loss, including the articular surface, greater and lesser tuberosities.
   - type 1C: calcar loss,
   - type 1G: loss or malunion of the greater tuberosity.
2. Type 2: bone loss of the metadiaphysis above the deltoid attachment.
   - type 2A: cortical thinning of the metadiaphysis greater than 50% of the expected cortical thickness,
   - type 2B: bone loss of both the metadiaphysis proximal to the deltoid and the epiphysis.
3. Type 3: diaphyseal bone loss extending below the deltoid attachment.
   - type 3A: cortical thinning of diaphysis greater than 50% of the expected cortical thickness.
   - type 3B: compromise of most of the diaphysis, along with loss of epiphyseal and metadiaphyseal bone.

Furthermore, a cut-off value of 5 cm has also been proposed as the threshold to define significant bone loss, with indication to a more aggressive reconstruction [2].

28.2.2 Management

Several treatment strategies have been described to address proximal humeral bone loss, which might be divided essentially in two broad categories based on the amount of proximal bone loss.

In case of shorter proximal humeral bone defects (≤ 5 cm), classified as A–B according to Boileau et al. [4] or 1 and 2A according to Chalmers et al. [5], the treatment options to restore length and obtain an adequate soft tissue tension include the use of thicker polyethylene/metal tray, cementing the stem proportionally proud to re-establish height or by implanting an inferior eccentric glenosphere [6]. In case of absence of greater tuberosity: a proximal cementoplasty or metaphyseal augments to increase soft tissue wrapping and if possible reattach the rotator cuff still present.

For type C–D according to Boileau et al. [4] and 2A-3 according to Chalmers et al. [5], the treatment strategy may require to reconstruct the proximal humerus with an allograft, the APC (Allograft Prosthetic Composite) construct or to use a proximal/total humeral replacement. Both options might include the use of a reverse shoulder or a hemiarthroplasty as replacement design.

It has been shown that modular implants may have a higher risk of mechanical failure in the setting of proximal humeral bone loss. Monoblock implants should be therefore preferred for reconstruction constructs in the setting of significant proximal humeral bone loss [1, 7].

Literature is lacking of trials comparing different treatment options in patients with shorter proximal humeral bone defects. Stephens et al. [7] evaluated the outcomes of 32 revision rTSA in patients with or without PHBL. Sixteen patients had PHBL with an average loss of 36.3 mm. Humeral bone deficiency was not associated with significant lower functional or subjective outcomes, except for active motion.

Budge et al. evaluated 15 patients undergoing revision for failed arthroplasty with an average PHBL of 38.4 mm at a minimum 2 years follow-up. The satisfaction rate was 87%. CS, ASES, VAS, forward flexion, and external rotation increased significantly. The authors reported a scapular notching rate of 20%, one humeral stem fracture, but no stem loosening, concluding that the use of RTSA for failed shoulder arthroplasty and deficient humeral bone stock provides a significant clinical benefit without the need for allograft augmentation [8].

The APC is a rare and challenging surgical procedure aiming at reconstruction of the proximal humeral bone stock with restoration of a functional glenohumeral joint. It was first described by Chacon et al. [9].

The restoration of proximal humeral bone stock improves stem fixation (neutralizing rotational forces exerted on it), decreases the risk of

shoulder instability (restoring the deltoid "wrapping" effect), and improves the cosmetic appearance of the shoulder.

It provides additional bone stock for needed future reconstructions and offers the possibility to reattach the rotator cuff tendons to the respective allograft insertions or perform an associated tendon transfer (L'Episcopo or latissimus dorsi), by fixing the tendons on the bone graft [4].

Several are the complications described for this procedure: delayed or no bone healing, humeral aseptic loosening, risk of de novo infection, allograft fragmentation, and/or resorption.

Different techniques to perform the APC have been described so far.

The first technique advocates a step-cut osteotomy within the allograft so that approximately 5 cm of bone remains laterally, resulting in a lateral bone plate and fixation to the humerus with cerclage wires [9] (Fig. 28.1).

The technique has been later modified by Boileau [4, 10], who suggested to perform a mirror step-cut osteotomy and use a long monoblock (cemented or uncemented) humeral reverse stem to create a construct functioning similarly to an intramedullary nail and preventing the need for plate fixation.

To achieve a compression at the graft-host junction, it has been suggested to use a 3.5-mm plate in compression mode associated to a simple cut osteotomy [6].

Apart from the differences described above, the technique follows the same steps. Both a humeral and femoral allograft might be used, and if possible it should have a diameter close to the one of the patient humerus.

In cases of severe PHBL, the allograft length needed is calculated preoperatively as the contralateral humeral length minus the operative humeral length. The proximal humeral allograft is then prepared for use by performing the distal humeral cut osteotomy and reaming/broaching the humeral canal.

The stem usually bypasses the host-graft junction, and a cemented fixation is more frequently

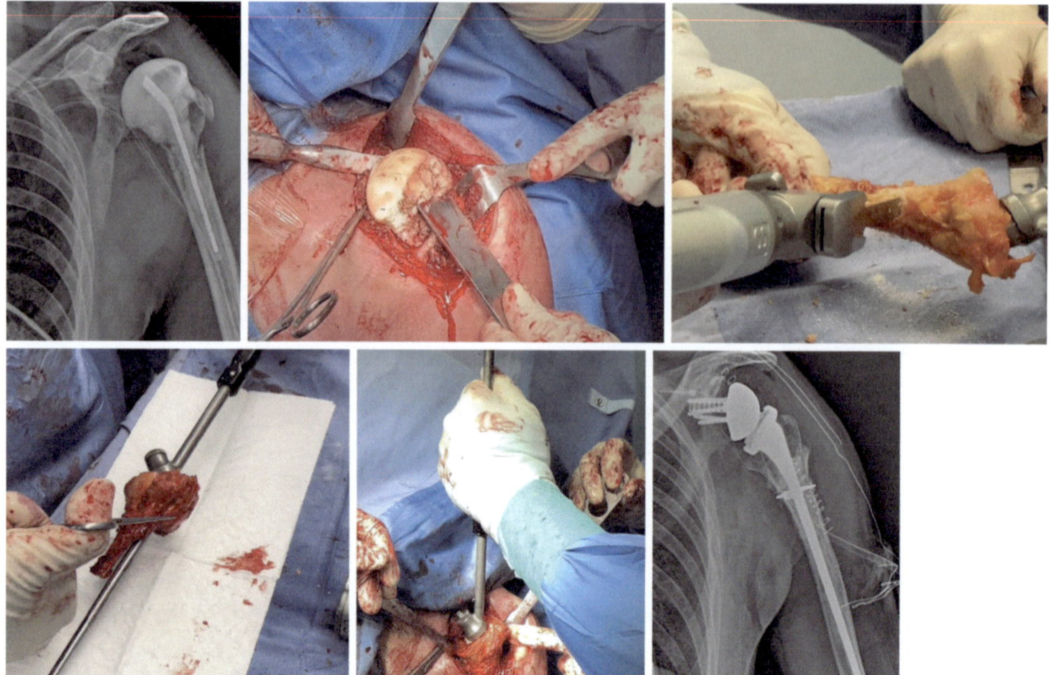

Fig. 28.1 The allograft prosthetic composite procedure

used. Any native tendons still present should then be repaired to their respective allograft tendon stumps.

In the absence of infection, the APC might be implanted with a cement-within-cement technique to avoid the need of removing, with potentially destructive consequences, the preexisting cement mantle.

Chacon et al. evaluated 25 patients receiving a proximal humeral allograft for the management of mean proximal humeral bone loss of 53.6 mm. 76% of patients reported a subjective good or excellent result, 20% a satisfactory result, and 4% an unsatisfactory result.

The radiographic incorporation rate at final follow-up was 84% and 76%, respectively, in the metaphyseal and diaphyseal region. Complication rate was reported as 16% [9].

Sanchez et al. [6] evaluated 8 primary and 18 revision APC rTSAs with a compression plate for graft fixation. The indications for the primary rTSAs included severe PHBL after trauma ($n = 5$) and tumor resection ($n = 3$). The indications for revision were failed hemiarthroplasty ($n = 11$),

aTSA ($n = 4$), and rTSA ($n = 3$). The most common cause of revision was instability ($n = 10$). This procedure leaded to significant improvements in pain scores and active ROM.

No significant differences in terms of clinical outcomes were outlined between primary and revision cases. The mean time to graft to host union was 7 months. The 2- and 5-year revision-free survival rate was 96%.

El Beaino et al. [11] reported 21 patients undergoing hemiarthroplasty APC after proximal humerus resection. At 5-year follow-up, the revision rate was 10.1%. Among complications are as follows: superior subluxation (12/21), delayed union (10/21), greater tuberosity resorption (9/21), and aseptic loosening (3/21).

Boileau et al. [4] assessed 25 consecutive patients undergoing rTSA-APC procedure for severe PHBL (>4 cm): 12 after failed reverse shoulder arthroplasty, 5 after failed hemiarthroplasty, 6 after failed mega-tumor prosthesis, and 2 after tumor resection. The satisfaction rate was 76%. The revision and incorporation rate at last follow-up were, respectively, 32% and 96%.

Cox et al. evaluated 73 patients undergoing a rTSA-APC at 2 years minimum follow-up. Good to excellent results were reported in 70%, satisfactory in 17%, and unsatisfactory in 13%. The reoperation-free survival rate was 88% at 5 years, 78% at 10 years, and 67% beyond 10 years. Among the causes for revision are periprosthetic fracture, instability, glenosphere dissociation, humeral loosening, and infection [3].

Although more frequently implanted after wide tumor resections, a mega-tumor prosthesis might be effectively used also to treat non-oncologic large bone defects. Although the healing of soft tissue to metal is controversial, native tendons might be sutured to the prosthesis [1].

Mengers et al. evaluated 13 patients undergoing an RSA tumor prosthesis for PHBL at 34 months follow-up. Six patients required wide excisions for proximal humerus tumors. Complications and revision rate were, respectively, 38% and 31% [12].

28.3 Glenoid Bone Deficiency

Glenoid bone deficiency is most frequently encountered in a revision setting but can also be present in patients with primary glenohumeral degeneration, CTA, rheumatoid arthritis, congenital deformations, and in post-traumatic cases.

The treatment of glenoid bone defects both in primary and revision total shoulder arthroplasty is challenging. The goal is to achieve the anatomic correction of glenoid version and inclination, preserve as much as possible of existing glenoid bone stock, and to have complete contact between the component and the underlying bone.

Failure to address this problem will lead to excessive joint line medialization (with altered soft tissue tensioning), baseplate malposition (superior inclination or excessive retroversion), and inadequate fixation, compromising the postoperative clinical outcomes and decreasing the implant survival [13]. Still debated is how to manage glenoid bone loss.

28.3.1 Evaluation and Classification

Glenoid bone deficiency and glenohumeral subluxation are evaluated with both radiographs (Grashey, scapular lateral and axillary views) and advanced imaging modalities as the CT scans, whether 2D or 3D. Recently the preoperative 3D modeling softwares have enabled a patient-specific planning, simulating ideal component positioning [14, 15] (Fig. 28.2).

Several classification systems have been proposed to describe glenoid bone defects.

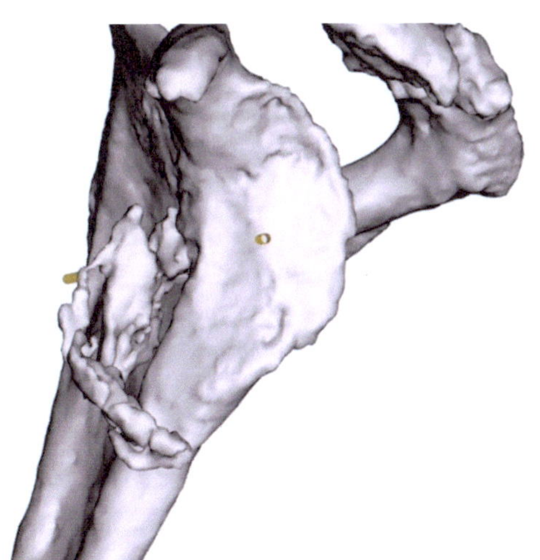
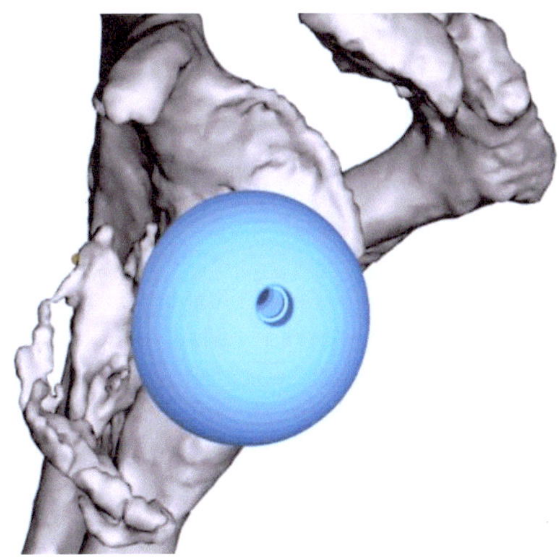

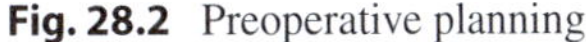

Fig. 28.2 Preoperative planning

Walch et al. introduced a classification system to identify patients with axial glenoid bone defects [16]. The classification system, which has been later modified, was based on three distinct parameters: glenoid retroversion, posterior glenoid wear, and posterior subluxation of the humeral head [16–18].

Glenoid bone loss is classified as follows

1. **Type A**: Concentric and symmetric erosion, well-centered humeral head, and absence of subluxation.
   - **A1**: minor erosion (without the native glenoid tangent line transecting the humeral head).
   - **A2**: major erosion (with the native glenoid tangent line transecting the humeral head).
2. **Type B**: Posterior wear pattern, posterior subluxation.
   - **B0**: uniconcave, pre-osteoarthritic posterior subluxation of the humeral head.
   - **B1**: uniconcave, posterior joint-space narrowing with subchondral sclerosis and osteophytes but no bone erosion.
   - **B2**: biconcave, retroverted glenoid with posterior rim erosion.
   - **B3**: uniconcave, with at least 15° of retroversion and/or 70% posterior humeral head subluxation.
3. **Type C**: uniconcave, glenoid retroversion of >25° not caused by erosion.
4. **Type D**: anteverted glenoid or anterior humeral subluxation measuring 40% or less.

Subluxation is referred to as greater than 55% or 45% respectively for posterior or anterior subluxation [19].

Iannotti et al. modified the Walch classification, utilizing the vault model theory, better defining the B3 and introducing the C2 [18].

The B3 glenoid has high pathologic retroversion with no paleoglenoid visible, normal premorbid version, and acquired central and posterior bone loss. Then a new subtype, the C2 glenoid, was introduced. The native morphology of a C2 glenoid is dysplastic (high premorbid version) and developed from further posterior erosion of a C1 glenoid, giving it the appearance of a biconcave glenoid with posterior translation

of the humeral head. The authors support the hypothesis that glenoid bone loss and humeral head posterior subluxation occurring in primary glenohumeral osteoarthritis are progressive: the B2 and C1 glenoids are the precursor to, respectively, the B3 and C2 glenoids ultimately forming when further posterior erosion eliminates the biconcavity.

It has been reported that humeral head subluxation and glenoid bone loss progress over time not always through the same pathway. In Logli et al. [20] 20% of type A developed eccentric wear whereas all B-type glenoids remained B type. Progression of bone loss from A1 to A2 and from B2 to B3 occurred, respectively, in 41% and 56% of the time.

Favard et al. introduced a classification system to identify patients with coronal glenoid bone defects [21]. The classification progresses from E0 to E4.

E0: no glenoid erosion

E1: concentric medialized glenoid erosion

E2: glenoid erosion predominantly in the superior pole

E3: global glenoid erosion more severe in the superior pole

E4: glenoid erosion predominantly in the anteroinferior pole

28.3.2 Management

The common strategies to manage patients with glenoid bone defects are eccentric reaming, bone grafting, augmented glenoid components, and salvage hemiarthroplasty.

Both Friedman line (or plane of the scapula) and the floor of the supraspinatus are used as references for the alignment of the baseplate. The goal is to implant the glenosphere within 10° of version and at 0° of inclination.

28.3.2.1 Reaming and Glenoid Augmentation

Asymmetric glenoid reaming is a commonly used technique to correct glenoid version and inclination [22]. It is not suitable for large bone defects as it may compromise the remaining

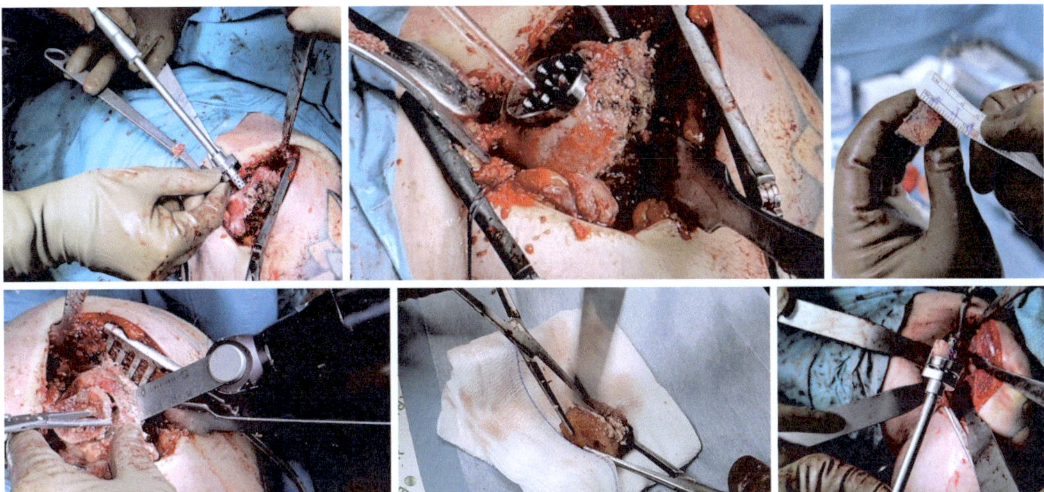

Fig. 28.3 The BIO-RSA technique modified by the senior author

glenoid bone stock, and it is mandatory to preserve as much native bone stock as possible; it is therefore favored for correction of small defects [22, 23]. More pronounced defects would require an associated bone graft or augmented component to correct the joint line with an appropriate fixation. Currently, it is suggested not to correct more than 10°–15° with asymmetric reaming [14].

Controversial is the amount of correction that can be safely obtained with eccentric reaming.

Before performing an eccentric reaming, also the quality of the bone should be considered. In B2 glenoids the posteroinferior quadrant contains substantially denser subchondral bone than the anterior quadrants. An eccentric reaming would create a flat surface with weak cancellous bone anteriorly and dense cancellous bone posteriorly, with unequal baseplate support.

Glenoid augmentation has been proposed in cases of glenoid defects where eccentric reaming would lead to excessive medialization, as it allows correction preserving the bone stock.

It is most frequently used for posterior and superior quadrants and often follows a minimal amount of asymmetric reaming. Glenoid augmentation is performed through bone grafting and polyethylene or metal component augments. The thickness of the augmentation should restore the glenoid bone stock to that of the native joint.

Glenoid bone grafting might be performed with a humeral head autograft, which can be symmetrical or trapezoidal (Bony Increased Off-Set BIO-RSA) or iliac crest bone graft (ICBG) [24] (Fig. 28.3).

Advantages of BIO-RSA include bone stock augmentation, lateralization, low donor-site morbidity, low relative cost, and flexibility as it might correct simultaneously posterior and superior glenoid defects. Glenoid bone grafting is easier to perform in rTSA than aTSA, due to the more robust baseplate fixation with both a long central peg and multiple locking screws. The rate of incorporation of both humeral and iliac bone graft has been reported to be satisfactory [25].

Polyethylene or metal-backed augments have been proposed to correct glenoid version, overcoming the issues of asymmetric reaming and bone grafts. Although augmented components have variable degrees of correction available, they cannot be used in very large defects.

28.3.2.2 Hemiarthroplasty

Glenoid implantation might be avoided with simple glenoid reaming and hemiarthroplasties, termed "ream and run" technique, but different authors have shown inferior results compared with total shoulder arthroplasties, due to continued bone erosion with increased pain, making it a final option in case of an inadequate bone stock support a glenoid component.

28.3.2.3 Anatomic Total Shoulder Arthroplasty

Treating severe glenoid retroversion and posterior humeral head subluxation with aTSA remains unpredictable with a high rate of polyethylene wear and glenoid loosening, due to the recurrence of humeral head subluxation.

Walch et al. [26] reported a loosening and revision rate of, respectively, 20.6 and 16.3% when using aTSA for biconcave glenoid. Patients with a neoglenoid retroversion of 27° and humeral head posterior subluxation of 80% had a higher risk for glenoid loosening, leading the authors to recommend rTSA, even in case of primary osteoarthritis, simply to correct the posterior subluxation using a semiconstrained arthroplasty. These values are still currently used within the treatment algorithm to decide whether to perform an aTSA or an rTSA in patients with primary OA.

As said, the glenoid altered version and inclination should be corrected to allow satisfactory implant positioning. Three are the techniques available: asymmetric reaming, posterior-augmented glenoid implant, and rarely a posterior bone graft (humeral head autograft, iliac crest, or femoral head allograft) [27–29]. Polyethylene component augments have been shown better clinical outcomes than metal-backed augments.

Rice et al. reported 13 patients undergoing an augmented glenoid aTSA to treat posterior glenoid bone deficiency at a minimum 2 years follow-up. 36% of patients had excellent, 50% satisfactory, and 14% unsatisfactory results, and no patients went through a revision [30].

Lenart et al. evaluated five patients undergoing an anterior augmented TSA [31]. The preoperative diagnosis were three anterior glenoid erosions, one glenoid fracture malunion, one glenoid fracture nonunion, and one post-traumatic arthritis. No glenoid component loosening, dislocation, or revision surgeries were

reported at an average of 33.2 months of follow-up.

Sandow and Schutz evaluated 10 patients who underwent an aTSA with a trabecular metal glenoid augment (15° or 30°) at a minimum 2 years follow-up [32]. No complication or hardware failure have been reported, and all components were implanted between 0° and 10° of version.

Sandow and Tu updated the previous series, evaluating 49 shoulders with a minimum follow-up of 2 years [33]. There were complications apart from one infection and one minor peg perforation. Good incorporation to bone of the wedge augment was highlighted. The average retroversion was corrected from 22° to 4°.

Zhang et al. in their systematic review evaluated the outcomes of aTSAs with bone graft [34]. The complications and revision rate at a mean follow-up of 6.3 years were respectively 12.6% and 5.4% (with glenoid loosening and infection listed as indications). Satisfaction rate was rated as 85% with function improvement and pain reduction. The authors emphasized the comparable revision rate in aTSA of bone grafting compared to augmented glenoid components.

During the last two decades, specialized components have been developed to address glenoid bone defects, with moderate results [35].

Cil et al. evaluated 38 patients who underwent a primary or revision aTSA, with one of 3 nonstandard glenoid components: a polyethylene component with an angled keel, a polyethylene component with 2 mm of extra thickness, or a posteriorly augmented metal-backed glenoid component. The loosening and revision rate were, respectively, 8 and 26% at an average 5.5 years of follow-up. The 10 years free revision rate was 73% for the angled keel component, 69% for of the extra thick component, and 31% for the posteriorly augmented metal-backed glenoid component [23]. Gunther et al. evaluated seven patients who underwent aTSA with an inset glenoid implant for severe glenoid bone deficiency. All implants were classified radiographically as "low risk" for glenoid loosening [36].

28.3.2.4   Reverse Total Shoulder Arthroplasty

Management of glenoid bone deficiency with rTSA has been suggested as an alternative, with good early results due to favorable biomechanics and a well-fixed baseplate. The rTSA design seems an appropriate way of treating posterior humeral head subluxation and resulted in excellent clinical outcomes [37, 38].

Mizuno et al. evaluated at 54 months follow-up the clinical outcomes of 27 rTSAs (10 with and 17 without bone grafts) performed for primary OA with biconcave glenoids [38]. The complication rate was 15% (4 patients), mainly due to neurologic complications (3/4). No radiolucent lines were observed around the glenoid component.

Collin et al. evaluated 49 shoulders with primary glenoid OA classified as B1, B2, B3, or C at 5-year minimum follow-up [37]. Bone grafting was performed in 16 cases and healed in all the shoulders. Patients had a significant increase of the Constant–Murley score from 30 to 68 points. Scapular notching and glenoid bone graft resorption had no influence on the CS.

Bone autograft, bone allograft, or augmented glenoid component might be used to correct glenoid defects, though bone autograft seems to be preferred in the current literature. Allografts are more frequently used in revision cases where local autograft options are limited.

Bone grafts are frequently classified as structural (e.g., iliac crest) and nonstructural (e.g., BIO-RSA).

It has been demonstrated that significant glenoid bone loss could be managed through bone grafting with a single-stage procedure with a high rate of graft incorporation and good to excellent clinical outcomes [39].

The Bony Increased Off-Set technique was described in 2011 by Boileau et al. [40]. The author reported then the outcomes of 143 consecutive patients treated with a BIO-RSA at 5–10 years follow-up. Both the revision free and the complete incorporation rate was 96% [13, 24].

The BIO-RSA is the technique to correct glenoid defects preferred at out institution as it has shown in our data to be more effective in ensuring a better baseplate inclination and in leading to better clinical outcomes [41, 42].

Werner et al. evaluated the clinical outcomes of 21 patients undergoing RSA with glenoid bone deficit due to neglected anterior dislocation treated with resected humeral head structural bone grafting. Two patients (9.5%) were revised due to baseplate loosening, respectively, with a hemiarthroplasty, and with a two-stage reconstruction using a tricortical iliac crest bone graft [43].

Holt and Throckmorton reported 49 patients undergoing rTSA for B2 or B3 glenoid bone defect [14]. In 92% of cases, the defect was managed with a bone graft (structural cortical bone grafting or impaction grafting). Neither mechanical failures nor reoperations were reported.

Italia et al. evaluating 21 patients undergoing rTSA with structural glenoid bone grafting (15 autografts, 6 allografts) confirmed the ability of this technique to restore the glenoid anatomy and bone stock [15].

Jones et al. reported 44 patients who underwent primary or revision rTSA with a structural bone graft (29 humeral head autograft, 1 iliac crest autograft, and 14 femoral head allografts) [44]. No significant differences were reported comparing allografts and autografts. The incorporation rate was 81%.

Mahylis et al. assessed the clinical outcomes of 30 patients undergoing revision rTSA with structural iliac crest bone autograft ($n = 15$) or nonstructural bone allograft NSBA ($n = 15$) at a minimum of 2 years follow-up [45]. No radiographic differences were found between the two groups in terms of implant position, graft integration, scapular notching, or failure of fixation.

Melis et al. reported the clinical outcomes of 37 patients undergoing revision rTSA for glenoid component loosening [46]. 78% of patients underwent glenoid bone grafting with structural iliac crest bone ($n = 21$), cancellous bone graft ($n = 5$), or allograft ($n = 3$). At the latest follow-up, the authors reported one bone graft lysis and a partial graft resorption rate of 21%.

Ernstbrunner et al. evaluated 41 primary rTSA with bone grafts (83% corticocancellous and

17% structural grafts) at a minimum follow-up of 2 years [47]. The rate of glenoid lucency, glenoid bone graft incorporation, and scapular notching were, respectively, 18%, 78%, and 30%. Each patient treated with a structural graft showed graft incorporation and no signs of glenoid lucency. No revision surgeries were reported.

Tashjian et al. evaluated 22 patients undergoing primary or revision rTSA with structural glenoid allografts [48]. The rate of complete graft incorporation at 1 year follow-up was 82%. Two patients showed baseplate loosening and migration, but no patients needed further surgeries.

Lopiz et al. reviewed 20 patients who underwent primary or revision rTSA with a glenoid bone graft (13 allografts and 7 autografts) at a minimum 2 years follow-up [49]. The rate of graft incorporation was 95%. No clinical or radiographic differences were showed while comparing the grafts. The postoperative complication rate was 20%: one aseptic glenoid component loosening, one surgical wound hematoma, one acromial fracture, and one symptomatic grade 3 scapular notching.

Recommendations have been made to achieve appropriate glenoid component stability in case of bone grafting with distorted glenoid geometry: the central peg device should traverse the graft and gain purchase in at least 10 mm of native glenoid bone and an altered screw trajectory might be used to maximize bony purchase [14, 43, 50].

Still debated is whether to use metal or bone to correct the glenoid defect. A recent systematic review by Lanham et al. compared glenoid bone grafting with augmented glenoid baseplates in rTSA [51]. The overall complication and revision rate, clinical outcomes, and ROM were similar for rTSA using either bone graft or augmented baseplates. However infections and scapular notching seemed to be higher in the bone grafting group.

Several with specific design implant, either custom or non-custom made have been proposed so far, to manage severe glenoid bone loss mainly in revision cases.

Valenti et al. proposed the use of a lateralized metal-backed keeled baseplate prolonged by a thin metallic post fixed directly in the subscapularis fossa [50]. Forty-four shoulders at a minimum 2 years follow-up were evaluated. The complication rate in primary and revision cases was, respectively, 12% and 25%.

The computer-aided design and computer-aided manufacturing (CAD–CAM) technology has gained popularity in the treatment of severe glenoid bone loss; it is used to design and manufacture products in different fields. In shoulder replacement, this technology enables surgeons to reconstruct the altered glenoid vault with a metallic patient-specific component.

A fine-cut 2D CT scan is used to construct a 3D model that is subsequently used to create a patient-specific glenoid implant.

Chammaa et al. proposed a custom-made CAD–CAM total shoulder replacement (TSR; Stanmore Implants Worldwide, Elstree, UK) resembling a total hip prosthesis, fixed to the scapula rather than to the glenoid itself, as an alternative for the most challenging severe glenoid bone loss cases, where glenoid component secure fixation cannot be achieved [52]. Thirty-seven patients at a mean follow-up of 5 years were evaluated and a statistically significant improvement in active ROM was reported. The revision rate reported was 16%.

Bodendorfer et al. [53] assessed 11 patients who underwent rTSAs using the glenoid vault reconstruction system (VRS; Zimmer-Biomet, Warsaw, IN) at an average follow-up time of 30 months. At final follow-up, all implants were radiographically stable without loosening.

Rangarajan et al. assessed the clinical outcomes of 19 patients with severe glenoid bone deficiency undergoing primary or revision rTSA using the VRS (Zimmer Biomet, Warsaw, IN, USA) [54]. The authors showed a complication rate of 21% but no radiographic evidence of component loosening, scapular notching, or hardware failure.

Debeer et al. evaluated ten patients with severe glenoid bone defect treated with the Glenius Glenoid Reconstruction System (Materialise NV, Leuven, Belgium), which is a custom-made porous coated metal component patient-specific implant, at an average follow-up of 30.5 months. The mean difference between the preoperative planned and the postoperative version and inclination were, respectively, 6° and 4°. Eight patients reported improved outcomes after the implant.

Custom glenoid baseplates are a novel and much more expensive solution for shoulder arthroplasties. The increased cost might be justified only in patients with severe glenoid bone loss and limited alternatives.

References

1. Kahn T, Chalmers PN. Proximal humeral bone loss in revision shoulder arthroplasty. Orthop Clin N Am. 2020;51(1):87–95. https://doi.org/10.1016/j.ocl.2019.08.003.
2. Cuff D, Levy JC, Gutierrez S, Frankle MA. Torsional stability of modular and non-modular reverse shoulder humeral components in a proximal humeral bone loss model. J Shoulder Elb Surg. 2011;20(4):646–51. https://doi.org/10.1016/j.jse.2010.10.026.
3. Cox JL, McLendon PB, Christmas KN, Simon P, Mighell MA, Frankle MA. Clinical outcomes following reverse shoulder arthroplasty-allograft composite for revision of failed arthroplasty associated with proximal humeral bone deficiency: 2–15-year follow-up. J Shoulder Elb Surg. 2019;28(5):900–7. https://doi.org/10.1016/j.jse.2018.10.023.
4. Boileau P, Raynier JL, Chelli M, Gonzalez JF, Galvin JW. Reverse shoulder-allograft prosthesis composite, with or without tendon transfer, for the treatment of severe proximal humeral bone loss. J Shoulder Elb Surg. 2020;29(11):e401–15. https://doi.org/10.1016/j.jse.2020.03.016.
5. Chalmers PN, Romeo AA, Nicholson GP, Boileau P, Keener JD, Gregory JM, Salazar DH, Tashjian RZ. Humeral bone loss in revision total shoulder arthroplasty: the proximal humeral arthroplasty revision osseous inSufficiency (PHAROS) classification system. Clin Orthop Relat Res. 2019;477(2):432–41. https://doi.org/10.1097/CORR.0000000000000590.
6. Sanchez-Sotelo J, Wagner ER, Sim FH, Houdek MT. Allograft-prosthetic composite reconstruction for massive proximal humeral bone loss in reverse shoulder arthroplasty. J Bone Jt Surg Am. 2017;99(24):2069–76. https://doi.org/10.2106/JBJS.16.01495.
7. Stephens SP, Paisley KC, Giveans MR, Wirth MA. The effect of proximal humeral bone loss on revision reverse total shoulder arthroplasty. J Shoulder Elb Surg. 2015;24(10):1519–26. https://doi.org/10.1016/j.jse.2015.02.020.
8. Budge MD, Moravek JE, Zimel MN, Nolan EM, Wiater JM. Reverse total shoulder arthroplasty for the management of failed shoulder arthroplasty with proximal humeral bone loss: is allograft augmentation necessary? J Shoulder Elb Surg. 2013;22(6):739–44. https://doi.org/10.1016/j.jse.2012.08.008.
9. Chacon A, Virani N, Shannon R, Levy JC, Pupello D, Frankle M. Revision arthroplasty with use of a reverse shoulder prosthesis-allograft composite. J Bone Jt Surg Am. 2009;91(1):119–27. https://doi.org/10.2106/JBJS.H.00094.
10. Boileau P. Complications and revision of reverse total shoulder arthroplasty. Orthop Traumatol Surg Res. 2016;102(1 Suppl):S33–43. https://doi.org/10.1016/j.otsr.2015.06.031.
11. El Beaino M, Liu J, Lewis VO, Lin PP. Do early results of proximal humeral allograft-prosthetic composite reconstructions persist at 5-year follow-up? Clin Orthop Relat Res. 2019;477(4):758–65. https://doi.org/10.1097/CORR.0000000000000354.
12. Mengers SR, Knapik D, Strony J, et al. The use of tumor prostheses for primary or revision reverse total shoulder arthroplasty with proximal humeral bone loss. J Shoulder Elb Arthroplast. 2022;6:24715492211063108. https://doi.org/10.1177/24715492211063108.
13. Boileau P, Morin-Salvo N, Bessiere C, Chelli M, Gauci MO, Lemmex DB. Bony increased-offset-reverse shoulder arthroplasty: 5–10 years' follow-up. J Shoulder Elb Surg. 2020;29(10):2111–22. https://doi.org/10.1016/j.jse.2020.02.008.
14. Holt AM, Throckmorton TW. Reverse shoulder arthroplasty for B2 glenoid deformity. J Shoulder Elb Arthroplast. 2019;3:2471549219897661. https://doi.org/10.1177/2471549219897661.
15. Italia KR, Green N, Maharaj J, Launay M, Gupta A. Computed tomographic evaluation of glenoid joint line restoration with glenoid bone grafting and reverse shoulder arthroplasty in patients with significant glenoid bone loss. J Shoulder Elb Surg. 2021;30(3):599–608. https://doi.org/10.1016/j.jse.2020.09.031.
16. Walch G, Badet R, Boulahia A, Khoury A. Morphologic study of the glenoid in primary glenohumeral osteoarthritis. J Arthroplast. 1999;14(6):756–60. https://doi.org/10.1016/s0883-5403(99)90232-2.
17. Domos P, Checchia CS, Walch G. Walch B0 glenoid: pre-osteoarthritic posterior subluxation of the humeral head. J Shoulder Elb Surg. 2018;27(1):181–8. https://doi.org/10.1016/j.jse.2017.08.014.
18. Iannotti JP, Jun BJ, Patterson TE, Ricchetti ET. Quantitative measurement of osseous pathology in advanced glenohumeral osteoarthritis. J Bone Jt Surg Am. 2017;99(17):1460–8. https://doi.org/10.2106/JBJS.16.00869.
19. Zimmer ZR, Carducci MP, Mahendraraj KA, Jawa A. Evolution of the Walch classification and its importance on the B2 glenoid. J Shoulder Elb Arthroplast. 2020;4:247154922090381. https://doi.org/10.1177/2471549220903815.
20. Logli AL, Pareek A, Nguyen NTV, Sanchez-Sotelo J. Natural history of glenoid bone loss in primary glenohumeral osteoarthritis: how does bone loss progress

over a decade? J Shoulder Elb Surg. 2021;30(2):324–30. https://doi.org/10.1016/j.jse.2020.05.021.

21. Favard L, Lautmann S, Sirveaux F, Oudet D, Kerjean Y, Huguet D. Hemiarthroplasty versus reverse arthroplasty in the treatment of osteoarthritis with massive rotator cuff tear. In: Walch G, Boileau P, Molé D, editors. Shoulder prostheses 2–10 years follow-up. Montpellier: Sauramps Medical; 2000. p. 261–8.

22. Gowda A, Pinkas D, Wiater JM. Treatment of glenoid bone deficiency in total shoulder arthroplasty: a critical analysis review. JBJS Rev. 2015;3(7):e2. https://doi.org/10.2106/JBJS.RVW.N.00097.

23. Cil A, Sperling JW, Cofield RH. Nonstandard glenoid components for bone deficiencies in shoulder arthroplasty. J Shoulder Elb Surg. 2014;23(7):e149–57. https://doi.org/10.1016/j.jse.2013.09.023.

24. Boileau P, Morin-Salvo N, Gauci MO, Seeto BL, Chalmers PN, Holzer N, Walch G. Angled BIO-RSA (bony-increased offset-reverse shoulder arthroplasty): a solution for the management of glenoid bone loss and erosion. J Shoulder Elb Surg. 2017;26(12):2133–42. https://doi.org/10.1016/j.jse.2017.05.024.

25. Singh J, Odak S, Neelakandan K, Walton MJ, Monga P, Bale S, Trail I. Survivorship of autologous structural bone graft at a minimum of 2 years when used to address significant glenoid bone loss in primary and revision shoulder arthroplasty: a computed tomographic and clinical review. J Shoulder Elb Surg. 2021;30(3):668–78. https://doi.org/10.1016/j.jse.2020.06.015.

26. Walch G, Moraga C, Young A, Castellanos-Rosas J. Results of anatomic nonconstrained prosthesis in primary osteoarthritis with biconcave glenoid. J Shoulder Elb Surg. 2012;21(11):1526–33. https://doi.org/10.1016/j.jse.2011.11.030.

27. Klika BJ, Wooten CW, Sperling JW, Steinmann SP, Schleck CD, Harmsen WS, Cofield RH. Structural bone grafting for glenoid deficiency in primary total shoulder arthroplasty. J Shoulder Elb Surg. 2014;23(7):1066–72. https://doi.org/10.1016/j.jse.2013.09.017.

28. Nicholson GP, Cvetanovich GL, Rao AJ, O'Donnell P. Posterior glenoid bone grafting in total shoulder arthroplasty for osteoarthritis with severe posterior glenoid wear. J Shoulder Elb Surg. 2017;26(10):1844–53. https://doi.org/10.1016/j.jse.2017.03.016.

29. Sabesan V, Callanan M, Ho J, Iannotti JP. Clinical and radiographic outcomes of total shoulder arthroplasty with bone graft for osteoarthritis with severe glenoid bone loss. J Bone Jt Surg Am. 2013;95(14):1290–6. https://doi.org/10.2106/JBJS.L.00097.

30. Rice RS, Sperling JW, Miletti J, Schleck C, Cofield RH. Augmented glenoid component for bone deficiency in shoulder arthroplasty. Clin Orthop Relat Res. 2008;466(3):579–83. https://doi.org/10.1007/s11999-007-0104-4.

31. Lenart BA, Namdari S, Williams GR. Total shoulder arthroplasty with an augmented component for anterior glenoid bone deficiency. J Shoulder Elb Surg. 2016;25(3):398–405. https://doi.org/10.1016/j.jse.2015.08.012.

32. Sandow M, Schutz C. Total shoulder arthroplasty using trabecular metal augments to address glenoid retroversion: the preliminary result of 10 patients with minimum 2-year follow-up. J Shoulder Elb Surg. 2016;25(4):598–607. https://doi.org/10.1016/j.jse.2016.01.001.

33. Sandow MJ, Tu CG. Porous metal wedge augments to address glenoid retroversion in anatomic shoulder arthroplasty: midterm update. J Shoulder Elb Surg. 2020;29(9):1821–30. https://doi.org/10.1016/j.jse.2020.01.101.

34. Zhang B, Niroopan G, Gohal C, Alolabi B, Leroux T, Khan M. Glenoid bone grafting in primary anatomic total shoulder arthroplasty: a systematic review. Shoulder Elb. 2021;13(5):509–17. https://doi.org/10.1177/1758573220917653.

35. Leafblad N, Asghar E, Tashjian RZ. Innovations in shoulder arthroplasty. J Clin Med. 2022;11(10):2799. https://doi.org/10.3390/jcm11102799.

36. Gunther SB, Lynch TL. Total shoulder replacement surgery with custom glenoid implants for severe bone deficiency. J Shoulder Elb Surg. 2012;21(5):675–84. https://doi.org/10.1016/j.jse.2011.03.023.

37. Collin P, Herve A, Walch G, Boileau P, Muniandy M, Chelli M. Mid-term results of reverse shoulder arthroplasty for glenohumeral osteoarthritis with posterior glenoid deficiency and humeral subluxation. J Shoulder Elb Surg. 2019;28(10):2023–30. https://doi.org/10.1016/j.jse.2019.03.002.

38. Mizuno N, Denard PJ, Raiss P, Walch G. Reverse total shoulder arthroplasty for primary glenohumeral osteoarthritis in patients with a biconcave glenoid. J Bone Jt Surg Am. 2013;95(14):1297–304. https://doi.org/10.2106/JBJS.L.00820.

39. Gupta A, Thussbas C, Koch M, Seebauer L. Management of glenoid bone defects with reverse shoulder arthroplasty-surgical technique and clinical outcomes. J Shoulder Elb Surg. 2018;27(5):853–62. https://doi.org/10.1016/j.jse.2017.10.004.

40. Boileau P, Moineau G, Roussanne Y, O'Shea K. Bony increased-offset reversed shoulder arthroplasty: minimizing scapular impingement while maximizing glenoid fixation. Clin Orthop Relat Res. 2011;469(9):2558–67. https://doi.org/10.1007/s11999-011-1775-4.

41. Franceschetti E, de Sanctis EG, Gregori P, Paciotti M, Palumbo A, Franceschi F. Angled BIO-RSA leads to better inclination and clinical outcomes compared to standard BIO-RSA and eccentric reaming: a comparative study. Shoulder Elb. 2021;2021:156. https://doi.org/10.1177/17585732211067156.

42. Franceschetti E, Ranieri R, de Sanctis EG, Palumbo A, Franceschi F. Clinical results of bony increased-offset reverse shoulder arthroplasty (BIO-RSA) associated with an onlay 145° curved stem in patients with cuff tear arthropathy: a comparative study. J Shoulder Elb Surg. 2020;29(1):58–67. https://doi.org/10.1016/j.jse.2019.05.023.

43. Werner BS, Bohm D, Abdelkawi A, Gohlke F. Glenoid bone grafting in reverse shoulder arthroplasty for long-standing anterior shoulder dislocation. J Shoulder Elb Surg. 2014;23(11):1655–61. https://doi.org/10.1016/j.jse.2014.02.017.

44. Jones RB, Wright TW, Zuckerman JD. Reverse total shoulder arthroplasty with structural bone grafting of large glenoid defects. J Shoulder Elb Surg. 2016;25(9):1425–32. https://doi.org/10.1016/j.jse.2016.01.016.

45. Mahylis JM, Puzzitiello RN, Ho JC, Amini MH, Iannotti JP, Ricchetti ET. Comparison of radiographic and clinical outcomes of revision reverse total shoulder arthroplasty with structural versus nonstructural bone graft. J Shoulder Elb Surg. 2019;28(1):e1–9. https://doi.org/10.1016/j.jse.2018.06.026.

46. Melis B, Bonnevialle N, Neyton L, Levigne C, Favard L, Walch G, Boileau P. Glenoid loosening and failure in anatomical total shoulder arthroplasty: is revision with a reverse shoulder arthroplasty a reliable option? J Shoulder Elb Surg. 2012;21(3):342–9. https://doi.org/10.1016/j.jse.2011.05.021.

47. Ernstbrunner L, Werthel JD, Wagner E, Hatta T, Sperling JW, Cofield RH. Glenoid bone grafting in primary reverse total shoulder arthroplasty. J Shoulder Elb Surg. 2017;26(8):1441–7. https://doi.org/10.1016/j.jse.2017.01.011.

48. Tashjian RZ, Broschinsky K, Stertz I, Chalmers PN. Structural glenoid allograft reconstruction during reverse shoulder arthroplasty. J Shoulder Elb Surg. 2020;29(3):534–40. https://doi.org/10.1016/j.jse.2019.07.011.

49. Lopiz Y, Garcia-Fernandez C, Arriaza A, Rizo B, Marcelo H, Marco F. Midterm outcomes of bone grafting in glenoid defects treated with reverse shoulder arthroplasty. J Shoulder Elb Surg. 2017;26(9):1581–8. https://doi.org/10.1016/j.jse.2017.01.017.

50. Valenti P, Sekri J, Kany J, Nidtahar I, Werthel JD. Benefits of a metallic lateralized baseplate prolonged by a long metallic post in reverse shoulder arthroplasty to address glenoid bone loss. Int Orthop. 2019;43(9):2131–9. https://doi.org/10.1007/s00264-018-4249-4.

51. Lanham NS, Peterson JR, Ahmed R, Jobin CM, Levine WN. Comparison of glenoid bone grafting versus augmented glenoid baseplates in reverse shoulder arthroplasty: a systematic review. J Shoulder Elb Surg. 2022;2022:22. https://doi.org/10.1016/j.jse.2022.02.022.

52. Chammaa R, Uri O, Lambert S. Primary shoulder arthroplasty using a custom-made hip-inspired implant for the treatment of advanced glenohumeral arthritis in the presence of severe glenoid bone loss. J Shoulder Elb Surg. 2017;26(1):101–7. https://doi.org/10.1016/j.jse.2016.05.027.

53. Bodendorfer BM, Loughran GJ, Looney AM, Velott AT, Stein JA, Lutton DM, Wiesel BB, Murthi AM. Short-term outcomes of reverse shoulder arthroplasty using a custom baseplate for severe glenoid deficiency. J Shoulder Elb Surg. 2021;30(5):1060–7. https://doi.org/10.1016/j.jse.2020.08.002.

54. Rangarajan R, Blout CK, Patel VV, Bastian SA, Lee BK, Itamura JM. Early results of reverse total shoulder arthroplasty using a patient-matched glenoid implant for severe glenoid bone deficiency. J Shoulder Elb Surg. 2020;29(7S):S139–48. https://doi.org/10.1016/j.jse.2020.04.024.

Rehabilitation Following Reverse Shoulder Arthroplasty

29

Nikolaos Platon Sachinis and Knut Beitzel

29.1 Introduction

There is currently no widespread consensus or guideline for the postoperative management of RSA in general or even for specific purposes. All relevant parameters, including the length of range of motion (ROM) restriction, or active ROM induction, are considerably different among protocols that are included in published studies. Thus, the fundamental elements and principles of rehabilitation are implemented and debated in many ways [1, 2].

Published data also suggests that patients having a RSA are willing to return to sports activities and many of them accomplish that goal [3]. Hence, establishing postoperative therapy models to safely increase patients' activities and satisfaction is crucial. Despite data sparsity, a review of published literature provides insight of therapy regimes that may improve patients' outcomes. By considering together all aspects of current knowledge, key components for patient-specific targeted rehabilitation and return to sports are presented in this chapter.

N. P. Sachinis
First Orthopaedic Department, Aristotle University of Thessaloniki, "Georgios Papanikolaou" Hospital, Thessaloniki, Greece

K. Beitzel (✉)
ATOS Orthoparc Klinik, Cologne, Germany
e-mail: beitzelknut@tum.de

29.2 What Do Patients Expect and Achieve

Due to the increasing heterogeneity of patients undergoing RSA, it is expected that a high percentage of them would like to be able to participate in recreational activities or sports. Past TSA and newer RSA studies support this hypothesis. Henn the Third et al. in 2011 [4], studied the preoperative expectations from 98 unilateral primary TSA cases. Mean age was 67.6 years (range, 30–86 years). Results of this study showed that 81/98 patients were expecting (to a variant degree) to be able to exercise or participate in sports and 83/98 to be able to engage in recreational activities. This expectation was found to be more significant in younger patients.

Likewise, Rauck et al. in 2019 [5] reviewed prospectively collected data of 333 RSA cases, 242 being performed for rotator cuff arthropathy (RCA), 68 for osteoarthritis (OA), and 23 for post-traumatic arthritis. By using the Hospital for Special Surgery's shoulder surgery expectations survey, they found a higher preoperative function, OA, and a history of no previous joint replacements to be correlated to greater RSA-related expectations. Specifically, 81.7% of patients were expecting to a variant importance of degree, to be able to perform recreational activities; 45.4% non-overhead sports; 37.7% over-head sports; and 56.5% professional sports. Regarding the last category, 24.9% of patients

A. D. Mazzocca et al. (eds.), *Shoulder Arthritis across the Life Span*,
https://doi.org/10.1007/978-3-031-33298-2_29

found it very important to be able to return to a professional sport, although the authors of this article argue that the reliability of this question, due to its varying interpretations, is debated.

Indeed, literature shows that a high number of patients manage to return to recreational activities and sports after RSA. Garcia et al. collected data from 76/132 consecutive patients who underwent RSA, from 2007 to 2013 [6]. Average follow-up was 31.6 months and the mean American Shoulder and Elbow Surgeons (ASES) scores improved from 34.30 preoperatively to 81.45. They also found that 85% of patients managed to return to sports at an average of 5.3 months after the operation. However they pointed that a decreased return to such activities was significantly related to age >70 years.

In a more recent systematic review in 2021, Francheschetti et al. searched for studies informing about the frequency of patients returning to sports after RSA [3]. The authors finally included six articles from 2015 to 2017 and a mean follow-up from 2.6 to 4.8 years [6–11]. The review revealed that the rate of return to sports ranged from 60 to 93% (mean 79%) with a mean ASES score of 78.8%, at a mean follow-up of 5.3 years. All studies included patients returning to overhead sports such as tennis, basketball, or volleyball.

29.3 Past Rehabilitation Protocols

Despite the huge number of publications regarding RSA, only few papers discuss in a general or specific way the rehabilitation protocol/mobilization process that patients have to follow and even fewer state if patients were able to return to their daily, recreational, or sports activities. The Rehabilitation Commission of the German Society of Shoulder and Elbow Surgery (RCGS) systematically searched for important aspects of rehabilitation in study protocols, from 01/1989 to 01/2016 [12]. Despite finding 22 articles that included at least a mobilization status depending on the postoperative week, due to a lack of detailed protocols, a survey between 63 RSA experts was conducted.

From these articles, Boudreau et al. review in 2007 was the only one to outline a structured rehabilitation protocol [1]. In summary, the authors proposed a four-stage rehabilitation process with the following postoperative time endpoints: 1st–6th week; 6th–12th week; 12th–16th week; and 16th week and onward. They proposed a sling to be worn for 3–4 weeks and no active shoulder ROM for the first 6 weeks, with subsequent gradual active ROM exercise initiation. Regarding shoulder immobilization, most other articles up to 2018 follow a consistent path of shoulder immobilization for two and up to 4 weeks [1, 13–26] and fewer advise for a sling to be worn for up to 6 weeks [27–32].

The protocol finally produced by RCGS, following the experts survey, pertained a four stage rehabilitation protocol, which by postoperative time frame was divided as follows: first stage, 1–6 weeks, with sling to be worn until 3 or 6 weeks (depending on the occasion) and passive, assistive exercises to be used for maintenance of ROM and scapula control; second stage, 6–12 weeks, with initiation of active ROM exercise and end goal of no scapula dyskinesia and full active ROM; third stage 12–16 weeks, commencement of strength increase exercises, management of pain free daily activities and achieving 75% of total strength and endurance; and fourth stage, 16 weeks and onward, with a final goal of symmetrical mobility and strength to the opposite side and return to sports activities, if desired [12].

29.4 Suggestions to Meet Higher Patient Expectations

As previously discussed, past rehabilitation protocols focused on immobilizing the shoulder on a sling or brace for the first few weeks, and prohibited patients from actively moving it for 6 weeks. The 6 week time point was presumably suggested especially in cases where the subscapularis tendon was refixed, thus giving it enough time to heal without increasing the chances of tendon repair failure. Past studies have shown a protective effect of subscapularis refixation to a RSA dislocation [33–35]. However, biomechanical studies revealed that a subscapularis repair increased the required deltoid and posterior cuff force and also the joint reaction forces [36].

Friedman et al. studied 340 patients undergoing RSA with refixation and 241 without refixation of the subscapularis tendon [37]. The authors found a significant degree of difference favoring the repaired group in some outcome scores and a significant difference favoring the non-repaired group on abduction and passive external rotation. They concluded that by not repairing the subscapularis, especially in lateralized reverse shoulder prostheses, similar outcomes may be achieved, without also finding a difference in dislocation/complication rates. However the rehabilitation process of these patients was dependent on each individual surgeon and not standardized for these two groups.

If the subscapularis tendon is not be repaired during RSA, then active ROM of the affected shoulder does not jeopardize any healing process, and patients may freely move their arm as much as their pain and apprehension allows them to do so. Van Essen et al. in 2020, published a protocol for fast track rehabilitation after RSA, without reattaching the subscapularis tendon, nor immobilizing the shoulder [38].

Likewise, Lee et al. in 2021 published a series of 357 consecutive RSA in 320 patients, from 2005 up to 2017 [2]. The senior author of this study changed the rehabilitation protocol throughout this period, from 6 weeks of immobilization with a sling (2005–2013), to 3 weeks (2013–2015), and finally to immediate mobilization (sling only for first 24/48 h until the interscalene block wears off). Arguably, advances in prosthesis implantation technique and learning curve attributed to this change. At 12 months follow-up, all three groups' outcome scores were significantly improved when compared to the preoperative status; no statistical differences were found between groups. The complications rate, which consisted of fractures and dislocations, was greater in the 6 week immobilization group. The authors reasoned that when patients are not wearing a sling, their proprioception improves, and they are less likely to fall. It should be noted that no revision or fracture cases were included in the study and that the senior author attempted to reattach the residual cuff to the metaphysis whenever possible.

29.5 Contraindications for Fast Track Rehabilitation Protocols

There are occasions where a RSA may need protection during the first 3–6 weeks, and a fast track protocol is contraindicated. Cho et al. revealed that reduced BMD, increased deltoid length, and revision surgery were risk factor for an acromial fracture, following RSA [39]. It has been demonstrated that female patients older than 60 have an increased risk of low BMD and especially after 70, a deteriorated balance and gait [40].

Outcomes of RSA differ between cases of RCA, revision arthroplasty, and fracture cases. Patients with rheumatoid arthritis have similar scores to those with primary RCA, but they are at a higher risk of intraoperative fractures and loosening due to poor bone quality [41, 42]. Boileau et al. demonstrated that tuberosity reattachment and healing in fracture cases improved active forward elevation, external rotation, and patient satisfaction [43]. Therefore, protection of shoulder movement for 6 weeks until tuberosities unite is advisable.

Particularly in revision surgery, it is necessary to assess each patient's soft tissue, bone, and neuromuscular function to develop a customized postoperative plan. Revision arthroplasty patients may have comparingly lower ASES and Constant Score [44]. Relative research indicates a high frequency of postoperative complications (loosening, instability) and supports the notion of personalized rehabilitation in revision RSA [45].

29.6 Conclusion

Based on current evidence, a standard and a fast track protocol are demonstrated in Tables 29.1 and 29.2, respectively. However, individual characteristics have to be taken in consideration for adapting a postoperative protocol.

Therefore, it is essential for the surgeon to communicate the individual changes to the patient, the treating physician, and the physiotherapist. Written postoperative treatment schedules may improve the communication in individual, complex cases.

Table 29.1 Standard rehabilitation protocol after a reverse shoulder arthroplasty [12]

Phases	Physiotherapy	Aim
First phase (week 1–6)	Immobilization (as a form of protection) in 15°–45° of abduction (ABD) for 3–6 weeks ABD brace/sling can be remove during showers, while eating and for physiotherapy Passive ROM training for 4 weeks, then gradual transition to active-assisted (AA) ROM Pendulum exercises Aquatic therapy if wounds are intact	Symmetrical and pain-free movement compared to opposite side: PROM flexion 90°; PROM ABD with adjacent scapula 90°
Second phase (week 6–12)	Full AAROM transitioning to active ROM against force of gravity Scar mobilization Aqua gymnastics/aquatic therapy CPM if favored Training in closed chain to avoid shearing forces Training in open chain to strengthen Muscles isolated Training on everyday movements (ADL) Limitation: up to the pain threshold No resistance or strengthening exercises	Active achievement of all possible active range of movements No scapulothoracic dysfunction Sufficient glenohumeral and scapulothoracic functionality
Third phase (week 12–16)	Further strengthening and an increase in daily activities plays an important role in this phase A special emphasis is based on proprioception and strength endurance	Free functional movement in a pain-free range ADL possible without pain/avoiding overhead exercises If enough strength in RC, phase 4 can start in order to carry out ADL cleanly and without pain 75% of normal strength and endurance
Fourth phase (>16 weeks)	Stretching Intensify functional training This phase includes the return to full daily activities and/or sports	Return to sports after 6 months Mobility and strength are symmetrical to the opposite side Scapulothoracic movement is present without significant side-to-side differences There is no pain at rest and during activity

Table 29.2 Fast track rehabilitation protocol after a reverse shoulder arthroplasty

Phases	Physiotherapy	Aim
First phase (week 0–2)	Sling for the first 24/48 h until the interscalene block wears off. Start physiotherapy from first day. Focus on elbow, wrist, hand function, and scapula setting first week, add ROM of glenohumeral joint second week, if possible active, guided by pain. Only restriction on forced adduction and extension of shoulder (push oneself off the chair)	Decrease swelling and pain. Recovery of ROM and muscle activation. Achieve if possible 60° of flexion and abduction
Second phase (week 2–6)	Retrieve ROM, isometric exercises of deltoid (when pain allows followed by isotonic, usually after third week). Strengthen scapulothoracic musculature	Recovery of ROM. Achieve 90° of flexion and abduction, if possible active
Third phase (week 6–12)	Mobilization of shoulder reaching preoperative values or contralateral side. Intensify deltoid and scapulothoracic strength and endurance. ADL training	Recovery of optimal ROM. >90° of flexion and abduction. No scapulothoracic dysfunction. Able to do most ADL
Fourth phase (>12 weeks)	Increase strengthening/endurance exercises. Intensify and optimize ADL, recreational/sport activities training	Do ADL pain-free. Start recreational activities. Start sport activities (caution is needed for overhead and professional sports, possible achievement if ROM and strength have reached approximately 90° of preoperative values)

References

1. Boudreau S, Boudreau ED, Higgins LD, Wilcox RB 3rd. Rehabilitation following reverse total shoulder arthroplasty. J Orthop Sports Phys Ther. 2007;37(12):734–43.
2. Lee J, Consigliere P, Fawzy E, Mariani L, Witney-Lagen C, Natera L, et al. Accelerated rehabilitation following reverse total shoulder arthroplasty. J Shoulder Elb Surg. 2021;30(9):e545–e57.
3. Franceschetti E, Giovannetti de Sanctis E, Gregori P, Palumbo A, Paciotti M, Di Giacomo G, et al. Return to sport after reverse total shoulder arthroplasty is highly frequent: a systematic review. J ISAKOS. 2021;6(6):363–6.
4. Henn RF 3rd, Ghomrawi H, Rutledge JR, Mazumdar M, Mancuso CA, Marx RG. Preoperative patient expectations of total shoulder arthroplasty. J Bone Jt Surg Am. 2011;93(22):2110–5.
5. Rauck RC, Swarup I, Chang B, Ruzbarsky JJ, Dines DM, Warren RF, et al. Preoperative patient expectations of elective reverse shoulder arthroplasty. J Shoulder Elb Surg. 2019;28(7):1217–22.
6. Garcia GH, Taylor SA, DePalma BJ, Mahony GT, Grawe BM, Nguyen J, et al. Patient activity levels after reverse total shoulder arthroplasty: what are patients doing? Am J Sports Med. 2015;43(11):2816–21.
7. Bulhoff M, Sattler P, Bruckner T, Loew M, Zeifang F, Raiss P. Do patients return to sports and work after total shoulder replacement surgery? Am J Sports Med. 2015;43(2):423–7.
8. Fink Barnes LA, Grantham WJ, Meadows MC, Bigliani LU, Levine WN, Ahmad CS. Sports activity after reverse total shoulder arthroplasty with minimum 2-year follow-up. Am J Orthop (Belle Mead NJ). 2015;44(2):68–72.
9. Simovitch RW, Gerard BK, Brees JA, Fullick R, Kearse JC. Outcomes of reverse total shoulder arthroplasty in a senior athletic population. J Shoulder Elb Surg. 2015;24(9):1481–5.
10. Liu JN, Garcia GH, Mahony G, Wu HH, Dines DM, Warren RF, et al. Sports after shoulder arthroplasty: a comparative analysis of hemiarthroplasty and reverse total shoulder replacement. J Shoulder Elb Surg. 2016;25(6):920–6.
11. Kolling C, Borovac M, Audige L, Mueller AM, Schwyzer HK. Return to sports after reverse shoulder arthroplasty—the Swiss perspective. Int Orthop. 2018;42(5):1129–35.
12. Buchmann S, Schoch C, Grim C, Jung C, Beitzel K, Klose M, et al. Rehabilitation following reverse shoulder arthroplasty. Obere Extremitat. 2019;14(4):269–83.
13. Rhee YG, Cho NS, Moon SC. Effects of humeral component retroversion on functional outcomes in reverse total shoulder arthroplasty for cuff tear arthropathy. J Shoulder Elb Surg. 2015;24(10):1574–81.

14. Gillespie RJ, Garrigues GE, Chang ES, Namdari S, Williams GR Jr. Surgical exposure for reverse total shoulder arthroplasty: differences in approaches and outcomes. Orthop Clin N Am. 2015;46(1):49–56.

15. Routman HD. Indications, technique, and pitfalls of reverse total shoulder arthroplasty for proximal humerus fractures. Bull Hosp Jt Dis. 2013;71(Suppl 2):64–7.

16. Castricini R, Gasparini G, Di Luggo F, De Benedetto M, De Gori M, Galasso O. Health-related quality of life and functionality after reverse shoulder arthroplasty. J Shoulder Elb Surg. 2013;22(12):1639–49.

17. Walch G, Bacle G, Ladermann A, Nove-Josserand L, Smithers CJ. Do the indications, results, and complications of reverse shoulder arthroplasty change with surgeon's experience? J Shoulder Elb Surg. 2012;21(11):1470–7.

18. Mizuno N, Denard PJ, Raiss P, Walch G. The clinical and radiographical results of reverse total shoulder arthroplasty with eccentric glenosphere. Int Orthop. 2012;36(8):1647–53.

19. Leung B, Horodyski M, Struk AM, Wright TW. Functional outcome of hemiarthroplasty compared with reverse total shoulder arthroplasty in the treatment of rotator cuff tear arthropathy. J Shoulder Elb Surg. 2012;21(3):319–23.

20. De Biase CF, Delcogliano M, Borroni M, Castagna A. Reverse total shoulder arthroplasty: radiological and clinical result using an eccentric glenosphere. Musculoskelet Surg. 2012;96(Suppl 1):S27–34.

21. Kempton LB, Balasubramaniam M, Ankerson E, Wiater JM. A radiographic analysis of the effects of prosthesis design on scapular notching following reverse total shoulder arthroplasty. J Shoulder Elb Surg. 2011;20(4):571–6.

22. Kempton LB, Balasubramaniam M, Ankerson E, Wiater JM. A radiographic analysis of the effects of glenosphere position on scapular notching following reverse total shoulder arthroplasty. J Shoulder Elb Surg. 2011;20(6):968–74.

23. Kalouche I, Sevivas N, Wahegaonker A, Sauzieres P, Katz D, Valenti P. Reverse shoulder arthroplasty: does reduced medialisation improve radiological and clinical results? Acta Orthop Belg. 2009;75(2):158–66.

24. Cazeneuve JF, Cristofari DJ. Delta III reverse shoulder arthroplasty: radiological outcome for acute complex fractures of the proximal humerus in elderly patients. Orthop Traumatol Surg Res OTSR. 2009;95(5):325–9.

25. Klein M, Juschka M, Hinkenjann B, Scherger B, Ostermann PA. Treatment of comminuted fractures of the proximal humerus in elderly patients with the Delta III reverse shoulder prosthesis. J Orthop Trauma. 2008;22(10):698–704.

26. Werner CM, Steinmann PA, Gilbart M, Gerber C. Treatment of painful pseudoparesis due to irreparable rotator cuff dysfunction with the Delta III reverse-ball-and-socket total shoulder prosthesis. J Bone Jt Surg Am. 2005;87(7):1476–86.

27. Ross M, Hope B, Stokes A, Peters SE, McLeod I, Duke PF. Reverse shoulder arthroplasty for the treatment of three-part and four-part proximal humeral fractures in the elderly. J Shoulder Elb Surg. 2015;24(2):215–22.

28. Walker M, Willis MP, Brooks JP, Pupello D, Mulieri PJ, Frankle MA. The use of the reverse shoulder arthroplasty for treatment of failed total shoulder arthroplasty. J Shoulder Elb Surg. 2012;21(4):514–22.

29. Sadoghi P, Vavken P, Leithner A, Hochreiter J, Weber G, Pietschmann MF, et al. Impact of previous rotator cuff repair on the outcome of reverse shoulder arthroplasty. J Shoulder Elb Surg. 2011;20(7):1138–46.

30. Reitman RD, Kerzhner E. Reverse shoulder arthroplasty as treatment for comminuted proximal humeral fractures in elderly patients. Am J Orthop (Belle Mead NJ). 2011;40(9):458–61.

31. Cuff D, Pupello D, Virani N, Levy J, Frankle M. Reverse shoulder arthroplasty for the treatment of rotator cuff deficiency. J Bone Jt Surg Am. 2008;90(6):1244–51.

32. Frankle M, Levy JC, Pupello D, Siegal S, Saleem A, Mighell M, et al. The reverse shoulder prosthesis for glenohumeral arthritis associated with severe rotator cuff deficiency. A minimum 2-year follow-up study of 60 patients surgical technique. J Bone Jt Surg Am. 2006;88(Suppl 1 Pt 2):178–90.

33. Edwards TB, Williams MD, Labriola JE, Elkousy HA, Gartsman GM, O'Connor DP. Subscapularis insufficiency and the risk of shoulder dislocation after reverse shoulder arthroplasty. J Shoulder Elb Surg. 2009;18(6):892–6.

34. Gallo RA, Gamradt SC, Mattern CJ, Cordasco FA, Craig EV, Dines DM, et al. Instability after reverse total shoulder replacement. J Shoulder Elb Surg. 2011;20(4):584–90.

35. Chalmers PN, Rahman Z, Romeo AA, Nicholson GP. Early dislocation after reverse total shoulder arthroplasty. J Shoulder Elb Surg. 2014;23(5):737–44.

36. Hansen ML, Nayak A, Narayanan MS, Worhacz K, Stowell R, Jacofsky MC, et al. Role of subscapularis repair on muscle force requirements with reverse shoulder arthroplasty. Bull Hosp Jt Dis. 2013;73(Suppl 1):S21–7.

37. Friedman RJ, Flurin PH, Wright TW, Zuckerman JD, Roche CP. Comparison of reverse total shoulder arthroplasty outcomes with and without subscapularis repair. J Shoulder Elb Surg. 2017;26(4):662–8.

38. van Essen T, Kornuijt A, de Vries LMA, Stokman R, van der Weegen W, Bogie R, et al. Fast track rehabilitation after reversed total shoulder arthroplasty: a protocol for an international multicentre prospective cohort study. BMJ Open. 2020;10(8):e034934.

39. Cho CH, Rhee YG, Yoo JC, Ji JH, Kim DS, Kim YS, et al. Incidence and risk factors of acromial fracture following reverse total shoulder arthroplasty. J Shoulder Elb Surg. 2021;30(1):57–64.

40. Daly RM, Rosengren BE, Alwis G, Ahlborg HG, Sernbo I, Karlsson MK. Gender specific age-related changes in bone density, muscle strength and functional performance in the elderly: a-10 year pro-

spective population-based study. BMC Geriatr. 2013;13:71.
41. Young AA, Smith MM, Bacle G, Moraga C, Walch G. Early results of reverse shoulder arthroplasty in patients with rheumatoid arthritis. J Bone Jt Surg Am. 2011;93(20):1915–23.
42. Khan WS, Longo UG, Ahrens PM, Denaro V, Maffulli N. A systematic review of the reverse shoulder replacement in rotator cuff arthropathy, rotator cuff tears, and rheumatoid arthritis. Sports Med Arthrosc Rev. 2011;19(4):366–79.
43. Boileau P, Alta TD, Decroocq L, Sirveaux F, Clavert P, Favard L, et al. Reverse shoulder arthro-plasty for acute fractures in the elderly: is it worth reattaching the tuberosities? J Shoulder Elb Surg. 2019;28(3):437–44.
44. Boileau P, Watkinson D, Hatzidakis AM, Hovorka I. Neer Award 2005: the Grammont reverse shoulder prosthesis: results in cuff tear arthritis, fracture sequelae, and revision arthroplasty. J Shoulder Elb Surg. 2006;15(5):527–40.
45. Flury MP, Frey P, Goldhahn J, Schwyzer HK, Simmen BR. Reverse shoulder arthroplasty as a salvage procedure for failed conventional shoulder replacement due to cuff failure—midterm results. Int Orthop. 2011;35(1):53–60.

Management of TSA and RSA Complications: Tips and Tricks to Avoid Them

Edoardo Giovannetti de Sanctis, Luca Saccone, Angelo Baldari, and Francesco Franceschi

30.1 Introduction

Anatomic (aTSA) and reverse (rTSA) total shoulder arthroplasties have shown to be successful in relieving pain and restoring shoulder function with increased joint mobility.

As with other total joint procedures, shoulder arthroplasty might be associated with a multitude of complications which are associated with catastrophic results, with reduced functional outcomes and a negative impact on the patient quality of life. Furthermore, complications might lead to revision shoulder replacement which is costly to both the patient and the healthcare system. Fortunately, revision surgery after prosthetic shoulder arthroplasty is rarely required.

Although the overall number of shoulder replacements performed each year has increased during the past two decades, the rate of complica-

tions has decreased. This might be due to a better understanding of shoulder biomechanics, more advanced implant designs with the widespread use of the reverse total shoulder arthroplasty and an increased surgeon experience gained during the years with those procedures.

Bohsali et al. [1] in their systematic review reported a complication rate after aTSA of 14.7% within the period 1995–2006. The same author [2] showed a decrease (7.4%) of the complication rate after both aTSA and rTSA within the period 2006–2015.

Parada et al. have analyzed a large database quantifying complication and revision rates for TSA and RSA [3]. The authors evaluated the outcomes of 2224 aTSA and 4158 rTSA.

Within the aTSA group, the complication and revision rate were, respectively, 10.7 and 5.6%.

The most frequent complication for aTSA was rotator cuff tears/failure, occurring in 6.2% of all patients and accounting for 57.7% of relative aTSA complications and 67.7% of relative aTSA revisions.

Aseptic glenoid loosening (complication rate = 2.5%, relative complication rate = 23%, revision rate = 1.9%, relative revision rate = 34.7%) and infection (complication rate = 1.3%, relative complication rate = 11.7%, revision rate = 0.8% relative revision rate = 14.5%) were, respectively, the second and third most common aTSA complications.

E. Giovannetti de Sanctis (✉) · A. Baldari
F. Franceschi
Department of Orthopaedic and Trauma Surgery, San Pietro Fatebenefratelli Hospital, Rome, Italy

UniCamillus-Saint Camillus International University of Health Sciences, Rome, Italy
e-mail: francesco.franceschi@unicamillus.org

L. Saccone
Department of Orthopaedic and Trauma Surgery, San Pietro Fatebenefratelli Hospital, Rome, Italy

Department of Orthopaedic and Trauma Surgery, Campus Biomedico University of Rome, Rome, Italy

© ISAKOS 2023
A. D. Mazzocca et al. (eds.), *Shoulder Arthritis across the Life Span*,
https://doi.org/10.1007/978-3-031-33298-2_30

Among the other aTSA complications: pain (complication rate = 1.8%, relative complication rate = 16.8%, revision rate = 0.1%, relative revision rate = 3.2%), nerve injury (complication rate = 0.7%, relative complication rate = 6.3%, revision rate = 0.1%, relative revision rate = 0.8%), instability (complication rate = 0.6%, relative complication rate = 5.9%, revision rate = 0.5%, relative revision rate = 8.1%), aseptic humeral loosening (complication rate = 0.4%, relative complication rate = 3.3%, revision rate = 0.2%, relative revision rate = 4.0%), and humeral fracture (complication rate = 0.4%, relative complication rate = 3.4%, revision rate = 0.1%, relative revision rate = 0.8%).

Within the rTSA group, the complication and revision rate were, respectively, 8.9 and 1.7%.

The most frequent complication was acromial and scapular fracture accounting for 18.5% of relative rTSA complications and 0.0% of relative rTSA revisions.

Pain (complication rate = 2%, relative complication rate = 22.1%, revision rate = 0.3%, relative revision rate = 10.6%) and instability (complication rate = 1.4%, relative complication rate = 16.1%, revision rate = 1%, relative revision rate = 38.5%) were, respectively, the second and third most common rTSA complication.

Among the other complications are as follows: infection (complication rate = 0.9%, relative complication rate = 9.7%, revision rate = 0.7%, relative revision rate = 26.9%), aseptic glenoid loosening (complication rate = 0.6%, relative complication rate = 6.5%, revision rate = 0.3%, relative revision rate = 12.5%), humeral fractures (complication rate = 0.8%, relative complication rate = 9.7%, revision rate = 0.0%, relative revision rate = 2%), nerve injury (complication rate = 0.4%, relative complication rate = 4%, revision rate = 0.0%, relative revision rate = 0.0%), and aseptic humeral loosening (complication rate = 0.1%, relative complication rate = 1.6%, revision rate = 0.1%, relative revision rate = 3.9%).

Scapular notching was assessed in 228 patients, with an overall rate of 7%. However, 91.7% of cases were classified as low grade according to Nerot-Sirveaux. Debated is whether there exists a correlation between scapular notching, often considered more as a problem than a complication, and clinical outcomes.

In rTSA, the incidence of complications has changed over time. In 2011 Zumstein et al. reported instability as the first cause (6.9%) of complications [4]. Ascione et al. in 2018 reported infection as first cause with a rate of 4.1% [5]. Therefore, with improvements in design and surgical skills, the rate of infection seems to be outpacing the rate of dislocation after rTSA.

In summary, the aTSA has a higher complication and revision rate than rTSA; the two most common complications for each of the group are unique to each device (aTSA: rotator cuff failure; rTSA: acromial/scapular fractures); the rate of infection is similar for both procedures.

As prevention is better than cure, the tips and tricks mentioned below might be helpful to minimize the risks of the most common complications.

30.2 Tips and Tricks to Avoid TSA Complications

30.2.1 Nerve Injury

Nerve injury in TSA might be due to direct or indirect causes [6]. A direct cause, such as transection during the surgical dissection and excessive compression with retractors, acts on the nerve itself.

Excessive traction, secondary to arm lengthening or intraoperative positioning, thermal injury from cement extrusion, and pressure from postoperative hematoma are the most common indirect causes, acting on a third party, which then acts on the nerve. These complications are generally reversible within 3 months from surgery.

The nerve structures at higher risk of injury during TSA are the axillary nerve, the radial nerve, the suprascapular nerve and the brachial plexus.

The axillary nerve injury causes deltoid dysfunction and persistent shoulder lateral pain. It is usually damaged during surgery at the inferior glenoid rim due to prolonged retraction or excessively wide exposure with electrocautery. Early diagnosis might be difficult as the shoulder is immobilized and the patient does not realize to have a deltoid deficit. Lateral hypoesthesia would help with the diagnosis.

In order to prevent this injury, caution should be used during periosteal detachment in glenoid preparation and when reaming the humeral metaphysis, as the axillary nerve has been shown to lie between 3.2 and 12.4 mm from inferior glenoid rim and at an average of 8.1 mm from the lesser edge of the humeral metaphysis [7, 8].

Lädermann et al. [9] observed a greater arm lengthening in patients with electromyography (EMG) subclinical changes indicating an axillary nerve lesion (4.2 cm vs 2.6 cm). Marion et al. [10] found that lowering the humeral center of rotation (CoR) beyond the middle of the glenoid should be avoided for not increasing nerve tension, whereas humeral lateralization had no effect on it.

Traction is the most common mechanism of brachial plexus injury in TSA [6]. Kam et al. [11] showed that a combination of excessive external rotation, extension, and abduction, respectively, greater than 60°, 50°, and 70° would increase the stress more than 10% at the brachial plexus.

The use of arm support during surgery would decrease the brachial plexus strain during the TSA procedure. It is therefore suggested to avoid excessive traction while placing the arm in those positions at risk (particularly during humeral preparation) and to use the arm support during the procedure.

The biggest risk factors for radial nerve injury in TSA are intraoperative periprosthetic humeral fracture, subsequent cement extravasation with both compressive and thermal damage, and direct damage due to wrong cerclage wire application [6]. It is recommended to ream and impact carefully the humeral component and once needed to place the cerclage proximal to the inferior edge of the latissimus dorsi tendon [12].

Glenoid baseplate fixation with screws during rTSA has been identified as the biggest risk factor for suprascapular nerve injury [6]. Posterior and superior screws could damage or overpenetrate the suprascapular nerve when drilling. During baseplate fixation in RSA, the distance of the posterior and superior screws should be carefully considered [13].

30.2.2 Periprosthetic Joint Infection

The rate of rTSA prosthetic infection has been reported by Ascione et al. to be 4.1% [5]. The predisposing factors are prior shoulder surgery (e.g., arthroscopic rotator cuff repair), obesity, rheumatoid arthritis, malnutrition, and long operation time [14]. The most common pathogen is the *Cutibacterium acnes* (formerly *Propionibacterium acnes*), which is normally present on the skin and takes up to 14 days to be detected from the culture [15]. The symptoms in case of *Cutibacterium* infection are unexplained pain with no other signs of infection and osteolysis at the radiographs or CT scan. Other commonly observed organisms are the *Staphylococcus epidermidis* and *Staphylococcus aureus*. Symptoms given by those bacteria normally are purulent joint fluid with pus discharge fistula.

Several are the strategies described to prevent periprosthetic infections: bathing with chlorhexidine gluconate on the day before surgery, administration of cephalosporin as a preventive antibiotic 1 h before surgery, changing surgical gloves regularly, changing the blade after skin incision, frequent surgical site irrigation (also with diluted povidone), injection of gentamicin at the time of closure, and use of antibiotic-loaded cement (1 g of vancomycin/bone cement) [16].

In low grade infection, intraoperative biopsy with arthroscopy and culture is mandatory for

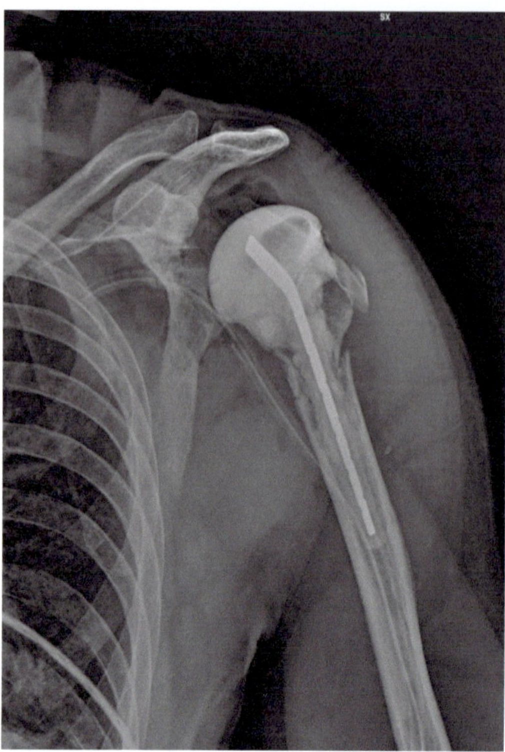

Fig. 30.1 Two-stage revision with use of antibiotic spacers

diagnosis. The biopsy is much more sensitive and specific than aspirate [17].

The preferred management strategy remains controversial. In acute infection (less than 6 weeks), open irrigation, debridement, and exchange of polyethylene could be a strategy, though it has shown a success rate of only 50%. In chronic infection, the two-stage revision is the gold standard at the moment with higher success rate (Fig. 30.1) [18]. One stage exchange has been proposed due to lower stress to soft tissues and decreased time and costs, showing good clinical outcomes in selected cases [19].

30.2.3 Intraoperative Fracture

Uncommon and difficult to manage, those fractures occur, more frequently on the humeral side, during impaction or arm positioning [20]. Broaching parallel to the humeral shaft and avoiding excessive fitting of the humeral stem might prevent these fractures.

While treating humeral fractures, it is mandatory to reach the stem stability. With a stable stem, the fracture might be fixed; otherwise the stem should be replaced with a longer cemented one [21].

Glenoid fractures occur most commonly during reaming or implant fixation and might be repaired with baseplate locking screws or external screws. Small fractures could be ignored, whereas catastrophic ones should be treated with a bone graft [22].

30.3 Tips and Tricks to Avoid rTSA Complications

30.3.1 Acromial and Scapular Fracture

Acromial and scapular fractures are relatively rare (Fig. 30.2). The cause of RSA-associated scapular spine fractures is still controversial. The etiopathogenesis is frequently classified as: traumatic (caused by another fall) or stress fractures due to increased deltoid strain.

Overtensioning the deltoid by lateralizing or distalizing the implant has been reported as a risk factor for acromial or scapular spine stress fractures [23].

Giles et al. [24] found that humeral lateralization, compared to glenoid lateralization and humeral lengthening, was the only parameter decreasing deltoid forces required for active abduction. Thus, humeral lateralization might reduce either deltoid fatigue or the risk of scapula-acromial fractures.

Lädermann et al. [25] evaluated the effects of arm lengthening on clinical outcomes. The amount of arm lengthening correlates with deltoid lengthening. A shortening of the arm and thus a lack of retensioning of the deltoid constantly lead to poor results, whereas excessive lengthening might increase the risk of complications such as acromial fracture. The arm lengthening is directly correlated to the thickness of the polyethylene insert, the size of the implant, the use of an eccentric

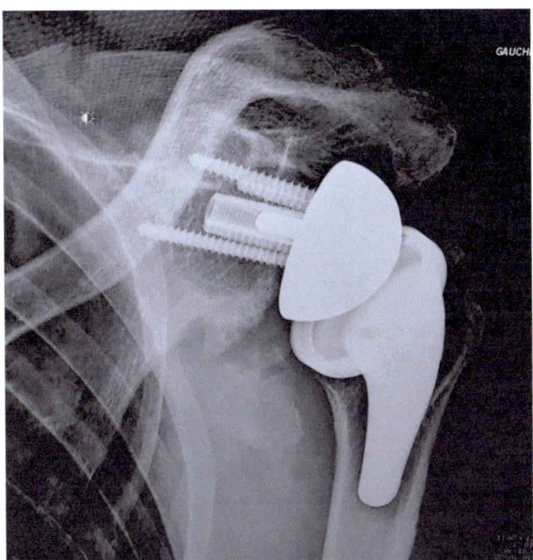

Fig. 30.2 Scapular fracture

glenosphere, and the position of the glenosphere in the vertical plane. The authors stated that arm lengthening above 2.5 cm compared with the contralateral side should be avoided, increasing the risk of complication without improving significantly the ROM. The goal should be to use the smallest-thinnest implant-insert with a good intraoperative stability.

Osteopenia due to both age and shoulder disuse might be taken into account, when deciding to implant a prosthesis with an increasing stress to the deltoid.

Lastly, attention must be paid while fixating the baseplate to avoid scapular fracture. The placement of the superior screw has been shown to be a risk factor for scapular fractures, when oriented posterosuperiorly toward the scapular spine; if oriented toward the coracoid, the risk of scapular spine fracture decreases dramatically [26].

Still debated is the preferred management strategy for scapular and acromial fractures in rTSA, as surgical treatment has not shown significantly better clinical outcomes. These fractures are more frequently treated nonoperatively (immobilization with an abduction sling for 4–6 weeks) and lead to inferior clinical and radiological results compared to RSA without an associated fractures [27]. Operative treatment with plate fixation of scapular spine fractures might be considered in younger patients with high functional demands.

30.3.2 Instability

Although the rTSA design has been proposed to improve joint stability, altering the shoulder biomechanics, the tensioning of the remaining muscles is mandatory in patients with poor soft tissue envelope to avoid anterior or posterior dislocations.

With improvements in designs, the incidence of early dislocations seems to be decreasing. Among the risk factors are as follows: previous surgery, lack of soft tissue tension (deltoid or subscapularis failure) due to implant malposition or tendon deficiency, improper version of the implant, and mechanical impingement [14].

The soft tissue tension might be decreased due to the design of the prosthesis (Grammont in rTSA) or to humerus proximalization (in proximal humeral bone loss—PHBL). The humeral height might be shortened, compared to the normal opposite side.

In rTSA the deltoid and cuff tension might be increased by lateralizing either the glenoid or humeral components using specific implants.

Debated is whether the glenosphere size has any effects in joint stability, modifying the force required to dislocate the shoulder [28–30]. It has been demonstrated that the humeral socket depth has higher effect than the glenosphere size; but the greater the constraint the higher the risk of impingement with decreased ROM [29, 31].

Glenosphere lateralization may have a role in increasing deltoid muscle compression forces and implant stability [24]. Henninger et al. [32] showed that glenoid lateralization leads to a progressive increase of forces required for the humerus to be dislocated anteriorly. The potential negative effects are an increased needed deltoid

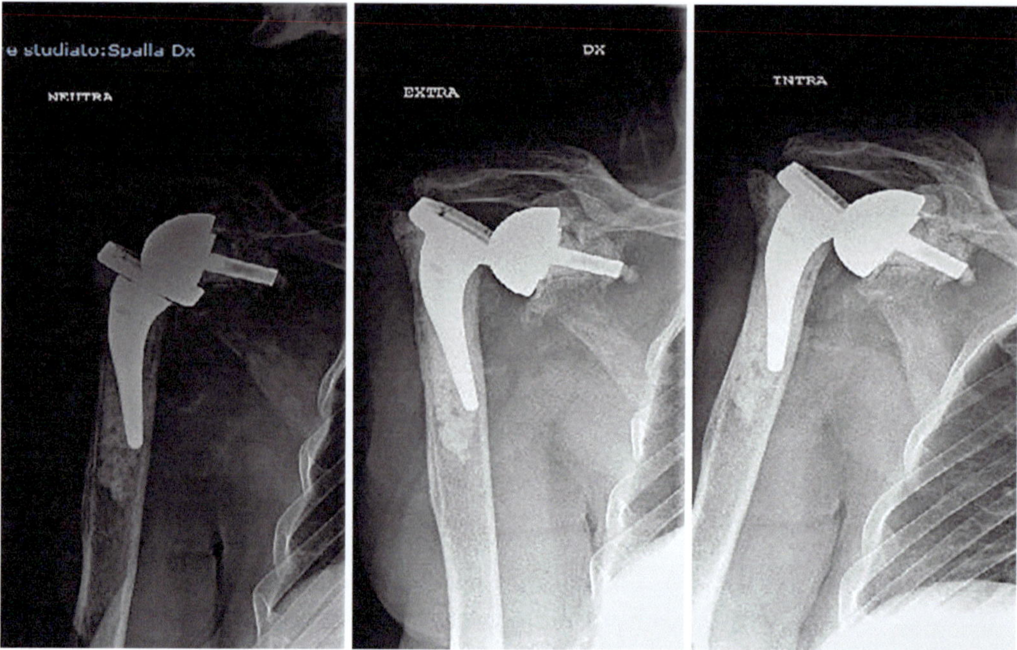

Fig. 30.3 rTSA instability caused by superior tilting of the baseplate

force for active ROM and a potential higher risk for acromial stress fractures.

Guarrella et al. [33], in a retrospective multicenter series of 1035 rTSA, confirmed that glenoid bony lateralization has a primary effect in preventing shoulder instability.

Both humeral and glenoid version have a role in the overall implant stability. Favre et al. [34] outlined a greater influence of the humeral component version in rTSA stability. Currently, the glenoid and humeral implant are recommended to be implanted, respectively, at 0°–10° and 0°–30° of retroversion to maximize stability [35].

Humeral lengthening is a crucial factor influencing rTSA stability. Lädermann et al. [36] have shown that humeral shortening is associated with an increased risk of dislocation. However, as mentioned previously, an excessive humeral lengthening might overstuff the joint, overtensioning the soft tissue envelope, with a decreased ROM [24, 37].

In case of PHBL, the aim should be distalizing the humerus to its correct height, which can be achieved by using a thicker polyethylene and/or metal tray or an inferior eccentric glenosphere.

Implanting an inferior eccentric glenosphere has been shown to prevent scapular notching and improve stability by 17% [28, 38]. Furthermore, the baseplate should be placed as inferior as possible for the same reasons mentioned above.

Inferior tilt of the glenoid has been proposed as a way of improving glenohumeral stability. In a biomechanical study, Gutiérrez et al. [39] concluded that an inferior tilt of 15°, compared to 0° and to a superior tilt of 15°, resulted in highest compressive forces with a reduced risk of instability. Those results were then confirmed by several authors [40, 41] (Fig. 30.3).

The subscapularis which is considered a protector against anterior dislocation in aTSA and medialized rTSA might be not necessary in lateralized rTSA implants, as the whole compression needed is carried out by the deltoid [42].

30.3.3 Aseptic Glenoid Loosening

Aseptic glenoid loosening may be related to poor bone stock, excessive version or superior inclination, the design of glenoid component, the technique of fixation used, and excessive joint reaction forces [43].

The compressive forces acting on the glenoid side have a stabilizing effect on the glenosphere, whereas the shear forces, acting in a direction parallel to the glenoid, might lead to the component loosening [44].

The correction of the glenoid version and inclination is mandatory and might be performed through an eccentric reaming and the use of bone grafts (e.g., Bony Increased Offset) or augmented baseplates [45]. Excessive reaming should be avoided as it is associated with weakening of the subchondral bone, loss of bone volume, and surface area. Bone grafts and augmented baseplates preserve bone stock enhancing the baseplate fixation, correct glenoid version and inclination, and increase the implant lateralization. In severe glenoid defect, a custom-made baseplate might be implanted.

The baseplate stability is due mainly to the central fixation element, which could be a modular central screw, a monoblock baseplate screw, a central peg, or central post. Debated is which among those elements improve the most implant stability.

The central screw offer enhanced initial fixation due to better compression, whereas a central post might have a higher long-term ingrowth potential.

After fixing the baseplate with the central fixation element, additional stability is achieved by peripheral screws. These might be either compression or locking screws. The failure rate of the glenoid component in rTSA have decreased significantly after the introduction of locking screws for baseplate fixation [46]. Formaini et al. [47], comparing a hybrid configuration of locking and compression screws with an all-locking screws configuration, reported no differences in terms of fixation failure rate.

The number of peripheral screws to be used depends on the implant design. Roche et al. [48] evaluated fixation strength comparing two, four, or six screws. Four screws led to an equal and higher fixation strength compared, respectively, to six and two screws. Furthermore, the authors showed that the longer the peripheral screws, the stronger the construct.

Optimal screw placement has been defined as that which maximized screw length, accomplished far cortical fixation, and attained screw purchase in good bone stock [49].

Humphrey et al. provided practical guidelines for surgeons and proposed the concept of the three major columns (the base of coracoid, the spine, and the pillar) to obtain optimal initial fixation of the glenoid component. Each column consists of bone that is suitable for achieving strong screw purchase. The trajectory of the superior screw should overlap with the first column (the base of the coracoid). The anterior screw should be placed through the second column (the scapular spine), and it should be aimed superiorly and posteriorly passing superior to the post of the baseplate. The inferior screw should be placed within the third column (the scapular pillar). The posterior screw might be placed anterosuperiorly toward the base of the scapular spine or anteroinferiorly toward the anterior prominence of the scapular pillar [49].

30.3.4 Scapular Notching

The scapular notching is a unique problem and a common radiographic finding after rTSA.

It refers to an erosive lesion of the inferior part of the scapular neck due to repetitive contact of the humeral component polyethylene during adduction and extension. It will also lead to polyethylene wear, joint inflammation, and a higher risk of implant loosening [50]. Frequently the impingement occurs with the arm in a resting position. Risk factors for scapular notching are low BMI, a small inferior overhang of the glenoid implant, a greater neck shaft angle, a superior tilt of the baseplate, and smaller implant size [38, 51].

Positioning the glenosphere with inferior overhang, inferior tilt, and lateralization has been proposed as the optimal combination on the glenoid side to reduce scapular notching risk [52–55].

In a 3D computer templating model, Werner and colleagues found that the 135° neck-shaft angle had a larger impingement-free ROM [56]. According to Gutierrez et al. the implant with the lowest rate of scapular notching would have a humeral neck-shaft angle of 130° and a 10 mm-lateralized 42 mm glenosphere with an inferior position (with 3.5 mm of inferior overhang [57]) and tilt.

In conclusion, to prevent this complication, the glenosphere should be implanted with both an inferior overhang and inferior tilt, the CoR should be lateralized, and the humeral NSA should be decreased.

30.4 Tips and Tricks to Avoid aTSA Complications

30.4.1 Rotator Cuff Tear and/or Subscapularis Failure

A well-functioning rotator cuff is necessary for successful anatomic total shoulder arthroplasty. Young et al. [58] suggested that secondary rotator cuff dysfunction is the natural progression and a recognized complication observed in aTSA long-term follow-up. The altered soft tissue envelope, as a consequence of surgery, the modified joint kinematics, and an increased rotator cuff demanding might be the causes of this complication. Postoperative rotator cuff failure, considered as a complication after aTSA, should be distinguished from incorrect indication (shoulder replacement performed in a patient with a preoperative RC alteration) and when surgery is not executed appropriately.

When performing an aTSA through a deltopectoral approach, preserving the integrity of the subscapularis tendon for final proper tenodesis and a clear visualization of the posterosuperior rotator cuff to reduce the risk of damage while resecting the humeral head is mandatory.

The glenoid component positioning is another crucial surgical step. The proper correction of

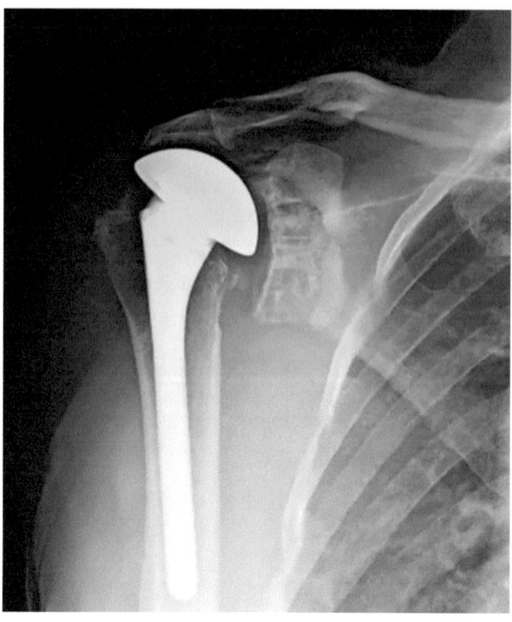

Fig. 30.4 A failed aTSA

glenoid version and inclination reduces the risk of joint kinematics alteration.

Furthermore, the glenoid and/or humeral implant overhang should also be avoided as it might increase the mechanical stress of the rotator cuff [59].

30.4.2 Aseptic Glenoid Loosening

Several factors have been proposed as causes of aseptic glenoid loosening in aTSA: the implant design, the surgical technique, patient characteristics, the preoperative integrity of the rotator cuff, and the static posterior subluxation of the humeral head (Fig. 30.4).

The "rocking horse" phenomenon has been proposed as explanation for glenoid component loosening [60]. The eccentric loading of the glenoid component, with repetitive compression on one side and distraction on the other side, leads to early mechanical failure at the bone-implant interface. This phenomenon might be worsened by GH instability, rotator cuff dysfunction, and glenoid component malposition [61].

The glenoid bone defect correction, avoiding excessive reaming to preserve bone stock and using augmented components or bone grafts, increases glenoid component fixation with a reduced risk of loosening [61, 62].

Several glenoid components for aTSA are available: anatomic pear-shaped vs elliptical, all-polyethylene vs metal backed, flat vs curved back design, inlay vs onlay, keels vs pegs, cemented vs uncemented. Still debated is which design has the lowest risk of loosening [63–65].

30.5 Conclusion

The number of shoulder arthroplasty performed has increased tremendously during the last decade, and it is estimated to rise by 322% by 2050 [66]; therefore a thorough understanding of the management of the main complications is mandatory. The relatively high complication rate, after aTSA, has led physician to shift to the "safer" rTSA. The reason for this is also a poor understanding of the cause of rotator cuff failure and glenohumeral posterior subluxation. Once a solution for those problems will be found, the rate of aTSA might increase significantly.

Lastly, surgical tips and tricks are useful once associated with a correct surgical indication, an exhaustive dialogue with the patient, and an accurate preoperative planning.

References

1. Bohsali KI, Wirth MA, Rockwood CA Jr. Complications of total shoulder arthroplasty. J Bone Jt Surg Am. 2006;88(10):2279–92. https://doi.org/10.2106/JBJS.F.00125.
2. Bohsali KI, Bois AJ, Wirth MA. Complications of shoulder arthroplasty. J Bone Jt Surg Am. 2017;99(3):256–69. https://doi.org/10.2106/JBJS.16.00935.
3. Parada SA, Flurin PH, Wright TW, Zuckerman JD, Elwell JA, Roche CP, Friedman RJ. Comparison of complication types and rates associated with anatomic and reverse total shoulder arthroplasty. J Shoulder Elb Surg. 2021;30(4):811–8. https://doi.org/10.1016/j.jse.2020.07.028.
4. Zumstein MA, Pinedo M, Old J, Boileau P. Problems, complications, reoperations, and revisions in reverse total shoulder arthroplasty: a systematic review. J Shoulder Elb Surg. 2011;20(1):146–57. https://doi.org/10.1016/j.jse.2010.08.001.
5. Ascione F, Domos P, Guarrella V, Chelli M, Boileau P, Walch G. Long-term humeral complications after Grammont-style reverse shoulder arthroplasty. J Shoulder Elb Surg. 2018;27(6):1065–71. https://doi.org/10.1016/j.jse.2017.11.028.
6. Vajapey SP, Contreras ES, Cvetanovich GL, Neviaser AS. Neurologic complications in primary anatomic and reverse total shoulder arthroplasty: a review. J Clin Orthop Trauma. 2021;20:101475. https://doi.org/10.1016/j.jcot.2021.06.005.
7. Leschinger T, Hackl M, Buess E, Lappen S, Scaal M, Muller LP, Wegmann K. The risk of suprascapular and axillary nerve injury in reverse total shoulder arthroplasty: an anatomic study. Injury. 2017;48(10):2042–9. https://doi.org/10.1016/j.injury.2017.06.024.
8. Loomer R, Graham B. Anatomy of the axillary nerve and its relation to inferior capsular shift. Clin Orthop Relat Res. 1989;243:100–5.
9. Ladermann A, Lubbeke A, Melis B, Stern R, Christofilopoulos P, Bacle G, Walch G. Prevalence of neurologic lesions after total shoulder arthroplasty. J Bone Jt Surg Am. 2011;93(14):1288–93. https://doi.org/10.2106/JBJS.J.00369.
10. Marion B, Leclere FM, Casoli V, Paganini F, Unglaub F, Spies C, Valenti P. Potential axillary nerve stretching during RSA implantation: an anatomical study. Anat Sci Int. 2014;89(4):232–7. https://doi.org/10.1007/s12565-014-0229-y.
11. Kam AW, Lam PH, Haen P, Tan M, Shamsudin A, Murrell GAC. Preventing brachial plexus injury during shoulder surgery: a real-time cadaveric study. J Shoulder Elb Surg. 2018;27(5):912–22. https://doi.org/10.1016/j.jse.2017.11.030.
12. Fu MC, Hendel MD, Chen X, Warren RF, Dines DM, Gulotta LV. Surgical anatomy of the radial nerve in the deltopectoral approach for revision shoulder arthroplasty and periprosthetic fracture fixation: a cadaveric study. J Shoulder Elb Surg. 2017;26(12):2173–6. https://doi.org/10.1016/j.jse.2017.07.021.
13. Yang Y, Zuo J, Liu T, Shao P, Wu H, Gao Z, Xiao J. Glenoid morphology and the safe zone for protecting the suprascapular nerve during baseplate fixation in reverse shoulder arthroplasty. Int Orthop. 2018;42(3):587–93. https://doi.org/10.1007/s00264-017-3646-4.
14. Boileau P. Complications and revision of reverse total shoulder arthroplasty. Orthop Traumatol Surg Res. 2016;102(1 Suppl):S33–43. https://doi.org/10.1016/j.otsr.2015.06.031.
15. Hsu JE, Gorbaty JD, Whitney IJ, Matsen FA 3rd. Single-stage revision is effective for failed shoulder arthroplasty with positive cultures

for Propionibacterium. J Bone Jt Surg Am. 2016;98(24):2047–51. https://doi.org/10.2106/JBJS.16.00149.

16. Kim SC, Kim IS, Jang MC, Yoo JC. Complications of reverse shoulder arthroplasty: a concise review. Clin Shoulder Elb. 2021;24(1):42–52. https://doi.org/10.5397/cise.2021.00066.

17. Dilisio MF, Miller LR, Warner JJ, Higgins LD. Arthroscopic tissue culture for the evaluation of periprosthetic shoulder infection. J Bone Jt Surg Am. 2014;96(23):1952–8. https://doi.org/10.2106/JBJS.M.01512.

18. Romanò CL, Borens O, Monti L, Meani E, Stuyck J. What treatment for periprosthetic shoulder infection? Results from a multicentre retrospective series. Int Orthop. 2012;36(5):1011–7. https://doi.org/10.1007/s00264-011-1467-4.

19. Mercurio M, Castioni D, Ianno B, Gasparini G, Galasso O. Outcomes of revision surgery after periprosthetic shoulder infection: a systematic review. J Shoulder Elb Surg. 2019;28(6):1193–203. https://doi.org/10.1016/j.jse.2019.02.014.

20. Brusalis CM, Taylor SA. Periprosthetic fractures in reverse total shoulder arthroplasty: current concepts and advances in management. Curr Rev Musculoskelet Med. 2020;13(4):509–19. https://doi.org/10.1007/s12178-020-09654-8.

21. Jarrett CD, Brown BT, Schmidt CC. Reverse shoulder arthroplasty. Orthop Clin N Am. 2013;44(3):389–408. https://doi.org/10.1016/j.ocl.2013.03.010.

22. Shah SS, Gaal BT, Roche AM, Namdari S, Grawe BM, Lawler M, Dalton S, King JJ, Helmkamp J, Garrigues GE, Wright TW, Schoch BS, Flik K, Otto RJ, Jones R, Jawa A, McCann P, Abboud J, Horneff G, Ross G, Friedman R, Ricchetti ET, Boardman D, Tashjian RZ, Gulotta LV. The modern reverse shoulder arthroplasty and an updated systematic review for each complication: part I. JSES Int. 2020;4(4):929–43. https://doi.org/10.1016/j.jseint.2020.07.017.

23. Lau SC, Large R. Acromial fracture after reverse total shoulder arthroplasty: a systematic review. Shoulder Elb. 2020;12(6):375–89. https://doi.org/10.1177/1758573219876486.

24. Giles JW, Langohr GD, Johnson JA, Athwal GS. Implant design variations in reverse total shoulder arthroplasty influence the required deltoid force and resultant joint load. Clin Orthop Relat Res. 2015;473(11):3615–26. https://doi.org/10.1007/s11999-015-4526-0.

25. Ladermann A, Walch G, Lubbeke A, Drake GN, Melis B, Bacle G, Collin P, Edwards TB, Sirveaux F. Influence of arm lengthening in reverse shoulder arthroplasty. J Shoulder Elb Surg. 2012;21(3):336–41. https://doi.org/10.1016/j.jse.2011.04.020.

26. Kennon JC, Lu C, McGee-Lawrence ME, Crosby LA. Scapula fracture incidence in reverse total shoulder arthroplasty using screws above or below metaglene central cage: clinical and biomechanical outcomes. J Shoulder Elb Surg. 2017;26(6):1023–30. https://doi.org/10.1016/j.jse.2016.10.018.

27. Sussiek J, Michel PA, Raschke MJ, Schliemann B, Katthagen JC. Treatment strategies for scapular spine fractures: a scoping review. EFORT Open Rev. 2021;6(9):788–96. https://doi.org/10.1302/2058-5241.6.200153.

28. Clouthier AL, Hetzler MA, Fedorak G, Bryant JT, Deluzio KJ, Bicknell RT. Factors affecting the stability of reverse shoulder arthroplasty: a biomechanical study. J Shoulder Elb Surg. 2013;22(4):439–44. https://doi.org/10.1016/j.jse.2012.05.032.

29. Gutierrez S, Keller TS, Levy JC, Lee WE 3rd, Luo ZP. Hierarchy of stability factors in reverse shoulder arthroplasty. Clin Orthop Relat Res. 2008;466(3):670–6. https://doi.org/10.1007/s11999-007-0096-0.

30. Langohr GD, Giles JW, Athwal GS, Johnson JA. The effect of glenosphere diameter in reverse shoulder arthroplasty on muscle force, joint load, and range of motion. J Shoulder Elb Surg. 2015;24(6):972–9. https://doi.org/10.1016/j.jse.2014.10.018.

31. Gutierrez S, Luo ZP, Levy J, Frankle MA. Arc of motion and socket depth in reverse shoulder implants. Clin Biomech (Bristol, Avon). 2009;24(6):473–9. https://doi.org/10.1016/j.clinbiomech.2009.02.008.

32. Henninger HB, Barg A, Anderson AE, Bachus KN, Burks RT, Tashjian RZ. Effect of lateral offset center of rotation in reverse total shoulder arthroplasty: a biomechanical study. J Shoulder Elb Surg. 2012;21(9):1128–35. https://doi.org/10.1016/j.jse.2011.07.034.

33. Guarrella V, Chelli M, Domos P, Ascione F, Boileau P, Walch G. Risk factors for instability after reverse shoulder arthroplasty. Shoulder Elb. 2021;13(1):51–7. https://doi.org/10.1177/1758573219864266.

34. Favre P, Sussmann PS, Gerber C. The effect of component positioning on intrinsic stability of the reverse shoulder arthroplasty. J Shoulder Elb Surg. 2010;19(4):550–6. https://doi.org/10.1016/j.jse.2009.11.044.

35. Henninger HB, Barg A, Anderson AE, Bachus KN, Tashjian RZ, Burks RT. Effect of deltoid tension and humeral version in reverse total shoulder arthroplasty: a biomechanical study. J Shoulder Elb Surg. 2012;21(4):483–90. https://doi.org/10.1016/j.jse.2011.01.040.

36. Ladermann A, Williams MD, Melis B, Hoffmeyer P, Walch G. Objective evaluation of lengthening in reverse shoulder arthroplasty. J Shoulder Elb Surg. 2009;18(4):588–95. https://doi.org/10.1016/j.jse.2009.03.012.

37. Tashjian RZ, Burks RT, Zhang Y, Henninger HB. Reverse total shoulder arthroplasty: a biomechanical evaluation of humeral and glenosphere hardware configuration. J Shoulder Elb Surg. 2015;24(3):e68–77. https://doi.org/10.1016/j.jse.2014.08.017.

38. Gutierrez S, Comiskey CA 4th, Luo ZP, Pupello DR, Frankle MA. Range of impingement-free abduction and adduction deficit after reverse shoulder arthroplasty. Hierarchy of surgical and

implant-design-related factors. J Bone Jt Surg Am. 2008;90(12):2606–15. https://doi.org/10.2106/JBJS.H.00012.

39. Gutierrez S, Greiwe RM, Frankle MA, Siegal S, Lee WE 3rd. Biomechanical comparison of component position and hardware failure in the reverse shoulder prosthesis. J Shoulder Elb Surg. 2007;16(3 Suppl):S9–S12. https://doi.org/10.1016/j.jse.2005.11.008.

40. Nyffeler RW, Werner CM, Gerber C. Biomechanical relevance of glenoid component positioning in the reverse Delta III total shoulder prosthesis. J Shoulder Elb Surg. 2005;14(5):524–8. https://doi.org/10.1016/j.jse.2004.09.010.

41. Randelli P, Randelli F, Arrigoni P, Ragone V, D'Ambrosi R, Masuzzo P, Cabitza P, Banfi G. Optimal glenoid component inclination in reverse shoulder arthroplasty. How to improve implant stability. Musculoskelet Surg. 2014;98(Suppl 1):15–8. https://doi.org/10.1007/s12306-014-0324-1.

42. Franceschetti E, de Sanctis EG, Ranieri R, Palumbo A, Paciotti M, Franceschi F. The role of the subscapularis tendon in a lateralized reverse total shoulder arthroplasty: repair versus nonrepair. Int Orthop. 2019;43(11):2579–86. https://doi.org/10.1007/s00264-018-4275-2.

43. Ladermann A, Schwitzguebel AJ, Edwards TB, Godeneche A, Favard L, Walch G, Sirveaux F, Boileau P, Gerber C. Glenoid loosening and migration in reverse shoulder arthroplasty. Bone Jt J. 2019;101-B(4):461–9. https://doi.org/10.1302/0301-620X.101B4.BJJ-2018-1275.R1.

44. Yang CC, Lu CL, Wu CH, Wu JJ, Huang TL, Chen R, Yeh MK. Stress analysis of glenoid component in design of reverse shoulder prosthesis using finite element method. J Shoulder Elb Surg. 2013;22(7):932–9. https://doi.org/10.1016/j.jse.2012.09.001.

45. Dilisio MF, Warner JJ, Walch G. Accuracy of the subchondral smile and surface referencing techniques in reverse shoulder arthroplasty. Orthopedics. 2016;39(4):e615–20. https://doi.org/10.3928/01477447-20160610-04.

46. Cuff D, Pupello D, Virani N, Levy J, Frankle M. Reverse shoulder arthroplasty for the treatment of rotator cuff deficiency. J Bone Jt Surg Am. 2008;90(6):1244–51. https://doi.org/10.2106/JBJS.G.00775.

47. Formaini NT, Everding NG, Levy JC, Santoni BG, Nayak AN, Wilson C. Glenoid baseplate fixation using hybrid configurations of locked and unlocked peripheral screws. J Orthop Traumatol. 2017;18(3):221–8. https://doi.org/10.1007/s10195-016-0438-3.

48. Roche C, DiGeorgio C, Yegres J, VanDeven J, Stroud N, Flurin PH, Wright T, Cheung E, Zuckerman JD. Impact of screw length and screw quantity on reverse total shoulder arthroplasty glenoid fixation for 2 different sizes of glenoid baseplates. JSES Open Access. 2019;3(4):296–303. https://doi.org/10.1016/j.jses.2019.08.006.

49. Humphrey CS, Kelly JD 2nd, Norris TR. Optimizing glenosphere position and fixation in reverse shoulder arthroplasty, part two: the three-column concept. J Shoulder Elb Surg. 2008;17(4):595–601. https://doi.org/10.1016/j.jse.2008.05.038.

50. Sirveaux F, Favard L, Oudet D, Huquet D, Walch G, Mole D. Grammont inverted total shoulder arthroplasty in the treatment of glenohumeral osteoarthritis with massive rupture of the cuff. Results of a multicentre study of 80 shoulders. J Bone Jt Surg Br. 2004;86(3):388–95. https://doi.org/10.1302/0301-620x.86b3.14024.

51. Falaise V, Levigne C, Favard L, Sofec. Scapular notching in reverse shoulder arthroplasties: the influence of glenometaphyseal angle. Orthop Traumatol Surg Res. 2011;97(6 Suppl):S131–7. https://doi.org/10.1016/j.otsr.2011.06.007.

52. Boileau P, Moineau G, Roussanne Y, O'Shea K. Bony increased-offset reversed shoulder arthroplasty: minimizing scapular impingement while maximizing glenoid fixation. Clin Orthop Relat Res. 2011;469(9):2558–67. https://doi.org/10.1007/s11999-011-1775-4.

53. Berhouet J, Garaud P, Favard L. Evaluation of the role of glenosphere design and humeral component retroversion in avoiding scapular notching during reverse shoulder arthroplasty. J Shoulder Elb Surg. 2014;23(2):151–8. https://doi.org/10.1016/j.jse.2013.05.009.

54. Frankle M, Levy JC, Pupello D, Siegal S, Saleem A, Mighell M, Vasey M. The reverse shoulder prosthesis for glenohumeral arthritis associated with severe rotator cuff deficiency. A minimum 2-year follow-up study of 60 patients surgical technique. J Bone Jt Surg Am. 2006;88(Suppl 1 Pt 2):178–90. https://doi.org/10.2106/JBJS.F.00123.

55. Valenti P, Sauzieres P, Katz D, Kalouche I, Kilinc AS. Do less medialized reverse shoulder prostheses increase motion and reduce notching? Clin Orthop Relat Res. 2011;469(9):2550–7. https://doi.org/10.1007/s11999-011-1844-8.

56. Werner BS, Chaoui J, Walch G. The influence of humeral neck shaft angle and glenoid lateralization on range of motion in reverse shoulder arthroplasty. J Shoulder Elb Surg. 2017;26(10):1726–31. https://doi.org/10.1016/j.jse.2017.03.032.

57. Collotte P, Bercik M, Vieira TD, Walch G. Long-term reverse total shoulder arthroplasty outcomes: the effect of the inferior shifting of glenoid component fixation. Clin Orthop Surg. 2021;13(4):505–12. https://doi.org/10.4055/cios20245.

58. Young AA, Walch G, Pape G, Gohlke F, Favard L. Secondary rotator cuff dysfunction following total shoulder arthroplasty for primary glenohumeral osteoarthritis: results of a multicenter study with more than 5 years of follow-up. J Bone Jt Surg Am. 2012;94(8):685–93. https://doi.org/10.2106/JBJS.J.00727.

59. Goetti P, Denard PJ, Collin P, Ibrahim M, Mazzolari A, Ladermann A. Biomechanics of anatomic and reverse shoulder arthroplasty. EFORT

Open Rev. 2021;6(10):918–31. https://doi.org/10.1302/2058-5241.6.210014.

60. Collins D, Tencer A, Sidles J, Matsen F 3rd. Edge displacement and deformation of glenoid components in response to eccentric loading. The effect of preparation of the glenoid bone. J Bone Jt Surg Am. 1992;74(4):501–7.

61. Pinkas D, Wiater B, Wiater JM. The glenoid component in anatomic shoulder arthroplasty. J Am Acad Orthop Surg. 2015;23(5):317–26. https://doi.org/10.5435/JAAOS-D-13-00208.

62. Gillespie R, Lyons R, Lazarus M. Eccentric reaming in total shoulder arthroplasty: a cadaveric study. Orthopedics. 2009;32(1):21. https://doi.org/10.3928/01477447-20090101-07.

63. Boileau P, Avidor C, Krishnan SG, Walch G, Kempf JF, Mole D. Cemented polyethylene versus uncemented metal-backed glenoid components in total shoulder arthroplasty: a prospective, double-blind, randomized study. J Shoulder Elb Surg. 2002;11(4):351–9. https://doi.org/10.1067/mse.2002.125807.

64. Gagliano JR, Helms SM, Colbath GP, Przestrzelski BT, Hawkins RJ, DesJardins JD. A comparison of onlay versus inlay glenoid component loosening in total shoulder arthroplasty. J Shoulder Elb Surg. 2017;26(7):1113–20. https://doi.org/10.1016/j.jse.2017.01.018.

65. Szabo I, Buscayret F, Edwards TB, Nemoz C, Boileau P, Walch G. Radiographic comparison of flat-back and convex-back glenoid components in total shoulder arthroplasty. J Shoulder Elb Surg. 2005;14(6):636–42. https://doi.org/10.1016/j.jse.2005.05.004.

66. Familiari F, Rojas J, Nedim Doral M, Huri G, McFarland EG. Reverse total shoulder arthroplasty. EFORT Open Rev. 2018;3(2):58–69. https://doi.org/10.1302/2058-5241.3.170044.

Clara de Campos Azevedo, Carlos Maia Dias, and Ana Catarina Ângelo

31.1 Introduction

Reverse total shoulder arthroplasty (RSA) was originally designed to improve the outcomes of patients who had glenohumeral osteoarthritis and a massive irreparable rotator cuff tear (RCT) and avoid the complications of anatomic total shoulder arthroplasty (aTSA) in this setting [1], whereas aTSA was the preferred treatment choice for patients with glenohumeral osteoarthritis and an intact rotator cuff. In recent years, the use of RSA has increased dramatically, and the good clinical outcomes have led surgeons to expand the indications beyond massive RCT arthropathy, including the treatment of massive irreparable RCTs without arthropathy, acute proximal humerus fractures, and fracture sequelae, revision surgery and revision shoulder arthroplasty, and the treatment of glenohumeral osteoarthritis with an intact rotator cuff.

In the present chapter, the rationale, results, and current indications for RSA in patients with primary glenohumeral osteoarthritis and an intact rotator cuff are reviewed and discussed.

C. de Campos Azevedo (✉) · A. C. Ângelo
Hospital dos SAMS de Lisboa, Lisbon, Portugal

Hospital CUF Tejo, Lisbon, Portugal

C. Maia Dias
Hospital CUF Tejo, Lisbon, Portugal

31.2 Biomechanical Rationale for Anatomic or Reverse Total Shoulder Arthroplasty in Patients with an Intact Rotator Cuff

The purpose of aTSA in the treatment of glenohumeral osteoarthritis is to replace the diseased glenohumeral joint, reestablish the anatomy, and restore painless shoulder function. One of the most important aspects that must be acknowledged when aiming to reestablish the anatomy of the glenohumeral joint is that the shoulder is an anatomically flawed joint, where the ball is too large for the socket, and therefore there is a high dependence on the labrum, capsule, ligaments, rotator cuff muscles, and scapular stabilizers to maintain glenohumeral stability. The surrounding soft tissues come into play together with the humerus, sternum, thorax, clavicle, and scapula, forming an anatomically complex joint, the "shoulder articular complex," that includes the glenohumeral joint, the acromioclavicular joint, the scapulothoracic joint, the sternoclavicular joint, and the subacromial space. To achieve maximum movement with minimum instability, the center of rotation (CoR) of the glenohumeral joint must remain in a "physiological box" throughout the range of motion (Fig. 31.1), which requires the preservation of (1) the combined action of the vertical and horizontal glenohumeral force couples, (2) the scapular force cou-

© ISAKOS 2023
A. D. Mazzocca et al. (eds.), *Shoulder Arthritis across the Life Span*,
https://doi.org/10.1007/978-3-031-33298-2_31

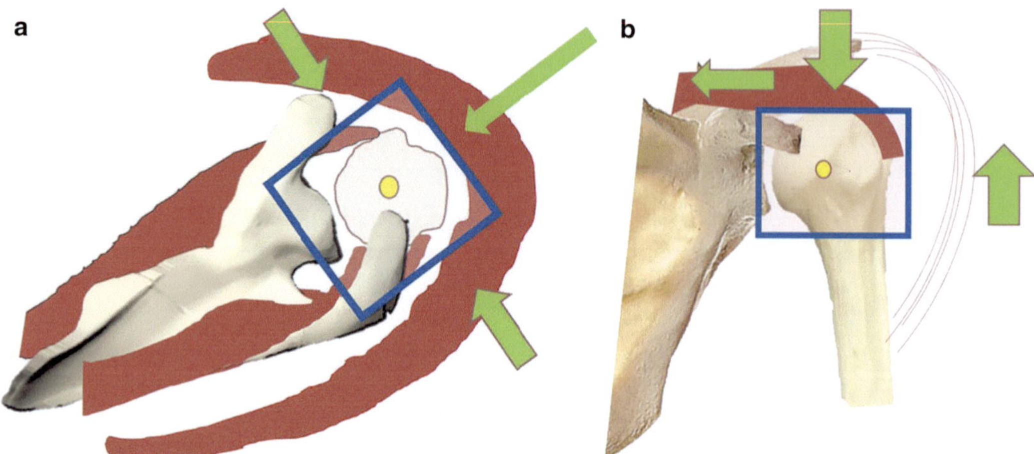

Fig. 31.1 Representation of the vertical and horizontal force couples. The green arrows represent the force couples in the coronal (**a**) and axial (**b**) planes that balance to keep the humeral head inside a "physiological box" (blue lined square). (**a**) **Vertical stability**—The upward deltoid pulling force is counteracted by the contracted superior cuff and by the superior capsule. Simultaneously, the rotator cuff pulls the head of the humerus toward the glenoid concavity, participating in the negative pressure generated by the surrounding labrum and capsuloligamentous structures. (**b**) **Horizontal stability**—The anterior cuff and capsule balance with the posterior cuff and capsule, keeping the humeral head centered in the glenoid, while simultaneously pulling the humeral head toward the center of the glenoid concavity

ples, (3) the scapulohumeral rhythm and scapular motion, and (4) the kinetic chain.

When aTSA is performed, only the glenohumeral bone and cartilage interface is replaced. Therefore, from the biomechanical and anatomical standpoints, the ideal indication for aTSA would be osteoarthritis of the glenohumeral joint in a patient with preserved vertical and horizontal force couples, with an intact rotator cuff and intact scapulohumeral rhythm. However, as Walch and colleagues previously acknowledged [2], there is a dynamic, progressive component in the natural history of glenohumeral osteoarthritis, which is probably related to rotator cuff muscular imbalance. Furthermore, the prevalence of RCTs increases with age, ranging from 30 to 80% for the population aged 60–80 years, respectively [3, 4]. Therefore, replacing the glenohumeral bony interface alone may be insufficient to effectively treat primary glenohumeral osteoarthritis, even in the setting of an intact rotator cuff

preoperatively. The high rate of complications of aTSA reported in the long-term follow-up study by Evans et al. [5] seems to further confirm this theory. This study showed a 100% rate of aseptic glenoid loosening and an 83.2% rate of RCTs 20 years after aTSA and high rates of glenoid loosening, humeral head migration, and declining patient outcomes 10 years after aTSA. The complication rate 20 years after aTSA may be less concerning in elderly patients who will probably not need a revision in their lifetime, whereas the 10-year complication rate of aTSA raises important concerns in younger patients who will probably require complex revision surgeries [5].

When RSA is performed, the glenohumeral bony interface alone is replaced as well, but the CoR of the new prosthetic glenohumeral joint is medialized and the humerus is distalized. The RSA restores the balance of the vertical force couples by providing a fulcrum to the deltoid pulling vector, and shoulder forward flexion is

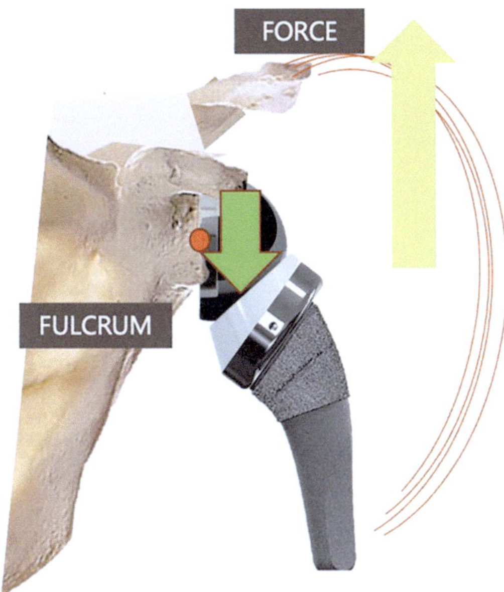

Fig. 31.2 Representation of the balanced vertical force couple in a reverse total shoulder arthroplasty (RSA). The vertical pulling vector (yellow arrow) of the deltoid muscle (orange curved lines) is counteracted by the fulcrum produced by the glenosphere-insert interface with the CoR (orange dot) of the new prosthetic glenohumeral joint and the distalized humerus

restored even in the setting of a RCT (Fig. 31.2). The semi-constrictive design of the RSA contributes to stabilize the joint throughout the range of motion (ROM). In studies using RSA designs that lateralize the humerus, increased internal rotation postoperatively has been reported, even in studies where no repair of the subscapularis tendon was performed.

Therefore, considering the biomechanics of the aTSA and RSA and the natural history of glenohumeral osteoarthritis, theoretically a more favorable and durable outcome might be achievable by using RSA compared to aTSA in the treatment of osteoarthritis in patients with an intact rotator cuff.

31.3 Clinical Rationale for RSA in Patients with an Intact Rotator Cuff

The trend toward RSA has increased in recent years, with the purpose of avoiding the most frequently reported complications after aTSA, and RSA has been advocated by several authors in the subsets of patients with an intact rotator cuff but who present a higher risk of complications after aTSA, particularly subscapularis or posterosuperior rotator cuff tendon failure and aseptic glenoid loosening. Indeed, aTSA has shown rates of clinical and subclinical subscapularis tendon failures as high as 50% [6], and several authors have shown the importance of subscapularis tendon-sparing approaches for achieving better outcomes after aTSA [7]. Conversely, modern lateralized RSA designs have been shown to be more forgiving regarding subscapularis tendon insufficiency, with reported decreased rates of instability compared to either classic Grammont RSA designs or aTSA [1]. Furthermore, RSA seems to perform better than aTSA in patients with an established glenoid deformity. Indeed, some studies have shown a tendency to less favorable outcomes after aTSA in patients who have an established glenoid bone deformity [8, 9], particularly in patients with Walch type B2 glenoids [10]. Therefore, the modified Walch classification for glenoid morphology in the setting of glenohumeral osteoarthritis [11] must be carefully considered when choosing between aTSA and RSA. Indeed, glenoid morphology has increasingly become one of the most consensual guides for the decision between aTSA and RSA, with primary glenohumeral osteoarthritis with advanced glenoid retroversion currently being the primary indication for RSA in patients with no RCTs (Fig. 31.3) [12].

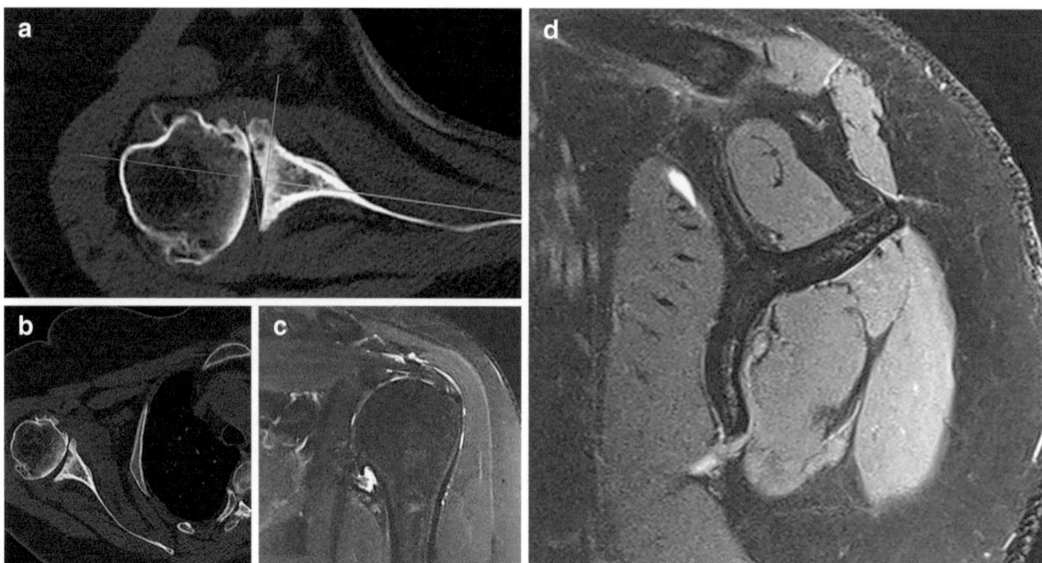

Fig. 31.3 Preoperative imaging study of a patient with a primary glenohumeral osteoarthritis and an intact rotator cuff. (**a**, **b**) Axial views of the preoperative computed tomography scan, showing a posteriorly decentered humeral head and a retroverted glenoid, as a result of an imbalanced horizontal force couple; (**c**) T2_fs coronal view of the magnetic resonance imaging (MRI) of the same shoulder, showing an intact superior rotator cuff; (**d**) T2_fs MRI sagittal view, showing the absence of muscle belly atrophy of each of the four rotator cuff muscles

31.4 Clinical Results of RSA in Patients with an Intact Rotator Cuff

Early clinical studies comparing patients treated with aTSA and RSA included different patient populations and different indications and either found that aTSA provided better outcomes than RSA [13–15] or that aTSA provided similar results than RSA [16–18]. However, recent studies comparing patients treated with aTSA and RSA in similar patient populations (similar average ages) and similar indications (glenohumeral osteoarthritis with an intact rotator cuff) have consistently shown that overall both procedures produce similar outcomes [19–22].

Merolla et al. [22] conducted a multicenter retrospective cohort study of 83 consecutive shoulders in patients with an average age of 71.6 years (range, 68–72 years), who had glenohumeral osteoarthritis and an intact rotator cuff. Forty-seven shoulders with aTSA (average age, 70 years; range 68–72) were compared with 36 shoulders with an RSA (average age, 74 years; range 69–75), at a minimum follow-up of 2 years (average follow-up, 28.8 months). The subgroup analysis of patients aged 70 years or older (26 patients with aTSA versus 32 patients with RSA) showed that the postoperative active forward elevation (170° versus 160°, $p = 0.072$), external rotation (22.5° versus 20°, $p = 0.269$), and internal rotation (6 versus 8 points, $p = 0.854$) were similar between the subgroups, whereas the postoperative active abduction was higher in the aTSA subgroup (160° versus 150°, $p = 0.006$). The RSA subgroup had significantly lower preoperative ROM scores except for external rotation (10° versus 7.5°, $p = 0.334$). The complication and revision rates did not significantly differ between the subgroups. The authors concluded that, overall, both aTSA and RSA produced good clinical midterm outcomes in patients aged 70 years or older, with an intact rotator cuff.

Haritinian et al. [19] conducted a single-surgeon retrospective cohort study that included patients with osteoarthritis and an intact rotator cuff. Thirty-nine patients treated with aTSA (average age, 68 years) were compared with 12 patients treated with RSA (average age, 71 years) at a minimum follow-up of 2 years. Preoperatively, the average external rotation, internal rotation, and Constant score (CS) were significantly higher in the aTSA group than in the RSA group (external rotation, +5° versus −4°, p = 0.037; internal rotation, 2.2 versus 0.8 points, p = 0.007; CS, 30 versus 22 points, p = 0.021, respectively). However, there were no significant differences between the aTSA and RSA groups in either the postoperative ROM or CS (71 versus 67 points) or in the improvements in the average ROM or CS (41 versus 45.5 points). The proportion of Walch type B glenoids was higher in the RSA group (Walch type A 33%, Walch type B 67%) compared with the aTSA group (Walch type A 51%, Walch type B 49%). In patients with Walch type B glenoids, the glenoid retroversion was significantly higher in the RSA group (25° versus 14°, p = 0.026). Patient satisfaction was similarly high in patients treated with aTSA and RSA, with 68% and 75% reporting being very satisfied and 28% and 17% reporting being satisfied, respectively.

Wright et al. [21] conducted a single-institution retrospective cohort study that included patients who had osteoarthritis with no full-thickness RCT and had less than 90° of forward elevation. One hundred and two patients treated with aTSA (average age, 77 years) were compared with 33 patients treated with RSA (average age, 78 years). There was a significant difference in the proportion of Walch type B3 glenoids between the RSA and aTSA groups (18% versus 2%, p = 0.001). At final follow-up, 30 patients were deceased (26 in the aTSA and 4 in the RSA group), others declined to participate in the clinical assessment or were lost to follow-up, and the patient-reported outcome measures (PROMs) were compared between 46 patients with aTSA (45% of all patients in the aTSA group) and 21 patients with RSA (64% of all patients in the RSA group). The authors found no significant difference in PROMs, complication rate, or revision surgery rate between patients treated with aTSA and RSA (complications, 13.7% versus 12.1%, p = 0.810; reoperations, 6.9% versus 3.0%, p = 0.418), at a minimum follow-up of 2 years (average, 81 months). The most frequent complication in the aTSA group was rotator cuff tear (11 cases), and most reoperations after aTSA were related to cuff dysfunction. The authors concluded that RSA can be considered to manage glenohumeral osteoarthritis in elderly patients with an intact rotator cuff and limited preoperative motion as it can achieve good clinical results, equivalent to aTSA. The authors highlighted the high rate of rotator cuff insufficiency at midterm follow-up in patients treated with aTSA and that this should be considered in the decision-making between the two treatment options because of the similar outcomes and patient satisfaction rates seen with RSA and aTSA.

Friedman et al. [20] conducted an international multi-institutional database study that compared 370 patients treated with aTSA with 370 patients treated with RSA who had an intact rotator cuff, osteoarthritis, and no previous surgery and who were matched for age (average, 73 years), sex, body mass index (BMI), and length of follow-up. No significant differences at a minimum follow-up of 2 years (average, 41 months) were found postoperatively between the aTSA and RSA group, either in the PROMs (CS, 71.0 versus 71.8; American Shoulder and Elbow Surgeons Score, 84.9 versus 86.7; University of California at Los Angeles Shoulder Score, 30.8 versus 31.1; and Simple Shoulder Test, 10.1 versus 10.5) or in active abduction and forward elevation, even though preoperatively the patients who underwent RSA had worse preoperative active abduction and forward elevation and increased glenoid bone deformity compared to patients who underwent aTSA. The authors reported that the average improvement in active forward elevation was significantly greater in the RSA than in the aTSA group (55.8° versus 47.5°, respectively; p = 0.0125) and, conversely, that the average postoperative active external rotation was significantly greater in the aTSA than in the RSA group (53° versus 38°, respectively; p = 0.0001), and this exceeded the minimal clinically importance difference (MCID). However, the clinical relevance of the average difference in active external rotation found between groups could be considered arguable. Furthermore, higher complication rates were found in the aTSA group (subscapularis tendon failure, RCTs, or aseptic glenoid loosening) compared to the RSA group (scapular and acromial fractures or instability), with statistical significance, and the revision rates were trending toward a statistical difference (3.2% versus 1.4%, $p = 0.08$). Nevertheless, pain relief was excellent, and patient satisfaction was high in both groups (94% and 93%), and the authors concluded that RSA is a viable treatment option in patients with an intact rotator cuff and offering similar clinical outcomes.

31.5 Summary

Early evidence suggested that RSA had higher complication and revision rates, but complication rates have decreased as RSA indications have expanded, experience has increased, and RSA designs have improved. The most recent studies comparing the outcomes of patients over 70 years of age with glenohumeral osteoarthritis and an intact rotator cuff treated with aTSA and RSA show that both procedures achieve similarly good clinical results, despite RSA being used in patients with worse preoperative outcome scores and more severe glenoid deformity. Therefore, RSA is a reasonable and reliable option to treat primary glenohumeral osteoarthritis in the elderly with an intact rotator cuff.

References

1. Kozak T, Bauer S, Walch G, Al-Karawi S, Blakeney W. An update on reverse total shoulder arthroplasty: current indications, new designs, same old problems. EFORT Open Rev. 2021;6(3):189–201.
2. Domos P, Checchia CS, Walch G. Walch B0 glenoid: pre-osteoarthritic posterior subluxation of the humeral head. J Shoulder Elb Surg. 2018;27(1):181–8.
3. Khatri C, Ahmed I, Parsons H, Smith NA, Lawrence TM, Modi CS, et al. The natural history of full-thickness rotator cuff tears in randomized controlled trials: a systematic review and meta-analysis. Am J Sports Med. 2019;47(7):1734–43.
4. Keener JD, Patterson BM, Orvets N, Chamberlain AM. Degenerative rotator cuff tears: refining surgical indications based on natural history data. J Am Acad Orthop Surg. 2019;27(5):156–65.
5. Evans JP, Batten T, Bird J, Thomas WJ, Kitson JB, Smith CD. Survival of the Aequalis total shoulder replacement at a minimum 20-year follow-up: a clinical and radiographic study. J Shoulder Elb Surg. 2021;30(10):2355–60.
6. Entezari V, Henry T, Zmistowski B, Sheth M, Nicholson T, Namdari S. Clinically significant subscapularis failure after anatomic shoulder arthroplasty: is it worth repairing? J Shoulder Elb Surg. 2020;29(9):1831–5.
7. Lee S, Sardar H, Horner NS, Al Mana L, Miller BS, Khan M, et al. Subscapularis-sparing approaches in shoulder arthroplasty: a systematic review. J Orthop. 2021;24:165–72.
8. Iannotti JP, Norris TR. Influence of preoperative factors on outcome of shoulder arthroplasty for glenohumeral osteoarthritis. J Bone Jt Surg Am. 2003;85(2):251–8.
9. Walch G, Moraga C, Young A, Castellanos-Rosas J. Results of anatomic nonconstrained prosthesis in primary osteoarthritis with biconcave glenoid. J Shoulder Elb Surg. 2012;21(11):1526–33.
10. Kleim BD, Garving C, Brunner UH. RSA, TSA and PyC hemi-prostheses: comparing indications and clinical outcomes using a second-generation modular short-stem shoulder prosthesis. Arch Orthop Trauma Surg. 2021;141(10):1639–48.
11. Bercik MJ, Kruse K 2nd, Yalizis M, Gauci MO, Chaoui J, Walch G. A modification to the Walch classification of the glenoid in primary glenohumeral osteoarthritis using three-dimensional imaging. J Shoulder Elb Surg. 2016;25(10):1601–6.
12. McClatchy SG, Heise GM, Mihalko WM, Azar FM, Smith RA, Witte DH, et al. Effect of deltoid volume on range of motion and patient-reported outcomes following reverse total shoulder arthroplasty in rotator cuff-intact and rotator cuff-deficient conditions. Shoulder Elb. 2022;14(1):24–9.
13. Ponce BA, Oladeji LO, Rogers ME, Menendez ME. Comparative analysis of anatomic and reverse total shoulder arthroplasty: in-hospital outcomes and costs. J Shoulder Elb Surg. 2015;24(3):460–7.
14. Flurin PH, Marczuk Y, Janout M, Wright TW, Zuckerman J, Roche CP. Comparison of outcomes using anatomic and reverse total shoulder arthroplasty. Bull Hosp Jt Dis. 2013;71(Suppl 2):101–7.
15. Friedman RJ, Eichinger J, Schoch B, Wright T, Zuckerman J, Flurin PH, et al. Preoperative parameters that predict postoperative patient-reported outcome measures and range of motion with anatomic and reverse total shoulder arthroplasty. JSES Open Access. 2019;3(4):266–72.

16. Kiet TK, Feeley BT, Naimark M, Gajiu T, Hall SL, Chung TT, et al. Outcomes after shoulder replacement: comparison between reverse and anatomic total shoulder arthroplasty. J Shoulder Elb Surg. 2015;24(2):179–85.
17. Flynn L, Patrick MR, Roche C, Zuckerman JD, Flurin PH, Crosby L, et al. Anatomical and reverse shoulder arthroplasty utilizing a single implant system with a platform stem: a prospective observational study with midterm follow-up. Shoulder Elb. 2020;12(5):330–7.
18. Parada SA, Flurin PH, Wright TW, Zuckerman JD, Elwell JA, Roche CP, et al. Comparison of complication types and rates associated with anatomic and reverse total shoulder arthroplasty. J Shoulder Elb Surg. 2021;30(4):811–8.
19. Haritinian EG, Belgaid V, Lino T, Nové-Josserand L. Reverse versus anatomical shoulder arthroplasty in patients with intact rotator cuff. Int Orthop. 2020;44(11):2395–405.
20. Friedman RJ, Schoch B, Eichinger JK, Flurin P, Wright T, Zuckerman J, et al. Anatomic and reverse total shoulder arthroplasty outcomes in patients with an intact rotator cuff and no previous surgery. J Shoulder Elb Surg. 2022;31(3):e132.
21. Wright MA, Keener JD, Chamberlain AM. Comparison of clinical outcomes after anatomic total shoulder arthroplasty and reverse shoulder arthroplasty in patients 70 years and older with glenohumeral osteoarthritis and an intact rotator cuff. J Am Acad Orthop Surg. 2020;28(5):e222–e9.
22. Merolla G, De Cupis M, Walch G, De Cupis V, Fabbri E, Franceschi F, et al. Pre-operative factors affecting the indications for anatomical and reverse total shoulder arthroplasty in primary osteoarthritis and outcome comparison in patients aged seventy years and older. Int Orthop. 2020;44(6):1131–41.

Tyler R. Johnston, Vivian Chen, and Ranjan Gupta

32.1 Introduction

Prior to the development of the reverse total shoulder arthroplasty (rTSA) prosthesis, anatomic shoulder replacement served as the only total shoulder arthroplasty option for treatment of advanced glenohumeral arthrosis, irrespective of patient age. In the elderly patient population particularly, concerns of patient selection, bone quality, bone loss, and soft tissue balancing come to a head, and anatomic total shoulder arthroplasty (aTSA) presents unique challenges that distinguish this surgical intervention as one of the most challenging surgeries confronted by upper extremity specialists.

On the other hand, since the introduction of rTSA, these designs have progressively gained acceptance and adoption with widespread implant availability as well as technical ease and implant refinements, corroborated by outcomes data. Accordingly, the threshold for performing a reverse has significantly decreased, resulting in more elderly patients receiving rTSAs over aTSAs. Nonetheless, aTSAs are still routinely performed in elderly patients and remain a powerful treatment option for the appropriately selected patient. Importantly, unlike an rTSA, in order for an aTSA to be successful, every aspect of the surgery, including patient selection, medical optimization, bone stock management, soft tissue integrity and handling, as well as postoperative patient compliance, must all be skillfully managed. Additionally, aTSA maintains important roles in specific patient subgroups including those with Parkinson's disease and/or history of stroke. Therefore, the ideal aTSA candidate is a carefully selected patient who the treating surgeon expects to benefit from the advantages of the implant design (compared to rTSA), diagnosed with primary osteoarthritis of the shoulder with minimal rotator cuff disease, healthy bone quality, few medical comorbidities, and robust rehabilitation capacity.

T. R. Johnston
Division of Sports Medicine, Department of Orthopaedic Surgery, Irvine Medical Center, University of California, Irvine, CA, USA
e-mail: tjohnst2@hs.uci.edu

V. Chen
Department of Orthopaedic Surgery, Irvine Medical Center, University of California, Irvine, CA, USA
e-mail: vychen1@hs.uci.edu

R. Gupta (✉)
Departments of Orthopaedic Surgery, Anatomy and Neurobiology, and Biomedical Engineering, Zeta Chapter of Alpha Omega Alpha Honor Medical Society, University of California, Irvine, CA, USA
e-mail: ranjang@hs.uci.edu

32.2 Concerns for aTSA

Primary considerations for aTSA in the elderly can be broken down into four principle categories: (1) medical comorbidities, (2) loss of bone mass, (3) soft tissue degeneration, and (4) patient compliance.

© ISAKOS 2023
A. D. Mazzocca et al. (eds.), *Shoulder Arthritis across the Life Span*,
https://doi.org/10.1007/978-3-031-33298-2_32

32.2.1 Medical Comorbidities

Due to decreased physiologic reserve across all organ systems, elderly patients are more predisposed to perioperative complications, even in the absence of any significant underlying pathology. Richetti et al. noted that although frank mortality of patients undergoing aTSA remains low even in the elderly demographic, they are susceptible to potentially debilitating systemic postoperative complications including delirium, urinary tract infections, pulmonary embolism, and myocardial infarction. Furthermore, elderly patients were noted to have increased transfusion requirements and longer length of hospital stay with a decreased number of direct to home discharges.

In 2014, Griffin et al. conducted a retrospective analysis of perioperative complications in 58,790 patients who had undergone shoulder arthroplasty (hemi and total) [1]. After stratifying patients by age, they observed that increased age was associated with higher rates of perioperative mortality, longer length of stay, as well as postoperative anemia. Koh et al. also published similar findings based on their review of 30-day postoperative complications in the NSQIP database that included 11,450 patients who underwent hemi, aTSA, or rTSA. Researchers found that increased age was a strong predictor for increased postoperative complications, length of stay, and unplanned readmissions across all types of shoulder arthroplasty, with an average postop hospital stay of 2.6 days and readmission rate of 5.5% for patients >80 years. These elderly patients exhibited a 15.3% 30-day postoperative complication rate, as compared to 8.2% and 6.8% in younger patient groups (51–79 years and < 50 years, respectively).

Thus, even relatively healthy elderly patients have a significantly increased perioperative risk profile and, therefore, necessitate thorough medical optimization prior to surgery. Elderly patients who have multiple comorbidities that delay healing or further increase risk of postoperative complications—such as history of cardiac and/or pulmonary disease, renal dysfunction, and poor diabetes control—are poor candidates for aTSA. While these perioperative risks by definition are present for all types of surgical treatments for shoulder arthritis to some degree (associated with anesthetic administration, surgical duration, fluid shifts, reduced mobility, and duration of hospital stay), they must be even more carefully considered in the case of aTSA in the elderly population given the significant postoperative recovery and rehabilitation required and in light of potential future need for return to the operating room for additional procedures such as conversion to rTSA in the event of rotator cuff failure or component revision/explant for technical complications or infection. Accordingly, the ideal elderly candidate for aTSA should be motivated and have few medical comorbidities so as to facilitate success after surgery, while potential tolerance of additional future surgeries must also be critically evaluated by the treating surgeon.

32.2.2 Loss of Bone Mass

In patients >50 years, particularly females, the incidence of osteoporosis and osteopenia continues to rise globally [2]. Several factors have been linked to increased osteoporosis including early menopause, age, low BMI, and vitamin D deficiency. Osteoporotic patients who undergo elective orthopedic surgeries are at higher risks for complications including aseptic loosening, periprosthetic fractures, and need for revision surgeries.

Although osteoporosis can be diagnosed with a dual-energy x-ray absorptiometry (DEXA) scan and other means, orthopedic patients do not routinely receive preoperative DEXA scans or formal osteoporosis evaluation. In a 2020 retrospective case review conducted at the University of Wisconsin, Bernatz et al. reported that osteoporosis is often underdiagnosed and undertreated in patients undergoing shoulder arthroplasty. While 68% of patients met criteria for bone mineral density screening, only 12% of patients received a DEXA scan. Similarly, while 32% of patients met National Osteoporosis Foundation (NOF) criteria for pharmacological treatment, only 7% were medically treated.

Maier et al. observed similar findings when they conducted a 14-question survey investigating orthopedic surgeon attitudes toward osteoporosis and hip arthroplasty. Although 60% of surgeons stated that low bone mineral density is a reason to re-evaluate preoperative planning, only 4% of surgeons routinely performed bone mineral density measurements preoperatively. This persistent gap between available evidence, surgeon beliefs, and clinical practice with regard to preoperative bone health management disproportionately impacts elderly patients undergoing arthroplasty procedures. Surgeons should work to bridge this practice gap by understanding risk factors for osteoporosis and critically examining proximal humerus cortical thickness (Tingart or Deltoid Tuberosity Index methods) of planned surgical patients, which has been shown to correlate with bone mineral density and decreases with age [3, 4].

Bone quality optimization can help reduce risk of surgical complications, especially in the elderly population already at increased risk of postoperative complications and implant failure in aTSA where implant bony integration is critical. Osteoporosis treatment guidelines should follow World Health Organization (WHO) and NOF recommendations. Current literature suggests that perioperative bisphosphonate use helps facilitate bony integration of prosthetics, reduces perioperative bone loss, and, by extension, reduces overall fracture risk [5]. Other medical treatments, such as denosumab and teriparatide, have not been sufficiently studied to determine their potential perioperative benefits. Thus, if patients meet criteria for bisphosphonate treatment, they should receive pharmacological treatment preoperatively to best help promote bony healing/fixation and reduce risk of complications.

Tailoring implants to accommodate bone loss can also further facilitate success of aTSA. Specifically, in terms of humeral implants, current guidelines (as published in the *Journal of Bone and Joint Surgery*) designate that stemless or canal-sparing implants are contraindicated in patients with metaphyseal bone deficiencies. Therefore, if there is clinical suspicion of osteoporosis, either evident on preoperative CT, X-ray, or DEXA scans, surgeons should utilize stemmed prosthesis. In patients with significant humeral bone loss or intraoperative surgeon concern for bone quality based on broach feel/stability, a cemented stemmed prosthesis should also be strongly considered.

With respect to the glenoid, while available literature has yet to describe a direct correlation between osteoporosis and glenoid bone stock or aTSA outcomes, an association is logical. Primary surgical concern for the glenoid in aTSA in the elderly patient, as in all patient subgroups, continues to be optimizing glenoid fixation and avoiding loosening in the setting of complex patterns of glenoid erosion/bone loss. Foruria et al. found that glenoid bone deficiency was common in their case series of shoulders over age 80 treated with aTSA, with 9/50 glenoids requiring bone grafting augmentation. Furthermore, posterior glenoid bone deficiency and treatment of glenoid defect with cancellous impaction grafting were associated with subsequent glenoid loosening. On the other hand, no glenoids treated with corticocancellous bone grafting demonstrated loosening during follow-up. Accordingly, although the authors noted sample size limitations, they highlighted the association of preoperative glenoid erosion and bone grafting technique (non-corticocancellous) with component loosening and poorer patient outcomes.

To ensure aTSA success in the elderly population, surgeons should carefully scrutinize patient selection and work to optimize patient factors as much as possible preoperatively. Furthermore, implant choice, bone preparation techniques, and fixation strategies should be carefully selected that are best able to compensate for osteoporotic bone and glenoid bone deficiencies.

32.2.3 Soft Tissue Balancing

Rotator cuff tears (RCTs) and disease are among the most widespread musculoskeletal problems, particularly among older patients. Some studies have found an incidence of RCTs as high as 80% in patients >80 years old. In addition to a higher prevalence of RCTs, advancing age is also associated with more severe tears as well as increased Goutallier grades of muscle fatty infiltration.

As aTSA implants rely on intact rotator cuff musculature to recreate native shoulder biomechanics and postoperative range of motion, patients with rotator cuff deficiency and advanced stages of fatty infiltration are unfortunately relegated to poor outcomes with this implant design. Rotator cuff muscles function as the dynamic stabilizers of the glenohumeral joint, responsible for humeral head centering. Accordingly, when there is insufficient functional rotator cuff to oppose deltoid forces, a stable center of humeral head rotation is not attainable, and the humeral head migrates superiorly. In prosthetic shoulders, this dynamic superior migration increases shear forces and eccentric loading on the glenoid component and can contribute to glenoid loosening via the so-called rocking-horse phenomenon [6].

Furthermore, available evidence has demonstrated significant rotator cuff tear susceptibility following aTSA. In a systematic review of aTSA across all age ranges, Levy et al. noted a 17.9% rate of moderate to severe humeral head radiographic superior migration at an average follow-up of 6.6 years in 1259 patients without preoperative tears, with an 11.3% rate of documented RCTs. This rate is similar to the 16.8% rate Young et al. found in a multicenter retrospective study that included 518 shoulders with 5-year radiographic follow-up. Due to this risk of subsequent rotator cuff dysfunction, particularly in the elderly population who have globally increased rates and severity of rotator cuff disease, aTSAs should be reserved for patients with minimal preexisting rotator cuff disease. With careful selection criteria, Jensen et al. recently demonstrated that patients 70 years of age and older have the capacity to have excellent clinical and radiographic outcomes at short-term (3.3-year average) follow-up, with only a 1.3% rate of symptomatic rotator cuff tears confirmed with advanced imaging and 0.5% rate of revision for cuff tear (2021). Thus, while it is imperative that patients are counseled preoperatively regarding risks and functional consequences of future rotator cuff disease in the setting of aTSA, appropriate patient selection and surgical technique can yield impressive results with dramatic improvements in pain, function, and motion.

It is also noteworthy that while larger preoperative RCTs often lead to aTSA clinical and radiographic failures, minor or incomplete RCTs have been shown to maintain shoulder ROM and implant integrity following aTSA. Simone et al. conducted a retrospective study of patients with a mean age of 73 years who had intraoperatively repaired RCTs during aTSA. Of the 33 patients, 5 patients experienced postoperative complications including radiographic evidence of loosening and symptomatic instability, with 4 patients requiring revision to rTSA. All five patients had medium or large rotator cuff tears (1–3 cm and 3–5 cm). Accordingly, the team concluded that aTSAs can still achieve acceptable postoperative outcomes in stable shoulders with repaired partial RCTs, but recommended rTSA consideration for those with tears larger than >1 cm and in older, less active patients.

These findings are consistent with work by Choate et al. and Edwards et al. evaluating the influence of rotator cuff disease on results of aTSA. Both retrospective studies reported that partial-thickness tears, especially those found in the supraspinatus, did not have a statistically significant negative impact on postoperative outcomes. Edwards et al. noted that even full-thickness tears confined to the supraspinatus only with minimal retraction performed similarly to shoulders without RCTs with regard to Constant and Murley scores. However, both studies noted that increased infraspinatus Goutallier grades were correlated with decreased postoperative ROM (forward elevation and external rotation), and Edwards reported that shoulders with moderate and severe infraspinatus fatty degeneration were associated with poorer functional results and patient satisfaction.

Overall, current literature suggests that aTSAs perform well if minimal rotator cuff dysfunction is present but can remain functional in the presence of partial and even small full-thickness tears of the supraspinatus. However, rotator cuff dysfunction is defined not only by presence/size of tears but also by amount of fatty tissue infiltration. Accordingly, elderly patients with significant rotator cuff muscle degeneration and/or presence/risk of large RCTs should instead be considered for rTSA.

32.2.4 Patient Compliance

Recovery and outcomes following aTSA are dependent on both surgeon- and patient-specific factors. Even with an optimal arthroplasty surgical technique, if patients are unable to consistently comply with postoperative protocols, recovery is typically limited. While surgeon-specific variations in postoperative aTSA rehabilitation protocols are common, most still follow a schedule divided into phases. The first phase, beginning immediately following surgery and lasting until 4–6 weeks post-op, limits active range of motion (ROM) and employs progressive passive ROM exercises protecting the subscapularis repair. The next phases gradually start full active ROM, followed by light and progressive strengthening beyond 12 weeks.

Patients who are unable to follow postoperative rehabilitation instructions and begin end-range active/resisted movements too soon are at risk of damaging newly repaired tissue (most notably subscapularis) and thereby impairing restoration of biomechanics, implant stability, and integration. The consequences of subscapularis repair failure have been well documented in the literature, correlating with prosthesis instability and worse patient outcome scores [7]. While optimal rehabilitation protocols have yet to be validated rigorously, available evidence points to the importance of adherence to postoperative rehabilitation programs for successful shoulder arthroplasty outcomes [8].

On the other hand, those who do not regularly participate in physical therapy or have difficulty performing ROM exercises postoperatively are at higher risk of stiffness. The latter scenario is commonly seen in stroke and Parkinson's patients who may have difficulty consistently following postoperative rehabilitation plans given neuro-

muscular decline. In these subsets of patients, aTSA is able to provide significant pain relief; however, ROM and functional recovery is highly variable and dependent on severity of patients' movement and neurocognitive impairments. While hemiarthroplasty, aTSA, and rTSA are all able to offer pain relief, Parkinson's patients have increased rates of postoperative infection, need for revision surgeries, component loosening, dislocations, and systemic complications [9]. rTSA is usually the preferred first-line treatment option due to the lower rates of postoperative complications and reoperations in these patient populations. In a similar vein, it is imperative that surgeons always account for postoperative weight-bearing status and patient-specific demands when considering shoulder arthroplasty (aTSA or otherwise), particularly in the elderly. While most implants will outlast elderly patients, the use of walker or cane may shorten prosthesis lifespan and increase risk of complications with repeated eccentric weight bearing.

32.3 Advantages of aTSA

Traditionally, aTSA is established as the benchmark treatment for patients with primary shoulder osteoarthritis with an intact rotator cuff. However, with recent improvements in rTSA surgical technique and implant design, complication rates for rTSA have decreased, leading to rTSAs being increasingly considered and used as a first-line treatment option for shoulder arthritis in elderly patients.

Theoretical advantages of aTSA over rTSA include preservation of native anatomic version and shoulder biomechanics, thereby enabling greater postoperative ROM, more "normal" shoulder function, as well as preserving shoulder symmetry. For both surgeries, reported complication rates vary between 5 and 15% with low mortality rates. Common complications are also similar and include infection, aseptic loosening, and instability. As previously described, aTSAs carry increased risk of developing clinically meaningful postoperative rotator cuff tears, while rTSAs do not. On the other hand, rTSAs are associated with increased risks of acromion and scapular fractures and scapular notching.

Historically, rTSAs maintained slightly higher complication rates than aTSAs (7.3% vs. 6.6%) [10]. However, it must be noted that such comparisons typically do not account for significantly different indications (and case complexity) for rTSA versus aTSA. Particularly, because rTSAs are indicated for revision surgeries, severe rotator cuff arthropathy, post-traumatic arthritis, and fractures and are appropriately referred to as "salvage-type procedures," rTSA patients often have more complex pathology and procedures compared to aTSA candidates.

Although few studies have directly compared outcomes and complication rates of aTSA and rTSA performed for the same indications, a recent systematic review included 6 studies with 447 total cases of shoulder arthroplasty performed in patients with osteoarthritis and intact rotator cuffs. Kim et al. reported that ROM was slightly improved in patients who received aTSA, although functional scores (Constant, SST, and ASES) remained similar across both groups. Regarding complications, aTSAs were noted to have higher rates of glenoid loosening, while rTSAs had higher rates of scapular notching. While these complications were present radiographically, most patients were asymptomatic and did not require further intervention, and revision rates were similar across both groups. Overall, while aTSA was shown to offer a minor advantage of increased ROM compared to rTSA, included studies demonstrated that aTSA carries significant risks of need for conversion to rTSA. Particularly, while Wright et al. reported no significant difference in complication or revision rates between rTSA and aTSA implanted in patients >70 years, they noted a 6.9% rate of revision at an average of 28 months after aTSA with the primary indication for revision being conversion to rTSA for posterior rotator cuff tear (2020).

A prospective study conducted by Flurin et al. with 778 patients and 8-year follow-up reported similar findings, with aTSAs demonstrating greater ROM but similar functional scores as rTSAs. Complication as well as revision rates were slightly higher in the aTSA group, but overall not statistically significantly different from the rTSA group. Overall, both surgeries yielded comparable outcomes and complication rates. On the other hand, in their prospective cohort of 95 consecutive elderly patients (>75 years old) with or without an intact rotator cuff who underwent either aTSA or rTSA based on rotator cuff status, Simon et al. found significantly better patient-reported outcome scores (PROs) in the aTSA group at 2-year follow-up, with a higher complication rate in the rTSA group due to scapular stress fractures (2022).

Thus, for patients with primary osteoarthritis with intact rotator cuff musculature, aTSA offers the potential advantage of increased ROM and PROs but carries risks of glenoid loosening and need for conversion to rTSA in the setting of symptomatic RCT. On the other hand, while outcomes and complications continue to improve, rTSA remains a "salvage-type operation" with risks of scapular stress fractures but is free from dependence on a functional rotator cuff. All these considerations must be carefully weighed for each individual patient, but certainly more so in the elderly demographic choosing to undergo elective shoulder surgery with associated risks including prolonged hospital stay, anesthetic risks, medical complications, and rehabilitation challenges.

32.4 Conclusion

For the appropriately selected patient, aTSA remains a gold standard for reconstructing native shoulder biomechanics, restoring motion, and alleviating pain of advanced arthrosis, irrespective of patient age. Furthermore, recent literature supports similar rates of complications and reoperations in the elderly patient population when compared to rTSA, with 5-year implant survival greater than 98%. However, as with anatomic shoulder arthroplasty in any age group, successful outcomes are highly contingent on sustained rotator cuff function as well as surgeon technical proficiency. Specifically, optimal soft tissue balancing and assessment/management of bone quality and bone loss is required to ensure appropriate implant fixation, shoulder stability and function, and prosthesis longevity. Beyond this precise application of the evolving "science" of aTSA surgical techniques, successful outcomes in elderly patients require surgeons to skillfully apply the "art" of surgical medicine. Principally, this entails careful patient selection to identify those who will actually benefit from the maximal postoperative shoulder ROM and the possibility of improved PROs associated with aTSA, allowing return to desired activities at the highest possible level. Also critical is a realistic assessment of patient risk tolerance for potential need for future operations for conversion to rTSA or other revision, as well as patient enthusiasm for both preoperative optimization and postoperative rehabilitation.

In conclusion, aTSA is best suited to optimally restore upper extremity ROM/function and decrease shoulder pain in healthy and motivated elderly patients with primary osteoarthritis, an intact rotator cuff, and minimal osteopenia or glenoid erosion. However, successful outcomes are significantly dependent on surgeon and patient factors. On the other hand, lower-demand patients with poorly controlled concomitant medical diseases, significant rotator cuff disease, and osteoporosis are poor aTSA candidates. In these patients, surgeons should strongly consider rTSA over an aTSA as a means to obtain more easily reproducible and consistent pain relief and adequate functional improvement.

References

1. Griffin JW, Hadeed MM, Novicoff WM, Browne JA, Brockmeier SF. Patient age is a factor in early outcomes after shoulder arthroplasty. J Shoulder Elbow Surg. 2014;23(12):1867–71. https://doi.org/10.1016/j.jse.2014.04.004.

2. Pisani P, Renna MD, Conversano F, et al. Major osteoporotic fragility fractures: risk factor updates and societal impact. World J Orthop. 2016;7(3):171–81. https://doi.org/10.5312/wjo.v7.i3.171.

3. Tingart MJ, Apreleva M, von Stechow D, Zurakowski D, Warner JJ. The cortical thickness of the proximal humeral diaphysis predicts bone mineral density of the proximal humerus. J Bone Joint Surgery Br. 2003;85(4):611–7. https://doi.org/10.1302/0301-620x.85b4.12843.

4. Spross C, Kaestle N, Benninger E, Fornaro J, Erhardt J, Zdravkovic V, Jost B. Deltoid tuberosity index: a simple radiographic tool to assess local bone quality in proximal humerus fractures. Clin Orthop Relat Res. 2015;473(9):3038–45. https://doi.org/10.1007/s11999-015-4322-x.

5. Wilkinson JM. The use of bisphosphonates to meet orthopaedic challenges. Bone. 2020;137:115443. https://doi.org/10.1016/j.bone.2020.115443. Epub 2020 May 20

6. Matsen F, Clinton J, Lynch J, Bertelsen A, Richardson M. Glenoid component failure in total shoulder arthroplasty. J Bone Joint Surg Am. 2008;90:885–96. https://doi.org/10.2106/JBJS.G.01263.

7. Shields E, Ho A, Wiater M. Management of the subscapularis tendon during total shoulder arthroplasty. J Shoulder Elbow Surg. 2017;26(4):723–31. https://doi.org/10.1016/j.jse.2016.11.006.

8. Kirsch, j, Namdari S. Rehabilitation after anatomic and reverse total shoulder arthroplasty; a critical analysis review. J Bone Joint Surg Rev. 2020;8(2):e0129. https://doi.org/10.2106/jbjs.rvw.19.00129.

9. Marigi EM, Shah H, Sperling JW Jr, Hassett LC, Schoch BS, Sanchez-Sotelo J, Sperling JW. Parkinson's disease and shoulder arthroplasty: a systematic review. JSES Int. 2021;6(2):241–6. https://doi.org/10.1016/j.jseint.2021.11.004. PMID: 35252920; PMCID: PMC8888176

10. Bohsali KI, Bois AJ, Wirth MA. Complications of shoulder arthroplasty. J Bone Joint Surg Am. 2017;99(3):256–69. https://doi.org/10.2106/JBJS.16.00935. Erratum in: J Bone Joint Surg Am 2017 Jun 21;99(12):e67

Revision Shoulder Arthroplasty

33

Ettore Taverna, Vincenzo Guarrella, and Marco Larghi

33.1 Revision of HA

HAs have a revision rate around 20%. HAs implanted for primary osteoarthritis are mainly revised for glenoid erosion and cuff insufficiency, whereas tuberosity migration, nonunion, or malunion are the main reasons to revise a HA implanted for acute fracture or fracture sequelae [1]. An oversized humeral head is frequently identified as a cause of glenoid erosion or cuff failure. In case of soft tissue or bone deficiency, revising a HA with a TSA leads to a failure 70% of surgeries; a revision with a RSA should be preferred in this clinical setting [1].

33.2 Revision of TSA

The two main reasons for revision surgery following TSA are glenoid loosening and instability, which often coexist. Glenoid radiolucencies appear at 5 years and progress over time. Neither polyethylene with cement nor metal-backed glenoid implants have passed the test of time [1, 2]. Similar to HAs, in case of soft tissue/bone deficiency, TSA revision should be performed with RSA to avoid multiple revisions.

33.3 Revision of RSA

The main reasons of failure of RSA are glenoid loosening, infection, and instability. Humeral complications (humeral loosening, disassembly, or fracture) increase with time and may become a major cause of revision surgery for RSA in the near future [1]. Revision of a failed RSA to another RSA, often combined with glenoid and/or humeral bone reconstruction, remains the treatment of choice. Revision of an RSA to a HA is rarely performed as it leads to a poor functional result [1].

33.4 Revision Shoulder Arthroplasty for Periprosthetic Joint Infection

Periprosthetic joint infection (PJI) is the most common reason for revision arthroplasty within 2 years of the index surgical procedure. Reports of periprosthetic joint infection's incidence commonly range from 3 to 4% in the literature, although rates as low as 0.5% and as high as 6.7% have been reported and over 15% after revision cases [4, 5]. As the utilization of shoulder arthroplasty continues to rise, shoulder surgeons must remain well versed in the diagnosis and treatment of these potentially devastating complications [4].

E. Taverna · V. Guarrella (✉) · M. Larghi
IRCCS Ospedale Galeazzi Sant'Ambrogio,
Milan, Italy
e-mail: ettore.taverna@eoc.ch

© ISAKOS 2023
A. D. Mazzocca et al. (eds.), *Shoulder Arthritis across the Life Span*,
https://doi.org/10.1007/978-3-031-33298-2_33

Less virulent organisms, such as *Cutibacterium acnes*, often cause periprosthetic joint infection following shoulder arthroplasty. *C. acnes* is associated with a nonspecific clinical presentation and traditional inflammatory markers less accurately identify its infection [4]. Similarly, the optimal treatment for shoulder periprosthetic joint infection remains unclear.

Treatment options include one-stage arthroplasty, two-stage arthroplasty, and resection arthroplasty, each with varying success rates.

33.4.1 Microbiology

The most frequently isolated organisms in shoulder periprosthetic joint infection are *C. acnes* (38.9%), *Staphylococcus epidermidis* (14.8%), and *Staphylococcus aureus* (14.5%). *C. acnes* appears also to be the most commonly isolated bacteria in patients undergoing revision shoulder arthroplasty (16.7%) [4].

33.4.1.1 *C. acnes*

Formerly known as *Propionibacterium acnes*, *C. acnes* is found around the sebaceous glands of moist skin regions.

The numerous sebaceous glands of the chest and back region produce large amounts of oily sebum, which creates an ideal environment for the lipophilic anaerobic bacterium to proliferate. The proximity of the incision site to the axilla is one proposed explanation for its role in between 31% and 70% of shoulder periprosthetic joint infection cases [4].

Furthermore, the increased quantity of sebaceous glands in male patients has also been implicated in the higher incidence of periprosthetic joint infection in this population. Anterolateral approach compared to deltopectoral approach was also associated with a higher risk of infection following open rotator cuff repair or open subacromial decompression, which may be because of the number of sebaceous glands transected [4].

C. acnes has been shown to form biofilm, especially in plasma-poor environments such as prosthetic joints, and their presence has been shown to put patients who undergo revision at a higher risk of reinfection, with rates reaching 20%. Of note, *C. acnes* can also form biofilm on gentamicin-containing bone cement [4].

33.4.2 Prevention of Periprosthetic Joint Infection

C. acnes has been shown to survive traditional superficial skin sterilization methods in the operating room, such as povidone-iodine or chlorhexidine gluconate [4].

As a result, there have been several studies exploring novel methods for reducing the *C. acnes* bacterial load.

Benzoyl peroxide is a bactericidal agent that has been shown in the dermatology literature to reduce the *C. acnes* load by penetrating sebaceous glands, and there have been promising results in the setting of shoulder surgical procedures as well. The application of benzoyl peroxide gel the night before the surgical procedure determined a decrease of *C. acnes* load (8% versus 28%) [4].

Of note, it is still unclear whether the organisms found in the skin cultures were causative of infection or merely commensal.

Furthermore, none of these studies evaluated the efficacy of these preparations for preventing periprosthetic joint infection, which limited their validity.

Other studies have examined the effectiveness of injecting intra-articular antibiotics in a revision surgical procedure.

Intra-articular injection of gentamicin at the time of closure also resulted to reduce periprosthetic joint infection after primary shoulder arthroplasty [4].

Cefazolin is currently the perioperative antibiotic of choice in shoulder arthroplasty in patients without a severe beta-lactam allergy. Currently, the 2018 ICM states postoperative antibiotics are not required, but, if given, should not be continued beyond 24 h postoperatively [6].

33.4.3 Diagnosis of Periprosthetic Joint Infection

33.4.3.1 Risk Factors

Major risk factors for PJI are male gender, younger patients, smoke, history of previous shoulder surgery, and revision shoulder arthroplasty [5]. Reverse shoulder arthroplasty and perioperative blood transfusion are also risk factors.

Exposure to cortisone injections can increase patients' risk of developing periprosthetic joint infection, especially within 3 months of the surgical procedure.

Extremity-specific risk factors include fracture, chronic lymphedema, venous stasis, vascular compromise, and radiation fibrosis. Postoperative hematoma has also been associated with infection. Interestingly, body mass index and race are not consistently associated with an increased risk of periprosthetic joint infection [4].

33.4.3.2 Clinical Presentation

The existence of a fistula that connects with the prosthesis is pathognomonic for periprosthetic joint infection. However, the majority of patients present without a sinus tract or the classic signs of infection (e.g., fever, chills, sweats, erythema, induration, wound drainage).

The most common symptoms are shoulder pain, followed by a draining sinus, stiffness, erythema, effusion, fever, night sweats, and chills. Other findings associated with infection include worsening physical examination findings, such as decreased range of motion.

Therefore, surgeons must have a heightened index of suspicion, and any deviation from normal postoperative findings should be considered infection until proven otherwise.

The 2018 ICM divided periprosthetic shoulder infection into four categories [7]: definite infection, probable infection, possible infection, and unlikely infection. A definite infection is defined by the presence of one or more of the following criteria: (1) presence of a sinus tract from the skin surface to the prosthesis, (2) intraarticular pus, or (3) two positive tissue cultures

Table 33.1 Minor criteria for shoulder PJI

Criteria	Weight
Unexpected wound drainage	4
Single positive tissue culture with a virulent organism	3
Single positive tissue culture with a low-virulent organism	1
Second positive tissue culture (identical low-virulence organism)	3
Humeral loosening	3
Positive frozen section (5 neutrophils in≥5 high-power fields)	3
Positive preoperative aspirate culture	3
Synovial neutrophil percentage > 80%	2
Synovial white blood cell count >3000 cells/μL beyond 6 weeks from surgery	2
ESR > 30 mm/h	2
CRP > 10 mg/L	2
Elevated synovial alpha-defensin	2
Cloudy synovial fluid	2

with phenotypically identical virulent organisms, such as *Staphylococcus aureus*. This is in contrast to low-virulence organisms, which include *C. acnes* and coagulase-negative *Staphylococcus* species. In addition to these definite criteria, the ICM also established a set of minor criteria for the definition of shoulder PJI.

A probable infection is defined as the presence of six or more minor criteria with an identified organism (Table 33.1).

A possible infection is defined as the one of the following: (1) presence of six or more minor criteria without an identified organism, (2) less than six minor criteria with a single positive culture with a virulent organism, or (3) less than six minor criteria with two positive cultures with a low-virulence organism. An unlikely infection is defined as the presence of less than six minor criteria with negative cultures or only a single positive culture with a low-virulence organism.

33.4.3.3 Radiographic Evaluation

Patients suspected to have a shoulder periprosthetic joint infection should receive radiographs, especially if they present with shoulder pain during postoperative follow-up. Although nonspecific for infection, radiographs show the overall alignment of the prosthesis and can show signs of loosening or osteolysis [5]. Serial radiographs over time that show progressive humeral osteolysis are highly suggestive of periprosthetic joint infection. Although nonspecific for the offending organism, progressive humeral osteolysis is associated with a tenfold increase in the risk of a *C. acnes* infection [4].

Computed tomography (CT), ultrasound, and magnetic resonance imaging (MRI) are not routinely utilized because they do not provide any diagnostic findings, except for the visualization of surrounding osteomyelitis or loculated abscesses. Technetium Tc-99 m bone scans are also not routinely used because they have limited sensitivity and specificity for a shoulder periprosthetic joint infection [4].

33.4.3.4 Laboratory Evaluation

Laboratory evaluation for suspected shoulder periprosthetic joint infection should include complete blood count with differential, CRP, and ESR. Unfortunately, ESR and CRP do not have reliable sensitivity and specificity following shoulder arthroplasty, especially in the setting of indolent infections caused by *C. acnes* or coagulase-negative *Staphylococcus* species.

The Infectious Diseases Society of America (IDSA) has endorsed diagnostic arthrocentesis in all patients with suspected acute periprosthetic joint infection unless the diagnosis is clinically evident, the surgical procedure is planned, and antimicrobials can be safely withheld prior to the surgical procedure. If the patient is clinically stable, the IDSA also recommended withholding antimicrobial therapy for at least 2 weeks prior to collection of synovial fluid to increase the likelihood of recovering an organism. It is recommended to perform aspiration under fluoroscopic or ultrasound guidance to improve accuracy and maximize the sample volume [4]. However, even when a sufficient volume is obtained, the cultures and cytology are often within normal limits.

Arthroscopic tissue biopsy seems to be substantially more reliable than aspiration in terms of sensitivity, specificity, positive predictive value, and negative predictive value.

Intraoperative open biopsy with culture remains the gold standard for the diagnosis of shoulder PJI. The sensitivity of intraoperative culture for shoulder periprosthetic joint infection has been reported to be 50% to 67%, depending on the organism. The IDSA currently recommends that surgeons obtain and send five intraoperative tissue specimens for microbiology culture. Currently, holding antibiotics prior to obtaining intraoperative cultures is not recommended.

These specimens should be grown on four to five media for a minimum of 13 to 14 days because of extended incubation period of *C. acnes* [5].

Frozen section at the time of revision surgery is an adjunct in the diagnosis of shoulder PJI; however, it requires an experienced pathologist and a negative result does not rule out infection.

The current literature does not support the use of routine implant sonication due to the low sensitivity as well as the lack of established diagnostic cutoffs for the quantification of bacteria in the obtained samples [5].

33.4.3.5 Recent Advances in Diagnosis

Recent efforts have been focused on finding innovative ways of diagnosing shoulder periprosthetic joint infection. Interleukin-6 (IL-6), a pro-inflammatory cytokine that mediates acute immune responses, has been identified as a potential indicator of periprosthetic joint infection because its serum concentration rises and falls to normal faster than CRP or ESR.

The synovial cytokine profiles of IL-6, tumor necrosis factor-a, alpha-defensin, and IL-2 are under investigation [5, 7].

33.4.4 Management

Shoulder periprosthetic joint infection is difficult to treat and the preferred management strategy remains controversial.

The treatment options for shoulder periprosthetic joint infection include intravenous antibiotics, tissue debridement with retention of the prosthesis, resection arthroplasty, one-stage and two-stage revision procedures, arthrodesis, and amputation [4].

Regardless of the ultimate treatment modality, all patients with suspected periprosthetic joint infection should receive perioperative antibiotics at the time of the revision surgical procedure.

Cefazolin is the agent most likely to provide optimal tissue concentrations for prophylaxis against the three most common causative organisms.

Antibiotic therapy alone is usually insufficient for the management of shoulder periprosthetic joint infection and has been shown to have a failure rate of 60% to 75% [4].

Previous studies have suggested that treating shoulder periprosthetic joint infection with debridement and retention of the prosthesis is possible only if the infection is identified within 30 days of the initial surgical procedure or after less than 3 weeks from the onset of symptoms, if the implant is stable, the isolated germ is of low virulence, and complete debridement is achieved [4]. More recent investigations showed unsatisfactory results with debridement and retention of the prosthesis in terms of infection eradication rate compared with other treatments, and previous studies have shown a failure rate of 50% to 63%. The 2018 ICM currently concluded that there is not enough evidence to support or discourage the use of irrigation and debridement with implant retention for acute or chronic shoulder PJI, but it may play a role in select patients [8].

Complete removal of the shoulder prosthesis is indicated in patients who present with infections after 4 weeks postoperatively; these patients are treated either with resection arthroplasty or with one-stage or two-stage revision.

The traditional treatment protocol for shoulder periprosthetic joint infection has consisted of complete prosthesis removal, implanting an antibiotic spacer, and a second stage consisting of a revision shoulder arthroplasty.

The literature has consistently supported the efficacy of two-stage revision, with infection recurrence rates reported to be 0% to 36% [4].

Cement spacers with vancomycin alone or in combination with an aminoglycoside have both been shown to be effective treatment options, can help to preserve the soft tissue envelope, and could be a permanent treatment option for patients with low functional demands.

Recent studies have focused on one-stage exchange because it involves less dissection and stress to the soft tissues, is quicker, and is more cost-effective. A systematic review of the shoulder arthroplasty literature found studies that showed that both one-stage and two-stage revisions provide >90% rates of eradication at a mean follow-up of 49 months. It suggested that single-stage treatment can result in less damage to the soft tissues, can avoid a second general anesthetic, and can reduce costs [9]. Another study showed almost one third of patients planned for two-stage revision did not undergo the second stage of the revision due to mortality, medical comorbidities, uncontrollable infection leading to amputation of the limb or lifetime antibiotic suppression, and unwillingness of patients to undergo a second surgery, as well as patient's satisfaction with the current status. Therefore, satisfactory results of a two-stage revision might not be achieved by almost one third of patients planned for revision [10].

Definitive treatment with an antibiotic spacer is another viable treatment option in select patients. Pellegrini et al. reported a case series of 19 shoulder PJI that were definitively treated with an antibiotic cement spacer. They reported no recurrent infections with good pain relief and improvement in outcome scores, but shoulder range of motion remained poor. They concluded that a definitive antibiotic spacer is a good option for low-demand, elderly individuals who do not wish to or are not otherwise able to undergo another operation [11]. Resection arthroplasty can provide substantial pain relief and excellent infection eradication. However, resection arthroplasty often results in functional deficits, especially with internal and external rotation. As such, resection arthroplasty is a good treatment option for elderly patients or patients with high-virulence germs, considerable tissue loss, or poor health [4].

33.5 Revision Shoulder Arthroplasty for Prosthetic Instability

Instability is one of the most frequent causes for reoperation after unconstrained shoulder prosthesis [12–14]. In literature, the rate of instability was found to be in range from 4.9% to 5.2% [15, 16]. Instability can occur in different patterns:

- Inferior Instability: Usually due to a shortened humerus or a failure to restore humeral length due a tumor or a fracture.
- Superior Instability: Usually results from a deficient superior rotator cuff.
- Anterior Instability: Usually from an insufficiency of the subscapularis or rotator interval with an excessively anteverted humeral component with a large head.
- Posterior Instability: Usually for a soft tissue deficiency associated with an incorrect version positioning of the humeral component; commonly a glenoid retroversion with elongation of the posterior capsule and excessive humeral retroversion [17].

A radiological study with an anteroposterior and axillary view is useful to categorize the direction of instability.

Depending on the instability pattern, specific revision procedures can be proposed such as repositioning or resizing the component, bone grafting procedures, and soft tissue repairs [17, 18]. A reduction of anteversion of the humeral component with repair or reconstruction of the anterior capsule and subscapularis could be proposed for anterior instability.

In case of posterior subluxation, a plication of the posterior capsule and rotator cuff and a posterior bone grafting have been proposed as surgical options. However, recurrent instability rate in case of soft tissue revision surgery is very high, and authors advocate considering revision to reverse shoulder arthroplasty [18].

Revision to a constrained design (RSA) provides better stability with good clinical outcomes and increased range of motion but worst results than those achieved with primary implantation of RSA [16, 17].

33.5.1 Instability in Reverse Shoulder Arthroplasty

Instability is the most common complication and main cause of revision surgery following RSA [3, 19–21]. It is a "difficult to manage" complication, with high risk of revision failure and recurrent instability [3, 22].

Risk factors for instability are younger age, revision surgery, male gender, scapular notching, and grater tuberosity absence or resorption [23]. Other factors to be considered prior to revision surgery are [20]:

Previous surgery: RSA for failure of osteosynthesis, hemiarthroplasty, anatomic prosthesis, or reverse prosthesis is three times more likely to show instability than primary RSA: 7% versus 2% [24].

Deltopectoral approach: seems to be associated with a higher risk of instability compared to superolateral deltoid approach [18, 24].

"Cam effect": mediated by soft tissue or bone block: obesity is protective against scapular notching, but induces a cam effect through fat in the upper limb and trunk [25]; humeral malunion or ossification may strike against the scapular pillar or glenosphere, inducing a leverage effect.

Bone loss or soft tissue deficiency: humeral or glenoid bone loss and soft tissue deficiency (subscapularis absent or non-inserted and/or anterior deltoid atrophy) [20].

Patients with shortened humerus due to a proximal bone loss have a higher risk of instability. Etiology of shortened humerus is various: implant migration, greater tuberosity lysis, or humeral resection that fails to restore humeral length (more frequently in tumor surgery, acute fracture, or previous hemiarthroplasty) [20]. A posterior greater tuberosity placement in setting of a RTSA for a proximal humerus fracture can also contribute to instability as the humeral component can be levered out of place with an impingement-like mechanism [26].

Glenosphere malpositioning can increase instability: excessive anteversion, retroversion, or superior inclination can place the patient at risk [27]. Glenoid medialization due to glenoid bone defect and the implantation of an excessively small glenosphere is also cause of instability [20].

33.5.1.1 Management of Instability

When facing RSA instability, it is essential to understand the etiology of instability and correct its causes.

Factors that need to be assessed are soft tissue deficiency or significant bone loss, components malposition, and impingement.

Another common cause of instability is inadequate deltoid tensioning. To restore the proper tension of the deltoid, the surgeon could increase the size of the glenosphere, increase the global amount of lateralization of the implant, and/or increase the amount of distalization on the humeral side [20, 28].

In early dislocation (within the first 3 months), without malrotation or bone defect, a closed reduction and a strict immobilization with an abduction splint is a good treatment option. The abduction splint promotes deltoid shortening and enhances the implant's cooptation force. Efficacy rates are between 30% and 50% [24].

In late dislocation (after 3 months), usually a revision surgery with correction of a technical mistakes is necessary. Restoring deltoid tension modifying the humeral shortening and/or excessive medialization is often needed. Humeral shortening can be managed by adding metal augmentation or increasing polyethylene height without changing the implants. When the shortening exceeds 15–20 mm, the humeral implant probably needs to be replaced [20].

Excessive medialization is often implicated in persistent instability despite restored humeral length. Management of excessive medialization could be achieved replacing the glenoid implant with a greater diameter glenosphere or using a bone grafting procedure (BIO-RSA) or a metallic-increased offset reverse shoulder arthroplasty (MIO-RSA) or both.

When functional subscapularis is present, reinsertion of the tendon and capsule should be performed.

33.6 Revision Arthroplasty for Prosthetic Loosening

33.6.1 Glenoid Loosening

Glenoid component loosening in shoulder arthroplasty is a leading complication and a common reason for implant failure and revision surgery [12, 14].

In the setting of anatomical shoulder arthroplasty [29], clinical presentations and x-ray with radiolucent lines are all important factors for the detection of implant loosening [30]. Patients affected by glenoid loosening often report pain and reduction of active range of motion and strength. Radiolucency around the implants has been discussed but there is no clear correlation with implant loosening [23]. Several publications showed that signs of radiolucency occurring shortly after surgery and their further progression are correlated with implant loosening [29]. Nevertheless, radiolucency can be very common especially after cemented polyethylene pegged glenoid component implantation [31]. Other radiographic signs of glenoid loosening have been proposed: superior shift of the humeral head and medialization due to erosion of the glenoid side [30, 32]. A loose glenoid component is frequently associated with a glenoid bone loss and may necessitate additional procedures to implant a new component. Bone augmentation with autograft or allograft or augmented glenoid components are necessary in a bone-deficient glenoid [33]. The reverse total shoulder arthroplasty is a useful reconstructive option capable of addressing bony and soft tissue problems [31–33].

Reverse total shoulder glenoid component loosening has a prevalence ranging from 1.7% to 3.5% [3]. To provide a stable fulcrum, the glenosphere needs a balance between compressive and shear forces. The compressive forces have a stabilizing effect on the glenosphere, while shear forces could contribute to destabilizing the component, leading to glenoid loosening [34]. Glenoid loosening usually appears at the interface between the baseplate and the native scapula and in rare cases may involve the interface between the scapula and any bone graft used or in the body of the scapula, medial to the baseplate screws. These different types of glenoid loosening are important as they dictate the type of revision needed [35]. Conservative and surgical treatments are both valid options in RSA failures due to glenoid loosening. Conservative treatment is suggested whenever possible [35]. Revision of the glenosphere could be considered if conservative fails. Conversion to hemiarthroplasty should remain a last salvage option [36].

Bone defect in glenoid loosening is very frequent and could be classified in three grades: cavity defect (A), uncontained wall defect (B), or complex defect (C) [20]. In cavity bone defect, it can be filled by impacted allograft or synthetic graft, without using iliac crest autograft. For complex defect and unconfined wall defect, it is suggested to use an iliac crest autograft to improve consolidation without resorption of the graft [20].

33.6.2 Humeral Loosening

Aseptic humeral loosening is an uncommon complication in shoulder arthroplasty. It occurred more commonly in cohorts with long-term follow-up at rates between 0.61% and 1.4% [37, 38]. Stem loosening is more frequent after RSA than anatomical shoulder arthroplasty, probably because constraint forces associated with Grammont RSA are predominantly located on the humeral side rather than the glenoid side [37, 38].

In anatomic shoulder arthroplasty, there is no correlation between bone resorption and the clinical results [39–42]. Also, after RSA bone resorption doesn't correlate to clinical results [42]. Nevertheless, proximal humeral bone loss is the main risk factor for humeral loosening, bone resorption affects more frequently the greater tuberosity area, and this could diminish the del-

toid wrapping angle and increasing risk of instability [42].

Risk factors for bone resorption in anatomical arthroplasty reported are age, secondary osteoarthritis, high filling ratio of the implant, low bone density, large implant size, on-grow-type stem coating, and hemiarthroplasty with rotator cuff tear [43].

In RSA risk factors are a high filling ratio, female sex, and an onlay-type stem [37]. Low bone quality because of osteoporosis could explain female sex risk factor. The more proximal osteotomy performed on inlay-type stems (compared to onlay type) leads to a more proximal fixation and possibly contributes to lower the rate of bone resorption [37].

Management of humeral loosening could be very difficult especially with a bone defect scenario. In this setting, the goal of a revision surgery should be to enhance implant stability, restore humeral length, and increase the deltoid wrapping angle.Boileau et al. for a humeral defect <5 cm in elderly patients with RSA recommend to create a cement collar around the implant (cementoplasty reconstruction) to fill the bone defect or implant a prosthesis used for tumor reconstruction surgery.

In humeral defects >5 cm, some authors recommend reconstruction by massive humeral allograft [20, 44].

33.7 Revision Arthroplasty for Periprosthetic Fractures

The incidence of periprosthetic fractures is reported between 1% and 3% [45, 46], and the number of revision arthroplasties is likely to rise over time with the increasing of the number of shoulder arthroplasties performed. In comparison to fractures associated with anatomic total shoulder arthroplasty, periprosthetic fractures in the setting of RSA occur more than three times as frequently [46].

Data on this topic is affected by considerable heterogeneity in the published literature especially in the classification and outcome measures; larger and more rigorous studies are needed [45].

33.7.1 Acromial and Scapular Spine Fractures

The acromion and scapular spine are anatomic sites uniquely predisposed to fracture in the setting of RSA with an incidence estimated between 1.3 and 4.3%. This prosthetic design distalizes and medializes the center of rotation of the shoulder increasing the forces transmitted across the acromion and scapula, including the scapular spine and coracoacromial ligament [46]. More recent RSA designs such as a short, lateralized humeral stem, and inferior glenosphere offset, were designed to counteract some of the commonly encountered complications associated with RSA, including implant instability and scapular notching. Newer design alterations, particularly humeral stems with increased offset, may effectively reduce the risk of scapular notching, yet they may also increase stresses seen at the acromion. To date, there is no clear evidence of implant design on acromial fractures [47, 48].

Acromial and scapular spine fractures can occur after a minor trauma or can have an insidious onset without history of trauma. Radiographs are very often unable to detect these fractures, and CT scan is recommended in all patients with acromial or scapular pain following RSA with radiographs negative for fractures [46].

Documented risk factors are osteoporosis, lateralized glenosphere, and decreased deltoid lengthening.

Controversial results are reported regarding the integrity of rotator cuff and subscapularis repair as it could act as deltoid antagonist, thereby increasing the workload of the deltoid with an increase of acromial stresses [46]. Positioning of the superior screw above the central glenoid axis appears to be a risk factor, especially if the tip of the screw engages the scapular spine. Other possible risk factors are an onlay humeral design, a short humeral stem, and the resection of coracoacromial ligament.

Acromial and scapular spine fractures after RSA are usually treated nonoperatively or with ORIF and rarely have been treated with revision with ORIF. In case of RSA revision associated with ORIF, the aim of revision was to eliminate risk factors related to RSA design substituting the implant with an inlay design, long humeral stem, and medialized glenosphere and without repairing the subscapularis tendon.

33.7.2 Humerus Fractures

A fracture of the humerus can occur intraoperatively or postoperatively. Major risk factors are osteopenia, female sex, post-traumatic arthritis, rheumatoid arthritis, osteonecrosis, the use of press-fit stems, and the setting of revision arthroplasty [46, 49].

The most commonly employed classification system for periprosthetic humeral fractures describes fractures in relation to the tip of the humeral stem. Type A comprised fractures proximal to the tip, type B comprised fractures at the tip and extending distally, and type C comprised fractures distal to the tip of the humeral stem [50]. Campbell et al. [51] proposed a classification system that incorporated fractures not restricted to the humeral diaphysis. In this four-part system, type 1 involves the lesser or greater tuberosity; type 2 involves the surgical neck; type 3, the metadiaphyseal junction; and type 4, the middle and distal humeral diaphysis.

The existing evidence basis to guide treatment decision-making relies on few published retrospective case series and expert opinion.

There are three main treatment strategies: the first is nonoperative treatment using orthoses, braces, or plaster casts; the second is fixation using wires, plates, and screws, external fixators, and strut cortical bone allografts with plates or customized intramedullary nail cut to size; and the third is revision arthroplasty using either a long stem to bypass the fracture, a revision stem with a strut allograft, a humeral endoprosthesis, a partial or total humeral prosthesis, or an allograft-prosthetic composite [45].

Wagner et al. [52] proposed a treatment algorithm for intraoperative humerus fracture in the setting of RSA. In this schema, fractures of the greater tuberosity are stabilized with a suture fixation construct, nondisplaced metaphyseal fractures are secured with multiple cerclage wires, and displaced fractures of the metaphysis are fixed using cables and strut allograft. Data on nonoperative treatment show a success rate of only 50%; it is suitable mainly for frail patients with little functional demand and unfit for surgery. Risk of complication in this group of patients is around 30% (mainly nonunion or malunion) [45].

ORIF is the most frequent strategy and has a mean success rate over 90% with better results if the prosthesis is well fixed. Complication rate of 17% is reported after ORIF (more frequently transient radial nerve palsy, infection and fracture extension, or fixation failure) [45]. In most cases of loose prosthesis, revision arthroplasty is preferred over ORIF; nevertheless ORIF shows a success rate of almost 90% even in cases of loose prosthesis [45].

Revision surgery can be necessary in the setting of a Campbell type 4 fracture with failure of nonoperative treatment. Revision can be achieved with placement of a long humeral stem and multiple cerclage wires.

Unstable stems should be revised with longer stems [46].

In the setting of a tuberosity fracture after anatomic replacement, conversion to RSA is suggested if tuberosities cannot be fixed [46].

Revision arthroplasty has a success rate over 80% with a complication rate of 29% (more frequently nonunion, dislocation, dissociations of prosthetic components, and transient or permanent nerve palsy) [45].

In case of extensive humeral bone loss, a strut allograft and additional plate fixation or the use of two hemicylinders of tibial allograft to form a "sarcophagus," used with cerclage wires but without a plate, should be used especially if the bone defect is over 5 cm [46].

Finally, a humeral endoprosthesis is an option for managing severe bone loss without allograft. Traditionally used in tumor surgery, these implants afford substantial modularity, allowing for reconstruction of large segmental defects [46].

References

1. Gauci MO, Cavalier M, Gonzalez JF, Holzer N, Baring T, Walch G, Boileau P. Revision of failed shoulder arthroplasty: epidemiology, etiology, and surgical options. J Shoulder Elbow Surg. 2020;29(3):541–9. https://doi.org/10.1016/j.jse.2019.07.034. Epub 2019 Oct 6. PMID: 31594726

2. Gonzalez JF, Alami GB, Baque F, Walch G, Boileau P. Complications of unconstrained shoulder prostheses. J Shoulder Elbow Surg. 2011;20(4):666–82. https://doi.org/10.1016/j.jse.2010.11.017. Epub 2011 Mar 21. PMID: 21419661

3. Zumstein MA, Pinedo M, Old J, Boileau P. Problems, complications, reoperations, and revisions in reverse total shoulder arthroplasty: a systematic review. J Shoulder Elbow Surg. 2011;20(1):146–57. https://doi.org/10.1016/j.jse.2010.08.001. PMID: 21134666

4. Cooper ME, Trivedi NN, Sivasundaram L, Karns MR, Voos JE, Gillespie RJ. Diagnosis and management of periprosthetic joint infection after shoulder arthroplasty. JBJS Rev. 2019;7(7):e3. https://doi.org/10.2106/JBJS.RVW.18.00152. PMID: 31291202

5. Contreras ES, Frantz TL, Bishop JY, Cvetanovich GL. Periprosthetic infection after reverse shoulder arthroplasty: a review. Curr Rev Musculoskelet Med. 2020;13(6):757–68. https://doi.org/10.1007/s12178-020-09670-8. PMID: 32827305; PMCID: PMC7661562

6. Garrigues GE, Zmistowski B, Cooper AM, Green A, ICM Shoulder Group. Proceedings from the 2018 international consensus meeting on orthopedic infections: prevention of periprosthetic shoulder infection. J Shoulder Elbow Surg. 2019;28(6S):S13–31. https://doi.org/10.1016/j.jse.2019.04.017. PMID: 31196506

7. Garrigues GE, Zmistowski B, Cooper AM, Green A, ICM Shoulder Group. Proceedings from the 2018 international consensus meeting on orthopedic infections: evaluation of periprosthetic shoulder infection. J Shoulder Elbow Surg. 2019;28(6S):S32–66. https://doi.org/10.1016/j.jse.2019.04.016. PMID: 31196514

8. Garrigues GE, Zmistowski B, Cooper AM, Green A, ICM Shoulder Group. Proceedings from the 2018 international consensus meeting on orthopedic infections: management of periprosthetic shoulder infection. J Shoulder Elbow Surg. 2019;28(6S):S67–99. https://doi.org/10.1016/j.jse.2019.04.015. PMID: 31196516

9. Nelson GN, Davis DE, Namdari S. Outcomes in the treatment of periprosthetic joint infection after shoulder arthroplasty: a systematic review. J Shoulder Elbow Surg. 2016;25(8):1337–45. https://doi.org/10.1016/j.jse.2015.11.064. Epub 2016 Mar 21. PMID: 27012542

10. Akgün D, Wiethölter M, Maziak N, Paksoy A, Karczewski D, Scheibel M, Moroder P. Two-stage exchange arthroplasty for periprosthetic shoulder infection is associated with high rate of failure to Reimplant and mortality. J Clin Med. 2021;10(21):5186. https://doi.org/10.3390/jcm10215186. PMID: 34768706; PMCID: PMC8584704

11. Pellegrini A, Legnani C, Macchi V, Meani E. Management of periprosthetic shoulder infections with the use of a permanent articulating antibiotic spacer. Arch Orthop Trauma Surg. 2018;138(5):605–9. https://doi.org/10.1007/s00402-018-2870-8. Epub 2018 Jan 15. PMID: 29335894

12. Kozak T, Bauer S, Walch G, Al-Karawi S, Blakeney W. An update on reverse total shoulder arthroplasty: current indications, new designs, same old problems. EFORT Open Rev. 2021;6(3):189–201. https://doi.org/10.1302/2058-5241.6.200085. PMID: 33841918; PMCID: PMC8025709

13. Best MJ, Aziz KT, Wilckens JH, McFarland EG, Srikumaran U. Increasing incidence of primary reverse and anatomic total shoulder arthroplasty in the United States. J Shoulder Elbow Surg. 2021;30(5):1159–66. https://doi.org/10.1016/j.jse.2020.08.010. Epub 2020 Aug 26. PMID: 32858194

14. Kircher J, Ohly B, Fal MF, Magosch P, Mauch F. Analysis of revision shoulder arthroplasty in the German nationwide registry from 2014 to 2018. JSES Int. 2021;5(3):382–90. https://doi.org/10.1016/j.jseint.2020.12.003. PMID: 34136844; PMCID: PMC8178607

15. Wirth MA, Rockwood CA Jr. Complications of total shoulder-replacement arthroplasty. J Bone Joint Surg Am. 1996;78(4):603–16. https://doi.org/10.2106/00004623-199604000-00018. PMID: 8609143

16. Bohsali KI, Wirth MA, Rockwood CA Jr. Complications of total shoulder arthroplasty. J Bone Joint Surg Am. 2006;88(10):2279–92. https://doi.org/10.2106/JBJS.F.00125. PMID: 17015609

17. Abdel MP, Hattrup SJ, Sperling JW, Cofield RH, Kreofsky CR, Sanchez-Sotelo J. Revision of an unstable hemiarthroplasty or anatomical total shoulder replacement using a reverse design prosthesis. Bone Joint J. 2013;95-B(5):668–72. https://doi.org/10.1302/0301-620X.95B5.30964. PMID: 23632679

18. Alentorn-Geli E, Wanderman NR, Assenmacher AT, Sperling JW, Cofield RH, Sánchez-Sotelo J. Revision anatomic shoulder arthroplasty with posterior capsular plication for correction of posterior instability. J Orthop Surg (Hong Kong). 2018;26(3):2309499018789527. https://doi.org/10.1177/2309499018789527. PMID: 30041574

19. Parada SA, Flurin PH, Wright TW, Zuckerman JD, Elwell JA, Roche CP, Friedman RJ. Comparison of complication types and rates associated with anatomic and reverse total shoulder arthroplasty. J Shoulder Elbow Surg. 2021;30(4):811–8. https://doi.org/10.1016/j.jse.2020.07.028. Epub 2020 Aug 4. PMID: 32763380

20. Boileau P. Complications and revision of reverse total shoulder arthroplasty. Orthop Traumatol Surg Res. 2016;102(1 Suppl):S33–43. https://doi.org/10.1016/j.otsr.2015.06.031. Epub 2016 Feb 12. PMID: 26879334

21. Kennedy J, Klifto CS, Ledbetter L, Bullock GS. Reverse total shoulder arthroplasty clinical and patient-reported outcomes and complications stratified by preoperative diagnosis: a systematic review. J Shoulder Elbow Surg. 2021;30(4):929–41. https://doi.org/10.1016/j.jse.2020.09.028. Epub 2020 Oct 22. PMID: 33558062

22. Ravi V, Murphy RJ, Moverley R, Derias M, Phadnis J. Outcome and complications following revision shoulder arthroplasty: a systematic review and meta-analysis. Bone Jt Open. 2021;2(8):618–30. https://doi.org/10.1302/2633-1462.28.BJO-2021-0092.R1. PMID: 34382837; PMCID: PMC8384442

23. Guarrella V, Chelli M, Domos P, Ascione F, Boileau P, Walch G. Risk factors for instability after reverse shoulder arthroplasty. Shoulder Elbowow. 2021;13(1):51–7. https://doi.org/10.1177/1758573219864266. Epub 2019 Jul 27. PMID: 33717218; PMCID: PMC7905521

24. Walch G, Wall B, Mottie F. Complications and revision of the reverse prosthesis: a multicenter study of 457 cases. Reverse shoulder arthroplasty. Montpellier: Sauramps Médical; 2006. p. 335–52.

25. Gupta AK, Chalmers PN, Rahman Z, Bruce B, Harris JD, McCormick F, Abrams GD, Nicholson GP. Reverse total shoulder arthroplasty in patients of varying body mass index. J Shoulder Elbow Surg. 2014;23(1):35–42. https://doi.org/10.1016/j.jse.2013.07.043. Epub 2013 Sep 30. PMID: 24090984

26. Erickson BJ, Shishani Y, Bishop ME, Romeo AA, Lederman E, Gobezie R. Tuberosity repair in reverse total shoulder arthroplasty for fracture using a stem-based double-row repair: a cadaveric biomechanical study. J Am Acad Orthop Surg. 2020;28(23):e1059–65. https://doi.org/10.5435/JAAOS-D-19-00667. PMID: 32195827

27. Black EM, Roberts SM, Siegel E, Yannopoulos P, Higgins LD, Warner JJ. Failure after reverse total shoulder arthroplasty: what is the success of component revision? J Shoulder Elbow Surg. 2015;24(12):1908–14. https://doi.org/10.1016/j.jse.2015.05.029. Epub 2015 Jul 7. PMID: 26163279

28. Erickson BJ. Failed reverse total shoulder arthroplasty: what are our bailouts? Curr Rev Musculoskelet Med. 2021;14(5):291–6. https://doi.org/10.1007/s12178-021-09712-9. Epub 2021 Aug 18. PMID: 34406603; PMCID: PMC8497668

29. Grob A, Freislederer F, Marzel A, Audigé L, Schwyzer HK, Scheibel M. Glenoid component loosening in anatomic total shoulder arthroplasty: association between radiological predictors and clinical parameters-an observational study. J Clin Med. 2021;10(2):234. https://doi.org/10.3390/jcm10020234. PMID: 33440646; PMCID: PMC7826694

30. Nagels J, Valstar ER, Stokdijk M, Rozing PM. Patterns of loosening of the glenoid component. J Bone Joint Surg Br. 2002;84(1):83–7. https://doi.org/10.1302/0301-620x.84b1.11951. PMID: 11837838

31. Collins D, Tencer A, Sidles J, Matsen F 3rd. Edge displacement and deformation of glenoid components in response to eccentric loading. The effect of preparation of the glenoid bone. J Bone Joint Surg Am. 1992;74(4):501–7. PMID: 1583044

32. Hawi N, Magosch P, Tauber M, Lichtenberg S, Habermeyer P. Nine-year outcome after anatomic stemless shoulder prosthesis: clinical and radiologic results. J Shoulder Elbow Surg. 2017;26(9):1609–15.

https://doi.org/10.1016/j.jse.2017.02.017. Epub 2017 Apr 11. PMID: 28410956

33. Flurin PH, Janout M, Roche CP, Wright TW, Zuckerman J. Revision of the loose glenoid component in anatomic total shoulder arthroplasty. Bull Hosp Jt Dis. 2013;71(Suppl 2):68–76. PMID: 24328585

34. Yang CC, Lu CL, Wu CH, Wu JJ, Huang TL, Chen R, Yeh MK. Stress analysis of glenoid component in design of reverse shoulder prosthesis using finite element method. J Shoulder Elbow Surg. 2013;22(7):932–9. https://doi.org/10.1016/j.jse.2012.09.001. Epub 2013 Jan 10. PMID: 23312816

35. Lädermann A, Schwitzguebel AJ, Edwards TB, Godeneche A, Favard L, Walch G, Sirveaux F, Boileau P, Gerber C. Glenoid loosening and migration in reverse shoulder arthroplasty. Bone Joint J. 2019;101-B(4):461–9. https://doi.org/10.1302/0301-620X.101B4.BJJ-2018-1275.R1. PMID: 30929497

36. Wagner ER, Hevesi M, Houdek MT, Cofield RH, Sperling JW, Sanchez-Sotelo J. Can a reverse shoulder arthroplasty be used to revise a failed primary reverse shoulder arthroplasty?: Revision reverse shoulder arthroplasty for failed reverse prosthesis. Bone Joint J. 2018;100-B(11):1493–8. https://doi.org/10.1302/0301-620X.100B11.BJJ-2018-0226.R2. PMID: 30418055

37. Inoue K, Suenaga N, Oizumi N, Yamaguchi H, Miyoshi N, Taniguchi N, Morita S, Munemoto M, Kurata S, Tanaka Y. Humeral bone resorption after reverse shoulder arthroplasty using uncemented stem. JSES Int. 2020;4(1):138–43. https://doi.org/10.1016/j.jses.2019.11.007. PMID: 32195476; PMCID: PMC7075776

38. Grey B, Rodseth RN, Roche SJ. Humeral stem loosening following reverse shoulder arthroplasty: a systematic review and meta-analysis. JBJS Rev. 2018;6(5):e5. https://doi.org/10.2106/JBJS.RVW.17.00129. PMID: 29762342

39. Raiss P, Edwards TB, Deutsch A, Shah A, Bruckner T, Loew M, Boileau P, Walch G. Radiographic changes around humeral components in shoulder arthroplasty. J Bone Joint Surg Am. 2014;96(7):e54. https://doi.org/10.2106/JBJS.M.00378. PMID: 24695931

40. Schnetzke M, Coda S, Raiss P, Walch G, Loew M. Radiologic bone adaptations on a cementless short-stem shoulder prosthesis. J Shoulder Elbow Surg. 2016;25(4):650–7. https://doi.org/10.1016/j.jse.2015.08.044. Epub 2015 Nov 7. PMID: 26560021

41. Schnetzke M, Rick S, Raiss P, Walch G, Loew M. Mid-term results of anatomical total shoulder arthroplasty for primary osteoarthritis using a short-stemmed cementless humeral component. Bone Joint J. 2018;100-B(5):603–9. https://doi.org/10.1302/0301-620X.100B5.BJJ-2017-1102.R2. PMID: 29701085

42. Melis B, DeFranco M, Lädermann A, Molé D, Favard L, Nérot C, Maynou C, Walch G. An evaluation of the radiological changes around the Grammont reverse geometry shoulder arthroplasty after eight to 12 years. J Bone Joint Surg Br. 2011;93(9):1240–6. https://doi.org/10.1302/0301-620X.93B9.25926. PMID: 21911536

43. Spormann C, Durchholz H, Audigé L, Flury M, Schwyzer HK, Simmen BR, Kolling C. Patterns of proximal humeral bone resorption after total shoulder arthroplasty with an uncemented rectangular stem. J Shoulder Elbow Surg. 2014;23(7):1028–35. https://doi.org/10.1016/j.jse.2014.02.024. PMID: 24929745

44. Chacon A, Virani N, Shannon R, Levy JC, Pupello D, Frankle M. Revision arthroplasty with use of a reverse shoulder prosthesis-allograft composite. J Bone Joint Surg Am. 2009;91(1):119–27. https://doi.org/10.2106/JBJS.H.00094. PMID: 19122086

45. Mourkus H, Phillips NJ, Rangan A, Peach CA. Management of periprosthetic fractures of the humerus: a systematic review. Bone Joint J. 2022;104-B(4):416–23. https://doi.org/10.1302/0301-620X.104B4.BJJ-2021-1334.R1. PMID: 35360951

46. Brusalis CM, Taylor SA. Periprosthetic fractures in reverse total shoulder arthroplasty: current concepts and advances in management. Curr Rev Musculoskelet Med. 2020;13(4):509–19. https://doi.org/10.1007/s12178-020-09654-8. PMID: 32506260; PMCID: PMC7340687

47. Colliton EM, Jawa A, Kirsch JM. Acromion and scapular spine fractures following reverse total shoulder arthroplasty. Orthop Clin North Am. 2021;52(3):257–68. https://doi.org/10.1016/j.ocl.2021.03.006. Epub 2021 May 7. PMID: 34053571

48. Ascione F, Kilian CM, Laughlin MS, Bugelli G, Domos P, Neyton L, Godeneche A, Edwards TB, Walch G. Increased scapular spine fractures after reverse shoulder arthroplasty with a humeral onlay short stem: an analysis of 485 consecutive cases. J Shoulder Elbow Surg. 2018;27(12):2183–90. https://doi.org/10.1016/j.jse.2018.06.007. Epub 2018 Aug 8. PMID: 30098923

49. Fram B, Elder A, Namdari S. Periprosthetic humeral fractures in shoulder arthroplasty. JBJS Rev. 2019;7(11):e6. https://doi.org/10.2106/JBJS.RVW.19.00017. PMID: 31770152

50. Kumar S, Sperling JW, Haidukewych GH, Cofield RH. Periprosthetic humeral fractures after shoulder arthroplasty. J Bone Joint Surg Am. 2004;86(4):680–9. https://doi.org/10.2106/00004623-200404000-00003. PMID: 15069130

51. Campbell JT, Moore RS, Iannotti JP, Norris TR, Williams GR. Periprosthetic humeral fractures: mechanisms of fracture and treatment options. J Shoulder Elbow Surg. 1998;7(4):406–13. https://doi.org/10.1016/s1058-2746(98)90033-7. PMID: 9752653

52. Wagner ER, Houdek MT, Elhassan BT, Sanchez-Sotelo J, Cofield RH, Sperling JW. What are risk factors for intraoperative humerus fractures during revision reverse shoulder arthroplasty and do they influence outcomes? Clin Orthop Relat Res. 2015;473(10):3228–34. https://doi.org/10.1007/s11999-015-4448-x. Epub 2015 Jul 11. PMID: 26162412; PMCID: PMC4562920

Alvaro Auñon, Prashant Meshram, Emilio Calvo, Edward G. McFarland, and Stephen C. Weber

The infected shoulder arthroplasty is a rare but devastating complication of shoulder replacement surgery. The mean incidence has been reported to be 1.1% but can be as high as 15% in reverse arthroplasty and up to 10% in a subset of high-risk, young, male patients [1]. Prosthetic joint infection (PJI) remains the most common cause of revision total shoulder surgery [2]. Risk factors for infection include posttraumatic osteoarthritis, previous surgery, steroid injection, rheumatoid arthritis, and diabetes mellitus. Other comorbidities associated with PJI are nutritional deficiency, drug abuse, and anemia from blood loss or iron deficiency. Demographic factors associated with PJI were younger age (OR, 1.020; 95% CI, 1.017–1.024; $P < 0.0001$) and male gender [1–4]. Management of the shoulder PJI continues to provoke controversy, with numerous options championed by various surgeons. Austin et al. in their review noted that septic procedures were further grouped as (1) debridement, antibiotics, irrigation, and implant retention (DAIR); (2) two-stage explant and delayed reimplantation with a temporary antibiotic spacer; (3) implant resection without reimplantation; or (4) unexpected positive cultures at revision surgery [4]. Single-stage reimplantation has also found increasing support in the literature [5, 6]. Austin et al. underscored the seriousness of PJI noting a 2.8% all-cause 1-year mortality, double that of noninfected patients [4]. Thus, choosing the correct management of the total shoulder PJI may be lifesaving as well as just limb-saving. While there is an understandable tendency to borrow from the hip and knee arthroplasty literature on this topic, PJI of the shoulder has different distributions of microorganisms and is less frequent compared to PJI of hip and knee arthroplasties [1]. Notably, *Cutibacterium acnes* is more common, especially in younger, male patients, and its slow-growing nature can make diagnosis of this pathogen especially difficult.

A. Auñon
Musculoskeletal Infections Unit, Department of Orthopedic Surgery and Traumatology, Fundación Jiménez Díaz, Universidad Autónoma, Madrid, Spain
e-mail: alvaro.aunon@fjd.es

P. Meshram
Orthocure Medical Center, Dubai, UAE

E. Calvo
Shoulder and Elbow Reconstructive Surgery Unit, Department of Orthopedic Surgery and Traumatology, Fundación Jiménez Díaz, Universidad Autónoma, Madrid, Spain
e-mail: ecalvo@fjd.es

E. G. McFarland · S. C. Weber (✉)
Shoulder Division, Department of Orthopedics, Johns Hopkins University, Baltimore, MD, USA
e-mail: emcfarl1@jhmi.edu

© ISAKOS 2023
A. D. Mazzocca et al. (eds.), *Shoulder Arthritis across the Life Span*,
https://doi.org/10.1007/978-3-031-33298-2_34

Furthermore, *C. acnes* has been suggested to play a role in the development of shoulder osteoarthritis [1, 7]. The management of the unexpected positive culture at revision shoulder surgery is complex and warrants a separate discussion of the controversies and treatment options. This paper will focus on the diagnosis and management of the more obviously infected primary and revision total shoulder arthroplasty.

34.1 Diagnosis

Diagnosis of the infected shoulder PJI remains challenging. Standard preoperative laboratory tests such as the complete blood count (CBC), erythrocyte sedimentation rate (ESR), and C-reactive protein are often negative in the face of obvious intraoperative findings of infection. Jauregui et al. [7] in a recent systematic review noted that synovial IL-6 and alpha-defensin may prove more useful, although other authors have disagreed [8]. Jauregui et al. noted relatively poor sensitivity and specificity with the CBC, sedimentation rate, and C-reactive protein in the preoperative diagnosis of PJI. Synovial fluid white cell counts have been widely employed, but the "dry tap" preoperatively remains a problem, even with image-guided aspiration. Moreover, even with successful aspiration, the reported positive result of synovial fluid, elevated white blood cell count, and microbiological culture is only in one third of the patients with PSI [9]. Paxton et al. [10] noted that "In contrast to the lower extremity, the relevance of aspiration in the evaluation of PJIS is less clear." Moroder et al. noted a cell count of greater than 2000/µL and/or more than 70% of polymorphonuclear leukocytes is indicative of a PJI [11]. Synovial leukocyte esterase strip testing has also been described [1, 8]. Ecker et al. however noted a sensitivity of 50% and a specificity of 87% using this technique [8].

Imaging has been similarly challenging. Plain radiographs are not usually useful; although there is an absence of infection, the loose uncemented humeral stem should raise suspicions for infection [10]. While technetium 99 m bone scanning has been widely employed in the imaging of lower extremity PJI, it has had only limited usefulness in the diagnosis of shoulder PJI. Technetium (Tc 99 m) bone scan is sensitive for identifying a failed arthroplasty but cannot differentiate between infection and aseptic failure [1]. Falstie-Jensen et al. noted that the WBC/BM scan results of 11 patients showed only 2 true positives along with 9 false negatives for a sensitivity of 18% [12]. Given the challenges of preoperative diagnosis of PSI, Meshram et al. evaluated the efficacy of metal artifact reduction sequence-magnetic resonance imaging (MARS-MRI) for diagnosis of PSI [13]. This study utilized the slice encoding for metal artifact correction (SEMAC) for MARS-MRI, and the radiological evaluation was done by two experienced radiologists trained in musculoskeletal imaging. The study reported that the MARS-MRI findings of lymphadenopathy, complex joint effusion, and edematous synovitis had the highest diagnostic performances with sensitivities >85%, specificities >90%, odds ratio > 3.6, and area under curve >0.9 for the diagnosis of PSI. These findings were limited to this specific SEMAC MRI sequence and to interpretation of the study by expert musculoskeletal radiologists, but it has potentially great value as an adjunct to making the diagnosis of shoulder PSI.

Arthroscopy can be an effective and accurate tool to identify low indolent causative organisms, thus detecting patients with infected shoulder arthroplasty in cases where classical preoperative workup to diagnose SPJI has been inconclusive. This could potentially reduce the number of unexpected ("surprise") intraoperative positive open cultures together with the non-true infected SA and consequently the number of unnecessary revision surgeries. Dilisio et al. found that culture of arthroscopically obtained tissue demonstrated 100% sensitivity, specificity, positive predictive value, and negative predictive value for identifying periprosthetic shoulder infection when one positive culture defined PSI concluding that arthroscopic tissue biopsy is a reliable method for diagnosing periprosthetic shoulder infection and identifying the causative organism [14]. Nevertheless, Akgun et al. were less optimistic and reported results a sensitivity and specificity of 80% and 94%, respectively, and the positive predictive value was 80% when two arthroscopically taken samples yielded positive cultures [15].

34.2 Intraoperative Findings

Gross purulence remains the most specific finding in shoulder PJI (Fig. 34.1). While intraoperative frozen sections of periprosthetic tissue have been used since the 1970s [16] and continue to be supported in the diagnosis of shoulder PJI [17], this technique can similarly be inconclusive, especially with low-virulence organisms [10]. Direct identification of infective agents at the time of revision is not practical, and some organisms, notably *C. acnes*, can take up to 26 days to grow in culture [7]. While promising, next-generation sequencing using polymerase chain reaction (PCR) has had problems with false-positive results, as it may identify nonclini-

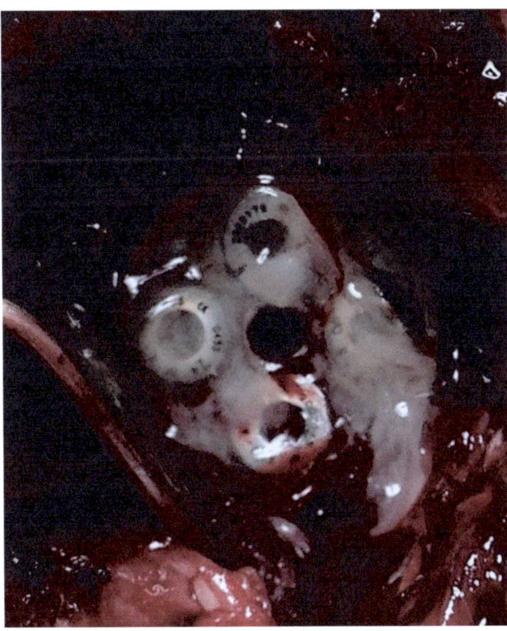

Fig. 34.1 Intraoperative photographs showing infected metaglene identified at the time of revision reverse shoulder arthroplasty. This type of visual appearance of gross purulence meets the major criteria in the 2018 International Consensus Meeting and would be categorized as "definite" PSI

cally relevant remnant DNA from dead bacteria [7, 18]. For these reasons, a high index of suspicion must be exercised in any revision, either primary or secondary for the subtle diagnosis of shoulder PJI.

34.3 Published Criteria for Defining Infection

Recognizing the challenge associated with the diagnosis of total joint infection, several scoring systems to standardize the diagnosis of shoulder PJI have been proposed. While several have been published, the 2018 International Consensus Meeting (ICM) on Musculoskeletal Infection has perhaps been the most widely adopted. The authors proposed a series of both major and minor criteria, similar to that of the MSIS criteria that have been consistently used for PJI diagnosis of the hip and knee. Meeting any one of the major criteria was determined to be diagnostic of a definite shoulder PJI and included "a sinus tract communicating with the prosthesis, gross intraarticular pus, or two positive cultures with phenotypically-identical virulent organisms." The minor criteria included many different diagnostic tests, as well as radiographic and exam findings, and placed a weighted value on each in order to categorize failed shoulder arthroplasties into different groups: probable PJI, possible PJI, and unlikely PJI [19]. Another widely referenced scoring system is that of Rangan et al. [17]. This scoring system represents the work of the British Elbow and Shoulder Society (BESS). Similar to the ICM scoring system, Rangan et al. had major criteria including a sinus tract or two positive separate cultures. Minor criteria were elevated ESR or C-reactive protein, synovial fluid leukocyte count greater than 1100/μL and/or 65% neutrophil percentage, gross purulence, one positive culture, or five neutrophils per high-power field observed from histologic analysis. The BESS scoring system is also proposed to recommend the urgency of referral. While other recent scoring systems have been proposed [8, 12, 18], the ICM scoring system remains the most useful and widely adopted. It should be noted that many of the criteria can only be applied postoperatively, and so its usefulness in the perioperative management of PJI remains challenging.

34.4 Treatment Options for Shoulder Prosthetic Joint Infection

34.4.1 Debridement, Antibiotics, Irrigation, and Implant Retention (DAIR)

Debridement, antibiotics, irrigation, and implant retention (DAIR) has been recommended in the management primarily within 6 weeks of surgery or those patients who have only experienced symptoms for 3 weeks [17]. This procedure requires that the positioning and execution of the prior arthroplasty remains good at the time of revision. Lower-virulence organisms have also been felt to be an indication [17]. The DAIR procedures have generally been performed open, as arthroscopic debridement has not provided consistently good results [20]. Rifampin has been recommended postoperatively due to its activity against nonresistant bacteria in the biofilm [1]. While tempting especially in older patients with significant comorbidities, the presence of a biofilm around the prosthesis quickly diminishes the effectiveness of concomitant antibiotics [21]. Chou et al. in their review of knee PJI showed double the rate of recurrent infection with DAIR compared to implant removal [22]. Eggleston et al. identified 12 primary studies using DAIR to treat shoulder PJI. They showed success rates of from 54% to 100%, but sample sizes of these studies were small [23]. Marcheggiani Muccioli et al. performed a systematic review of the treatment of infected shoulder arthroplasty [24]. These authors noted a 29.6% rate of persistent infection with debridement and felt that debridement should not be recommended for the management of infected shoulder arthroplasty. Ludwick et al. evaluated the risk factors for recurrent infection and sepsis in DAIR procedures for hip and knee procedures [25]. These authors felt that sepsis was a contraindication to use of a DAIR procedure, recommending instead a two-stage procedure. For all these reasons, DAIR procedures should be used with caution, due to the high risk of recurrent infection.

34.5 Single-Stage Revision of Infected Prostheses

Single-stage revision of infected shoulder prostheses has shown increased interest in the last decade. The advantages of decreased surgical morbidity, cost, and potential improvement in the outcome of the revision all seem obvious [10]. The equally obvious concern has been with recurrent infection with single-stage procedures. Several studies have sought to explore this topic. Mercurio et al. [26] performed a systematic review of the outcome of revision surgery for shoulder PJI. In their review, the infection eradication rate was 96% with one stage, 93% with permanent spacers, 86% with two stages, 85% with resection arthroplasty, and 65% with irrigation and debridement. One-stage revision was the best treatment, considering postoperative flexion and abduction, compared with resection arthroplasty, permanent spacers, and two-stage revision. One-stage revision showed fewer postoperative complications than irrigation and debridement, resection arthroplasty, and two-stage surgery. These authors favored one-stage revision for all cases except those where the bacterium involved was unknown. Interestingly, only 45% were revised to RTSA, although this number was high in two-stage procedures, respectively. There were no significant postoperative Constant and Simple Shoulder Test (SST) score differences between the one- and two-stage procedures. Eggleston et al. [23] in their systematic review noted that "we are unable to comment on what variables are more likely to produce a successful outcome following single-stage revision." Rangan et al. in their review proposed a more conservative approach to single-stage revision: "The indications for a one-stage revision are where the bacterium is known to be of low virulence or easily treatable; and where multiple operative procedures are contra-indicated due to risk to patient and/or the limb" [17]. Kunutson et al. noted that "New evidence suggests one-stage revision is at least equally as effective as the two-stage in controlling infection, maintaining joint function, and improving complications in shoulder PJI"; however "clinical measures of function and pain were not significantly different between the two revision strategies." Belay et al. noted that "shoulder surgeons treating PJI can be reassured of a low recurrence rate (6.3%) for single-stage and 10.1% for two-stage revision, but this was not significant." Paxton et al. [10] noted similar rates of recurrent infection for both procedures, but that "more research is needed to determine when each approach is appropriate." Nelson et al. [27] noted in their systematic review that "When outcomes were pooled, no statistical difference was found in the success rates of 1-stage, 2-stage, or resection arthroplasty revision; each displayed a success rate >90%. However, single-stage revision produced the highest mean Constant score."

Overall, the literature regarding one-stage revision remains inconclusive. While eradication of infection can occur, the conclusion that single-stage revision is as effective as two-stage revision is often biased by the selection of single-stage revision in less complex situations with less-virulent organisms [10]. There is only minimal data to suggest that single-stage revision improves functional outcomes by any measure, best summarized by Belay et al., who stated that "There are underwhelming data with patient-reported outcomes and functional outcomes to support single-stage over 2-stage revision" [5].

34.5.1 Two-Stage Explant and Delayed Reimplantation with a Temporary Antibiotic Spacer

Based on the early experience with the management of lower extremity PJI, two-stage explant and delayed reimplantation with a temporary antibiotic spacer has long been considered the gold standard. While the above argument regarding single-stage revision has been widely circu-lated, the morbidity and more rarely mortality of recurrent infection have caused many surgeons to exercise caution in their choice of revision proce-dure. That said, the cost and morbidity of two large surgical procedures and extensive antibiotic therapy cannot be overstated. This issue is per-haps best expressed in the large number of patients who ultimately select permanent treat-ment with an implanted spacer to avoid the mor-bidity of a second procedure, with a reasonable rate of patient satisfaction [28]. At least one study showed that definitive treatment without implant revision showed only modest diminution in out-come over secondary revision surgery using an implant [29]. Increasingly the toxicity of both systematic antibiotics and that of antibiotics delivered by the spacer has been described [30, 31]. Edelstein et al. clearly described nephrotox-icity with high-dose spacer use in the lower extremity and the difficulty of removing the source of the nephrotoxicity when this issue is established [27].

Spacers themselves are not without complica-tions. McFarland et al. [32] described their expe-rience with 50 implanted spacers. A total of 18 complications in 14 patients occurred, including bone erosion ($n = 8$), spacer fracture ($n = 4$), spacer rotation ($n = 3$), and humeral fracture ($n = 3$). Both prefabricated and intraoperatively molded spacers were used. Ten patients in this group were treated definitively with spacers, with four complications in three patients.

All of the data regarding recurrent infection using any treatment algorithm is confounded by the lack of mid- and long-term follow-up. The above studies have no more than 2-year mini-mum follow-up and many less than this. Our group reviewed the results of 17 revisions for infection at a minimum of 5-year follow-up [9]. In this review a recurrent infection developed in 3 (18%) of the 17 patients. Two of these were ini-tially infected with *C. acnes* and one with *Staphylococcus aureus*, only one of which had the same organism at re-revision as the initial organism at revision. The cumulative incidence of recurrence of infection was 0% at 1 year, 6% at 2 years, and 18% at 5 years. There were six (36%) other complications, including four periprosthetic fractures, one spacer fracture, and one dislocation. This study also retroactively applied the ICM criteria for infection. Using the ICM 2018 criteria at first-stage revision surgery, the category of PSI for ten (59%) patients was "definite PSI," four (23%) patients was "probable PSI," and three (18%) patients was "possible PSI." All of these patients had a positive frozen-section pathology report. This data gives one pause in regard to accepting 2-year data as definitively cleared of infection, although it appears that two of three with recurrent infection had clearance of their initial organism. Three patients were excluded because they were definitively treated with a spacer, as was one of the patients with recurrent infection.

34.5.2 Resection Arthroplasty Without Reimplantation

There are limited studies in the literature about the efficacy of resection arthroplasty for treatment of PSI. Stone et al. stated that "Resection arthroplasty is an option for low demand patients when revision arthroplasty is not possible" [33]. These authors described a recurrence rate of from 0 to 30% [33]. Other authors have noted similar results [34–37]. In this group's experience, resection arthroplasty is efficient in eradication of infection, but the functional outcomes are generally poor. Nonetheless, resection arthroplasty could be of value to treat patients with high suspicion of infection but who are medically unfit for a major surgery like single- or two-stage revision.

In summary, progress in the treatment of shoulder PJI remains slow. There is no single best test for diagnosis of PSI, and it should be based on multiple clinical, laboratory, and radiological investigations. MARS-MRI is an emerging investigation for diagnosing PSI and needs further investigation for its efficacy. Single- versus two-stage revision for chronic PSI should be individualized based on severity of clinical findings and ability to identify and the virulence of the causative organism of PSI. While the last decade has shown some improvements, challenges with both diagnosis and treatment of this increasingly important problem remain. Continued exploration of new options and further rigorous clinical study of these options will be the cornerstone of progress in this challenging area.

References

1. Fink B, Sevelda F. Periprosthetic joint infection of shoulder arthroplasties: diagnostic and treatment options. Biomed Res Int. 2017;2017:4582756.
2. Richards J, et al. Patient and procedure-specific risk factors for deep infection after primary shoulder arthroplasty. Clin Orthop Relat Res. 2014;472(9):2809–15.
3. Wirth MA, Rockwood CA Jr. Complications of shoulder arthroplasty. Clin Orthop Relat Res. 1994;307:47–69.
4. Austin DC, et al. Shoulder periprosthetic joint infection and all-cause mortality: a worrisome association. JB JS Open Access. 2022;7(1):e21.00118.
5. Belay ES, et al. Single-stage versus two-stage revision for shoulder periprosthetic joint infection: a systematic review and meta-analysis. J Shoulder Elbow Surg. 2020;29(12):2476–86.
6. Kunutsor SK, et al. One- and two-stage surgical revision of infected shoulder prostheses following arthroplasty surgery: a systematic review and meta-analysis. Sci Rep. 2019;9(1):232.
7. Jauregui JJ, et al. Diagnosing a periprosthetic shoulder infection: a systematic review. J Orthop. 2021;26:58–66.
8. Unter Ecker N, et al. What is the diagnostic accuracy of alpha-defensin and leukocyte esterase test in periprosthetic shoulder infection? Clin Orthop Relat Res. 2019;477(7):1712–8.
9. Meshram P, et al. Midterm results of two-stage revision surgery for periprosthetic shoulder infection. Sem Arthrop JSES. 2021;31(3):402–11.
10. Paxton ES, Green A, Krueger VS. Periprosthetic infections of the shoulder: diagnosis and management. J Am Acad Orthop Surg. 2019;27(21):e935–44.
11. Moroder P, et al. Diagnostik und Management des Endoprotheseninfekts am Schultergelenk. Obere Extremität. 2016;11(2):78–87.
12. Falstie-Jensen T, et al. Labeled white blood cell/bone marrow single-photon emission computed tomography with computed tomography fails in diagnosing chronic periprosthetic shoulder joint infection. J Shoulder Elbow Surg. 2019;28(6):1040–8.
13. Meshram P, et al. Can metal artifact reduction sequence magnetic resonance imaging (MARS-MRI) help in the diagnosis of Periprosthetic shoulder infection? J Shoulder Elbow Surg. 2022;31(3):e149–50.
14. Dilisio MF, et al. Arthroscopic tissue culture for the evaluation of periprosthetic shoulder infection. J Bone Joint Surg Am. 2014;96(23):1952–8.

15. Akgün D, et al. Diagnostic arthroscopy for detection of Periprosthetic infection in painful shoulder arthroplasty. Arthroscopy. 2019;35(9):2571–7.

16. Mirra JM, et al. The pathology of the joint tissues and its clinical relevance in prosthesis failure. Clin Orthop Relat Res. 1976;117:221–40.

17. Rangan A, et al. Investigation and management of periprosthetic joint infection in the shoulder and elbow: evidence and consensus based guidelines of the British elbow and shoulder society. Shoulder Elbow. 2018;10(1 Suppl):S5–s19.

18. Namdari S, et al. Comparative study of cultures and next-generation sequencing in the diagnosis of shoulder prosthetic joint infections. J Shoulder Elbow Surg. 2019;28(1):1–8.

19. Garrigues GE, et al. Proceedings from the 2018 international consensus meeting on orthopedic infections: the definition of periprosthetic shoulder infection. J Shoulder Elbow Surg. 2019;28(6s):S8–s12.

20. Jeon IH, et al. Arthroscopic management of septic arthritis of the shoulder joint. J Bone Joint Surg Am. 2006;88(8):1802–6.

21. Gbejuade HO, Lovering AM, Webb JC. The role of microbial biofilms in prosthetic joint infections. Acta Orthop. 2015;86(2):147–58.

22. Choi H-R, et al. Can implant retention be recommended for treatment of infected TKA? Clin Orthop Relat Res. 2011;469(4):961–9.

23. Egglestone A, et al. Scoping review: diagnosis and management of periprosthetic joint infection in shoulder arthroplasty. Shoulder Elbow. 2019;11(3):167–81.

24. Marcheggiani Muccioli GM, et al. Surgical treatment of infected shoulder arthroplasty. A systematic review. Int Orthop. 2017;41(4):823–30.

25. Ludwick L, et al. For patients with acute PJI treated with debridement, antibiotics, and implant retention, what factors are associated with systemic sepsis and recurrent or persistent infection in septic patients? Clin Orthop Relat Res. 2022;480:1491.

26. Mercurio M, et al. Outcomes of revision surgery after periprosthetic shoulder infection: a systematic review. J Shoulder Elbow Surg. 2019;28(6):1193–203.

27. Nelson GN, Davis DE, Namdari S. Outcomes in the treatment of periprosthetic joint infection after shoulder arthroplasty: a systematic review. J Shoulder Elbow Surg. 2016;25(8):1337–45.

28. Pellegrini A, et al. Management of periprosthetic shoulder infections with the use of a permanent articulating antibiotic spacer. Arch Orthop Trauma Surg. 2018;138(5):605–9.

29. Black EM, et al. Failure after reverse total shoulder arthroplasty: what is the success of component revision? J Shoulder Elbow Surg. 2015;24(12):1908–14.

30. Edelstein AI, et al. Nephrotoxicity after the treatment of Periprosthetic joint infection with antibiotic-loaded cement spacers. J Arthroplast. 2018;33(7):2225–9.

31. Luu A, et al. Two-stage arthroplasty for prosthetic joint infection: a systematic review of acute kidney injury, systemic toxicity and infection control. J Arthroplast. 2013;28(9):1490–8.e1.

32. McFarland EG, et al. Complications of antibiotic cement spacers used for shoulder infections. J Shoulder Elbow Surg. 2018;27(11):1996–2005.

33. Stone MA, Namdari S. Reverse shoulder arthroplasty: diagnostic and treatment options for the infected reverse. Ann Jt. 2018;3:3.

34. Jacquot A, et al. Surgical management of the infected reversed shoulder arthroplasty: a French multicenter study of reoperation in 32 patients. J Shoulder Elbow Surg. 2015;24(11):1713–22.

35. Ortmaier R, et al. Treatment strategies for infection after reverse shoulder arthroplasty. Eur J Orthop Surg Traumatol. 2014;24(5):723–31.

36. Braman JP, et al. The outcome of resection shoulder arthroplasty for recalcitrant shoulder infections. J Shoulder Elbow Surg. 2006;15(5):549–53.

37. Muh SJ, et al. Resection arthroplasty for failed shoulder arthroplasty. J Shoulder Elbow Surg. 2013;22(2):247–52.

Periprosthetic Humerus Fractures After Shoulder Arthroplasty

35

Casey L. Wright, Maria A. Theodore, Richard Smith, and Evan A. O'Donnell

Periprosthetic humerus fractures adjacent to shoulder arthroplasty pose a challenging problem for orthopedic surgeons and patients alike. Recent decades have seen a substantial increase in the prevalence of shoulder arthroplasty, which increased by approximately 730% between 1995 and 2017 [1]. In 2017, approximately 2% of the population over the age of 80 was living with a shoulder arthroplasty. As the prevalence of shoulder arthroplasty increases, so too does the population at risk of periprosthetic complications. Although overall complication rates may be downtrending with improvements in surgical technique and implant design [2, 3], estimates of the complication rates of anatomic and reverse total shoulder arthroplasty are variable and may be as high as 25% [3–6]. Complications include instability, periprosthetic fracture, infection, implant loosening, neurologic injury, acromial or scapular spine fracture, hematoma, deltoid injury, rotator cuff injury, and venous thromboembolism. Periprosthetic humerus fractures account for approximately 20% of all complications, with the majority of fractures occurring intraopera-

tively [3, 7]. Fractures are significantly more likely to occur in cases of reverse (OR 4.01) [3, 8] and revision arthroplasty (RR 2.8) [9, 10]; the prevalence of both of which can be expected to increase in coming years.

While humeral shaft fractures in the absence of an implant demonstrate reliable healing, periprosthetic fractures are associated with greater rates of nonunion [11, 12]. The presence of a prosthesis may disrupt endosteal blood supply, cause persistent distraction at the fracture site, and alter the mechanical environment at the fracture by altering glenohumeral joint motion [11, 13]. Patient factors predisposing to fracture, such as medical comorbidities in the aging population, rheumatoid arthritis, and osteopenia, may also hinder healing [13]. Further complicating shared decision-making among patients and surgeons is the relative lack of evidence-based guidance on management of periprosthetic humerus fractures, with most recommendations limited to expert opinion and small case series [12].

C. L. Wright · R. Smith · E. A. O'Donnell (✉)
Department of Orthopaedic Surgery, Massachusetts General Hospital, Boston, MA, USA
e-mail: clwright@partners.org;
rsmith21@partners.org; eodonnell4@partners.org

M. A. Theodore
Harvard College, Cambridge, MA, USA
e-mail: mtheodore@college.harvard.edu

35.1 Classification Schemes

Several classification schemes for periprosthetic humerus fractures have been proposed, primarily based on fracture location. Successive classification systems have attempted to improve the utility of fracture classification in guiding management by incorporating factors such as

© ISAKOS 2023
A. D. Mazzocca et al. (eds.), *Shoulder Arthritis across the Life Span*,
https://doi.org/10.1007/978-3-031-33298-2_35

fracture pattern, available bone stock, and implant loosening. Only the most recent classification schemes, which were developed after the widespread adoption of reverse, short-stem, and stemless implants, consider implant design.

One of the most widely accepted periprosthetic humerus fracture classification schemes was proposed by Wright and Cofield in 1995, which utilized the tip of the implant as a reference point (Fig. 35.1) [14]. Wright and Cofield Type A and B fractures both originate at the tip of the stem, with Type A fractures demonstrating proximal extension greater than one-third the length of the stem, Type B fractures extending proximally to a lesser extent, and Type C fractures located entirely distal to the stem.

In 1998, Campbell et al. classified fractures based on the *anatomic* location of the fracture [15]. Fractures are classified based on their location within the greater and/or lesser tuberosities (region 1), metaphysis (region 2), proximal diaphysis (region 3), or mid- to distal humeral diaphysis (region 4).

Similar to the original Wright and Cofield classification, Worland et al. proposed a classification scheme centered around the location of the fracture relative to the stem, with a subclassification based on fracture pattern and stability of the implant [16]. In the Worland classification, Type A fractures involve the tuberosities, Type B occur at the level of the stem, and Type C occur distal to the implant. Type B fractures are further subdivided into spiral fractures (Type B1), oblique fractures near the stem tip (Type B2), and fractures associated with an unstable implant (Type B3). Such subclassification is designed to reduce the ambiguity in treatment of Type B fractures, as Type B2 can typically be treated nonoperatively and Type B3 fractures should be managed surgically.

In 2008, Groh et al. developed a classification scheme for both intra- and postoperative fractures, utilizing the stem as a reference point, which could guide management [17]. Type I fractures exist entirely proximal to the stem tip and are amenable to cerclage if occurring intraoperatively. Type II fractures, which extend distal to the stem tip, and Type III fractures, occurring entirely distal to the stem, are amenable to cerclage and conversion to a long-stem prosthesis when occurring intraoperatively. When occurring postoperatively, Type III fractures involving a stable implant are amenable to a trial of nonoperative management.

The above classification schemes have demonstrated only moderate interobserver agreement, with Fleiss' kappa values between 0.483 (Groh classification) and 0.583 (Wright and Cofield classification) for fracture classification and in guiding management [18]. Fractures of the humeral diaphysis at or proximal to the stem tip, including Wright and Cofield Type A, Campbell Region 3, Worland Type B, and Groh Type II fractures, present a significant challenge to surgeons evidenced by variability in preferred management. The variability could result from degree of fracture displacement, implant instability, and/or remaining bone stock, which are not well-accounted for in the available classification schemes, as well as surgeon preference.

Recently, Kirchoff et al. proposed a more comprehensive classification system and treatment algorithm inclusive of some of these factors

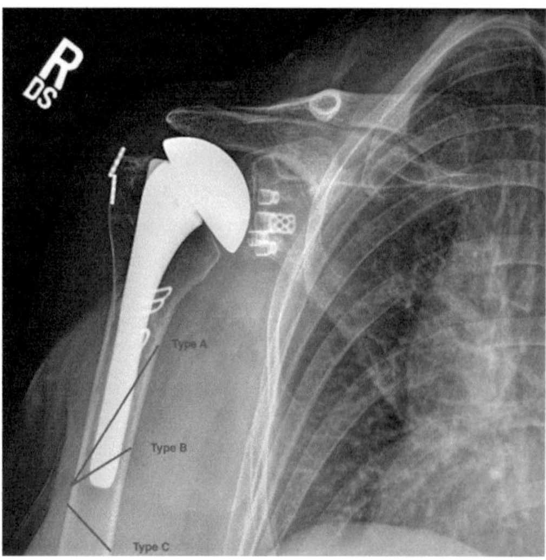

Fig. 35.1 AP x-ray of the right shoulder with an anatomic total shoulder replacement. Lines demonstrate the Wright and Cofield fracture classification. Type A fractures originate at the stem tip and extend proximally greater than one-third the length of the stem. Type B fractures originate at the stem tip and extend proximally to a lesser extent. Type C fractures occur distal to the stem tip

[19]. The system takes into consideration the type of prosthesis (anatomic, stemless, reverse), anatomic fracture location (acromion, glenoid, humerus), location of the fracture in relation to the implant, presence of a glenoid prosthesis, integrity of the rotator cuff, and implant stability. In a subsequent retrospective validation study, they found high inter-rater reliability between two board-certified trauma surgeons (Cohen's kappa of 0.94) with the sole discrepancy resulting from disagreement classifying a stem as loose or stable [20]. Eighty-four percent of the fractures were treated in accordance with the proposed treatment algorithm, and 94% of these cases (15 of 16) had a good outcome. Conversely, in all three cases in which the surgeon deviated from the proposed treatment, the patient experienced a poor outcome.

To date, however, no classification scheme has been universally adopted. The lack of a standardized classification system hinders both the creation of larger data repositories on periprosthetic humerus fractures and the development of management guidelines.

35.2 Risk Factors

Proximal humerus periprosthetic fractures are best considered in two broad groups, intra- and postoperative, each of which has its own risk factor profile, management options, and clinical outcomes.

Intraoperative periprosthetic humerus fractures largely occur during implant removal in revision cases (up to 81%), during reaming and broaching (up to 31%), during trialing or implant insertion (up to 19%), or due to excessive torque or retraction (up to 13–15%) [10, 15, 21, 22]. Risk factors include both modifiable and non-modifiable patient factors, including female sex (RR 3.3 [9] – 4.19 [23]), post-traumatic arthritis (RR 1.9 [9] – 2.55 [23]) [15, 21], instability (RR 2.65 [10]), osteoporosis [14, 15, 24, 25], and rheumatoid arthritis [13, 14, 26–28]; implant factors, such as the use of press-fit stems (RR 2.9 [9]) or prior hemiarthroplasties in revision cases (OR 2.34 [10]); and surgical factors, such as revi-

sion cases (RR 2.8 [9]). Revision cases pose a particular challenge due to the scar tissue encountered during the approach, the need to remove the previous implant, and stress shielding of the greater tuberosity in uncemented and diaphyseal-fitting stems [15, 22]. Excessive scar tissue may necessitate increased torque to obtain adequate exposure, whereas stress shielding predisposes the tuberosities to fracture.

A comprehensive understanding of a patient's risk factors for periprosthetic fracture is imperative to preoperative planning and informed consent discussions. In high-risk patients, the possible need for intraoperative fixation or conversion to reverse total shoulder arthroplasty should be discussed preoperatively. Surgeons may also ensure additional equipment, such as cerclage wires, plates, screws, long-stem implants, reverse components, and cement, are available.

Several mitigation techniques exist to reduce the risk of intraoperative fracture, and start with patient positioning. The patient should be positioned to allow for full extension and adduction of the humerus, which allows for adequate humeral canal preparation without levering of the distal humerus. Surgeons should ensure adequate capsular release, especially in cases of severe osteoarthritis, significant medial glenoid wear, and revision cases with soft tissue contracture, to allow for adequate exposure without excessive torque on the humerus. The humerus is at particular risk of fracture due to torque and excessive external rotation during initial dislocation and glenoid preparation. Appreciating preexisting humeral deformity in the case of post-traumatic arthritis or revision surgery is important to ensure a correct entry point and trajectory for reaming, avoiding perforation. Intraoperative fluoroscopy may be useful to plan and confirm the appropriate positioning of reamer, broaches, or implants. Overzealous reaming and endosteal notching predispose to both intra- and postoperative fractures by creating a stress riser at the tip of the implant stem. Hand reaming is particularly useful in mitigating this risk, especially in osteoporotic bone in which it allows for compression of cancellous bone. Finally, appropriate preoperative templating may mitigate the risk of fracture associated with underreaming and placement of an oversized prosthesis. Intraoperative radiographs taken prior to leaving the OR are useful in identifying unrecognized fractures or risk factors for postoperative periprosthetic fracture.

In revision cases, implant removal and disruption of the bone-implant or cement-implant interface may result in significant bone loss and are typically associated with fractures involving the greater tuberosity. The greater tuberosity is at particular risk with metaphyseal-filling ingrowth stems or cemented stems with proximal fins, which result in significant proximal bone loss during removal. Preventative measures include utilization of implant-specific removal devices and decreasing the force necessary to remove the implant by performing a corticotomy [22].

Some surgeons utilize prophylactic placement of heavy, nonabsorbable sutures or cerclage wires around the tuberosities or metaphysis. This may be especially useful in patients at high risk of fracture during stem removal, reaming, or insertion, including those with a thin greater tuberosity.

The vast majority of postoperative fractures occur after a fall [13, 14, 16, 24] or through an area of cortical weakening due to a stress riser or prosthetic loosening [14, 24]. Risk factors for postoperative fractures include osteonecrosis and increased Charlson medical comorbidity index [23]. Generally, postoperative fractures occur at the tip of the stem or cement mantle. However, with short-stem or canal-sparing implants, fractures may involve the tuberosities and proximal humeral shafts.

35.3 Patient Evaluation

Evaluation of patients with periprosthetic humeral fractures involves a thorough history, physical examination, and radiographic evaluation. A thorough history should elicit the mechanism of injury, risk factors for periprosthetic fracture as detailed above, and review of prior operative reports. Review of operative reports should note the preoperative diagnosis and implants used. Note should also be made of any prior complications and revision surgeries. During the physical examination, it is imperative to note neurovascular status particularly of the axillary and radial nerves, as well as distal perfusion, as revision shoulder arthroplasty and open reduction and internal fixation (ORIF) of periprosthetic fractures are higher-risk operations for neurovascular complication.

X-rays of the shoulder (AP, true AP (Grashey), scapular Y, and axillary views) and full-length humerus (AP and lateral) should be assessed for previous implant, implant loosening, stress shielding, available bone stock, fracture pattern, and any preexisting humeral deformity. Metal suppression CT is useful for assessing remaining bone stock, implant stability, fracture pattern, glenoid version, and rotator cuff integrity [29]. Axial imaging also aids the surgeon in planning the feasibility and trajectory of possible "skive" screws, or bicortical non-locking screws angled to skirt around the implant, in cases of planned ORIF.

35.4 Management and Outcomes

Management of periprosthetic humeral fractures is dependent on several factors including timing of fracture (intraoperative vs postoperative); implant type and stability; fracture location and morphology; and patient factors, such as bone quality, rotator cuff integrity, and medical comorbidities. Treatment options vary and include nonoperative treatment, open reduction and internal fixation, and revision arthroplasty. The goals of fracture management are pain relief, early range of motion, preservation of shoulder function, and promotion of fracture union while maintaining implant stability.

35.5 Intraoperative Fractures

Management of intraoperative fractures is highly dependent on fracture location. Metaphyseal, calcar, and proximal humeral diaphyseal fractures are generally amenable to bypassing the fracture by two [24] to three [15] cortical diameters with either a standard-length or long-stem prosthesis, with supplemental cerclage, tape/suture, and plate and screw fixation as needed. Tuberosity fractures may be managed with transosseous suture fixation to secure the rotator cuff attachments, with or without screw augmentation. If unable to attain stable fixation, conversion to a fracture or revision stem may improve stability by improving proximal ingrowth and providing more options for fixation through the stem. In cases in which there is persistent inability to attain stable fixation, conversion to a reverse arthroplasty may be necessary.

Intraoperative shaft fractures can similarly be managed with conversion to a longer-stemmed prosthesis, bypassing the fracture site by at least two cortical diameters. Placement of cement in the distal canal to engage the tip of the prosthesis may improve stability. When a fracture is sustained prior to cementation, it is imperative to prevent cement from escaping through the fracture site, which can impede healing and result in nerve injury. If a fracture occurs after cementation and the stem is determined to be stable, plate fixation may avoid the risk of fracture propagation and increased morbidity associated with stem removal [11]. If unable to bypass the fracture site by a sufficient length or in the setting of severe osteopenia, additional fracture fixation with cerclage cables, suture fixation, plate and screw fixation, and/or strut allograft is advisable. Supplementary fixation allows for earlier range of motion and higher union rates [11, 15].

In their report of intraoperative fractures, Athwal and colleagues noted all fractures demonstrated radiographic healing at a mean of 17 weeks postoperatively (range, 6–56 weeks) [9]. Non-displaced greater tuberosity fractures healed at a mean of 6.5 weeks, whereas displaced tuberosity fractures healed at a mean of 13.5 weeks. Humeral shaft fractures healed at a mean of 22.5 weeks.

35.6 Postoperative Fractures

35.6.1 Nonoperative Management

Many surgeons advocate for a trial of nonoperative management for postoperative shaft fractures

in acceptable alignment without evidence of implant loosening [17, 24, 26, 30]. Acceptable alignment is generally defined as less than 20 degrees of flexion/extension, 15–20 degrees of rotation, and 30 degrees of varus/valgus deformity [11, 31, 32]. Long oblique and spiral fractures are most amenable to nonoperative treatment [14], unless overlapping a significant portion of the stem compromising implant stability. Nonoperative management generally involves immobilization with a shoulder immobilizer, cast, or Sarmiento brace, depending on the fracture location.

Although many authors advocate for a trial of nonoperative management, it is important to understand the low success and high complication rates associated with nonoperative treatment (Table 35.1) [5, 13–17, 24, 26, 33–35]. A recent systematic review of management of periprosthetic humerus fractures found a 50% failure rate of nonoperative treatment [12]. Of the 32 patients identified in their study who were treated entirely nonoperatively, 10 (31%) developed complications including malunion/nonunion, radial nerve palsy, shoulder stiffness, and skin necrosis from the orthosis.

35.6.2 Open Reduction and Internal Fixation

Indications for fracture fixation include failure of nonoperative management for a humeral shaft fracture surrounding a stable implant and tuberosity fracture near a hemiarthroplasty or anatomic total shoulder arthroplasty [36]. Failure of nonoperative treatment can be assumed when there is failure to maintain adequate reduction or there is nonunion of an unstable fracture after at least 3 months of attempted nonoperative management [11, 24]. Transverse and short oblique fractures are more likely to fail nonoperative management [14]. Tuberosity fractures can be repaired via transosseous sutures, tape, cerclage, or conversion to reverse total shoulder arthroplasty. Fixation of periprosthetic shaft fractures around a well-fixed implant can be achieved with either a plate, strut allograft, or both. The plate may be secured around the stem with either cer-

Table 35.1 Outcomes of periprosthetic humerus fractures managed conservatively

Study	No. of fractures managed non-operatively	No. of fractures that healed with non-operative management	Mean time to radiographic healing	Complications (%)	Complications
Boyd (1992) [13]	7	1 (14.3%)	3 months	1 (100%)	Union with pain
Krakauer (1994) [26]	11	6 (54.5%)	11–13 weeks[a]	Not specified	Not specified
Wright (1995) [14]	8	4 (50%)	5.3 months	1 (12.5%)	Persistent pain
Campbell (1998) [15]	5	5 (100%)	3.1 months	2 (40%)	Frozen shoulder, skin slough and cellulitis
Worland (1999) [16]	2	1 (50%)	3 months	1 (100%)	Death
Kumar (2004) [24]	11	6 (54.5%)	180 days	None reported	None reported
Groh (2008) [17]	4	4 (100%)	11 weeks[b]	None reported	None reported
Wolf (2012) [33]	2	0 (0%)	N/A	1 (100%)	Nonunion, persistent pain
Garcia-Fernandez (2015) [34]	1	1 (100%)	18 weeks[b]	None reported	None reported
Ascione (2018) [5]	5	5 (100%)	Not specified	None reported	None reported
Ragusa (2020) [35]	5	4 (80%)	4.4 months	3 (60%)	Acromial stress fracture, second fracture, hypertrophic nonunion

[a] Range, mean value not provided
[b] Inclusive of all fractures, treated operatively and non-operatively

clage wires, short unicortical locking screws, or bicortical "skive" screws. To avoid the creation of a stress riser, the plate should overlap the prosthesis by at least two cortical diameters. Locking plates, which may be particularly useful in osteopenic bone, have the benefit of increased bone-implant stability and screw pullout [11]. Contraindications to operative management include medical comorbidities precluding general anesthesia and active infection.

Operative management with internal fixation has demonstrated good outcomes with respect to healing among appropriately selected patient cohorts. In 2022, Mourkus and colleagues published a systematic review of clinical outcomes following periprosthetic humerus fractures [12]. The review included 99 patients who underwent open reduction and internal fixation, in which union was achieved in 93.07% (95% CI 87.15–97.45) without further intervention. Eighty-four of these patients underwent fixation acutely, whereas 15 had previously failed a trial of nonoperative management. The overwhelming majority (95%) involved a well-fixed prosthesis, and fracture healing, which was reported for 75.7% of the patients, occurred at a mean of 5.5 months (range, 2–10). Of those studies which reported patient satisfaction scores, 72% of patients reported being satisfied with their outcome. Complications included hardware irritation, transient nerve palsies, deep infection, fracture extension or failure of fixation, and nonunion.

Despite reliable radiographic healing, functional deficits may persist. Among five patients treated with open reduction and internal fixation using a locking plate, Kurowicki et al. noted a mean time to radiographic union of 19 weeks (range, 9–53 weeks) with only one patient reporting a VAS pain score above 0 (average 0.5) [37]. However, functionally limiting range of motion deficits were not uncommon. The average active shoulder flexion was 86 degrees (range, 60–130), abduction 70 degrees (range, 50–90 degrees), and external rotation 18 degrees (range, −10–60 degrees). The mean ASES total score was 75 (range, 62–100), while the mean ASES function score was 28 (range, 15–50).

The largest case series to date, published by Andersen et al., included 17 fractures treated with ORIF occurring after anatomic (9) or reverse (8) shoulder arthroplasties [38]. Eight of the fractures were augmented with strut allograft. All fractures demonstrated radiographic healing at a mean 6.8 months postoperatively (range, 3.25 to 12 months). Mean ASES score at time of final follow-up was 45.1 (95% CI, 26.8 to 63.5). Five of six patients in whom pre-fracture ASES scores were available returned to their pre-fracture score. Seven of the 17 fractures experienced complications, 4 of which required subsequent reoperation. These included a remote broken anatomic humeral stem due to recurrent trauma, failure of glenosphere baseplate fixation and the humeral socket, distal plate fixation failure, and distal fracture-line extension. The latter two occurred shortly postoperatively and required extension of fixation with an additional locking plate. Radial nerve palsies occurred in three additional cases and were managed nonoperatively.

35.6.3 Revision Arthroplasty

Revision arthroplasty is indicated in fractures involving a loose implant or those in which surrounding bone stock is insufficient for fracture fixation. Implant loosening can be assessed by changes in implant positioning on serial radiographs or when radiolucency is noted in at least three of eight humeral zones [39, 40]. Traumatic loosening can occur when a fracture line extends along a significant portion of the implant, destabilizing it [11]. Revision arthroplasty typically involves conversion to a long-stemmed implant that bypasses the fracture by at least two to three cortical diameters. The long-stem implant can be either press fit or cemented, dependent on the implant chosen and available bone stock [11, 14, 16, 24]. Implant revision is often accompanied by additional fixation, usually with a strut allograft and cerclage or a plate and screws. Osteolysis and loss of available bone stock may complicate management of periprosthetic humeral fractures and may necessitate component-allograft composites or humeral endoprostheses.

Andersen and colleagues reported on 19 periprosthetic fractures involving 9 reverse and 10 anatomic implants treated with revision arthroplasty [38]. All stems were loose at the time of surgery. Fourteen were treated with a long-stem prosthesis, whereas five were treated with a short stem supplemented by ORIF. They noted an average time to radiographic union of 7.7 months (range, 3.5 to 13.5 months). Allograft augmentation was utilized in 17 of the cases and 18 went on to union. Pre-fracture ASES scores were available for five of the patients (32.0 (95% CI, 14.0–50.0)), with all postfracture ASES scores exceeding pre-injury scores (54.4 (95% CI, 44.6 to 64.2)). Complications occurred in seven cases, three of which required reoperation. These included subsequent periprosthetic fracture, nonunion following multiple surgeries, and dissociation of the humeral socket-stem Morse taper. Complications treated nonoperatively included a transient radial nerve palsy, loosening of the stem, postoperative hematoma, and dislocation.

35.7 Conclusion

Periprosthetic humeral fractures are increasing in their incidence and represent a challenging clinical problem. A thorough preoperative evaluation including previous operative notes with implant specifics, radiographs, and axial imaging are necessary. Classification systems remain cumbersome and complex. Nonoperative management can be considered, though with high rates of nonunion and malunion. Surgical interventions include ORIF and revision shoulder arthroplasty and should be tailored to patient and fracture morphology.

References

1. Farley KX, Wilson JM, Kumar A, Gottschalk MB, Daly C, Sanchez-Sotelo J, et al. Prevalence of shoulder arthroplasty in the United States and the increasing burden of revision shoulder arthroplasty. JBJS Open Access. 2021;6(3) https://doi.org/10.2106/JBJS.OA.20.00156.

2. Bohsali KI, Wirth MA, Rockwood CA. Complications of total shoulder arthroplasty. J Bone Joint Surg Am. 2006;88(10):2279–92.

3. Bohsali KI, Bois AJ, Wirth MA. Complications of shoulder arthroplasty. J Bone Joint Surg Am. 2017;99(3):256–69.

4. Kristensen MR, Rasmussen JV, Elmengaard B, Jensen SL, Olsen BS, Brorson S. High risk for revision after shoulder arthroplasty for failed osteosynthesis of proximal humeral fractures. Acta Orthop. 2018;89(3):345–50.

5. Ascione F, Domos P, Guarrella V, Chelli M, Boileau P, Walch G. Long-term humeral complications after Grammont-style reverse shoulder arthroplasty. J Shoulder Elbow Surg. 2018;27(6):1065–71. https://doi.org/10.1016/j.jse.2017.11.028.

6. Saltzman BM, Chalmers PN, Gupta AK, Romeo AA, Nicholson GP. Complication rates comparing primary with revision reverse total shoulder arthroplasty. J Shoulder Elbow Surg. 2014;23(11):1647–54.

7. Gombera MM, Laughlin MS, Vidal EA, Brown BS, Morris BJ, Bradley Edwards T, et al. The impact of fellowship type on trends and complications following total shoulder arthroplasty for osteoarthrosis by recently trained board-eligible orthopedic surgeons. J Shoulder Elbow Surg. 2020;29(7):e279–86. https://doi.org/10.1016/j.jse.2019.11.023.

8. Ross BJ, Wu VJ, McCluskey LC, O'Brien MJ, Sherman WJ, Savoie FH. Postoperative complication rates following total shoulder arthroplasty (TSA) vs. reverse shoulder arthroplasty (RSA): a nationwide analysis. Semin Arthrop JSES. 2020;30(2):83–8.

9. Athwal GS, Sperling JW, Rispoli DM, Cofield RH. Periprosthetic humeral fractures during shoulder arthroplasty. J Bone Joint Surg Am. 2009;91(3):594–603.

10. Wagner ER, Houdek MT, Elhassan BT, Sanchez-Sotelo J, Cofield RH, Sperling JW. What are risk factors for intraoperative humerus fractures during revision reverse shoulder arthroplasty and do they influence outcomes? Clin Orthop Relat Res. 2015;473(10):3228–34.

11. Steinmann SP, Cheung E. Treatment of periprosthetic humerus fractures associated with shoulder arthroplasty. J Am Acad Orthop Surg. 2008;16(4):199–207.

12. Mourkus H, Phillips NJ, Rangan A, Peach CA. Management of periprosthetic fractures of the humerus: a systematic review. Bone Joint J. 2022;104-B(4):416–23.

13. Boyd AD, Thornhill TS, Barnes CL. Fractures adjacent to humeral prostheses. J Bone Joint Surg Am. 1992;74(10):1498–504.

14. Wright TW, Cofield RH. Humeral fractures after shoulder arthroplasty. J Bone Joint Surg Am. 1995;77(9):1340–6.

15. Campbell JT, Moore RS, Iannotti JP, Norris TR, Williams GR. Periprosthetic humeral fractures: mechanisms of fracture and treatment options. J Shoulder Elbow Surg. 1998;7(4):406–13.

16. Worland RL, Kim DY, Arredondo J. Periprosthetic humeral fractures: management and classification. J Shoulder Elbow Surg. 1999;8(6):590–4.

17. Groh GI, Heckman MM, Wirth MA, Curtis RJ, Rockwood CA, Antonio S. Treatment of fractures adjacent to humeral prostheses. J Shoulder Elbow Surg. 2008;17(1):85–9.

18. Kuhn MZ, King JJ, Wright TW, Farmer KW, Levy JC, Hao KA, et al. Periprosthetic humerus fractures after shoulder arthroplasty: an evaluation of available classification systems. J Shoulder Elbow Surg. 2022;S1058-2746(22):00439–6. https://doi.org/10.1016/j.jse.2022.05.011. Epub ahead of print

19. Kirchhoff C, Kirchhoff S, Biberthaler P. Classification of periprosthetic shoulder fractures. Unfallchirurg. 2016;119(4):264–72.

20. Kirchhoff C, Beirer M, Brunner U, Buchholz A, Biberthaler P, Crönlein M. Validation of a new classification for periprosthetic shoulder fractures. Int Orthop. 2018;42(6):1371–7.

21. Williams GR, Iannotti JP. Management of periprosthetic fractures: the shoulder. J Arthroplast. 2002;17(4):14–6.

22. Fram B, Elder A, Namdari S. Periprosthetic humeral fractures in shoulder arthroplasty. JBJS Rev. 2019;7(11):e6. https://doi.org/10.2106/JBJS.RVW.19.00017.

23. Singh JA, Sperling J, Schleck C, Harmsen W, Cofield R. Periprosthetic fractures associated with primary total shoulder arthroplasty and primary humeral head replacement: a thirty-three-year study. J Bone Joint Surg Am. 2012;94(19):1777–85.

24. Kumar S, Sperling JW, Haidukewych GH, Cofield RH. Periprosthetic humeral fractures after shoulder arthroplasty. J Bone Joint Surg Am. 2004;86(4):680–9.

25. Bonutti PM, Hawkins RJ. Fracture of the humeral shaft associated with total replacement arthroplasty of the shoulder: a case report. J Bone Joint Surg Am. 1992;74(4):617–8.

26. Krakauer JD, Cofield RH. Periprosthetic fractures in total shoulder replacement. Oper Tech Orthop. 1994;4(4):243–52.

27. Brenner BC, Ferlic DC, Clayton ML, Dennis DA. Survivorship of unconstrained total shoulder arthroplasty. J Bone Joint Surg Am. 1989;71(9):1289–96.

28. Barrett WP, Franklin JL, Jackins SE, Wyss CR, Matsen FA 3rd. Total shoulder arthroplasty. J Bone Joint Surg Am. 1987;69(6):865–72.

29. Buck FM, Jost B, Hodler J. Shoulder arthroplasty. Eur Radiol. 2008;18(12):2937–48.

30. Updegrove GF, Mourad W, Abboud JA. Humeral shaft fractures. J Shoulder Elbow Surg. 2018;27:87–97.

31. Klenerman L. Fractures of the shaft of the humerus. Bone Joint J. 1966;48(1):105–11.
32. Shields E, Sundem L, Childs S, Maceroli M, Humphrey C, Ketz JP, et al. The impact of residual angulation on patient reported functional outcome scores after non-operative treatment for humeral shaft fractures. Injury. 2016;47(4):914–8.
33. Wolf H, Pajenda G, Sarahrudi K. Analysis of factors predicting success and failure of treatment after type B periprosthetic humeral fractures: a case series study. Eur J Trauma Emerg Surg. 2012;38(2):177–83.
34. García-Fernández C, Lópiz-Morales Y, Rodríguez A, López-Durán L, Martínez FM. Periprosthetic humeral fractures associated with reverse total shoulder arthroplasty: incidence and management. Int Orthop. 2015;39(10):1965–9.
35. Ragusa PS, Vadhera A, Jang JM, Ali I, McFarland EG, Srikumaran U. Nonoperative treatment of periprosthetic humeral shaft fractures after reverse total shoulder arthroplasty. Orthopedics. 2020;43(6):E553–60. https://doi.org/10.3928/01477447-20200910-06.
36. Sanchez-Sotelo J, Athwal GS. Periprosthetic postoperative humeral fractures after shoulder arthroplasty. J Am Acad Orthop Surg. 2022;30:e1227. https://doi.org/10.5435/JAAOS-D-21-01001. Epub ahead of print.
37. Kurowicki J, Momoh E, Levy JC. Treatment of periprosthetic humerus fractures with open reduction and internal fixation. J Orthop Trauma. 2016;30(11):e369–74. https://doi.org/10.1097/BOT.0000000000000646.
38. Andersen JR, Williams CD, Cain R, Mighell M, Frankle M. Surgically treated humeral shaft fractures following shoulder arthroplasty. J Bone Joint Surg Am. 2013;95(1):9–18.
39. Sanchez-Sotelo J, Wright TW, O'Driscoll SW, Cofield RH, Rowland CM. Radiographic assessment of uncemented humeral components in total shoulder arthroplasty. J Arthroplast. 2001;16(2):180–7.
40. Sperling JW, Cofield RH, O'Driscoll SW, Torchia ME, Rowland CM. Radiographic assessment of ingrowth total shoulder arthroplasty. J Shoulder Elbow Surg. 2000;9(6):507–13.

Tendon Transfers and Shoulder Arthroplasty

Ryan Lohre and Bassem Elhassan

36.1 Paralysis, Pseudoparalysis, and Pseudopareses: A Spectrum of Motion Loss

Etiology of deficiencies in range of motion (ROM) requires clear definitions prior to treatment. Active loss of forward elevation or rotation at the glenohumeral joint can occur secondary to traumatic or compressive neuropathies or dystrophies such as neuralgic amyotrophy (Parsonage-Turner syndrome). A C5 compressive radiculopathy may defunction the deltoid and be associated with traumatic or degenerative rotator cuff disorders. These patients will present with extremely reduced ROM of the shoulder secondary to weakness of the deltoid muscle from proximal neuropathy. Axillary nerve palsies will similarly present with true paralysis of the shoulder, showing extremely limited glenohumeral joint ROM including forward elevation and external rotation. Brachial plexopathies will also provide a truly paralytic shoulder and, depending on location of neurologic injury, allow for motion only to occur through the scapulothoracic articulation. Spinoglenoid notch cysts can cause variable compression of the suprascapular nerve resulting in weakness and eventual degeneration of the supraspinatus and infraspinatus musculature, presenting as weakness in forward elevation or external rotation, or combined weakness. True paralysis secondary to neurologic injury should be clearly diagnosed as the etiology of weakness and loss of function requires distinct and separate surgical treatments with differing expectations of recovery.

Pseudoparalysis has varying definitions though it is best considered through understanding patient active motion losses, extent of rotator cuff deficiency, chronicity, presence of stiffness/adhesive capsulitis, arthritic changes, and neurologic and functional status of the deltoid. A recent consensus statement by Hawkins et al. defined pseudoparalysis as a lack of active elevation with maintained passive elevation, chronic, and with physical exam findings of anterosuperior escape of the proximal humerus with no pain relief on intra-articular local anesthetic injection [1]. Pseudoparalysis has also been described as active forward elevation <45 degrees with preserved passive ROM and chronic in nature without traumatic origin [2]. Pseudoparalysis can also similarly occur in multiple planes of motion depending on rotator cuff deficiency. Active motion loss in ER when tested at 20 degrees of abduction results in passive lagging toward the abdomen and measured as a negative angle. Active motion loss in IR is best assessed by a modified belly press test, seen by wrist flexion of

R. Lohre · B. Elhassan (✉)
Department of Orthopaedic Surgery, Harvard Medical School, Massachusetts General Hospital, Boston Shoulder Institute, Boston, MA, USA
e-mail: rlohre@mgh.harvard.edu;
belhassan@mgh.harvard.edu

© ISAKOS 2023
A. D. Mazzocca et al. (eds.), *Shoulder Arthritis across the Life Span*,
https://doi.org/10.1007/978-3-031-33298-2_36

around 90 degrees with inability to maintain a neutral wrist position if the elbow is passively moved away from the body. Collin et al. described rotator cuff tear patterns predictive of pseudoparalysis (defined as an inability to elevate the arm to 90 degrees) as anterosuperior tears (upper and lower subscapularis plus supraspinatus), posterosuperior tears (teres minor, infraspinatus, and supraspinatus), or infraspinatus, supraspinatus, and upper subscapularis [3]. Weiser et al. and Ernstbrunner et al. additionally provided evidence that the lower, muscular portion of the subscapularis is the most important predictor of pseudoparalysis [4, 5]. The teres minor is also important in constraining the anteroposterior force couple of the humeral head during elevation and external rotation as shown by Collin et al. [3]. To appropriately balance the cranially directed force of the deltoid, at least one unit in the anterior, posterior, and superior cuff must be present; otherwise the humerus will likely translate and escape anterosuperiorly.

Pseudoparesis occurs similarly to pseudoparalysis; however it lacks frank anterosuperior escape. In pseudoparesis as described by Gerber et al., forward elevation is limited to 90 degrees when not secondary to pain [6]. External rotation pseudoparesis is limited with active ER to neutral, full passive ROM and a lag sign back to neutral. Similarly, in pseudoparesis of internal rotation, modified belly press test shows wrist flexion angles of 30 and 60 degrees. A lag sign is present and occurs to these flexion angles when the elbow is moved passively away from the patient. Pseudoparesis occurs on a spectrum of rotator cuff insufficiency along with pseudoparalysis; however the check-rein effect of the anterior and posterior cuff is sufficient to prevent frank escape.

36.2 Radiographic Considerations

Without constraint of the rotator cuff, the glenohumeral joint undergoes progressive degeneration over time in variable arthritic patterns. Initially, proximal migration of the humerus is seen and can progress through acetabularization of the coracoacromial arch with humeral head collapse. Hamada et al. classified this progression secondary to loss of dynamic constraint due to chronic rotator cuff deficiency, termed cuff tear arthropathy (CTA) [7]. The typical glenoid wear pattern seen in these circumstances is in a posterosuperior orientation, though a small group of patients have anteroinferior glenoid erosion and subluxation. These patterns have been described by Favard et al. in their classification system of glenoid erosion secondary to CTA [8]. Seebauer et al. produced a biomechanical classification of CTA, incorporating morphologic and radiographic features of proximal migration with clinical findings of pseudoparalysis in advanced stages secondary to loss of constraint by the coracoacromial arch [9]. Radiographs assist the surgeon predominantly in indicating the patient for arthroplasty secondary to degenerative changes and assist in prosthesis preoperative planning. It is through a combination of radiography and careful physical examination that MTTs are indicated for shoulder arthroplasty based on notable deficiencies.

36.3 Tendon Transfers Prior to Shoulder Arthroplasty and Outcomes

Muscle tendon transfers (MTTs) for rotator cuff deficiency without significant arthritic changes have been increasing in popularity. For younger, more active patients, tendon transfers to nonanatomically recreate the glenohumeral force coupling have shown consistent improvements in patient-reported outcome measures (PROMs) and do not show advancement of arthritic changes in early follow-up. For those patients requiring reoperation and conversion to RSA, survivorship is estimated at 71.2% at 5 years [10]. Dislocation remained the largest complication in a series of 33 patients receiving RSA for failed tendon transfers (9.1%). Patients receiving this salvage operation do however consistently improve their PROMs above minimal clinically important difference (MCID) thresholds and improve upon their measured forward elevation [10].

Technically, it is important for surgeons to obtain prior operative records or be familiar with their prior cases and techniques to understand the location of transferred tendons. For posterosuperior rotator cuff reconstructions using lower trapezius transfers, the surgeon should be aware that this may result in tight posterior structures, resulting in a difficulty to translate the humerus for glenoid preparation and reduction maneuvers. Considering the risk of dislocation in these revision surgeries, appropriate implant sizing, positioning, and soft tissue tensioning are key. Though debate remains about repairing the subscapularis during RSA, for patients with prior anterior tendon transfers, it may be beneficial to respect these and repair them to their nonanatomic transfer site, rather than release to provide soft tissue tension and added constraint to the implant.

36.4 Concepts and Indications for Tendon Transfers During Reverse Shoulder Arthroplasty

36.4.1 CLEER

Combined loss of elevation and external rotation (CLEER) is an early concept developed by Boileau et al. to describe patients with pseudoparalytic symptoms undergoing RSA with loss of force coupling in both vertical and horizontal planes [11]. Though some describe adequate resolution of ER loss with a lateralized implant alone, patients with true pseudoparalysis in forward elevation and ER would likely obtain the greatest benefit from an additional tendon transfer. In a comparative study of patients with a diagnosis of CLEER preoperatively, 73.3% of patients receiving a combined latissimus dorsi and teres major transfer achieved resolution of their hornblower sign compared to 58.3% in those that received a lateralized implant only [12]. Studies examining patients with pseudoparesis in elevation and ER also show improvements in PROMs, elevation, and external rotation with low failure rates [13, 14]. It appears that

there may be a requirement to distinguish patients into categories of having true pseudoparalysis or pseudoparesis, as many studies likely vary on their inclusion criteria [15]. Indications for an RSA in patients with combined pseudoparesis or pseudoparalysis in multiple planes include glenohumeral arthritis, shoulder instability, and irreparability of rotator cuff tear.

In patients with true pseudoparalysis and loss of active forward elevation and active external rotation, with an ER lag sign and positive hornblower, our preferred treatment is a lateralized RSA implant with an isolated latissimus dorsi tendon transfer to the posterolateral greater tuberosity.

36.4.2 CLEIR

Internal rotation pseudoparalysis is corrected through nonanatomic RSA. Given the change in center of rotation, it is likely that the pectoralis major, latissimus dorsi, teres major, and anterior deltoid account for improved internal rotation through implant biomechanics alone. Repair of the subscapularis is variably reported after RSA with variably reported differences in outcomes. There may be a subset of patients however with combined loss of internal rotation musculature including the subscapularis and pectoralis major (through extensive intraoperative release) that may have appreciable weakness with internal rotation that may be improved by an anterior latissimus dorsi tendon transfer, though these are rare circumstances and currently have limited indications. The concept of combined loss of elevation and internal rotation (CLEIR) has also been described, with anterior tendon transfers showing improvements in functional toileting capacity in short-term follow-up [16]. Though this study utilized transfer of the conjoint (latissimus dorsi and teres major) tendon, biomechanically this can compress the axillary nerve, and tendons should ideally be mobilized separately as shown by Elhassan et al. to minimize this occurrence [17].

For patients with failed anatomic TSA secondary to subscapularis deficiency, with or without anterior subluxation of the humeral head, RSA is the standard treatment. Anterior latissimus dorsi tendon transfer alone or in combination with the teres major as a double tendon transfer (for dynamic or static subluxation) performed open or arthroscopically assisted can reconstruct the deficient subscapularis. There is no published data on the long-term outcomes of these treatments, and caution should be taken with clear patient shared decision-making before performing any salvage/reconstructions rather than conversion to RSA. The concepts of anterior latissimus dorsi tendon transfers in the setting of RSA are evolving and may prove to be beneficial in patients with preoperative CLEIR or at high risk of dislocation.

36.4.3 Deltoid Deficiency

Indications for a pedicled pectoralis major transfer include true paralysis with atrophic deltoid musculature (particularly anterior and middle deltoid). Contraindications include active infection, tumor, or axillary neuropraxia with expected recovery. Additional nerve transfer options should be considered prior to reconstructive efforts. The pedicled pectoralis major transfer attempts to reconstruct the deficient anterior deltoid musculature to improve forward elevation of the arm. The pectoralis major sternal and clavicular heads are detached from their origins and insertion, allowing for the muscle to be rotated on its neurovascular pedicle and reattached to the lateral clavicle and anterior acromion. Reorienting the pectoralis major muscle fibers allows for a vertical line of pull similar to the deltoid. Remaining posterior and middle deltoid that is contractile and non-atrophic can additionally be detached and mobilized anteriorly to assist in forward elevation strength. Performing the pedicled pectoralis major transfer around an RSA allows for improved biomechanics through medializing the center of rotation.

Another MTT option for deltoid deficiency includes a pedicled latissimus dorsi transfer. The broad nature of this muscle may cover greater deltoid defects [18]. A pedicled latissimus dorsi

transfer does not provide as much strength or improvements in range of motion (ROM) as reliably as a pedicle pectoralis major transfer, though it provides excellent soft tissue coverage including skin flaps if necessary. A glenohumeral fusion may also be a treatment option for this patient population.

36.5 Techniques

36.5.1 L'Episcopo

The L'Episcopo technique involves transferring the conjoint or combined tendons of both the latissimus dorsi and the teres major from their insertion medial to the bicipital groove to the lateral aspect of the humerus. Published results have described resolution of abduction external rotation and neutral external rotation pseudoparalysis [13, 14]. The technique involves harvesting the tendons as a single unit inferior to the subscapularis and deep to the sternal head of the pectoralis major. The upper third to half of the pectoralis major is frequently released for later repair to access the broad (~33–37 mm) latissimus dorsi tendon [19]. Care must be taken to identify and protect the radial nerve and plexus superficial and medial to the conjoint during harvest. Proximally and superiorly, the axillary nerve traverses through the quadrilateral space around 27 mm from the humeral insertion of the latissimus dorsi [19]. Both nerves are closer to the surgical field while the arm is in adduction. Fascial reflections are found to the triceps and should be removed proximally and distally to assist in excursion. Once harvested, the tendon can be transferred most easily during dislocation and prior to reduction of final humeral implants. The tendon can be secured through several methods including bone tunnels or the use of fixation devices such as buttons or tenodesis screws. With a standard, stemmed RSA component, this may impede fixation, and repair methods must be directed around the stem. We prefer to tubularize the tendon during transfer in the setting of RSA to provide a more robust tendonous insertion and affix the tendon using buttons and nonabsorbable suture.

The tendon is most frequently transferred directly laterally without proximal or distal translation to the humeral shaft. The line of pull thus biomechanically favors an external rotation vector with the arm in abduction. Other biomechanical studies provide evidence that inserting the tendon onto the posterolateral aspect of the greater tuberosity at the footprint of the teres minor produces greater moment arms [20].

36.5.2 Latissimus Dorsi

36.5.2.1 Posterior

The isolated latissimus dorsi tendon transfer has shown improvements in multiple retrospective series of patients in combination with RSA noted to have CLEER preoperatively [14, 21]. The isolated transfer differs when compared to the L'Episcopo technique by its relevant surgical anatomy. Approximately 10% of patients will have a conjoint tendon between the latissimus dorsi and teres major at its humeral insertion which must be carefully divided through its extent to adequately separate and provide excursion [19, 22]. Aside from a true conjoint tendon, there are two areas of fascial tissue that require release to maximize excursion of the latissimus dorsi. Approximately 36 mm proximal to the humeral insertion of the latissimus dorsi is a distal fibrous band existing between the latissimus and teres major that requires dissection, though the radial nerve passes directly inferior at this location. Additionally, there is a fibrous band that connects the latissimus to the triceps, which normally helps to anchor the brachial plexus to the proximal humerus [23]. Once released, adequate excursion can occur. Once released, the latissimus dorsi tendon can be transferred through the muscle of the teres major or, ideally, distal and below the muscle. A curved clamp is used to accomplish this with care to avoid the radial nerve medially, popping through the posterior capsular tissues adjacent to the humeral metaphysis and posterolateral greater tuberosity. This tendon can be affixed through bone tunnels or with the use of a button and nonabsorbable sutures after the humeral canal has been pre-

pared. The tendon may be attached directly posteriorly on the humeral metaphysis adjacent to the pectoralis major insertion or at the level of the teres minor insertion on the metaphysis. Biomechanically, the more proximal insertion may provide more rotational strength [20].

An additional incision may be produced in the axillary crease adjacent to the deltopectoral incision along the anterior border of the palpable latissimus dorsi with the arm in an abducted and internally rotated position. Dissection is carried down directly to the latissimus dorsi and teres major and followed to their insertion on the humerus. In this orientation, visible tendon equates to the latissimus dorsi, while muscle encountered is that of the teres major. Both the distal fibrous band and connection to the triceps must again be released in this position, though in this orientation, the radial nerve will be deep and lateral. Once released, a clamp is directed through the deltopectoral incision on the posterior aspect of the humerus between the teres minor and posterior deltoid through the subdeltoid space. Care must be taken to pass the clamp such that the axillary nerve coursing along the posterior deltoid fascia is respected, and the latissimus tendon again does not pierce the teres major and passes below. It has been described to affix the tendon in a position of external rotation and hyperextension; however this is a dynamic muscle transfer, and if adequately released, there should be enough excursion of this large muscle to accommodate fixing in any arm position. Postoperatively however, it is recommended that the patient be placed in a neutral-to-ER shoulder immobilizer for a period of 6–8 weeks to allow for tendon incorporation before progressive therapy.

36.5.2.2 Anterior

The anterior latissimus dorsi transfer involves similar harvest as the single-incision approach for a posterior transfer. Once the isolated tendon has been harvested and adequate excursion has been achieved, the tendon is affixed on the footprint of the subscapularis on the anterior aspect of the lesser tuberosity. Releasing the distal fibrous band and the triceps fascial reflections should provide enough muscle excursion to transfer the tendon proximally without significant tension. Again, buttons, anchors, or bone tunnels may be used to affix the tendon and should be done after preparing the humerus for implantation. Baek et al. demonstrated improved outcomes in patients with CLEIR receiving an anterior conjoint (latissimus dorsi and teres major) tendon transfer, with the tendon transferred proximally from its insertion and lateral to the bicipital groove. Two transient axillary neuropraxias developed though were reported to resolve [16]. We caution on the combined transfer of these muscles anteriorly as a unit as this may compress the axillary nerve in the quadrilateral space, and both should be released if a double tendon transfer is required. In settings of RSA and an intact deltoid, anterior latissimus transfer to the lesser tuberosity alone likely suffices and may reduce risk of neurologic injury. Immobilization should be a standard shoulder immobilizer in internal rotation for a period of

6–8 weeks before progressive therapy to allow tendon healing. How these muscles function longitudinally after anterior transfer alongside RSA is unknown.

36.5.3 Pectoralis Major Transfer

The pectoralis major has broad origins on the sternum and manubrium as well as the clavicle. The goal of the pectoralis major transfer is to reconstruct the function of the anterior deltoid, and as such, muscular contraction must change from an adductor moment to a flexor moment, requiring a bipolar transfer to be most effective. A large curvilinear incision is produced extending from just proximal to the xiphoid process and medial to the sternocostal junction, over the sternoclavicular joint and extending just distal to the clavicle (Fig. 36.1). The incision crosses the AC joint and then proceeds to the anterolateral acro-

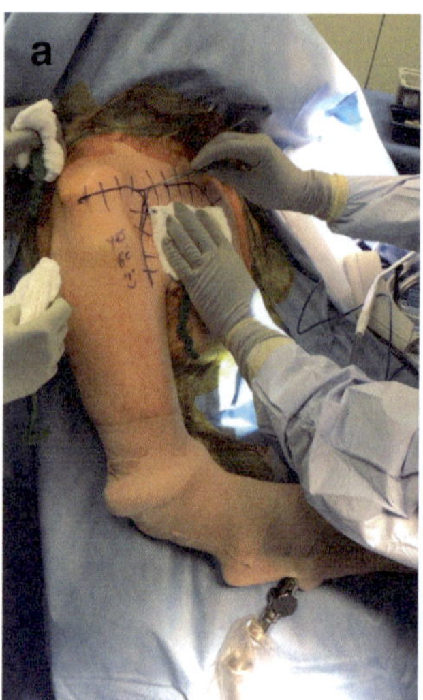
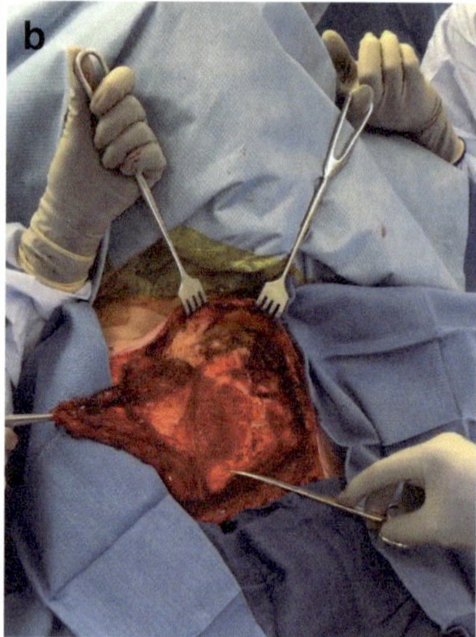
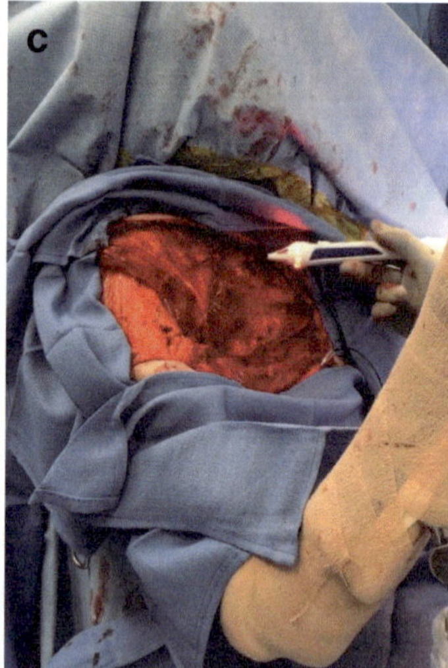

Fig. 36.1 (**a**) A patient positioned in a beach chair with an arm holder. Deltoid deficiency is seen by the visible acromion and greater tuberosity of the proximal humerus. The incision extends from proximal to the xiphoid process and traverses laterally along the inferior border of the clavicle. Typically, this then extends along a deltopectoral interval; however in this patient, the incision has been also extended laterally for additional planned middle deltoid mobilization. (**b**) The upper two-thirds of the pectoralis major muscle innervated by the lateral pectoral nerve and differentiated from the lower sternocostal head innervated by the medial pectoral nerve is clamped and retracted laterally. Fascial tissue is seen on the undersurface of the muscle which was overlying the pectoralis minor, also innervated by the medial pectoral nerve. The pectoralis minor is retained on the chest wall and ribs 3–5. (**c**) The pedicled pectoralis major transfer has been completed, with the muscle attached to the lateral third of the clavicle and acromion proximally, and distally inserted at the original deltoid insertion. A reverse shoulder arthroplasty underlies the tendon transfer. A nerve and muscle stimulator is utilized with the arm in 30–45 degrees of forward elevation to test the contractility of the pectoralis major and its ability to flex the arm at the shoulder

mion before extending distally, or a "T" incision can be performed, with one limb traversing distally along a standard deltopectoral incision, while the other limb proceeds to the posterolateral acromion. The decision to perform either of these is based on prior incisions in the area as well as if transfer of the middle or posterior heads of the deltoid is to be additionally performed. The origin of the pectoralis major is detached using electrocautery from the sternum and clavicle. Costal arterial branches are encountered, and care should be taken to cauterize these as they may retract deep and continue to bleed. The pectoralis minor is encountered originating from ribs 3–5. As dissection is continued lateral, the neurovascular pedicle of the pectoralis major is encountered near the middle of the clavicle, distal to the subclavius muscle near the subclavian artery and vein and brachial plexus. Any atrophic anterior deltoid muscle is excised and the anterolateral acromion is cleared of tissue. The insertion of the pectoralis major sternal and clavicular heads is released to allow for proper orientation of the muscle. The muscle proximally is folded on itself and the distal insertion is rotated so there is no twist in the muscle. In this orientation, the muscle fibers are all traversing in the long axis of the arm. Using buttons, the pectoralis major tendon is fixed to the clavicle and acromion. The most important fixation point is the medial/lateral extent of the new origin which should occur at the medial/lateral distance of the neurovascular pedicle so it does not tether this structure. Fixation proceeds distally to the anterolateral acromion. We typically use seven to eight buttons with double loaded sutures tied in a cow-hitch fashion to secure the muscle and tendon to bone. Once the new origin and insertion have been attached, checking the muscular contraction using a nerve and muscle stimulator device will show flexion of the arm at the shoulder and is indicative of appropriate muscle tension. The interval between the pectoralis major and remaining deltoid if approximated can be oversewn for added fixation. Postoperatively, we prefer to place patients' arms in a flexed position of 45–60 degrees with slight internal rotation, held in a shoulder spica cast.

36.6 Emerging Techniques

36.6.1 Lower Trapezius

Concurrent lower trapezius tendon transfer at the time of RSA for pseudoparalysis may be an option for patients with compromised latissimus dorsi/teres major tendons. A biomechanical analysis of lower trapezius versus latissimus dorsi tendon transfers showed that the lower trapezius provided a greater moment arm and was more resistant to effects of arm position in producing effective ER than the isolated latissimus dorsi transfer. Using a contemporary lateralized implant also provided significantly greater ER moment arms for lower trapezius transfers [24]. This technique has been limited secondary to requiring an additional posterior incision, allograft, and the unknown biomechanical effects on the prosthesis. Practically, the patient requires a standard beach chair position with access to the medial border of the ipsilateral scapula for tendon harvest. The lower trapezius tendon attaches on the undersurface of the scapular spine approximately 3 cm from the medial border of the scapula. The muscle traverses from its spinal origin in an oblique orientation through the surgical field (Fig. 36.2). The lower trapezius tendon harvest is best achieved through a longitudinal incision in line with the scapular spine, approximately 3 cm below the scapular spine and aimed toward the posterior glenohumeral joint. There is a thickened layer of fat surrounding the muscle and tendon which can be excised. Deep to the lower trapezius is the infraspinatus fascia which can be used as a landmark. Care must be taken to not harvest this fascia instead of the tendon. The tendon is then released from bone, and dissection is carried medial along a fatty demarcation between the lower and middle trapezius muscle heads. The spinal accessory nerve lies in the fascia on the undersurface of the trapezius musculature approximately 2 cm from the border of the medial scapular body, and careful dissection from superficial to deep must therefore be used. The muscle should be freed of adhesions and have adequate excursion prior to graft incorporation. The infraspinatus fascia should then be opened in line with

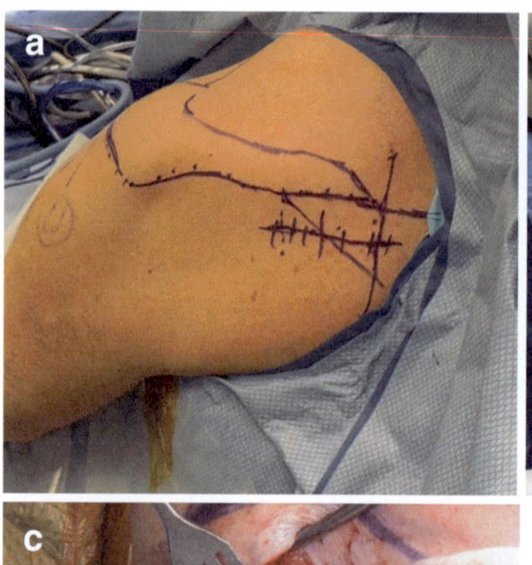
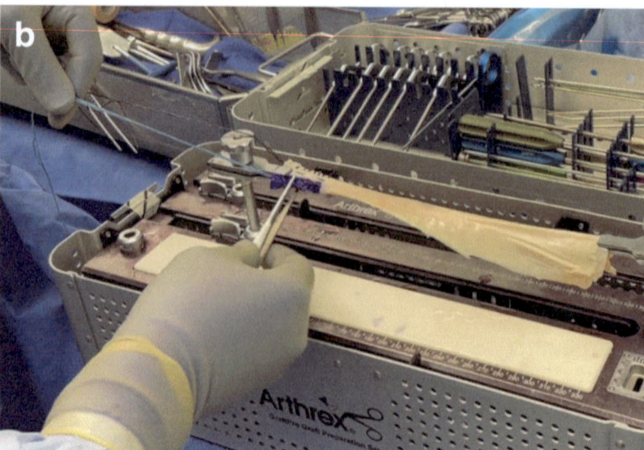
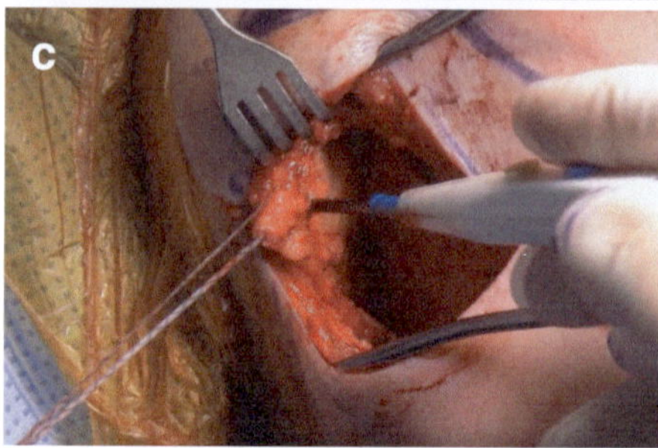

Fig. 36.2 (**a**) A patient positioned in a beach chair with the scapular spine, medial scapular border, planned incision, and obliquely crossing lower trapezius muscle landmarked. (**b**) An Achilles tendon allograft being prepared. One side is colored along with the use of different colored suture to ensure the graft does not twist on passage. (**c**) A lower trapezius tendon harvested from the scapular spine. The electrocautery is pointing at the fascial (deep) undersurface of the tendon. The tendon has been tagged with retracting sutures

the incision with blunt palpation occurring under the fascia and the posterior deltoid toward the joint. Looking anteriorly through a deltopectoral incision, access to this plane can be achieved posterior to the glenoid in the subdeltoid space. An Achilles tendon allograft (typically greater than 18 cm) is affixed to the posterolateral greater tuberosity near the footprint of the teres minor and infraspinatus using buttons or suture anchors and nonabsorbable suture on the calcaneal end. This should occur after humeral preparation and prior to reduction. The gastrocnemius end of the tendon is then grasped through the soft tissue tunnel previously described and pulled into the posterior incision. The implant can be reduced and the graft is then attached to the lower trapezius tendon. Our preferred method is to split the Achilles tendon, removing approximately half. The remaining tendon is then passed through the musculotendinous junction of the lower trapezius from deep to superficial and then pulled back laterally and tied on itself again with nonabsorbable suture. Care is taken to assure that any trapezius fascia or posterior deltoid fascia/muscle are not incarcerated in the transfer. Postoperatively, an external rotation shoulder immobilizer or brace providing neutral rotation of the arm and slight abduction should be used for a period of 6–8 weeks to allow graft incorporation.

36.6.2 Combined Lower Trapezius and Latissimus Dorsi (Anterior)

In settings of complete rotator cuff deficiency and cuff tear arthropathy, patients have up to 30% reductions in their PROMs and are at higher risk of dislocation [25]. Aside from optimizing implant position and size, providing soft tissue for added dynamic constraint to the prosthesis may aid in reducing this complication. In these

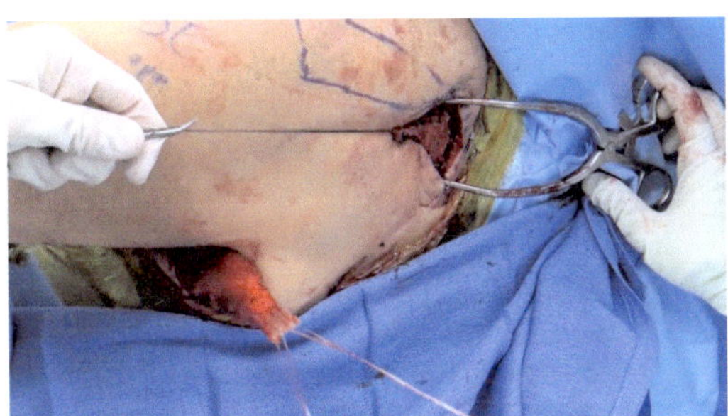

Fig. 36.3 A lower trapezius tendon is visualized in the posterior incision, and a latissimus dorsi tendon has been harvested and is visualized with tagging sutures coming from an axillary incision. Latissimus graft harvest can occur through a deltopectoral approach or through a separate axillary incision. The two tendons are harvested in preparation for an anterior latissimus dorsi and posterior lower trapezius tendon transfer with a reverse shoulder arthroplasty prosthesis

circumstances, combining a lower trapezius tendon transfer as previously described in conjunction with an anterior latissimus dorsi transfer can been performed (Fig. 36.3). Care should be taken to transfer the latissimus dorsi in isolation, leaving the teres major for adduction strength, particularly if the pectoralis major has been released. Though transfer of the pectoralis major tendon more proximally to the most anterior aspect of the lesser tuberosity has been described for subscapularis deficiency, biomechanically this may remain unfavorable. The angle of the pectoralis major and its line of pull is nearly 90 degrees to the action of the native subscapularis. Though the overall center of rotation is medialized during RSA, the transfer more superficially relative to its insertion on the diaphysis is quite minimal and likely does not alter the line of pull significantly and may actually produce an anterior translative force and contribute to implant stability. The latissimus dorsi, on the other hand, when transferred to the most anterior segment of the lesser tuberosity would have an effective posterior translative force combined with IR given its line of pull. No comparative biomechanical or clinical studies have examined the effectiveness of these transfers in contemporary RSA designs. For all emerging treatment options, further study is required on the longitudinal effects and survivorship.

36.7 Summary

Distinguishing paralysis, pseudoparalysis, and pseudoparesis in patients defines treatment and provides reconstructive options through MTTs and RSA. Distinguishing deficits in forward elevation or rotation assists in determining the most appropriate MTT. Patients presenting with pseudoparalysis in a CLEER pattern with CTA show improvements in range of motion and PROMs with latissimus dorsi or latissimus dorsi and teres major posterior transfers. Patients with CLEIR may improve strength with anterior latissimus or anterior latissimus and teres major transfers, though further research is required. For patients with deltoid deficiency, a pedicled pectoralis major transfer provides a reconstructive deltoid option aside from fusion. More novel transfers including lower trapezius tendon transfers or combined lower trapezius and anterior latissimus dorsi tendon transfers alongside RSA require further study.

References

1. Tokish JM, Alexander TC, Kissenberth MJ, Hawkins RJ. Pseudoparalysis: a systematic review of term definitions, treatment approaches, and outcomes of management techniques. J Shoulder Elbow Surg. 2017;26(6):e177–87.
2. Burks RT, Tashjian RZ. Should we have a better definition of Pseudoparalysis in patients with rotator cuff tears? Arthroscopy. 2017;33(12):2281–3.
3. Collin P, Matsumura N, Lädermann A, Denard PJ, Walch G. Relationship between massive chronic rotator cuff tear pattern and loss of active shoulder range of motion. J Shoulder Elbow Surg. 2014;23(8):1195–202.
4. Wieser K, Rahm S, Schubert M, Fischer MA, Farshad M, Gerber C, et al. Fluoroscopic, magnetic resonance imaging, and electrophysiologic assessment of shoulders with massive tears of the rotator cuff. J Shoulder Elbow Surg. 2015;24(2):288–94.
5. Ernstbrunner L, El Nashar R, Favre P, Bouaicha S, Wieser K, Gerber C. Chronic Pseudoparalysis needs to be distinguished from Pseudoparesis: a structural and biomechanical analysis. Am J Sports Med. 2021;49(2):291–7.
6. Werner CML, Steinmann PA, Gilbart M, Gerber C. Treatment of painful pseudoparesis due to irreparable rotator cuff dysfunction with the Delta III reverse-ball-and-socket total shoulder prosthesis. J Bone Joint Surg Am. 2005;87(7):1476–86.

7. Hamada K, Fukuda H, Mikasa M, Kobayashi Y. Roentgenographic findings in massive rotator cuff tears. A long-term observation. Clin Orthop Relat Res. 1990;254):92–6:92???96.

8. Sirveaux F, Favard L, Oudet D, Huquet D, Walch G, Mole D. Grammont inverted total shoulder arthroplasty in the treatment of glenohumeral osteoarthritis with massive rupture of the cuff: results of a multicentre study of 80 shoulders. J Bone Jt Surg Br. 2004;86:388–95.

9. Visotsky JL, Basamania C, Seebauer L, Rockwood CA, Jensen KL. Cuff tear arthropathy: pathogenesis, classification, and algorithm for treatment. J Bone Joint Surg Am. 2004;86(Suppl):35–40.

10. Marigi EM, Harstad C, Elhassan B, Sanchez-Sotelo J, Wieser K, Kriechling P. Reverse shoulder arthroplasty after failed tendon transfer for irreparable posterosuperior rotator cuff tears. J Shoulder Elbow Surg. 2022;31(4):763–71. https://www.sciencedirect.com/science/article/pii/S1058274621006984

11. Boileau P, Rumian AP, Zumstein MA. Reversed shoulder arthroplasty with modified L'Episcopo for combined loss of active elevation and external rotation. J Shoulder Elbow Surg. 2010;19(2 Suppl):20–30.

12. Young BL, Connor PM, Schiffern SC, Roberts KM, Hamid N. Reverse shoulder arthroplasty with and without latissimus and teres major transfer for patients with combined loss of elevation and external rotation: a prospective, randomized investigation. J Shoulder Elbow Surg. 2020;29(5):874–81.

13. Puskas GJ, Catanzaro S, Gerber C. Clinical outcome of reverse total shoulder arthroplasty combined with latissimus dorsi transfer for the treatment of chronic combined pseudoparesis of elevation and external rotation of the shoulder. J Shoulder Elbow Surg. 2014;23(1):49–57.

14. Shi LL, Cahill KE, Ek ET, Tompson JD, Higgins LD, Warner JJP. Latissimus Dorsi and Teres major transfer with reverse shoulder arthroplasty restores active motion and reduces pain for Posterosuperior cuff dysfunction. Clin Orthop Relat Res. 2015;473(10):3212–7.

15. Bauer S, Okamoto T, Babic SM, Coward JC, Coron CMPL, Blakeney WG. Understanding shoulder pseudoparalysis: part I: definition to diagnosis. EFORT Open Rev. 2022;7(3):214–26.

16. Baek CH, Kim JG, Baek GR. Restoration of active internal rotation following reverse shoulder arthroplasty: anterior latissimus dorsi and teres major combined transfer. J Shoulder Elbow Surg. 2022;31(6):1154–65. https://doi.org/10.1016/j.jse.2021.11.008.

17. Elhassan B, Christensen TJ, Wagner ER. Feasibility of latissimus and teres major transfer to reconstruct irreparable subscapularis tendon tear: an anatomic study. J Shoulder Elbow Surg. 2014;23(4):492–9.

18. Le Hanneur M, Lee J, Wagner ER, Elhassan BT. Options of bipolar muscle transfers to restore deltoid function: an anatomical study. Surg Radiol Anat. 2019;41(8):911–9.

19. Goldberg BA, Elhassan B, Marciniak S, Dunn JH. Surgical anatomy of latissimus dorsi muscle in transfers about the shoulder. Am J Orthop (Belle Mead NJ). 2009;38(3):E64–7.

20. Chan K, Langohr GDG, Welsh M, Johnson JA, Athwal GS. Latissimus dorsi tendon transfer in reverse shoulder arthroplasty: transfer location affects strength. JSES Int. 2021;5(2):277–81.

21. Popescu I-A, Bihel T, Henderson D, Martin Becerra J, Agneskirchner J, Lafosse L. Functional improvements in active elevation, external rotation, and internal rotation after reverse total shoulder arthroplasty with isolated latissimus dorsi transfer: surgical technique and midterm follow-up. J Shoulder Elbow Surg. 2019;28(12):2356–63.

22. Ranade AV, Rai R, Rai AR, Dass PM, Pai MM, Vadgaonkar R. Variants of latissimus dorsi with a perspective on tendon transfer surgery: an anatomic study. J Shoulder Elbow Surg. 2018;27(1):167–71. https://doi.org/10.1016/j.jse.2017.06.046.

23. Morelli M, Nagamori J, Gilbart M, Miniaci A. Latissimus dorsi tendon transfer for massive irreparable cuff tears: an anatomic study. J Shoulder Elbow Surg. 2008;17(1):139–43.

24. Chan K, Langohr GDG, Athwal GS, Johnson JA. The biomechanical effectiveness of tendon transfers to restore rotation after reverse shoulder arthroplasty: latissimus versus lower trapezius. Shoulder Elbow. 2022;14(1):48–54.

25. Saini SS, Pettit R, Puzzitiello RN, Hart P-A, Shah SS, Jawa A, et al. Clinical outcomes after reverse total shoulder arthroplasty in patients with primary glenohumeral osteoarthritis compared with rotator cuff tear arthropathy: does preoperative diagnosis make a difference? J Am Acad Orthop Surg. 2022;30(3):e415–22.

Influence of Biomechanics in RSA (Reverse Shoulder Arthroplasty) and Its Implication in Surgical Decision-Making Process

Giovanni Di Giacomo, Leonardo Moreno R, and Mattia Pugliese

37.1 Introduction

Due to degenerative pathologies of the shoulder, the arthroplasty was seen years before as a salvage procedure. The advent of good results in joints as the hip and knee tends the orthopedic field to try to recreate some characteristics of this prosthesis to the glenohumeral joint without acknowledging the biomechanics of this technique [1].

From the very beginning, the anatomic shoulder arthroplasty was used as the primary treatment for patients with glenohumeral arthrosis and massive rotator cuffs. The results were not satisfactory due to high failure rates related to excessive edge loading and the rocking horse phenomenon [2, 3]. Patients with osteoarthritis and a rotator cuff deficiency were grouped by Neer himself as patients with "limited goals surgery" [4]. Around the early 1980s, options like hemiarthroplasty provided pain relief, but functionally the range of motion

G. Di Giacomo
Department of Shoulder Surgery, Concordia Hospital, Rome, Italy

L. Moreno R (✉)
Department of Shoulder Surgery, Concordia Hospital, Rome, Italy

Hospital Occidente de Kennedy, Bogotá, Colombia

M. Pugliese
Trauma and Orthopaedic Surgery Department, Ospedale Maggiore C.A. Pizzardi, Bologna, Italy

postoperatively was poor, and loosening of the glenoid component was quite common with total unconstrained shoulder arthroplasty which led to unacceptable results and unsatisfactory outcomes for patients [5].

Paul Grammont developed the concept of functional surgery of the shoulder and with this the principles of the actual reverse shoulder arthroplasty in order to mitigate the undesired results of previous prosthesis. This concept is aimed to allow the person to be able to exert the function of the shoulder in his/her environment [5]. The impossibility to obtain good results with the anatomic total shoulder arthroplasty without anatomic repair of the torn cuff makes Grammont break the normal anatomy and restore the effective function through a novel morphology of the joint [5].

In 1977 Grammont and Lelaurain developed the "Acropole" prosthesis which introduced a subacromial joint to resurface and use the subacromial space to oppose the upward migration of the head and center it back in front of the glenoid [6] prosthesis that years later was abandoned due to coracoacromial impingement and glenoid loosening. These problems made them realize that the main problem they were facing was the inability to counter the deltoids subluxating effect in the absence of the cuff [5].

In 1985 he described his original reverse prosthesis that revolutionized shoulder arthroplasty with its novel design [1]. After several

© ISAKOS 2023

A. D. Mazzocca et al. (eds.), *Shoulder Arthritis across the Life Span*,
https://doi.org/10.1007/978-3-031-33298-2_37

attempts Grammont settled on an uncemented glenoid prosthesis. Central peg fixed with four divergent peripheral screws, glenoid component comprised of a third of a sphere with a large diameter, and removing the neck that was adapted from other joint prosthesis thus reversing the concavity of the glenoid which became convex and placed a nonanatomic inclination on the humeral component which went from convex to concave [7].

Nowadays with the development of different types of prosthesis and worldwide experience implantation of this type of elements, we know that the ability to generate power in the shoulder after reverse shoulder arthroplasty (RSA) is dependent upon several factors such as muscle physiological cross-sectional area, neural activity, length-tension relationship of soft tissues, atrophy, and/or fatty infiltration so beyond the inherent characteristics of the prosthesis, the patient selection keeps being a fundamental step to get the best results possible [8].

37.2 Grammont Principles

In order to contrast the effects of the deltoid and recreate a stable construct, two basic biomechanical principles were introduced in Grammont RSA: medialization of the glenohumeral center of rotation and a lowering of the humerus [9].

In practice these principles are represented by four items: (1) the center of rotation must be fixed, distalized, and medialized to the level of the glenoid surface, (2) the lever arm of the deltoid must be effective from the start of movement, (3) the prosthesis must be inherently stable, and (4) create a semiconstrained articulation [1].

37.2.1 Medialized and Fixed Center of Rotation

RSA components create a fixed center of rotation secondary to increased constraint and matched radii of curvature. Movements of the shoulder produce a resultant force vector, composed of both compressive and shear forces that varies throughout the range of motion but that consistently passes through the joints' fixed center of rotation [1]. Medialization of the center of rotation converts the mechanical torque at the glenosphere into more compressive forces across the prosthesis-bone interface and decreases the peak shear forces experienced by the glenoid component fixation [1, 10, 11].

The center of rotation in a ball and socket joint is kept at the center of the convex surface. Thus RSA shifts the center of rotation from the humeral head to the glenosphere. Since the glenosphere is fixed to the native glenoid surface, the distance from the glenoid surface to the center of rotation is directly proportional to the mechanical torque about the component and the shear forces at the glenoid bone-prosthesis interface [7, 11]. The effect of lateralizing the joint center of rotation is an increase in the distance between this point and the bone-implant interface; this distance is equal to the lever arm through which destabilizing forces act on the glenosphere resulting in increased torque [1].

Medialization of the center of rotation also brings inferomedial aspect of the humeral socket against the scapula neck which can also increase polyethylene component erosion and inferior scapular notching [12, 13]; for this reason an inferior overhang of the glenosphere provides a space between the glenosphere and the scapular neck that may decrease notching and also creates additional clearance between the greater tuberosity and coracoacromial arch decreasing the risk of impingement during abduction, goal also achieved by using a humeral implant with a non-anatomic inclination of 155 grades increasing the acromial-humeral distance [1, 7].

Lateralizing the center of rotation may improve shoulder range of motion by increasing the efficiency of external rotators lengthening [1, 14].

Nevertheless to address the problems of the medialized design, bony increased offset reverse shoulder arthroplasty (BIO-RSA) emerged to harness the potential advantages of component lateralization while limiting the known disadvantages of distancing the rotational center from the bone-implant interface [14].

37.2.2 Lever Arm of the Deltoid

Also medializing the center of rotation, an increase in lever arm of the deltoid is achieved allowing the deltoid to produce a large torque to rotate the humerus and elevate the arm, thanks to the increase of the abductor moment for the anterior, middle deltoid and posterior muscle; the latter acts in contrast to its physiologic role as an adductor in normal shoulders [15]. Muscularly not all the periscapular muscles show an increase in his efficiency; as the deltoid lever arm increases, medialization decreases the efficiency of the external rotators as the infraspinatus and teres minor [16].

Another way to increase the lever arm of the deltoid muscle without jeopardizing external rotators efficiency is by distalizing the humerus. Since the overall tension produced by a muscle is the sum of active and resting tension, the deltoid can produce more torque without increasing muscle contraction solely by increasing its resting length; this resting length is increased by distalizing the humeral insertion of the deltoid further away from its origin [7, 17]; be aware to not over-length it; this can decrease the resting tension and has also been correlated with postoperative neuropraxia and potentially with acromial stress fracture [7, 18].

37.2.3 Semiconstrained Articulation and Inherently Stable

Due to the absent rotator cuff and the impossibility of the dynamic stabilizers to provide stability, the relative position of the humerus against the glenoid must be maintained by the prosthesis [1, 7]; in order to maintain the relative position of the humerus against the glenoid, the reverse shoulder arthroplasty (RSA) places the convex surface on the glenoid and the concave surface on the humerus; this constrains the joint and prevents the humerus of translating superiorly against glenoid even during deltoid contraction. The fixed fulcrum of the RSA is then achieved by matching the radius of curvature between the convex and concave surfaces of the implant imposing con-

centric motion [7]. The intrinsic stability of the two prosthetic components depends on the ratio between their depth and diameter, also increasing the humeral socket depth is proportional to stability, but it is inversely proportional to impingement and notching-free range of motion [12, 19].

As we said before, increasing deltoid tension may help to stabilize the joint; as seen with an eccentric glenosphere, this increase in stability is based on larger muscle forces. The net compressive force acting on the glenohumeral articulation is the most significant element of stability [7, 20, 21] and also indicates that active rehabilitation can be more beneficial for patients than passive rehabilitation as the muscle activity could reduce the risk of instability, thus increasing muscular compressive force [20].

A quantitative measure of joint stability is the stability ratio, defined as the maximum allowable subluxation force/joint compression force. The normal glenohumeral joint has a stability ratio of approximately 0.5, whereas total shoulder arthroplasty has a ratio of approximately 1.0 [7, 22, 23]. In contrast, RTSA has a stability ratio > 2.0. With the glenohumeral joint in 90% of abduction, the reverse total shoulder is approximately 4–5 times more stable than a normal joint and 2–3 times more stable than a conventional total shoulder prosthesis [22]. The stability ratio increases approximately 60% with the glenohumeral joint at 90% of abduction and decreases with the arm in a fully adducted position [20].

37.3 Reverse Shoulder Arthroplasty Prosthesis Design Classification System

Routman et al. propose a RSA prosthesis design classification system to objectively identify and categorize different designs based upon their specific glenoid and humeral prosthesis characteristics for the purpose of standardizing nomenclature and a better understanding by the orthopedic surgeon for the different combinations and to help the decision-making in determined clinical scenario.

Glenoid components can be either medialized or lateralized depending on the center of rotation related to the glenoid face. For a typical glenosphere and a baseplate configuration, the position of the center of rotation is determined by the spherical radius and thickness of the glenosphere. For humeral prosthesis classification, humeral offset is defined as the horizontal distance between intramedullary canal and humeral stem axis to the center of the humeral liner; the offset determines the amount of humeral lateralization and is influenced by humeral neck angle, humeral osteotomy, humeral tray, and stem design [24]. Each of the configurations has pros and cons of which the surgeon should be aware at the moment of implantation.

37.3.1 Medialized Glenosphere (MedG)

This configuration is associated with a greater medial shift in the center of rotation relative to the native anatomic joint which increases the deltoid abductor moment arm requiring less muscle force to elevate the arm [15, 25] and also experience lesser shear force at the glenoid-baseplate interface improving glenoid fixation. Keep in mind that this configuration impacts negatively by shortening the residual rotator cuff [26]; has less deltoid wrapping, thus reducing the horizontal stabilizing compressive force vector of the deltoid; and may increase the risk of dislocation if not addressed on the humeral side and increased risk of scapular notching [25, 27].

37.3.2 Lateralized Glenosphere (LatG)

Lateralized design of the glenoid also medializes the center of rotation relative to the native anatomic joint by placing the center of rotation on the convex surface. The center of rotation in this situation is laterally shifted from the glenoid face by an amount equivalent to the difference between its thickness and radius. LatG designs have better residual rotator cuff muscles due to increased lever arm of infraspinatus and teres minor which

potentially improves internal and external rotation; nevertheless these are also associated with less humeral and scapular impingement and therefore with lower scapular notching rates [25]; also this design improves deltoid wrapping which increases the horizontal stabilizing compressive force vector of the deltoid and may decrease the risk of dislocation [25, 28].

The lateral shift of the glenoid component makes the deltoid less efficient compared with the MedG decreasing his abductor moment. Therefore the deltoid force must be greater in order to elevate the arm; this may be related to negative implications to range of motion, stable glenoid fixation, and acromial stress fracture due to increased shear force generated by the deltoid [25, 29].

37.3.3 Medialized Humeral Design (MedH)

Classically described by Grammont after a non-anatomic 155* osteotomy. It distally shifts the humerus relative to the native anatomic joint to increase deltoid tensioning. MedH designs have larger medial shift position of the humerus relative to native shoulders, thus decreasing deltoid wrapping which affects negatively the deltoid abductor moment so it is necessary to increase the deltoid force to elevate the arm; also as it happens with the MedG, it shortens the residual rotator cuff muscle length affecting postoperative internal and external rotation [12, 26].

37.3.4 Lateralized Humeral Designs (LatH)

Lateralized humeral designs are typically onset to place the humeral tray and liner on top of an anatomic neck osteotomy increasing the deltoid tensioning. This results in better residual rotator cuff tensioning and better deltoid wrapping to improve stability which also lengthens the deltoid moment arm to improve joint efficiency [12, 26, 28].

37.4　Effect of RSA Design Parameters on Rotator Cuff and Deltoid Muscle Torques

Due to the intrinsic characteristics of the nonanatomic design of the RSA and the biomechanics behind this design, the ideal configuration of his components is still in the making. Some limitations of the classic Grammont reverse shoulder arthroplasty design have been described above as scapular notching, instability, and decreased range of motion [24, 30]. These biomechanical differences between configurations have increased the seeking of effects of varying RSA design parameters.

Several configurations are available in terms of medialization and lateralization of the humeral and glenoid components and their effects on moment arms of the rotator cuff and deltoid muscles, in order to bring corroborating evidence on the most advantageous configuration of RSA implant helping surgeons worldwide make more conscious choices when a decision is made on implant positioning. Di Giacomo et al. (2021) conduct a computational biomechanical analysis assessing the moment arms of different implant configurations to provide a systematic understanding of the fundamental effects of glenosphere and humeral component design parameters on deltoid, infraspinatus, and teres minor forces required to achieve elevation and external rotation in adduction and abduction.

For a better understanding, it must be clear that the force required to produce active motion through a joint is resolved into two components: one perpendicular to the lever arm (rotatory component) and the other one parallel to the lever arm (stabilizing component). There is a line of action of the force (muscles) applied to the lever arm (bones) intended as the distance between the center of rotation and the point where the force is applied. And in order to measure the effectiveness of a muscle contribution to a specific motion over a range of configurations exist the torque and moment arm which are directly proportional (Fig. 37.1) [8].

When talking about torque and moment arm, it is fundamental to understand their defi

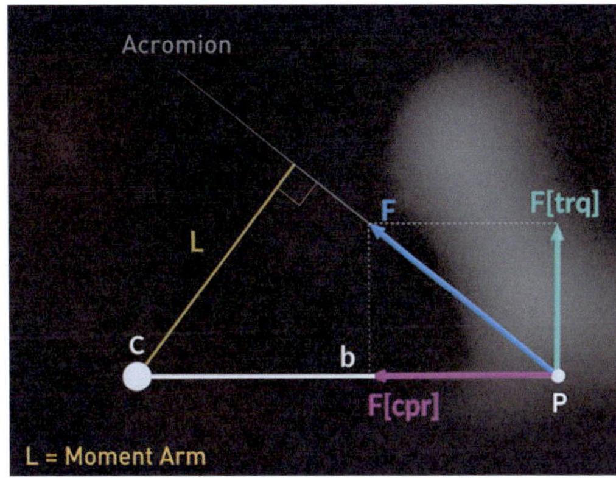

Fig. 37.1 Force required to produce active motion through a joint. C (center of rotation), F (force), trq (torque), P (point where the force is applied)

nition: The magnitude of torque depends on the force applied and the lever arm vector connecting the point about which the torque is being measured (CoR) to the point of force application, and the angle between the force and lever arm vectors and the moment of arm is the length of the shortest distance of a line that starts at the center of rotation that is perpendicular to the line of action where the force comes from [8].

The deltoid and rotator cuff muscle torque necessary to produce active motion in different planes are influenced by the configuration of the RSA implant. Four different RSA configurations are possible: medialized glenosphere and medialized humerus (MedG/MedH), medialized glenosphere and lateralized humerus (MedG/LatH), lateralized glenosphere and medial humerus (LatG/MedH), and both components lateralized (LatG/LatH).

In this study four categories were compared in terms of torque variation with respect to the native shoulder; three planes of motion were considered for the study of torque values, scapular plane when considering abduction by action of the deltoid muscle, axial plane when considering external rotation by the action of the deltoid and infraspinatus (Fig. 37.2), and sagittal oblique plane when considering external rotation by action of the teres minor muscle [8].

A procedural modeling software was used to create an anatomical model of the shoulder in

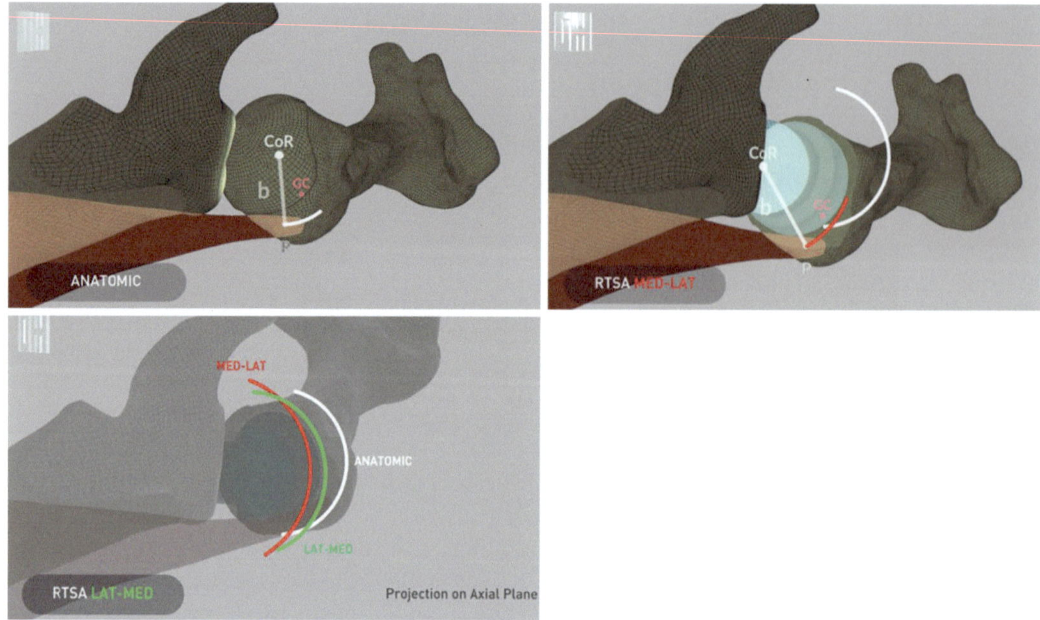

Fig. 37.2 CoR (center of rotation), GC (geometric center)

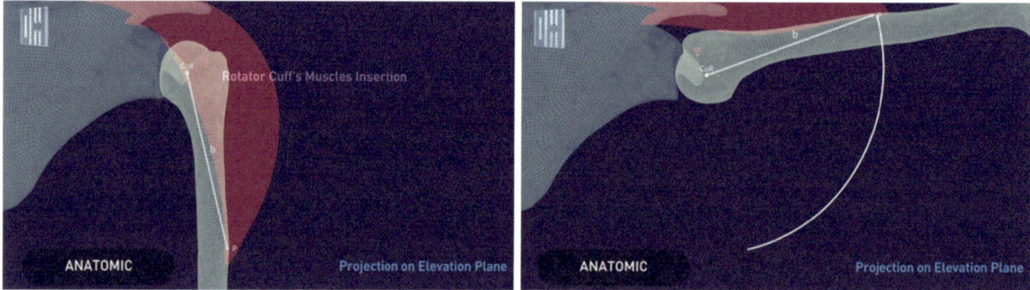

Fig. 37.3 Center of rotation projection on elevation plane of the native shoulder

order to calculate torque intensity. This study confirms that the moment arms of all four different configurations of reverse shoulder arthroplasty configuration were longer than the native shoulder because of the lateral offset of the native humerus and his proper center of rotation (Fig. 37.3). The lateralized glenosphere and medial humerus (LatG/MedH) displayed the most similar torque pattern to the native shoulder because of the shorter distance between the center of rotation and the humeral muscles insertion when compared to other designs of RSA (Fig. 37.4) [8].

When assessing the infraspinatus and teres minor for external rotation, mean torque in MedG/LatH and LatG/LatH configurations during range of motion was significantly higher than MedG/MedH and LatG/MedH. This study also showed that medialized glenoid and lateralized humeral component (MedG/LatH configuration) (Fig. 37.4) leads to the best torque on the three different planes under the action of deltoid as elevator on scapular plane and external rotator in adduction on the axial plane, infraspinatus and teres minor as external rotators, respectively, on axial and sagittal oblique planes [8].

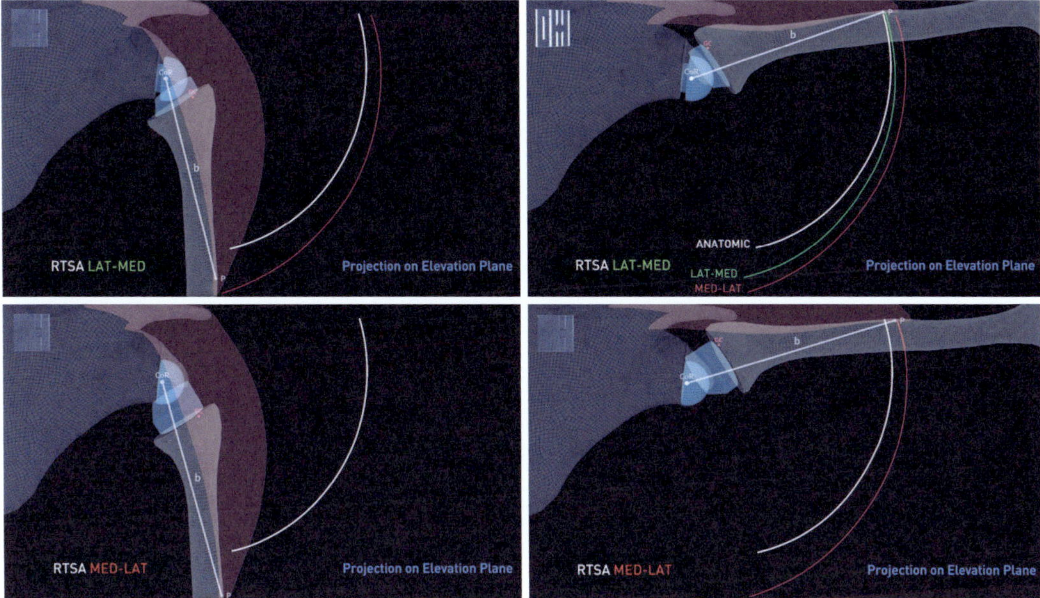

Fig. 37.4 RTSA (reverse total shoulder arthroplasty), LAT-MED (lateralized glenosphere and medial humerus), MED-LAT (medialized glenosphere and lateralized humerus)

37.5 Rotator Cuff Repair After Reverse Shoulder Arthroplasty

The RSA has been indicated for the treatment of rotator cuff tear arthropathy or massive rotator cuff tears that are deemed irreparable [31, 32], and due to these there has been disagreement regarding whether, when possible, repaired in conjunction with RSA. But also these indications have expanded to include surgical conditions with an intact rotator cuff such as the management of A2, B2, or C glenoid erosion; thus the surgeon has the option to preserve or release the rotator cuff [33–35].

The discussion around the repair of the rotator cuff has been focused on postoperative prosthesis stability, but this idea cannot leave behind the outcomes related with the effects of the muscles in range of motion postoperatively [33].

The repair of the rotator cuff theoretically should improve stability and decrease the incidence of dislocation. The internal rotation improves significantly if the subscapularis tendon is repaired, but some studies have reported that this repair may be detrimental for external rotation outcomes postoperatively through antagonistic loading against the already weakened posterior cuff [36, 37]. Also it has been described in literature where subscapularis muscle after being repaired markedly shifted toward adduction instead of keeping his internal rotation native role, thus resisting abduction increasing muscle and joint loading [15].

A biomechanical study was conducted to identify the kinetic effects of rotator cuff repair and how this is affected by RSA configuration. Giles et al. (2016) found that rotator cuff repair increases the demands on the deltoid during abduction, increasing joint loading. LatG exacerbated this effect; instead LatH reduced the deltoid muscles' required force which decreases joint loading caused by rotator cuff repair; this biomechanical effect is due to the wrap of the deltoid around the greater tuberosity, redirecting tension through the humeral head producing a more compressive joint load, effectively stabilizing the joint without introducing additional force into the joint [33].

References

1. Berliner JL, Regalado-magdos A, Ma CB, Feeley BT. Biomechanics of reverse total shoulder arthroplasty. J Shoulder Elb Surg. 2014;24:1–11. https://doi.org/10.1016/j.jse.2014.08.003.
2. Franklin JL, Barrett WP, Jackins SE, Matsen FA III. Glenoid loosening in total shoulder arthroplasty: associated with rotator cuff deficiency. J Arthroplast. 1988;3:39–46.
3. Pollock RG, Deliz ED, McIlveen SJ, Flatow EL, Bigliani LU. Prosthetic replacement in rotator cuff deficient shoulders. J Shoulder Elb Surg. 1992;1:173–86.
4. Neer C, Craig E, Fukuda H. Cuff tear arthropathy. J Bone Joint Surg Am. 1983;65:1232–44.
5. Story T, Grammont P, Concept FS, Principle R. Grammont's idea. 2011;2425–2423.
6. Grammont PM, Lelaurain G. Osteotomy of the scapula and the Acropole prosthesis (author's transl). Orthopade. 1981;10:219–29.
7. Rossy WH, Kwon YW. Biomechanics of the reverse shoulder arthroplasty. 2016;31–37.
8. Di Giacomo G, Athwal G, Pugliese M. The effect of Reverse Shoulder Arthroplasty design parameters on rotator cuff and deltoid muscles torques: a computational biomechanical analysis.
9. Boileau P, Watkinson D, Hatzidakis AM, Hovorka I. Neer award 2005: the Grammont reverse shoulder prosthesis: results in cuff tear arthritis, fracture sequelae, and revision arthroplasty. J Shoulder Elb Surg. 2006;15:527–40.
10. Kwon YW, Forman RE, Walker PS, Zuckerman JD. Analysis of reverse total shoulder joint forces and glenoid fixation. Bull NYU Hosp Joint Dis. 2010;68(4):273–80.
11. Harman M, Frankle M, Vasey M. Initial glenoid component fixation in "reverse" total shoulder arthroplasty: a biomechanical evaluation. J Shoulder Elb Surg. 2005;14(1 Suppl S):162S–7S.
12. Boileau P, Watkinson DJ, Harzidakis AM, Balg F. Grammont reverse prosthesis: design, rationale and biomechanics. J Shoulder Elb Surg. 2005;14:147s–61s.
13. Sirveaux F, Favard L, Oudet D, Huquet D, Walch G, Mole D. Grammont inverted total shoulder arthroplasty in the treatment of glenohumeral osteoarthritis with massive rupture of the cuff: results of a multicentre study of 80 shoulders. J Bone Joint Surg Br. 2004;86:388–95.
14. Boileau P, Moineau G, Roussanne Y, O'Shea K. Bony increased-offset reversed shoulder arthroplasty: minimizing scapular impingement while maximizing glenoid fixation. Clin Orthop Relat Res. 2011;469:2558–67. https://doi.org/10.1007/s11999-011-1775-4.
15. Ackland DC, Roshan-Zamir S, Richardson M, Pandy MG. Moment arms of the shoulder musculature after reverse total shoulder arthroplasty. J Bone Joint Surg Am. 2010;92(5):1221–30.
16. Walker M, Brooks J, Willis M, Frankle M. How reverse shoulder arthroplasty works. Clin Orthop Relat Res. 2011;469:2440–51.
17. Gerber C, Pennington SD, Nyffeler RW. Reverse total shoulder arthroplasty. J Am Acad Orthop Surg. 2009;17(5):284–95.
18. Ladermann A, Walch G, Lubbeke A, Drake GN, Melis B, Bacle G, Collin P, Edwards TB, Sirveaux F. Influence of arm lengthening in reverse shoulder arthroplasty. J Shoulder Elb Surg. 2012;21(3):336–41.
19. Gutierrez S, Luo Z-P, Levy JC, Frankle MA. Arc of motion and socket depth in reverse shoulder implants. Clin Biomech. 2009;24(6):473–9.
20. Clouthier AL, Hetzler MA, Fedorak G, Bryant JT, Deluzio KJ, Bicknell RT. Factors affecting the stability of reverse shoulder arthroplasty: a biomechanical study. J Shoulder Elb Surg. 2013;22(4):439–44. https://doi.org/10.1016/j.jse.2012.05.032.
21. Gutierrez S, Keller TS, Levy JC, Lee WE 3rd, Luo ZP. Hierarchy of 024 stability factors in reverse shoulder arthroplasty. Clin Orthop Relat Res. 2008;466:670–6. https://doi.org/10.1007/s11999-007-0096-0.
22. Favre P, Sussmann PS, Gerber C. The effect of component positioning on intrinsic stability of the reverse shoulder arthroplasty. J Shoulder Elb Surg. 2010;19:550–6. https://doi.org/10.1016/j.jse.2009.11.044.
23. Halder A, Kuhl S, Zobitz M, Larson D, An K. Effects of the glenoid labrum and glenohumeral abduction on stability of the shoulder joint through concavity-compression: an in vitro study. J Bone Joint Surg Am. 2001;83:1062–9.
24. Routman HD, Flurin PH, Wright TW, Zuckerman JD, Hamilton MA, Roche CP. Reverse shoulder arthroplasty prosthesis design classification system. Bull Hosp Jt Dis (2013). 2015;73(Suppl 1):S5–14. PMID: 266311
25. Terrier A, Reist A, Merlini F, Farron A. Simulated joint and muscle forces in reversed and anatomic shoulder prostheses. J Bone Joint Surg Br. 2008;90(6):751–6.
26. Hamilton MA, Roche CP, Diep P, et al. Effect of prosthesis design on muscle length and moment arms in reverse total shoulder arthroplasty. Bull Hosp Jt Dis (2013). 2013;71(Suppl 2):S31–5.
27. Hamilton MA, Diep P, Roche C, et al. Effect of reverse shoulder design philosophy on muscle moment arms. J Orthop Res. 2015;33(4):605–13.
28. Roche C, Crosby L. Kinematics and biomechanics of reverse total shoulder arthroplasty. In: Nicholson GP, editor. Orthopaedic knowledge update: shoulder and elbow. Rosemont, IL: American Academy of Orthopaedic Surgeons; 2013. p. 45–54.
29. Herrmann S, König C, Heller M, et al. Reverse shoulder arthroplasty leads to significant biomechanical changes in the remaining rotator cuff. J Orthop Surg Res. 2011;6:42.
30. Wall B, Nove-Josserand L, O'Connor DP, Edwards TB, Walch G. Reverse total shoulder arthroplasty: a review of results according to etiology. J Bone Joint

Surg Am. 2007;89:1476–85. https://doi.org/10.2106/JBJS.F.00666.

31. Drake GN, O'Connor DP, Edwards TB. Indications for reverse total shoulder arthroplasty in rotator cuff disease. Clin Orthop Relat Res. 2010;468:1526–33. https://doi.org/10.1007/s11999-009-1188-9.

32. Harreld KL, Puskas BL, Frankle M. Massive rotator cuff tears without arthropathy: when to consider reverse shoulder arthroplasty. J Bone Joint Surg Am. 2011;93:973–84.

33. Giles JW, Langohr GDG, Johnson JA, Athwal GS. The rotator cuff muscles are antagonists after reverse total shoulder arthroplasty. J Shoulder Elb Surg. 2016;25:1592–600. https://doi.org/10.1016/j.jse.2016.02.028.

34. Sears BW, Johnston PS, Ramsey ML, Williams GR. Glenoid bone loss in primary total shoulder arthroplasty: evaluation and management. J Am Acad Orthop Surg. 2012;20:604–13. https://doi.org/10.5435/JAAOS-20-09-60.

35. Denard PJ, Walch G. Current concepts in the surgical management of primary glenohumeral arthritis with a biconcave glenoid. J Shoulder Elb Surg. 2013;22:1589–98. https://doi.org/10.1016/j.jse.2013.06.017.

36. Wall B, Nové-Josserand L, O'Connor DP, Edwards TB, Walch G. Reverse total shoulder arthroplasty: a review of results according to etiology. J Bone Joint Surg Am. 2007;89:1476–85. https://doi.org/10.2106/JBJS.F.0066.

37. Boulahia A, Edwards TB, Walch G, Baratta RV. Early results of a reverse design prosthesis in the treatment of arthritis of the shoulder in elderly patients with a large rotator cuff tear. Orthopedics. 2002;25:129–33.

Arthroscopy and Shoulder Arthroplasty

Juan Sebastián Vázquez, Maria Valencia, and Emilio Calvo

38.1 Introduction

Total shoulder arthroplasty (TSA) has been established as the treatment of choice for end-stage glenohumeral arthritis and has demonstrated durability and effectiveness. Most patients obtain durable shoulder comfort and function following SA, but postoperative problems may occur, including instability, component loosening, malposition, infection, neurovascular injury, stiffness, impingement, periprosthetic fracture, and rotator cuff and biceps injury [1]. The number of revision surgeries is expected to increase as more patients undergo TSA to alleviate shoulder pain and functional impairment. This will eventually occur despite improvement in prosthetic design and surgical technique, and indication as TSA has a limited durability.

Shoulder arthroscopy has become a potent diagnostic and therapeutic tool that has transformed the diagnosis and management of shoulder pathology. Clear indications for patients with symptomatic TSA have not been established clearly. Arthroscopic well-known advantages (i.e., minimal invasiveness; improved visualization in some cases; less hospital stay, blood loss, and surgery time; lower complication rates; no image artifact, among others) could be applied among these patients [2–5].

Nevertheless, potential drawbacks and technical challenges should be taken into consideration. It could add an extra procedure in patients who anyhow end up having open revision surgery. Iatrogenic component damage or loosening and other arthroscopic-related complications, like infection, neurovascular damage, bleeding, and prosthetic component damage, among others, are best avoided by meticulous attention to detail, including precise portal placement, careful navigation, and proper use of instruments around the prosthesis.

The number of potential indications of arthroscopy in symptomatic patients with TSA is increasing (Table 38.1). In this chapter the indications, general principles, and surgical technique of arthroscopy in shoulder arthroplasty will be described.

38.1.1 General Surgical Principles of Arthroscopy on Shoulder Arthroplasty

Arthroscopy for shoulder arthroplasty can be performed either in the lateral decubitus or beach chair positions. Beach chair offers the possibility to convert to an open approach if needed. Gentle traction on the humerus is recommended. It is important to insert the trocar carefully into the

J. S. Vázquez · M. Valencia · E. Calvo (✉)
Shoulder and Elbow Reconstructive Surgery Unit, Department of Orthopedic Surgery and Traumatology, Hospital Universitario Fundación Jiménez Díaz, Universidad Autónoma, Madrid, Spain
e-mail: svazquez@alumni.unav.es;
maria.valencia@quironsalud.es; ecalvo@fjd.es

© ISAKOS 2023
A. D. Mazzocca et al. (eds.), *Shoulder Arthritis across the Life Span*,
https://doi.org/10.1007/978-3-031-33298-2_38

Table 38.1 Indications for arthroscopy in prosthetic shoulders

1. High clinical suspicion for periprosthetic joint infection without confirmation by exam or diagnostic tests. Septic arthritis acute treatment.
2. Implant loosening assessment and glenoid loose component removal.
3. Shoulder stiffness.
4. Subacromial impingement, bursitis, and acromioclavicular pathology.
5. Rotator cuff tear.
6. Long head of biceps (LHB) pathology.
7. Periprosthetic shoulder Instability.
8. Scapular notching.
9. Loose bodies.

Table 38.2 General surgical tips for performing arthroscopy on shoulder arthroplasty

- Use Lateral decubitus or beach chair position (preferred by author due to the).
- Gentle lateral traction on the humerus with the arm adducted and internally rotated.
- Cautiously enter the joint (to prevent iatrogenic prosthetic component loosening or damage), and manipulate instruments carefully.
- More proximally placed posterior portal (1 cm inferior the undersurface of the posterolateral acromial corner) avoids the thickest portion of the prosthetic humeral head.
- Avoid sharp-tipped trocars.
- Create new portals or enlarge preexisting portals if needed.
- Use cannulas every time if possible.
- Turn the 30° arthroscope away from the metal prosthetic component, or use the novel needle-sized 0° arthroscope to prevent mirror phenomenon.

joint to prevent iatrogenic prosthetic component loosening or damage and manipulate instruments carefully. Sharp-tipped trocars should be avoided. For anatomic TSA, a posterior entry portal is used, but it should be placed more proximally (1 cm inferior the undersurface of the posterolateral acromial corner) in order to avoid the thickest portion of the prosthetic humeral head. In the case of reverse shoulder arthroplasty (RSA), the same posterior portal can be followed to enter the joint. However, a lateral portal located 1 cm lateral to the acromial edge and midway between the anterior and posterolateral acromial aspects is frequently safer. The trocar should be directed 45 degrees inferiorly to enter the joint.

Once into the joint, the humeral head in the case of anatomic TSA or the glenosphere if RSA is easily identified, and the "mirror" phenomenon consisting of the reflection off the humeral head or glenosphere can cause technical difficulties. Turning the 30° arthroscope away from the metal prosthetic component or using the novel needle-sized 0° arthroscope is useful to prevent mirror phenomenon.

Scar tissue and synovitis are frequently encountered in the joint. This tissue should be removed as much as possible to visualize the components and to gain full access to implant to bone interfaces. A shaver introduced through a conventional anterior portal can be used for this purpose (Table 38.2).

38.1.2 Arthroscopy for Diagnosis and Treatment of Shoulder Periprosthetic Joint Infection After SA

Periprosthetic shoulder joint infection (PSJI) can be a devastating complication of arthroplasty, with considerable associated morbidity and cost. It occurs in approximately 1% of cases after primary and up to 15% after revision arthroplasty [6–8]. The true incidence could possibly be even higher due to frequent low-grade-type clinical appearance imitating an aseptic failure [9]. The ideal treatment of PSJI is unclear, and no reliable algorithm for acute or chronic PSJI has been established [10–12]. Diagnosis has traditionally been based on the clinical history and examination, in combination with laboratory analysis in peripheral blood, radiologic findings, and aspiration culture results. However, signs can be subtle and investigations equivocal [4]. Low-virulence organism's infection such as *Cutibacterium acnes* [8, 9] can present with lack of typical features of infection such as fever and erythema delaying diagnosis and therefore worsening the prognosis by late treatment. Many authors stated that routine investigations for infection have a low efficacy in confirming PSJI in these cases [13–15].

In regard to classical preoperative workup to diagnose PSJI, synovial fluid culture and analysis has been the most accurate tool to date, but infections caused by indolent organisms may still be missed. Cell count and biomarker assays such as alpha-defensin may aid in these cases [16, 17]. However its overall utility has been questioned [18]. In addition, 14 days of incubation and different media are needed to identify these organisms [19]. Sperling found that approximately 50% of all joint aspirations fail to recover any fluid ("dry tap"); therefore, neither biomarker assays nor culture of specimens is possible in these cases [6, 20]. Dilisio et al. found that fluoroscopically guided glenohumeral aspiration yielded a sensitivity of 16.7%, specificity of 100%, positive predictive value of 100%, and negative predictive value of 58.3% [21].

On account of this, arthroscopic management could be the next step in cases where there is a high clinical suspicion of PSJI along with no clear clinical evidence of infection, nonconclusive image studies, negative joint aspiration cultures, and normal/subtle inflammatory laboratory markers. Dilisio et al. found that culture of arthroscopically obtained tissue demonstrated 100% sensitivity, specificity, positive predictive value, and negative predictive value for identifying periprosthetic shoulder infection when one positive culture defined PSJI, concluding that arthroscopic tissue biopsy is a reliable method for diagnosing periprosthetic shoulder infection and identifying the causative organism [21]. Nevertheless, Akgun et al. found a sensitivity and specificity of 80% and 94%, respectively, and the positive predictive value was 80% when two arthroscopically taken samples yielded positive cultures. Histopathologic cultures have shown low sensitivity, and no clear advantages of sonification over conventional cultures have been found [22, 23].

Arthroscopically identified synovitis has not been found to be an accurate finding to diagnose PSJI due to the low virulence of *C. acnes* together with the concomitant macroscopic signs of synovitis secondary to noninfectious process initiated by polyethylene, cement, or metal debris synovitis [24].

In regard to antibiotic prophylaxis for arthroscopy, the International Consensus Meeting recommends that preoperative antibiotics should not be held until cultures are obtained in revision shoulder arthroplasty. It was also stated that antibiotics can be continued up until final culture results are obtained in revision cases if there is some suspicion of infection while awaiting the final culture results [25].

In summary, arthroscopic management is an effective and accurate tool to identify low-indolent causative organisms, thus detecting patients with infected shoulder arthroplasty in cases where classical preoperative workup to diagnose PSJI has been unconclusive despite high clinical suspicion. This could potentially reduce the number of unexpected intraoperative positive open cultures together with the non-true infected shoulder arthroplasty and consequently the number of unnecessary revision surgeries. The main disadvantage of diagnostic arthroscopy is that it can potentially result in an additional surgical procedure. Although the main treatment for a chronic PSJI would be one- or two-stage open revision surgery, arthroscopic management could benefit poor major surgery candidates. In regard to acute PSJI, arthroscopic management could be used to diagnose and treat septic arthritis in the acute setting but not as a definitive treatment. Likewise, if mobile component removal is needed, unless the component is loose, it could not be done arthroscopically.

38.2 Surgical Technique for Assessing PSJI

Prior to arthroscopy, aspiration with a spinal needle from posterior portal could be done. Any fluid egress throughout the initial dry arthroscope sheath should be collected and sent for culture. Abnormal appearance synovial and tissue biopsies are obtained through working portal using a tissue punch, pituitary rongeur, or grasper (Fig. 38.1). To improve diagnostic accuracy, samples should be obtained from a minimum of three different sites. We recommend five biopsies, including component-bone-cement interface. A

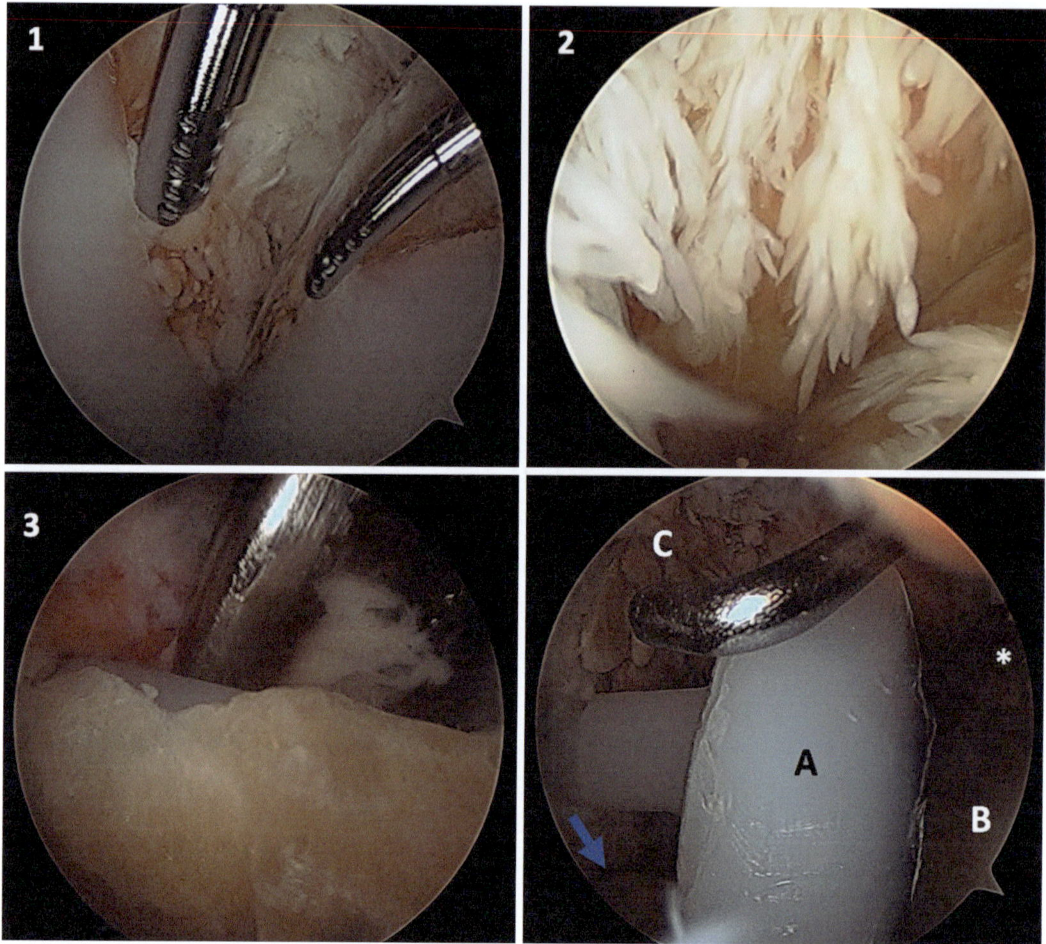

Fig. 38.1 Arthroscopy in a patient with painful total shoulder arthroplasty with high index of suspicion for PSJI despite normal studies. 1. Posterior view of a TSA. Note the "mirror" phenomenon reflecting the tip of the shaver on the humeral head. 2. Synovitis. 3. Samples taken from glenoid component-bone interface. 4. Loose all-polyethylene glenoid component (**a**), humeral component (**b**), synovitis (**c**), and cement mantle (arrow)

"no-touch" technique can be applied by using new sterile instruments each time. A cannula may be used to prevent skin flora contamination of samples. This is followed by irrigation and debridement of articular and subacromial space. Samples are immediately sent to microbiological analysis (gram staining and aerobic, anaerobic, and fungal culture assessment), and a minimum of 14 days of incubation is preferred to increase the likelihood of detecting *C. acnes* [1, 26].

38.2.1 Arthroscopy and Implant Loosening After Shoulder Arthroplasty

Loosening of glenoid component is one of the most likely causes on painful and late failure following shoulder arthroplasty; specifically, the most common following an anatomic TSA [27, 28], it may be the consequence of the "rocking horse phenomenon" or eccentric glenoid component loading, imperfect glenoid preparation and cementing technique, poor glenoid bone quality, or defective component design [29]. Symptoms are nonspecific, but worsening pain together with gradual loss of motion or mechanical symptoms during arm movement should awaken concern [30]. If these symptoms are present and implant loosening suspected, image studies should be taken. Radiolucent lines or gross shifts in component position should be looked through [31]. Computed tomography (CT), with or without intra-articular contrast, may aid in detecting glenoid component loosening [32], but its reliability has been questioned. Arthroscopy can identify gross glenoid loosening initially missed by conventional imaging studies [33].

Although image studies may be helpful in diagnosing loosening, arthroscopy has been described as a useful adjunct when radiographs are equivocal. Arthroscopic techniques have been found to be more sensitive than radiologic studies in the evaluation of component loosening. Therefore, loosening could be established even in the absence of radiographic evidence [33] (Fig. 38.1).

Arthroscopic therapeutic management for loose glenoid component has also been described [34, 35]. Removing the loose glenoid component could leave bone defects which should be assessed and treated if necessary. These may be small or large contained or uncontained, the latter being more difficult to treat by arthroscopy. This scenario may require open structural bone grafting with or without revision to RSA. Defined indications for bone grafting of peg holes or larger contained defects remain unclear [36, 37].

38.3 Surgical Technique to Evaluate and Remove Implant Loosening

Glenoid component is assessed using a probe or any other device to gently manipulate the glenoid or humeral component evaluating for component loosening. Flexible plastic cannulas and trocars may be used to reduce iatrogenic harm [35]. The glenoid component extraction can be achieved in two ways. The first is performing as complete removal of the component in grossly loose by completely releasing the rotator interval, enlarging the anterior portal by 1–2 cm immediately prior to removal by using an arthroscopic grasper to firmly grasp and lift up the glenoid component (Fig. 38.2). The other option is to sequentially cut the component surface into smaller fragments to facilitate extraction using arthroscopic graspers.

The remaining cement can be broken and removed by curettes or graspers. Debriding the cement with a high-speed burr is also an option in cases of poor glenoid bone quality [1, 34]. Bone defect after removal should be assessed. Removal of a pegged component may leave contained or uncontained holes in the glenoid subchondral bone. Impaction on allograft bone chips may be performed in larger bone defects using cannulas or trephines through accessory or standard portals (Fig. 38.2). Dermal allografts patches could be used with knotless sutures on glenoid to contain the bone graft as it articulates with the humeral component [1, 35]. Smaller defects may be left untreated.

38.3.1 Arthroscopy and Shoulder Stiffness After SA

Postoperative stiffness after TSA is a common cause of pain and is the most frequent cause of patient dissatisfaction [38]. The etiology is multifactorial but is mainly associated with technical factors depending on the surgeon (component malpositioning and overstuffing) and patient factors (noncompliance with postoperative rehabilitation, prolonged shoulder immobilization, exuberant scar formation, infection, among others) [1].

Pain and stiffness after shoulder arthroplasty should be evaluated with careful physical examination. Component malpositioning and soft-tissue contracture should be differentiated by physical exam determining whether there is a firm versus rubbery range-of-motion end point, respectively. If component malpositioning or wrong sizing is confirmed by image studies, open revision surgery should be performed. If early

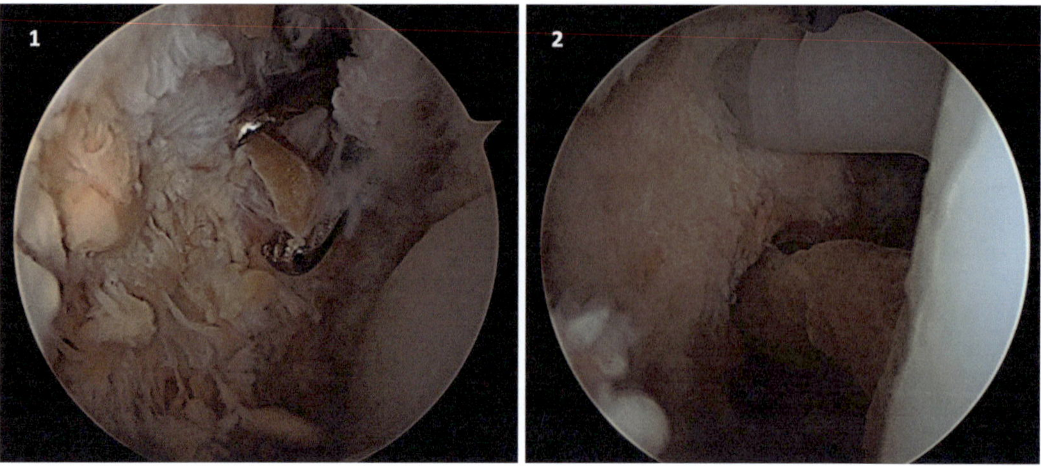

Fig. 38.2 Arthroscopic image of a loose all-polyethylene glenoid component. 1. Removal of cement. 2. Loose glenoid component removal

postoperative stiffness not associated with component malpositioning is present, initial physical therapy may be effective; nonetheless care should be taken to avoid scapular fracture or subscapularis failure [1].

If any of these problems is diagnosed, it should be assessed either by conservative or surgical treatment. Arthroscopic management will take place when pain and limited range of motion compromise shoulder function with or without the presence of obvious PSJI or component-related issues and despite extended rehabilitation. In these cases, arthroscopic contracture release and lysis of adhesions may be indicated [1]. Reports of arthroscopic treatment of stiffness and impingement following shoulder arthroplasty are limited to retrospective case series, but successful outcomes have been reported [39].

38.4 Surgical Technique of Arthroscopic Release for Stiff Shoulder Arthroplasty

Barth and Burkhart described the technique of arthroscopic capsular release after hemiarthroplasty of the shoulder [40]. Scar tissue and adhesions are debrided to improve visualization and to clearly evaluate prosthesis components. Rotator interval and middle glenohumeral ligament are released. Subscapularis is separated from anterior capsule. Care should be taken not to damage subscapularis. Using an anterior viewing portal, posterior capsule and adhesions are released.

After intra-articular release is done, subdeltoid and subacromial adhesions are resected, and bursectomy is done using a posterior vision portal and a peripheral lateral working portal to avoid injury to the cuff. At this point, inferior capsule release is done if contracture remains after subacromial and subdeltoid release. The preferred author's method for inferior capsular release is by using scissors to palpate thickness and quality of tissue preventing damage to axillar nerve. Finally, passive range of motion is evaluated.

Aguilar-Gonzalez et al. described the technique to perform a circumferential release to treat a stiff RSA [41]. For stiff RSA multiple portals performed under direct visualization from posterior to anterior can be used if needed, but four portals (i.e., modified posterior, posterolateral, anterolateral, and anterior) are usually enough. It is important to visualize the entire circumference of the prosthetic humeral platform and polyethylene resecting all subacromial adhesions and scar tissue (Fig. 38.3). A circumferential release procedure performing an anterior capsulotomy that

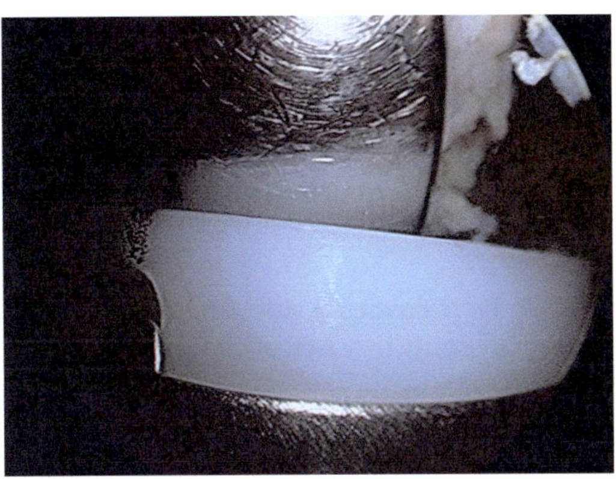

Fig. 38.3 Arthroscopic view of a reverse shoulder arthroplasty from a posterolateral portal. The contact and movement between the glenosphere and the humeral component should be examined circumferentially

should be extended medially and posteriorly as far as possible should be carried out. The surgical assistant can help performing arm rotations to gain access to the periprosthetic soft tissue as needed during the procedure.

38.4.1 Arthroscopy and Subacromial Impingement and Acromioclavicular Pathology After SA

Subacromial impingement after SA is unusual, and it is often related to head overstuffing or malposition of humeral component. Primary subacromial impingement has to be ruled out first and treated if found [42].

If secondary impingement pain is suspected, diagnosis should be made. Acromial or scapular spine changes in position due to previous fractures or abutment of greater tuberosity excrescences (secondary to cuff tear arthropathy in RSA or fracture sequelae) should be ruled out prior contemplating arthroscopic treatment. In these cases, arthroscopic tuberoplasty or subacromial flattening could be performed [43].

The surgical technique is the same as for nonprosthesis-associated subacromial impingement. Acromioplasty should also release the coracoacromial ligament and adjacent bursa underneath the anterior aspect of the acromion.

38.4.2 Arthroscopy and Rotator Cuff Repair After SA

Acute or chronic rotator cuff tears may be encountered following an anatomic TSA. The overall incidence is 2–3%, being the third most common complication requiring revision surgery after anatomic TSA. The most typical scenario may be an acute subscapularis tear or a chronic rotator cuff tear, being either traumatic or atraumatic in etiology [44, 45].

In young active patients with anatomic TSA, acute traumatic or atraumatic tears are more frequent. If clinical impairment or instability is present, they may benefit from arthroscopic rotator cuff repair rather than nonoperative treatment which could lead to future tear propagation and possible revision to RSA [1, 46].

In contrast, chronic retracted tears may not heal after surgical repair due to irreparability factors such as anterior or superior glenohumeral subluxation, fatty atrophy, or muscle fatty infiltration. In these patients, revision to RSA may be reasonable when symptoms remain despite nonoperative treatment.

There is lack of reports on the outcome of arthroscopic rotator cuff repair after TSA. Tytherleigh et al. found that 4 of 29 patients undergoing arthroscopy after SA had rotator cuff tear; 1 had a large full-thickness tear treated with subacromial decompression and a mini-open repair, whereas the other 3 patients had partial tears treated with arthroscopic debridement. Other study recognized 8 rotator cuff tears out of 14 patients (57%) who undergone diagnostic arthroscopy due to possible infection. Nevertheless, some patients underwent revision to RSA, and none of them had arthroscopic cuff repair [47].

Subscapularis tendon failure is an early recognized complication following anatomic TSA which could lead to impair active motion and shoulder instability. Open repair using the deltopectoral incision facilitates direct access to the tear; therefore arthroscopic subscapularis repair may not have a proper indication. There is lack of reports on arthroscopic subscapularis repair following aSA. However, clinical results have been disappointing even when open prompt repair has been done resulting in tendon transfer or revision to RSA [1, 48].

## 38.5	Surgical Technique of Rotator Cuff Tear Repair After TSA

After diagnostic arthroscopy and intra-articular debridement are done, subacromial space is assessed by bursal and scar tissue debridement. Care should be taken to preserve the coracoacromial arch since it acts as a static restraint to anterosuperior escape [1, 45]. The underlying prosthetic humeral head may be revealed in presence of a large, retracted tear. At this point, careful abrasion of the greater tuberosity at the footprint is done to promote healing of the repair.

To achieve a secure suture anchor without damaging the prosthesis, lateral placement of a single row for suture anchors may be used. In this step, transosseous suture repair may also be possible [1].

### 38.5.1	Arthroscopy and Biceps Tendon Injury After SA

The long head of the biceps (LHB) can be managed either by tenotomy or tenodesis or left untreated during TSA. Tethering, perching, or incarceration between the prosthetic humeral head and the tuberosities may lead to residual postoperative stiffness and pain if the LHB is retained [39].

Arthroscopic tenotomy could be helpful in patients with retained LHB-associated pain, especially in shoulder prosthesis implanted to treat humeral fractures. In these patients, the fracture pattern or the tuberosity repair around the prosthesis could potentially harm the LHB causing pain.

Alternatively, arthroscopic tenotomy could be followed by arthroscopic or open LHB tenodesis. Arthroscopically it can be done suprapectoral. High suprapectoral arthroscopic tenodesis at the bicipital groove may be performed using suture anchors [1]. If not possible, it should be done with an open approach through a small portion of the previous deltopectoral incision.

Concerning surgical technique, tenotomy should be done as in a non-arthroplasty shoulder. In regard to tenodesis, high or low suprapectoral tenodesis may be performed using suture anchors preventing damage to prosthetic components.

### 38.5.2	Arthroscopy and Shoulder Instability After SA

Shoulder anterosuperior instability after TSA usually results from acute or degenerative rotator cuff tear. On the other hand, posterior shoulder instability often relates to preoperative glenoid retroversion and posterior joint subluxation. If confirmation of RC injury or problems related to component malpositioning is made, surgical RC repair (open or arthroscopically) or revision surgery should be done to correct these complications. Few case reports have been published regarding shoulder instability treated with arthroscopic management. Grieshaber-Bouyer et al. reported on a 53-year-old patient who underwent arthroscopic posterior capsule reefing for recurrent posterior instability following aSA. The patient coped well for 9 years until the instability recurred, prompting revision to RSA [49].

Gee et al. reported a 74-year-old patient who developed atraumatic recurrent posterior instability 3 years after an aTSA for glenohumeral arthritis [48]. After discarding other causes of pain and instability related to aTSA, using the beach chair position, two suture anchors were placed posteroinferiorly on the glenoid and just medial to the glenoid component. The patient underwent arthroscopic posterior capsular plication in the beach chair position using two suture anchors that were placed posteroinferiorly on the glenoid and just medial to the glenoid component. The arthroscopy was followed by 6 weeks of immobilization and graduated physical therapy.

### 38.5.3	Arthroscopy and Diagnosis of Scapular Notching

To evaluate scapular notching, a passive arthroscopic evaluation can be done by alternating different positions of shoulder mobility (rota-

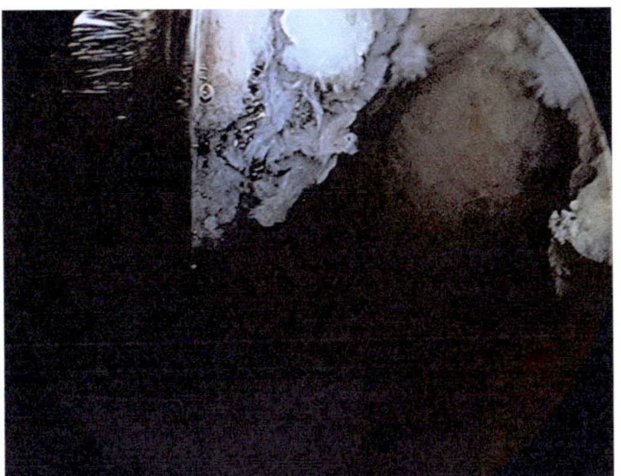

Fig. 38.4 Sirvaux grade 2 scapular notching and medial polyethylene wear

tions, abduction and adduction in different rotation angles) in order to find osteolysis of the inferior scapular edge. Scapular notching is frequently associated with medial polyethylene wear (Fig. 38.4) [41, 49, 50].

38.5.4 Arthroscopy and Loose Bodies Extraction

Loose bodies causing pain or mechanical symptoms after SA could be managed by arthroscopic removal plus diagnosing associated conditions.

38.6 Conclusions

Altogether, arthroscopic applications in patients with painful shoulder arthroplasty may be considered and applied if appropriate patient and pathology is present when other clinical tools fail; arthroscopic management could potentially avoid open surgeries together with its associated complications. The learning curve is not unreasonable but considerable when advanced therapeutic techniques are used.

Patients should be informed and accept the risk of arthroscopic treatment failure as well as the possibility of an eventual open revision surgery ending in an additional surgical intervention. Although arthroscopic management has a low complication rate, it should be carefully done to prevent iatrogenic harm.

Shoulder arthroscopy in patients after arthroplasty is safe and effective when used as a diagnostic tool. Regarding treatment of associated pathologies, available literature has demonstrated its utility. Patient satisfaction after shoulder arthroscopy is usually high, standardized outcome scores generally improve, and there is an overall low risk of complications.

References

1. Parker DB, Smith AC, Fleckenstein CM, Hasan SS. Arthroscopic evaluation and treatment of complications that arise following prosthetic shoulder arthroplasty. JBJS Rev. 2020;8(8):e20.
2. Fuerst M, Fink B, Ruther W. The value of preoperative knee aspiration and arthroscopic biopsy in revision total knee arthroplasty (German). Z Orthop Ihre Grenzgeb. 2005;143(1):36–41.
3. Horner NS, et al. Indications and outcomes of shoulder arthroscopy after shoulder arthroplasty. J Shoulder Elbow Surg. 2016;25:510–8.
4. Mallo GC, Burton L, Coats-Thomas M, Daniels SD, Sinz NJ, Warner JJP. Assessment of painful total shoulder arthroplasty using computed tomography arthrography. J Shoulder Elbow Surg. 2015;24:1507–11.
5. Heaven S, de Sa D, Simunovic N, Williams DS, Naudie D, Ayeni OR. Hip arthroscopy in the setting of hip arthroplasty. Knee Surg Sports Traumatol Arthrosc. 2016;24(1):287–94. Epub 2014 Nov 20
6. Sperling JW, Kozak TK, Hanssen AD, Cofield RH. Infection after shoulder arthroplasty. Clin Orthop Relat Res. 2001;382:206–16.
7. Singh JA, Sperling JW, Schleck C, Harmsen WS, Cofield RH. Periprosthetic infections after total shoulder arthroplasty: a 33-year perspective. J Shoulder Elbow Surg. 2012;21(11):1534–41.
8. Padegimas EM, et al. Periprosthetic infection in the United States: incidence and economic burden. J Shoulder Elbow Surg. 1015;24:741–6.
9. Hsu JE, Somerson JS, Vo KV, Matsen FA 3rd. What is periprosthetic shoulder infection? A Systematic review of two decades of publications. Int Orthop. 2017;41:813–22.
10. Klatte TO, et al. Single-stage revision for periprosthetic shoulder infection: outcomes and results. Bone Joint J. 2013;95(3):391–5.
11. Ince A, Seemann K, Frommelt L, Katzer A, Loehr JF. One-stage Exchange shoulder arthroplasty for peri-prosthetic infection. J Bone Joint Surg Br. 2005;87(6):814–8.

12. Saltzman MD, Marecek GS, Edwards SL, Kalainov DM. Infection after shoulder surgery. J Am Acad Orthop Surg. 2011;19(4):208–18.

13. Pottinger P 3rd, et al. Prognostic factors for bacterial cultures positive for Propionibacterium acnes and other organisms in a large series of revision shoulder arthroplasties performed for stiffness, pain, or loosening. J Bone Joint Surg Am. 2012;94(22):2075–83.

14. Lutz MF, et al. Arthroplastic and osteosynthetic infections due to Propionibacterium acnes: a retrospective study of 52 cases, 1995-2002. Eur J Clin Microbiol Infect Dis. 2005;24(11):739–44.

15. Levy O, et al. Propionibacterium acnes: an underestimated etiology in the pathogenesis of osteoarthritis? J Shoulder Elbow Surg. 2013;22(4):505–11.

16. Garrigues GE, Zmistowski B, Cooper AM, Green A; ICM Shoulder Group. Proceedings from the 2018 International Consensus Meeting on Orthopedic Infections: management of periprosthetic shoulder infection. J Shoulder Elbow Surg. 2019;28(6S):S67–S99.

17. Frangiamore SJ, et al. a-defensin as a predictor of periprosthetic shoulder infection. J Shoulder Elbow Surg. 2015;24(7):1021–7.

18. Weigelt L, et al. Alpha-defensin lateral flow test does not appear to be useful in predicting shoulder periprosthetic joint infections. Int Orthop. 2020;44(6):1023–9.

19. Richards J, et al. Patient and procedure-specific risk factors for deep infection after primary shoulder arthroplasty. Clin Orthop Relat Res. 2014;472(9):2809–15.

20. Piper KE, et al. Microbiologic diagnosis of prosthetic shoulder infection by use of implant sonication. J Clin Microbiol. 2009;47(6):1878–84.

21. Dilisio MF, Miller LR, Warner JJP, Higgins LD. Arthroscopic tissue culture for the evaluation of periprosthetic shoulder infection. J Bone Joint Surg Am. 2014;96(23):1952–8.

22. Akgun D, Maziak N, Plachel F, Minkus M, Scheibel M, Perka C, Moroder P. Diagnostic arthroscopy for detection of periprosthetic infection in painful shoulder arthroplasty. Arthroscopy. 2019;35(9):2571–7.

23. Grosso MJ, et al. Performance of implant sonication culture for the diagnosis of periprosthetic shoulder infection. J Shoulder Elbow Surg. 2018;27:211–6.

24. Gorbaty JD, Lucas RM, Matsen FA 3rd. Detritic synovitis can mimic a Propionibacterium periprosthetic infection. Int Orthop. 2016;40:95–8.

25. Parvizi J, Gehrke T. Proceedings of the Second International Consensus Meeting on Musculoskeletal Infection. Brooklandville, MD: Data Trace Publishing; 2018.

26. Guild T, et al. The role of arthroscopy in painful shoulder arthroplasty: is revision always necessary? Arthroscopy. 2020;36(6):1508–14.

27. Schoch B, Schleck C, Cofield RH, Sperling JW. Shoulder arthroplasty in patients younger than 50 years: minimum 20-year follow-up. J Shoulder Elbow Surg. 2015;24(5):705–10.

28. Wilde AH. Shoulder arthroplasty: what is it good for and how good is it? In: Matsen III FA, Fu FH, Hawkins RJ, editors. The shoulder: a balance of mobility and stability. Rosemont, IL: American Academy of Orthopaedic Surgeons; 1993. p. 459–81.

29. Brems J. The glenoid component in total shoulder arthroplasty. J Shoulder Elbow Surg. 1993;2(1):47–54.

30. Hawkins RJ, Greis PE, Bonutti PM. Treatment of symptomatic glenoid loosening following unconstrained shoulder arthroplasty. Orthopedics. 1999;22(2):229–34.

31. Mileti J, Boardman ND 3rd, Sperling JW, Cofield RH, Torchia ME, O'driscoll SW, Rowland CM. Radiographic analysis of polyethylene glenoid components using modern cementing techniques. J Shoulder Elbow Surg. 2004;13(5):492–8.

32. Wiater BP, Moravek JE Jr, Wiater JM. The evaluation of the failed shoulder arthroplasty. J Shoulder Elbow Surg. 2014;23(5):745–58.

33. Bonuti PM. Et all, arthroscopic assessment of glenoid component loosening after TSA. Arthroscopy. 1993;9:272–6.

34. O'Driscoll SW, Petrie RS, Torchia ME. Arthroscopic removal of the glenoid component for failed total shoulder arthroplasty. A report of five cases. J Bone Joint Surg Am. 2005;87(4):858–63.

35. Abildgaard JT, Bentley JC, Hawkins RJ, Tokish JM. Arthroscopic removal of a loose polyethylene glenoid component with bone grafting and patch augmentation for glenoid osseous defect. Arthrosc Tech. 2017;6(3):29–35.

36. Namdari S, Glaser D. Arthroscopically assisted conversion of total shoulder arthroplasty to hemiarthroplasty with glenoid bone grafting. Orthopedics. 2011;34(11):862–5.

37. Iannotti JP, Frangiamore SJ. Fate of large structural allograft for treatment of severe uncontained glenoid bone deficiency. J Shoulder Elbow Surg. 2012;21(6):765–71.

38. Hasan SS, Leith JM, Campbell B, Kapil R, Smith KL, Matsen FA 3rd. Characteristics of unsatisfactory shoulder arthroplasties. J Shoulder Elbow Surg. 2002;11(5):431–41.

39. Hersch JC, Dines DM. Arthroscopy for failed shoulder arthroplasty. Arthroscopy. 2000;16(6):606–12.

40. Barth JR, Burkhart SS. Arthroscopic capsular release after hemiarthroplasty of the shoulder for fracture: a new treatment paradigm. Arthroscopy. 2005;21(9):1150.

41. Aguilar-Gonzalez J, Luengo-Alonso G, Calvo E. Arthroscopic circumferential release for stiff reverse total shoulder arthroplasty. Arthrosc Tech. 2020;9(9):e1369–74.

42. Freedman KB, Williams GR, Iannotti JP. Impingement syndrome following total shoulder arthroplasty and humeral hemiarthroplasty: treatment with arthroscopic acromioplasty. Arthroscopy. 1998;14(7):665–70.

43. Sperling JW, Hawkins RJ, Walch G, Mahoney AP, Zuckerman JD. Complications in total shoulder arthroplasty. Instr Course Lect. 2013;62:135.

44. Wirth MA, Rockwood CA Jr. Complications of total shoulder-replacement arthroplasty. J Bone Joint Surg Am. 1996;78(4):603–16.

45. Mahony GT, et al. Risk factors for failing to achieve improvement after anatomic total shoulder arthroplasty for glenohumeral osteoarthritis. J Shoulder Elbow Surg. 2018;27(6):968–75.

46. Abboud JA, Anakwenze OA, Hsu JE. Soft-tissue management in revision total shoulder arthroplasty. J Am Acad Orthop Surg. 2013;21(1):23–31.

47. Tytherleigh-Strong GM, Levy O, Sforza G, Copeland SA. The role of arthroscopy for the problem shoulder arthroplasty. J Shoulder Elbow Surg. 2002;11(3):230–4.

48. Gee AO, Angeline ME, Dines JS, Dines DM. Shoulder instability after total shoulder arthroplasty: a case of arthroscopic repair. HSS J. 2014;10(1):88–91.

49. Grieshaber-Bouyer R, Gerber C. Arthroscopic repair of recurrent posterior shoulder subluxation after total shoulder arthroplasty: a case report. JBJS Case Connect. 2017;7(3):e71.

50. Boughebri O, Duparc F, Adam J-M, Valenti P. Arthroscopic dynamic analysis of scapular notching in reverse shoulder arthroplasty RSS. Orthop Traumatol Surg Res. 2011;97(8):779–84.

Preoperative Planning and Plan Execution in Shoulder Arthroplasty

Moby Parsons, Rick F. Papandrea, and Alexander T. Greene

39.1 Introduction

Shoulder arthroplasty has greatly increased in frequency over the past two decades. As the indications for its utilization have broadened, surgeons have developed a much greater understanding of shoulder pathoanatomy and pathomechanics and their impacts on shoulder reconstruction. 3D imaging is now the gold standard in preoperative assessment of degenerative shoulder problems, which gives surgeons a greater understanding of how to measure bone morphology and how differences may influence surgical decision-making. Preoperative planning based on 3D imaging has increased in popularity as most shoulder implant manufacturers now offer planning software to assist surgeons in preferred implant selection and placement.

Research to date in the field of preoperative planning and glenoid reconstruction has yielded several findings:

1. There is variability in how pathoanatomy is measured between planning platforms that may influence surgical decision-making.
2. There is variability in how surgeons plan shoulder arthroplasty, and this variability increases as the complexity of pathoanatomy increases.
3. Some method of plan execution is necessary as free-hand instrumentation is inaccurate.

This chapter will address each of these issues as well as discuss novel technologies and future directions in planning and navigation in shoulder arthroplasty.

39.2 Assessment of Glenoid Morphology

Much has been written about measurement of glenoid version and inclination in the degenerative shoulder including the description of different image-based planes that are used to reference these measurements. Some of the first studies looking at 2D CT-based measurements of glenoid version date back to Friedman's original description of the axis that bears his name [1]. Subsequent advancements in 3D imaging have shown that 2D measurements are less accurate due to variability of the scapular position relative to the alignment of the CT plane [2]. Several studies have shown that scapular rotation, as may occur due to posi-

M. Parsons (✉)
The Knee Hip and Shoulder Center,
Portsmouth, NH, USA

R. F. Papandrea
Orthopedic Associates of Wisconsin,
Pewaukee, WI, USA
e-mail: rick@papandrea.net

A. T. Greene
RSQ Technologies, Poznari, Poland
e-mail: Alex.greene@rsqtechnologies.com

© ISAKOS 2023
A. D. Mazzocca et al. (eds.), *Shoulder Arthritis across the Life Span*,
https://doi.org/10.1007/978-3-031-33298-2_39

tion on the thorax and patient position in the CT gantry, may influence version measurements by up to 10° [2–4].

3D imaging techniques have the advantage of correcting image orientation relative to the scapular plane, thereby reducing errors associated with off-axis acquisition [5, 6]. Reid et al. compared 2D to 3D version measurement and found that 3D techniques yield a greater retroversion value in 73% of cases with an average difference of 3.5° [7]. Chalmers et al. demonstrated that in B2 glenoids, failure to correct 2D CT images to the scapular plane led to an overestimation of version measurement of >5° in a substantial number of cases [5]. These findings demonstrate that failure to correct image rotation on 2D slices may impact surgical decision-making if there is overestimation of the measured version [8].

Determination of the axis of measurement relative to glenoid deformity also presents a challenge. Kim et al. showed that glenoid version is measured differently at different superior/inferior levels on the glenoid face [9]. This may be particularly important in the case of the B2 glenoid where the wear pattern changes in the superior-inferior plane [10]. As glenoid deformity increases, determining the center of the glenoid face becomes more subject to variability in defining the measurement plane [11]. As such, there is no consensus on the definition of the optimal plane of measurement for version, and surgeons must recognize these limitations when planning with the goal of correcting glenoid deformity.

Inclination can also vary by method of measurement. Correction of images to the scapular plane is also important for accurate measurement. The accuracy of inclination measurement may also be affected by the severity of the deformity, particularly when methods are based off an axis that references the center of the glenoid. The Maurer method defined the beta angle, which is the angle between the superior and inferior glenoid tubercle and the floor of the supraspinatus fossa [12]. This has proven the most reproducible method that is more resistant to scapular rotation. Daggett et al. showed that the beta angle is best measured on CT slices corrected to the scapular

plane as measurement on uncorrected CT slices and on plain radiographs is inaccurate [13].

Boileau described the reverse shoulder arthroplasty (RSA) angle recognizing that in cuff tear arthropathy cases with certain patterns of central erosion, the inclination of the inferior glenoid is greater than that of the whole glenoid face [14]. He found that placement of the baseplate must be orthogonal to the floor of the supraspinatus fossa for proper inclination correction, and correction based on the beta angle may lead to superiorly inclined baseplate placement in these cases of central wear.

Finally, posterior humeral subluxation or decentering is another measurement parameter that surgeons may use when planning shoulder arthroplasty. Terrier et al. have shown that this measurement is also subject to variation between the alignment of the scapular plane and plane of image capture [15]. Further, there is no consensus on whether this is best measured relative to the axis of the scapular body or relative to a perpendicular to the glenoid face. These different methods of assessing subluxation can yield different degrees of apparent severity. Sabesan et al. have suggested that displacements relative to the glenoid fossa and relative to the scapular plane are independent values and may have different pathologic impacts [16]. In addition, static orientation of the humerus in the CT scanner may lead to the appearance of subluxation since the arm is positioned passively in internal rotation where the articular surface is directed posteriorly. Further research is needed to determine the impact of these factors on subluxation measurement and its importance in surgical decision-making.

39.3 Preoperative Planning: Glenoid Side

The growing popularity of 3D CT-based preoperative planning software is predicated on the recognition that glenoid deformity is more common than previously appreciated and that correction of glenoid deformity through optimal bone preparation and implant placement may be important to the long-term outcomes of shoulder arthroplasty. However, work to date suggests that there are no set standards by which to measure glenoid deformity, and different planning software may provide different information based on the measurement technique and plane of reference used.

Planning software use both manual and automated measurement techniques. Manual techniques can be surgeon-based or technician-based. Erickson et al. compared surgeon to software measurement of glenoid deformity and found significant differences between the two [17]. Shukla et al. compared manual versus automated measurement of glenoid morphology and found that automation resulted in greater retroversion by an average of 4° as well as greater subluxation and lesser inclination [18]. Shah et al. also found that automated measurement techniques using the best-fit sphere method tended to result in higher values for retroversion [19].

Surgeons must recognize that their decision-making relative to implant choice and deformity correction may be biased by how the software they use measures glenoid pathoanatomy (Fig. 39.1). Denard et al. compared two different commonly used planning platforms and found that more than a 5° difference was measured in 30% of cases for version and 45% of cases for inclination. The authors concluded, "Given that implant choice and desired component positioning are based on preoperative measurements, further study is needed to evaluate the differences between the measurements obtained with different techniques" [20]. Erickson et al. also found little agreement when comparing glenoid deformity measurement between four commercially available planning software systems [17].

Differences in the measurement of glenoid wear may impact how surgeons plan, including (1) correcting pathologic retroversion and inclination, (2) minimizing bone loss through corrective reaming, (3) maximizing implant contact with bone, (4) minimizing vault perforation of fixation pegs, (5) maximizing impingement-free range of motion, and (6) restoring anatomical relationships.

Despite the perceived benefits of planning, there are yet no consensus standards to guide plan optimization. Surgeons must rely on varying degrees of gestalt, experience, and scientific information to inform their choices based on what their system offers. Guidelines such as correcting retroversion to <10° are based largely on finite element or biomechanical models that do not reflect modern implant technology [21, 22]. Surgeons' perception that reverse shoulder arthroplasty is more forgiving of residual retroversion is largely subjective which has resulted in the increased use of reverse shoulders in patients with higher degrees of pathologic retroversion such as Walch B2 and B3 glenoids.

Variability in preoperative planning has been studied for both anatomic and reverse shoulder arthroplasty. Parsons et al. showed substantial variability in how nine different surgeons planned a series of shoulder arthroplasty cases [23, 24]. Variability was significant across frequency of and threshold for augment use, degree of correction, and implant size and placement on the glenoid face. Surgeons even differed from themselves when planning the same case on separate occasions, which suggests that there are significant gaps in our current knowledge based on patient-specific plan optimization and that each surgeon is subject to experiential bias.

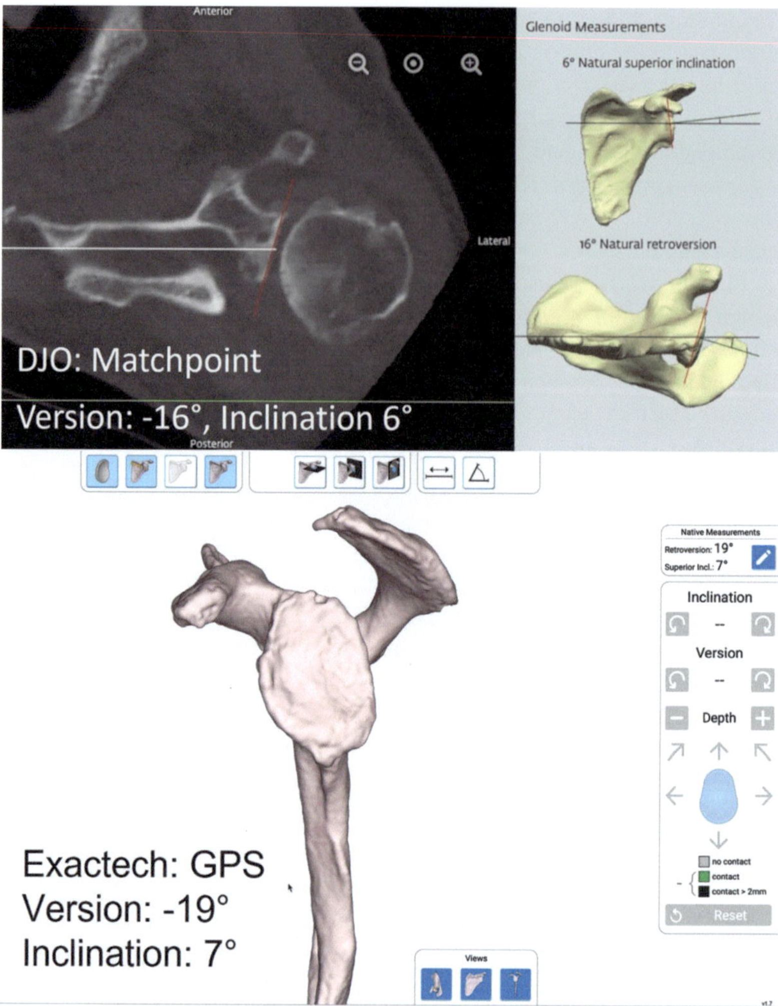

Fig. 39.1 The same CT imported into different commercially available planning platforms (Matchpoint, DJO, and Exactech, Inc). Different values for version and inclination are measured by different platforms

39.4 Preoperative Planning: Humeral Side

While planning has largely focused on the glenoid side to date, most systems are now incorporating humeral planning with a view toward providing a more complete picture of proposed implant selection as well as its impact on anatomic parameters such as center of rotation, lateralization, distalization, and range of motion. Lima et al. have demonstrated that different software platforms measure head height and diameter with better concordance than glenoid parameters [25]. Accurate determination of humeral retroversion must be defined either relative to the transepicondylar axis of the elbow or the bicipital groove [26]. Planning can help surgeons determine the level and orientation of the humeral osteotomy plane and how this impacts placement of the implant. As planning software can now simulate virtual range of motion as a function of implant configuration, humeral-sided planning is an important step forward in providing actionable insights. To date however, motion simulation in these softwares does not account for scapulothoracic rotation and other issues such as thoracic kyphosis

39.5 Preoperative Planning: Deficiencies and Future Opportunities

While planning platforms can inform surgeons on how implant choice and position affect anatomical relationships in shoulder arthroplasty, they remain a passive tool that cannot replicate many features of native shoulder biomechanics. Perhaps the most important of these is the role of the soft tissues. For anatomic shoulder replacement, preoperative stiffness due to muscle atrophy and contracture may influence decisions such as head diameter and height to optimize postoperative motion while balancing the need for stability. In addition, joint line lateralization may occur with placement of a prosthetic glenoid, which can affect soft tissue tension. As current planning software cannot accurately model this information, surgeons must still rely on qualitative intraoperative assessment.

Similarly in reverse shoulder arthroplasty, residual cuff integrity, prior cuff surgery, and degree of static proximal humeral migration may all impact the balance between stability and tension and how these may contribute to complications such as dislocation and scapular spine fractures. While CT scans can provide radiographic information on cuff integrity and muscle atrophy and fatty degeneration, the ability of current software systems to integrate this information into planning requires further study. Pitocchi et al. have used statistical shape modeling to study the impact of implant configuration on muscle elongation [27]. Other authors have determined ways to segment muscle volume and fatty infiltration on CT scans to better understand how these are affected by diagnosis and how they relate to other elements of the pathoanatomy such as version and subluxation [28, 29]. Further research and development is needed to incorporate this information into actionable decision-making insights.

Another opportunity is the incorporation of scapulothoracic motion in planning software. Current platforms look only at glenohumeral motion when predicting postoperative range and boney impingement as a function of implant configuration and presence of osteophytes. Actual shoulder motion is more complex after shoulder arthroplasty and may be influenced by extra-articular factors such as posture, kyphosis, and scoliosis [30]. Articular factors such as implant design and position, residual cuff integrity, repair of the subscapularis muscle, use of muscle transfer techniques, and other factors may also influence in vivo range of motion. Further research is necessary to better predict how implant and technique-related factors can impact postoperative function.

Finally, in the era of big data, planning platforms will eventually include machine learning-based, predictive analytical tools to help automate planning based on selected data inputs, such as demographic, diagnostic, radiographic, and clinical information. Efforts to build out data ecosystems will eventually better automate the capture of postoperative clinical data which can be fed into machine learning tools to reconcile implant configuration and placement with outcomes. Data science has the ability to identify and account for biases in datasets, which also improves the predictive capacity of these tools.

The successful deployment of artificial intelligence-based planning tools will require systems to capture final implant placement at surgery, postoperative range of motion, and patient-reported outcomes in a manner that is accurate, reliable, and efficient. As these platforms grow in the breadth and depth of their datasets, the goal is to eventually have preoperative planning software provide surgeons with an optimal plan that is data-driven rather than experience-driven and patient-specific rather than convention-based. This allows for all surgeons regardless of experience or skill to leverage the collective experience of a wider shoulder arthroplasty community via machine learning.

39.6 From Planning to Placement

Preoperative planning does not guarantee precise or accurate implant placement. Traditional free-hand instruments combined with limited ability to visualize scapular anatomy intraoperatively can lead to significant deviation from the planned implant placement. While Raiss et al. have shown a high concordance between planned and implanted glenoid type and size, Schoch et al. found that planning without some form of intra-operative guidance would leave 48% of components malpositioned relative to the plan [31, 32]. Schoch's study found a mean error between plan and placement of 3.2 ± 2.0 mm for translation, 6.4° ± 5.6° for version, and 6.6° ± 4.9° for inclination. Sadoghi et al. also found an average error in glenoid version of 10.6° with standard instrumentation. Iannotti et al., comparing standard instruments with 2D imaging to patient-specific instrumentation based on a 3D plan, found a difference of 8.2° ± 0.9° in version, 11.4° ± 1.2° in inclination, and 1.7 ± 0.2 mm in translation, which were all statistically significant [33]. Other studies have demonstrated that free-handing the humeral head osteotomy relative to a preoperative plan is not reliably accurate and may lead to problems such as overstuffing and varus angulation [34, 35]. Collectively, these studies demonstrate that methods to improve implant placement are necessary to translate the benefits of preoperative planning into the actual surgical procedure.

39.6.1 Patient-Specific Instrumentation (PSI)

PSI entails the use of 3D printed guides to aid in identifying the entry point and trajectory for K-wire placement which is used to align glenoid reaming. Numerous studies have looked at the accuracy of different PSI systems with variability in reported results [33, 36–40]. A meta-analysis summarizing the results of the current literature on this topic determined that PSI improves glenoid component positioning for all parameters except implant rotation. The number of outliers, as defined by >10° or 4 mm of deviation from the plan, was 15% with PSI versus 69% with standard instruments [41]. The principal advantage of PSI is relative ease of use without the need for fiducial-based navigation. Disadvantages include the cost and time of manufacturing, reports of difficulty determining proper guide placement on the boney anatomy, and the requirement of K-wire-based reaming which is not the preferred surgical technique for all surgeons.

39.6.2 Augmented and Mixed Reality (AR/MR)

Augmented reality (AR) combines elements of both the real and virtual world superimposed in a visual field. Mixed reality (MR) is an extension of AR that allows real and virtual data to interact. This has been used to allow the surgeon to position a virtual model of the preoperative plan into the surgical field of view and thus has the potential in aiding the guidance of surgical tools to execute a preoperative plan (Fig. 39.2). Based on a head-mounted display, MR in shoulder arthroplasty has

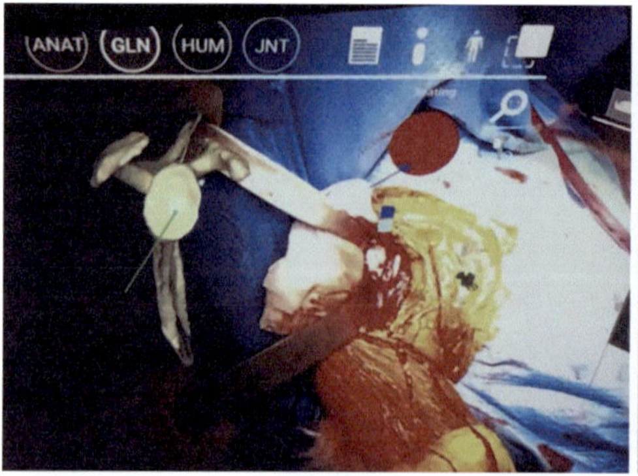

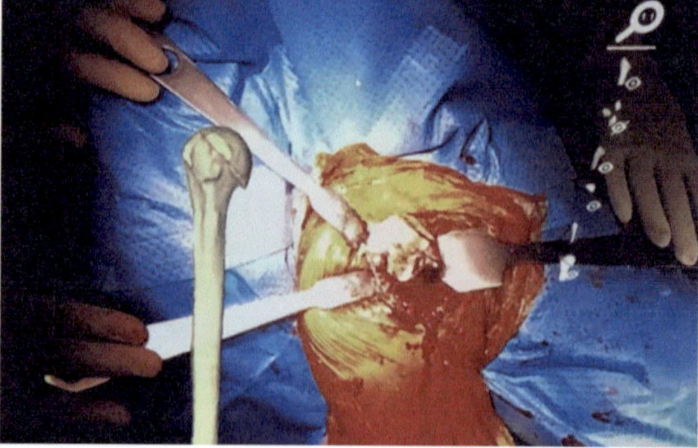

Fig. 39.2 Mixed reality allows for a virtual overlay of a preoperative plan in the surgical field. The surgeon can interact with this plan in the operative environment

the potential to allow surgical navigation without a larger geographic footprint of robotic systems.

The accuracy of this technology is somewhat dependent on the computing power and optical capabilities of the software and hardware. Gu et al. have shown that alignment of the preoperative plan and intraoperative anatomy can be challenging and when used to guide pin placement for glenoid reaming, the accuracy was 3.8 ± 1.3 mm for translation and 4.7° ± 2.9° for angulation [42]. Similarly, Kriechling et al. used MR to assist in K-wire placement and found a mean deviation from the preoperative plan of 3.5 ± 1.7 mm for translation and a mean trajectory deviation of 3.8° ± 1.7° [43]. These numbers are a significant improvement over free-hand instrumentation and demonstrate promise, but until the accuracy approaches that of traditional navigation and robotics, the clinical efficacy remains uncertain.

39.6.3 Computer-Assisted Surgical Navigation

Computer-assisted surgery has existed for decades, but early systems were limited by the available computing technology of the time. Advancements in processing power and software engineering have greatly improved navigation in shoulder arthroplasty. These systems use tracker-based technology to register the preoperative plan to both the patient's osseous anatomy and the surgical instruments. Once registered, surgeons can visualize in real time the entry point and trajectory for all surgical tools used to prepare the glenoid. "Intelligent" instruments can also be used to guide rotation and impaction of the final implant as well as to register final implant position for later correlation with outcomes and complications (Fig. 39.3).

Jones et al. studied the accuracy of baseplate placement in RTSA using navigation and found an average deviation from the plan of 1.9° for version and 2.4° for inclination [44]. Nashikar et al. demonstrated that computer-aided navigation led to greater accuracy in restoring neutral

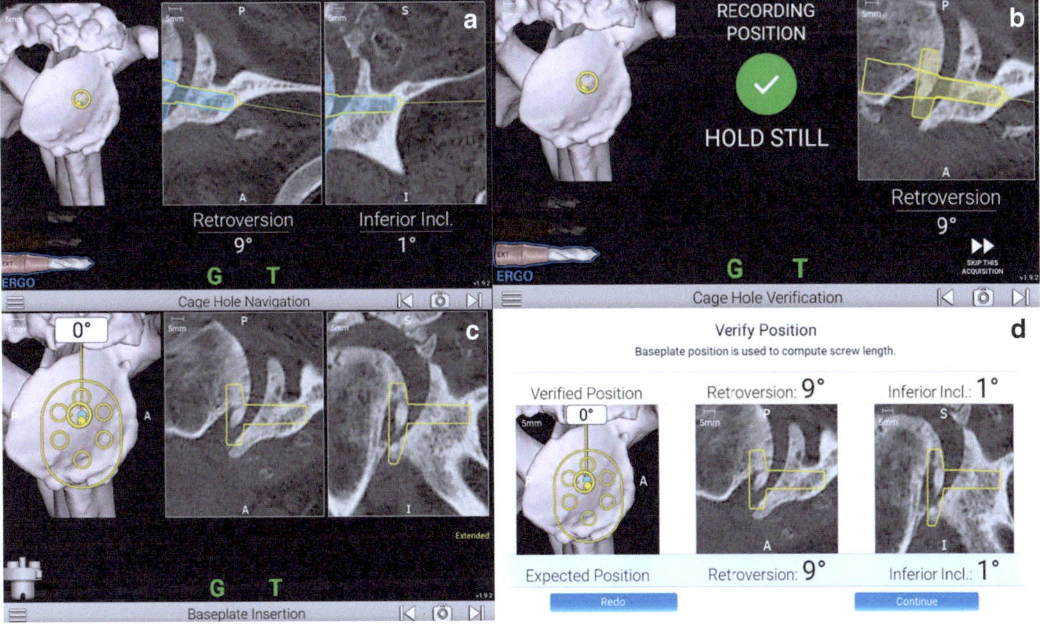

Fig. 39.3 Surgical navigation allows real-time visualization and verification of drill trajectory (**a** and **b**) and rotation, orientation, and verification of baseplate impaction (**c** and **d**)

version with the use of augmented glenoids with 40% of plans replicated perfectly and 70% of plans within 5° [45]. Similarly, they showed that navigation led to improved reverse baseplate screw purchase and length with markedly reduced central peg perforation [46]. Hones et al. also found that the use of navigation in RSA led to longer fixation screws and the need for fewer screws to achieve adequate fixation [47]. Trackerless navigation to improve surgical workflow and avoid line of sight issues is in development and, if validated, may improve the ease of use of this technology. This may be combined with AR headsets to optimize surgical workflow [42].

39.7 Future Directions: From Planning to Placement

39.7.1 Robotic-Assisted Shoulder Arthroplasty

Arthroplasty of the lower extremities has seen an explosion in robotic assistance. The technology has several potential benefits. Similar to computer navigation, registration of the osseous anatomy with the robot allows the surgeon to precisely replicate the preoperative plan. Haptic feedback and boundary-stop programming provide the potential for increased precision and safety by having the system auto-stop when the surgical tools reach a planned degree of bone preparation or migrate outside of a predefined boundary.

Like navigation, robotics also has the potential to improve the precision of the humeral osteotomy which may aid in replication of the center of rotation of the humeral implant and prevent common errors of varus/valgus malalignment and overstuffing. Similarly, robotic systems can capture information on final implant placement so that configuration and placement data can be combined with a larger data ecosystem to provide data-driven and patient-specific future planning. This may eventually allow surgeons to better understand the relationship between implant design, configuration, placement, and clinical outcomes like impingement-free range of motion, stability, notching, and stress fracture.

There are not yet any commercially available systems that allow for a robotic-assisted shoulder arthroplasty, though several companies are working toward this goal. As with any new technology, the incremental cost of robotics should be weighed against the clinical benefits its use provides. This has proven a matter of debate in the lower extremity where there is a dearth of unbiased clinical data from well-designed studies that proves a short- or long-term benefit that is solely attributable to the use of robotics in isolation from all other variables that may influence outcomes. The substantial market penetration of robotic knee and hip replacement in the absence of robust outcomes data supporting its value has led several knee arthroplasty thought leaders to question whether the marketing power of robotics has gotten ahead of the impact of its innovation on outcomes [48]. Thus, shoulder surgeons need to be mindful of the value equation when considering the adoption of innovative but cost-increasing technology.

39.8 Conclusion

Technology that assists in planning and execution of shoulder arthroplasty has witnessed a significant evolution in the past decade. This has fostered a much greater understanding of glenohumeral pathoanatomy and has equally raised other questions about what the best plan for a given patient may be. Advancements in hardware and software will continue to shepherd innovation in fields like AR, navigation, robotics, and artificial intelligence with the ultimate goal of achieving patient-specific, data-driven plans to reduce complications and improve outcomes while preserving cost. Such technology needs careful assessment and stewardship of its value particularly in light of the growing prevalence of shoulder arthroplasty.

References

1. Friedman RJ, Hawthorne KB, Genez BM. The use of computerized tomography in the measurement of glenoid version. J Bone Joint Surg Am. 1992;74(7):1032–7.
2. Hoenecke HR, Hermida JC, Flores-Hernandez C, D'Lima DD. Accuracy of CT-based measurements of glenoid version for total shoulder arthroplasty. J Shoulder Elbow Surg. 2010;19(2):166–71.
3. Bokor DJ, O'Sullivan MD, Hazan GJ. Variability of measurement of glenoid version on computed tomography scan. J Shoulder Elbow Surg. 1999;8(6):595–8.
4. Bryce CD, Davison AC, Lewis GS, Wang L, Flemming DJ, Armstrong AD. Two-dimensional glenoid version measurements vary with coronal and sagittal scapular rotation. J Bone Joint Surg Am. 2010;92(3):692–9.
5. Chalmers PN, Salazar D, Chamberlain A, Keener JD. Radiographic characterization of the B2 glenoid: is inclusion of the entirety of the scapula necessary? J Shoulder Elbow Surg. 2017;26(5):855–60.
6. Budge MD, Lewis GS, Schaefer E, Coquia S, Flemming DJ, Armstrong AD. Comparison of standard two-dimensional and three-dimensional corrected glenoid version measurements. J Shoulder Elbow Surg. 2011;20(4):577–83.
7. Reid JJ, Kunkle BF, Greene AT, Eichinger JK, Friedman RJ. Variability and reliability of 2-dimensional vs. 3-dimensional glenoid version measurements with 3-dimensional preoperative planning software. J Shoulder Elbow Surg. 2022;31(2):302–9.
8. Werner BS, Hudek R, Burkhart KJ, Gohlke F. The influence of three-dimensional planning on decision-making in total shoulder arthroplasty. J Shoulder Elbow Surg. 2017;26(8):1477–83.
9. Kim H, Yoo CH, Park SB, Song HS. Difference in glenoid retroversion between two-dimensional axial computed tomography and three-dimensional reconstructed images. Clin Shoulder Elbow. 2020;23(2):71–9.
10. Knowles NK, Keener JD, Ferreira LM, Athwal GS. Quantification of the position, orientation, and surface area of bone loss in type B2 glenoids. J Shoulder Elbow Surg. 2015;24(4):503–10.
11. Scalise JJ, Codsi MJ, Bryan J, Brems JJ, Iannotti JP. The influence of three-dimensional computed tomography images of the shoulder in preoperative planning for total shoulder arthroplasty. J Bone Joint Surg Am. 2008;90(11):2438–45.
12. Maurer A, Fucentese SF, Pfirrmann CWA, Wirth SH, Djahangiri A, Jost B, et al. Assessment of glenoid inclination on routine clinical radiographs and computed tomography examinations of the shoulder. J Shoulder Elbow Surg. 2012;21(8):1096–103.
13. Daggett M, Werner B, Gauci MO, Chaoui J, Walch G. Comparison of glenoid inclination angle using different clinical imaging modalities. J Shoulder Elbow Surg. 2016;25(2):180–5.
14. Boileau P, Gauci MO, Wagner ER, Clowez G, Chaoui J, Chelli M, et al. The reverse shoulder arthroplasty angle: a new measurement of glenoid inclination for reverse shoulder arthroplasty. J Shoulder Elbow Surg. 2019;28(7):1281–90.
15. Terrier A, Ston J, Farron A. Importance of a three-dimensional measure of humeral head subluxation in osteoarthritic shoulders. J Shoulder Elbow Surg. 2015;24(2):295–301.
16. Sabesan VJ, Callanan M, Youderian A, Iannotti JP. 3D CT assessment of the relationship between humeral head alignment and glenoid retroversion in glenohumeral osteoarthritis. J Bone Joint Surg Am. 2014;96(8):e64.
17. Erickson BJ, Chalmers PN, Denard P, Lederman E, Horneff G, Werner BC, et al. Does commercially available shoulder arthroplasty preoperative planning software agree with surgeon measurements of version, inclination, and subluxation? J Shoulder Elbow Surg. 2021;30(2):413–20.
18. Shukla DR, McLaughlin RJ, Lee J, Nguyen NTV, Sanchez-Sotelo J. Automated three-dimensional measurements of version, inclination, and subluxation. Shoulder Elbow. 2020;12(1):31–7.
19. Shah SS, Sahota S, Denard PJ, Provencher MT, Parsons BO, Hartzler RU, et al. Variability in total shoulder arthroplasty planning software compared to a control CT-derived 3D printed scapula. Shoulder Elbow. 2021;13(3):268–75.
20. Denard PJ, Provencher MT, Lädermann A, Romeo AA, Parsons BO, Dines JS. Version and inclination obtained with 3-dimensional planning in total shoulder arthroplasty: do different programs produce the same results? JSES Open Access. 2018;2(4):200–4.
21. Shapiro TA, McGarry MH, Gupta R, Lee YS, Lee TQ. Biomechanical effects of glenoid retroversion in total shoulder arthroplasty. J Shoulder Elbow Surg. 2007;16(3 Suppl):S90–5.
22. Farron A, Terrier A, Büchler P. Risks of loosening of a prosthetic glenoid implanted in retroversion. J Shoulder Elbow Surg. 2006;15(4):521–6.
23. Parsons M, Greene A, Polakovic S, Byram I, Cheung E, Jones R, et al. Assessment of surgeon variability in preoperative planning of reverse total shoulder arthroplasty: a quantitative comparison of 49 cases planned by 9 surgeons. J Shoulder Elbow Surg. 2020;29(10):2080–8.
24. Parsons M, Greene A, Polakovic S, Rohrs E, Byram I, Cheung E, et al. Intersurgeon and intrasurgeon variability in preoperative planning of anatomic total shoulder arthroplasty: a quantitative comparison of 49 cases planned by 9 surgeons. J Shoulder Elbow Surg. 2020;29(12):2610–8.
25. Lima DJL, Markel J, Yawman JP, Whaley JD, Sabesan VJ. 3D preoperative planning for humeral head selection in total shoulder arthroplasty. Musculoskelet Surg. 2020;104(2):155–61.
26. Johnson JW, Thostenson JD, Suva LJ, Hasan SA. Relationship of bicipital groove rotation with humeral head retroversion: a three-dimensional com-

puted tomographic analysis. J Bone Joint Surg Am. 2013;95(8):719–24.

27. Pitocchi J, Plessers K, Wirix-Speetjens R, Debeer P, van Lenthe GH, Jonkers I, et al. Automated muscle elongation measurement during reverse shoulder arthroplasty planning. J Shoulder Elbow Surg. 2021;30(3):561–71.

28. Terrier A, Ston J, Dewarrat A, Becce F, Farron A. A semi-automated quantitative CT method for measuring rotator cuff muscle degeneration in shoulders with primary osteoarthritis. Orthop Traumatol Surg Res. 2017;103(2):151–7.

29. Werthel JD, Boux de Casson F, Burdin V, Athwal GS, Favard L, Chaoui J, et al. CT-based volumetric assessment of rotator cuff muscle in shoulder arthroplasty preoperative planning. Bone Jt Open. 2021;2(7):552–61.

30. Moroder P, Urvoy M, Raiss P, Werthel JD, Akgün D, Chaoui J, et al. Patient posture affects simulated ROM in reverse total shoulder arthroplasty: a modeling study using preoperative planning software. Clin Orthop Relat Res. 2022;480(3):619–31.

31. Raiss P, Walch G, Wittmann T, Athwal GS. Is preoperative planning effective for intraoperative glenoid implant size and type selection during anatomic and reverse shoulder arthroplasty? J Shoulder Elbow Surg. 2020;29(10):2123–7.

32. Schoch BS, Haupt E, Leonor T, Farmer KW, Wright TW, King JJ. Computer navigation leads to more accurate glenoid targeting during total shoulder arthroplasty compared with 3-dimensional preoperative planning alone. J Shoulder Elbow Surg. 2020;29(11):2257–63.

33. Iannotti J, Baker J, Rodriguez E, Brems J, Ricchetti E, Mesiha M, et al. Three-dimensional preoperative planning software and a novel information transfer technology improve glenoid component positioning. J Bone Joint Surg Am. 2014;96(9):e71.

34. Suter T, Gerber Popp A, Kolz CW, Tashjian RZ, Henninger HB. Accuracy of free-hand humeral head resection planned on 3D-CT models in shoulder arthroplasty: an in vitro analysis. Arch Orthop Trauma Surg. 2022;142(11):3141–7.

35. Grubhofer F, Muniz Martinez AR, Haberli J, Selig ME, Ernstbrunner L, Price MD, et al. Does computerized CT-based 3D planning of the humeral head cut help to restore the anatomy of the proximal humerus after stemless total shoulder arthroplasty? J Shoulder Elbow Surg. 2021;30(6):e309–16.

36. Levy JC, Everding NG, Frankle MA, Keppler LJ. Accuracy of patient-specific guided glenoid baseplate positioning for reverse shoulder arthroplasty. J Shoulder Elbow Surg. 2014;23(10):1563–7.

37. Dallalana RJ, McMahon RA, East B, Geraghty L. Accuracy of patient-specific instrumentation in anatomic and reverse total shoulder arthroplasty. Int J Shoulder Surg. 2016;10(2):59–66.

38. Walch G, Vezeridis PS, Boileau P, Deransart P, Chaoui J. Three-dimensional planning and use of patient-specific guides improve glenoid component position: an in vitro study. J Shoulder Elbow Surg. 2015;24(2):302–9.

39. Iannotti JP, Walker K, Rodriguez E, Patterson TE, Jun BJ, Ricchetti ET. Accuracy of 3-dimensional planning, implant templating, and patient-specific instrumentation in anatomic total shoulder arthroplasty. J Bone Joint Surg Am. 2019;101(5):446–57.

40. Verborgt O, Hachem AI, Eid K, Vuylsteke K, Ferrand M, Hardy P. Accuracy of patient-specific guided implantation of the glenoid component in reversed shoulder arthroplasty. Orthop Traumatol Surg Res. 2018;104(6):767–72.

41. Villatte G, Muller AS, Pereira B, Mulliez A, Reilly P, Emery R. Use of patient-specific instrumentation (PSI) for glenoid component positioning in shoulder arthroplasty. A systematic review and meta-analysis. PLoS One. 2018;13(8):e0201759.

42. Gu W, Shah K, Knopf J, Josewski C, Unberath M. A calibration-free workflow for image-based mixed reality navigation of total shoulder arthroplasty. Comput Methods Biomech Biomed Eng. 2021;10:243–51.

43. Kriechling P, Roner S, Liebmann F, Casari F, Fürnstahl P, Wieser K. Augmented reality for base plate component placement in reverse total shoulder arthroplasty: a feasibility study. Arch Orthop Trauma Surg. 2021;141(9):1447–53.

44. Jones RB, Greene AT, Polakovic SV, Hamilton MA, Mohajer NJ, Youderian AR, et al. Accuracy and precision of placement of the glenoid baseplate in reverse total shoulder arthroplasty using a novel computer assisted navigation system combined with preoperative planning: a controlled cadaveric study. Sem Arthrop JSES. 2020;30(1):73–82.

45. Nashikkar PS, Scholes CJ, Haber MD. Computer navigation re-creates planned glenoid placement and reduces correction variability in total shoulder arthroplasty: an in vivo case-control study. J Shoulder Elbow Surg. 2019;28(12):e398–409.

46. Nashikkar PS, Scholes CJ, Haber MD. Role of intraoperative navigation in the fixation of the glenoid component in reverse total shoulder arthroplasty: a clinical case-control study. J Shoulder Elbow Surg. 2019;28(9):1685–91.

47. Hones KM, King JJ, Schoch BS, Struk AM, Farmer KW, Wright TW. The in vivo impact of computer navigation on screw number and length in reverse total shoulder arthroplasty. J Shoulder Elbow Surg. 2021;30(10):e629–35.

48. Booth RE, Sharkey PF, Parvizi J. Robotics in hip and knee arthroplasty: real innovation or marketing Ruse. J Arthroplast. 2019;34(10):2197–8.

Past, Present, and Future of Robotic Surgery in Shoulder Arthroplasty

40

Lacee K. Collins, Matthew W. Cole, William F. Sherman, Michael J. O'Brien, and Felix H. Savoie

40.1 Background and History of Robotics

Total shoulder arthroplasty (TSA) is a highly successful procedure for restoring joint function and alleviating pain in the treatment of end-stage osteoarthritis with a survivorship of 93% at 10 years and 85% at 20 years [1–3]. In the United States (US), the annual demand for TSA procedures is increasing every year. From 2011 to 2017, the annual number of primary TSA procedures increased by 103.7%, and the total number of procedures is expected to top 350,000 by 2025 [4]. While the number of elective TSA per year has increased over the past decade, reverse total shoulder utilization for fracture management has also increased by 1841.4% from 2010 to 2019 [5]. With the increasing demand for shoulder arthroplasty, technological advances to assist the surgeon and mitigate the risk for complications are also increasing. As technology continues to advance, robotic surgeries are becoming more mainstream in attempt to deliver more precision, better surgical planning, and complication prevention.

Over the past several decades, technological advances such as computed tomography (CT)- and magnetic resonance imaging (MRI)-based patient-specific cutting guides, computer navigation, and patient-specific implants have been developed to improve patient-reported outcome measures and patient satisfaction. Robotics has emerged as a leader in the frontier of total joint arthroplasties, specifically the hip and knee [6]. Robotics is still a novel tool in the field of orthopedics; however it has been used in general surgery, neurosurgery, and urology for nearly three decades [7]. The first documented use of a robot-assisted surgical procedure occurred in 1985 when a robotic surgical arm (PUMA) was used to perform a neurosurgical biopsy [8].

Orthopedic robotic-assisted surgeries were originally designed to improve the precision of total hip arthroplasties, with the first procedures occurring in the 1990s [9, 10]. ROBODOC (THINK Surgical, CA) was the original robotic-assisted system developed for total hip arthroplasties (THAs) in 1994, but was not cleared by the US Food and Drug Administration until 2008 [11]. This system was used in Europe demonstrating radiographic improvements in joint alignment using robot arm-assisted total joint arthroplasty (TJA) [12, 13]. However, systematic and meta-analyses indicate that patient satisfaction for patients undergoing active robot arm-assisted THA and total knee arthroplasty (TKA) are comparable with conventional surgery [14, 15].

L. K. Collins (✉) · M. W. Cole · W. F. Sherman · M. J. O'Brien · F. H. Savoie
Department of Orthopaedic Surgery, Tulane University School of Medicine,
New Orleans, LA, USA
e-mail: lcollins2@tulane.edu; mcole8@tulane.edu; swilliam1@tulane.edu; mobrien@tulane.edu; fsavoie@tulane.edu

© ISAKOS 2023
A. D. Mazzocca et al. (eds.), *Shoulder Arthritis across the Life Span*,
https://doi.org/10.1007/978-3-031-33298-2_40

As of 2018, over 17,000 THAs have been performed using the ROBODOC system worldwide. MAKO robotic-assisted devices (MAKO Stryker, Fort Lauderdale, Florida) are another common orthopedic robotic system with over 700 systems in use across the United States in 2020 [16, 17]. As of 2020, the MAKO system is the only FDA-approved robotic-assisted device for both THA and TKA [16]. Currently, four other robots are available for robot-assisted orthopedic procedures. Smith & Nephew's Navio (Smith & Nephew, Inc., Memphis, TN, USA), introduced in 2017, uses a probe to map out the bony anatomy of the patient [18]. Zimmer Biomet's Rosa robot was introduced in Australia in 2018 and recently gained FDA approval in the United States [18]. OMNIBotics knee system (OMNIlife Science, Inc., Raynham, MA, USA) is also a semi-active system [18]. TSolution One (Think Surgical Inc., Fremont, CA, USA) is an image-dependent active robotic system that incorporates technology originally developed for ROBODOC [18].

Robotic-assisted surgeries have added to previously used orthopedic surgical technologies using computer-assisted devices and three-dimensional planning [19]. The robotic arm provides tactile, visual, and auditory feedback to assist orthopedic surgeons in achieving desired orientation and provides greater stability and mobility intraoperatively [17]. The three types of robotics platforms that are currently in use are active system, semi-active system, and tele-surgical system. Active system, or supervisory-controlled, robots work autonomously and undergo pre-programmed tasks [9, 20]. Semi-active, or shared-controlled, systems have combined pre-programmed elements with surgeon-drive elements [9, 20]. Tele-surgical robotic systems are under complete control of the surgeon, which includes the popular Da Vinci robotic systems [20].

Robotic-assisted surgeries have become a tool to help surgeons minimize human error and maximize accuracy [10]. In orthopedics, robotic-assisted total joint replacements are aimed to improve specific aspects of the surgery, such as bone cuts and prosthesis alignment [10]. Robotic surgery has demonstrated accuracy in orthopedic implant placement, resulting in less intraoperative radiation exposure, postoperative bleeding, and pain [21]. Such procedures use preoperative advanced imaging to create three-dimensional reconstructions of the preoperative joint, which assist in the measurements for implant size, positioning, and balancing of ligaments [10] (Fig. 40.1). THAs and TKAs have adopted the use of robotic-assisted surgeries; however, data has yet to show consistently improved outcome scores [22]. When exploring the use of robotic-assisted surgeries in the shoulder, even less data is available. Facca et al. demonstrated in 2014 successful brachial plexus repair using robotic-assisted surgery in cadavers [23]. As such, strides in the use of robotics in total shoulder arthroplasties have not caught up to that of total hip and knee arthroplasties.

Although the use of robotics potentially improves accuracy and reproducibility of the implant in the glenoid, complications specific to the shoulder may be the underlying reason for such lack of advancements in the use of robots in TSAs [24]. The instrumentation in the shoulder becomes more complicated when attempting to obtain sufficient exposure of the glenoid, as well as the risks of coracoid fracture and neurovascular injuries from the pins used [24]. As such, recent studies have aimed to develop safer techniques in order to utilize the use of robotics for TSAs. A cadaveric study published in 2021 attempted to resolve some concerns, with the approach producing reliable guidewires placements and accurate results [25]. As of July 2022, commercial use of robotics for TSAs is not available [24]. With this, it is apparent that further studies and trials must be conducted to evaluate for optimal use of robotics during total shoulder arthroplasties.

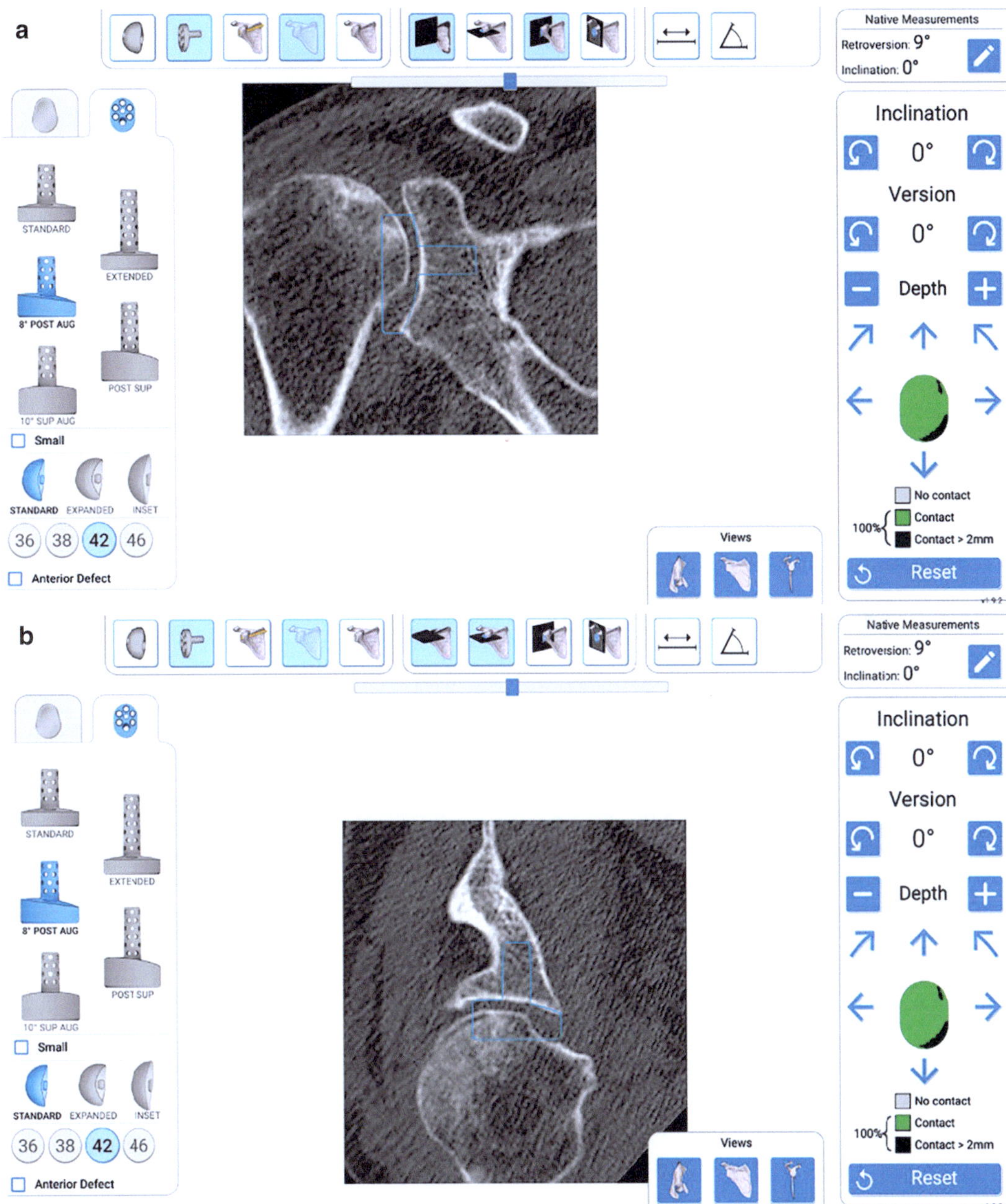

Fig. 40.1 (**a–d**) Preoperative templating software utilizes three-dimensional reconstructions of the joint to choose the best size implants to match the patient's anatomy and place the components in the optimal position to appropriately tension soft tissues to maximize patient function. All figures are original and obtained with permission from Dr. Michael O'Brien, who is an author on this manuscript

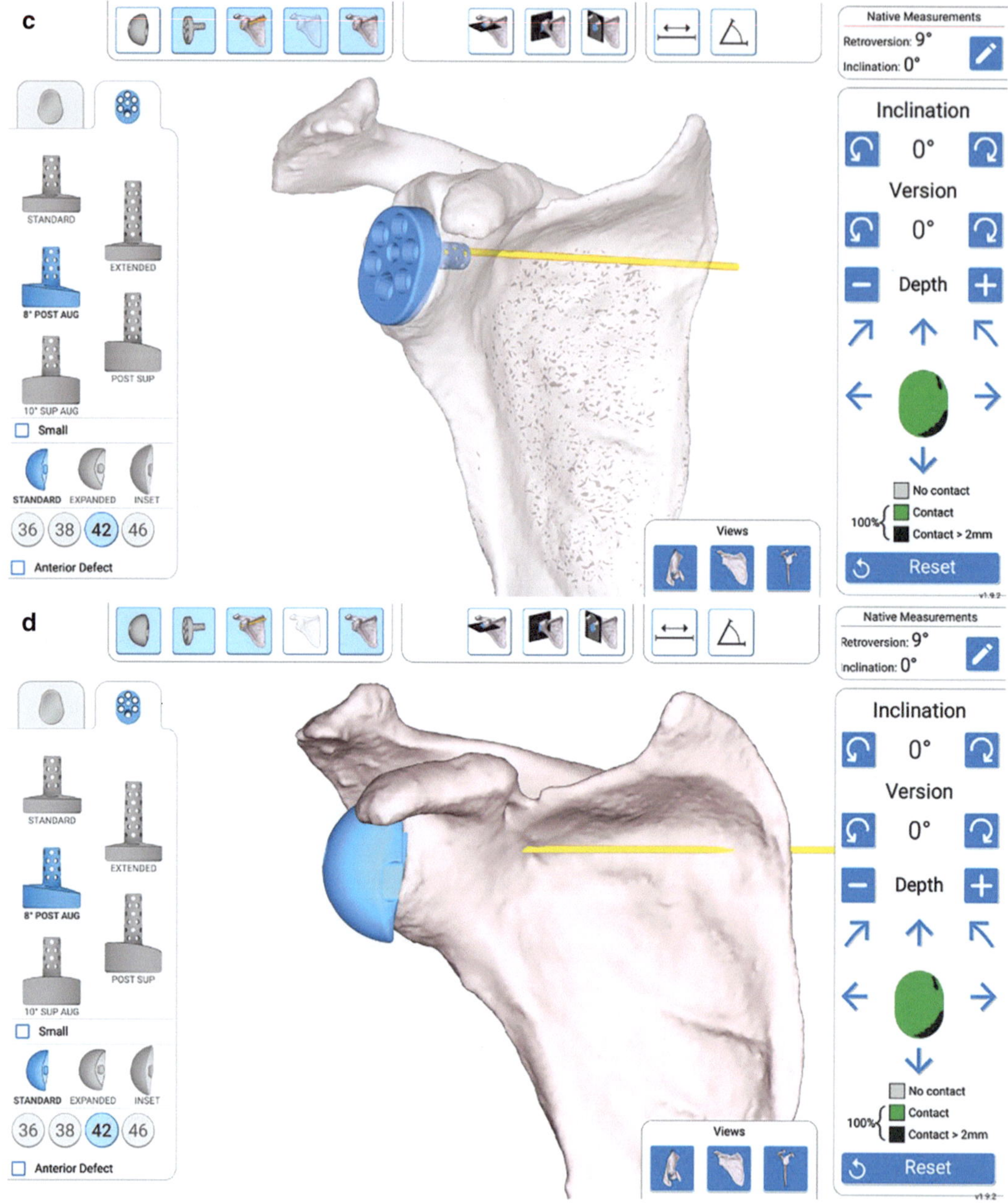

Fig. 40.1 (continued)

40.2 History and Application of Augmented and Virtual Reality

The emergence of the use of augmented and virtual reality has enhanced surgical procedures. Augmented reality is specifically achieved by superimposing images using video or computer-generated models onto the patient's anatomic body part [26]. Virtual reality (VR), originally coined in 1986 in the entertainment industry, has now expanded to clinical medicine by generating a completely artificial computer-simulated image and environment with real-time interaction [26,

27]. Since the development of VR, efforts to incorporate the human body into the virtual experience have driven significant advances in VR and augmented reality (AR), which consist of input devices, output displays, and hardware and software parts [28]. The American Board of Orthopaedic Surgery in 1997 and the American Academy of Orthopaedic Surgeons in 1998 each created task forces to explore adapting this technology for application in orthopedics [29].

Orthopedic surgical procedures require geometric information, such as angles of deformity and anatomic relations for instrumentation and implantation, all of which can be optimized using augmented reality [30]. The use and development of augmented reality has continued to evolve since it became utilized in the medical field. In June 2022, the VisAR, an augmented reality navigation system, received FDA approval for precision-guided intraoperative spine surgery [30]. Schleuter-Brust et al. demonstrated that augmented reality use in reversed shoulder arthroplasty provided better component placement accuracy, reduced operative time, and improved outcomes [31]. Both augmented reality and virtual reality have also proved to be effective learning tools for orthopedic surgery residents, with improving procedural skills for various scenarios and procedures, aiding to help teach crucial decision-making skills [27, 32].

Virtual reality is readily available for both shoulder and knee arthroscopies and total joint arthroplasties [33]. Virtual reality has played an important role in surgical planning, which is crucial to stability and longevity in total shoulder arthroplasty implants [27]. While standard radiographs and 2D CT scans provide some assistance to preoperative planning, virtual reality provides more immersive information for operative plans [27]. Additionally, virtual reality provides the option to practice a procedure prior to the actual surgery, aiding in improving surgical techniques and confidence of the surgeon and residents, thereby improving outcomes [34].

As such, virtual reality training has moved to the forefront of education and training for orthopedic surgery residents. Lohre et al. demonstrated that orthopedic surgery residents who used vir-tual reality as a component of their training had greater improvements of knowledge and procedural skills compared to residents taught primarily with video instruction [27].

40.3 Computer Navigation and Patient-Specific Instrumentation

Glenoid component position is an important factor for both function and implant survival in both anatomic and reverse TSA [35]. The glenoid malposition can lead to inferior clinical outcomes, humeral instability, implant loosening, and early failure due to increased stresses at the bone-prosthesis interface [36, 37]. Since the advent of computer-assisted navigation for TKA, which was first introduced and validated on cadavers in total knee arthroplasty in 1996 and the first computer-assisted prosthesis implanted in a live patient in 1997 [38], this technology has been adapted to TSA.

Additional techniques for improving glenoid component position are patient-specific instrumentation (PSI) guides and computer navigation. PSI systems involve the use of custom-made guides constructed from CT-based 3D preoperative computer templating [39]. The PSI guide is placed on the native glenoid intraoperatively to assist with accurate glenoid component placement. Computer navigation allows synchronization of the preoperative CT scan to enact real-time intraoperative feedback to the surgeon while placing components to improve accuracy and execute the preoperative plan (Fig. 40.2). Numerous studies have demonstrated navigation and PSI to improve the accuracy of glenoid positioning in both anatomic and reverse TSA [25, 39–41]. While the improvement in glenoid position with computer-assisted navigation has been well documented, there is little direct data on the extent that the use of computer-assisted navigation helps with prosthesis survivorship or patient functional outcomes [42]. The Blueprint system was among the first to incorporate PSI guides to use within surgery based on CT models [39]. The Exactech system similarly was among the first to

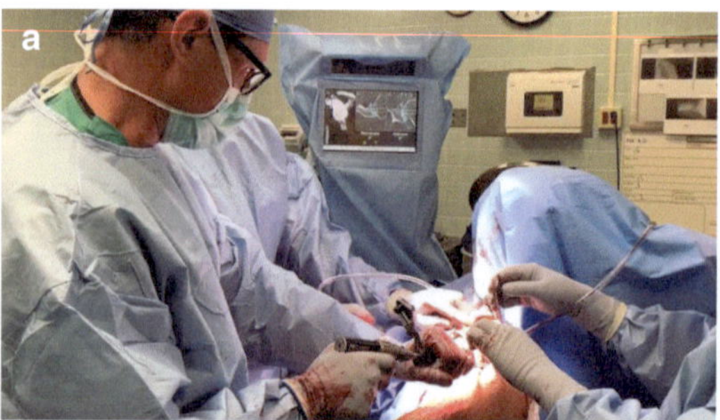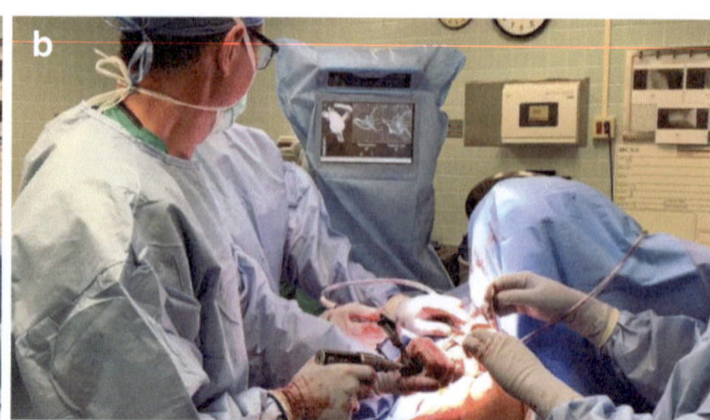

Fig. 40.2 (**a** and **b**) Computer-assisted navigation allows real-time intraoperative feedback to the surgeon to assist with component position and execute the preoperative plan. All figures are original and obtained with permission from Dr. Michael O'Brien, who is an author on this manuscript

generate "GPS"-guided instrumentation [43]. In this system, the surgeon plans the glenoid intervention as in the computer program, and then sensors on the shoulder create virtual anatomic, real-time views of instrument and implant position [43].

Computer-assisted navigation (CAN) may come with some drawbacks. There is a learning curve to the technique. In a case series of 16 patients, it was demonstrated that navigation was aborted in 6 patients due to technical problems and that operating time was prolonged by 31 min compared to standard technique [44]. The additional operative time can decrease to 11 min after a sufficient learning curve has been reached and the surgeon becomes more proficient with the operative technique [45]. In addition, corocoid fractures have been described with placement of the navigation tracker on the corocoid process [46]. Computer-assisted navigation is gaining popularity but has not yet become widespread for use in TSA procedures [47, 48].

patient-specific intraoperative guides and was designed to be portable [25]. This technology will require extensive in vivo trials. However, this does represent the beginning of adaptation of robotic technology to TSA.

Sherman and Wu studied the willingness of orthopedic surgeons to adopt a new innovation or technology using Rogers' diffusion of innovations principle which categorizes groups that adopt a new idea as innovators, early adopters, early majority, late majority, and laggards [50]. This study demonstrated a left shift in the total joint surgeon population compared to the general population suggesting orthopedic surgeons will embrace new technology and was independent of age or years in practice [51].

Factors driving the emergence of robotics for shoulder arthroplasty include a search for technology to provide better and more reproducible clinical outcomes. As robotic technology evolves, it will likely play a larger role in shoulder arthroplasty as it has in knee and hip arthroplasty as well as other fields in medicine.

40.4 Future Directions and Surgeon Adaptation

Currently robotic-assisted TSA is not commercially available, but it is an emerging technology [49]. In 2022, a cadaveric study on a novel TSA robotics platform by Darwood et al. was published in the *Journal of Shoulder and Elbow Surgery* [25]. The authors demonstrated this new robotics platform to be able to reliably produce

References

1. Puzzitiello RN, Agarwalla A, Liu JN, Cvetanovich GL, Romeo AA, Forsythe B, et al. Establishing maximal medical improvement after anatomic total shoulder arthroplasty. J Shoulder Elbow Surg. 2018;27(9):1711–20.
2. Raiss P, Bruckner T, Rickert M, Walch G. Longitudinal observational study of total shoulder replacements with cement: fifteen to twenty-year follow-up. J Bone Joint Surg Am. 2014;96(3):198–205.

3. Deshmukh AV, Koris M, Zurakowski D, Thornhill TS. Total shoulder arthroplasty: long-term survivorship, functional outcome, and quality of life. J Shoulder Elbow Surg. 2005;14(5):471–9.

4. Wagner ER, Farley KX, Higgins I, Wilson JM, Daly CA, Gottschalk MB. The incidence of shoulder arthroplasty: rise and future projections compared with hip and knee arthroplasty. J Shoulder Elbow Surg. 2020;29(12):2601–9.

5. Patel AH, Wilder JH, Ofa SA, Lee OC, Savoie FH, O'Brien MJ, et al. Trending a decade of proximal humerus fracture management in older adults. JSES Int. 2022;6(1):137–43.

6. Antonios JK, Korber S, Sivasundaram L, Mayfield C, Kang HP, Oakes DA, et al. Trends in computer navigation and robotic assistance for total knee arthroplasty in the United States: an analysis of patient and hospital factors. Arthroplast Today. 2019;5(1):88–95.

7. Leung T, Vyas D. Robotic surgery: applications. Am J Robot Surg. 2014;1(1):1–64.

8. Bargar WL. Robots in orthopaedic surgery: past, present, and future. Clin Orthop Relat Res. 2007;463:31–6.

9. Lane T. A short history of robotic surgery. Ann R Coll Surg Engl. 2018;100(6_sup):5–7.

10. Saber AY, Marappa-Ganeshan R, Mabrouk A. Robotic assisted total knee arthroplasty. In: StatPearls [Internet]. Treasure Island, FL: StatPearls Publishing; 2022. [cited 2022 Jul 12]. http://www.ncbi.nlm.nih.gov/books/NBK564396/

11. Bargar WL, Parise CA, Hankins A, Marlen NA, Campanelli V, Netravali NA. Fourteen year follow-up of randomized clinical trials of active robotic-assisted total hip arthroplasty. J Arthroplast. 2018;33(3):810–4.

12. Konan S, Maden C, Robbins A. Robotic surgery in hip and knee arthroplasty. Br J Hosp Med (Lond). 2017;78(7):378–84.

13. Elson L, Dounchis J, Illgen R, Marchand RC, Padgett DE, Bragdon CR, et al. Precision of acetabular cup placement in robotic integrated total hip arthroplasty. Hip Int. 2015;25(6):531–6.

14. Karunaratne S, Duan M, Pappas E, Fritsch B, Boyle R, Gupta S, et al. The effectiveness of robotic hip and knee arthroplasty on patient-reported outcomes: a systematic review and meta-analysis. Int Orthop. 2019;43(6):1283–95.

15. Agarwal N, To K, McDonnell S, Khan W. Clinical and radiological outcomes in robotic-assisted total knee arthroplasty: a systematic review and meta-analysis. J Arthroplast. 2020;35(11):3393–3409.e2.

16. Kalavrytinos D, Koutserimpas C, Kalavrytinos I, Dretakis K. Expanding robotic arm-assisted knee surgery: the first attempt to use the system for knee revision arthroplasty. Case Rep Orthop. 2020;2020:4806987.

17. Robotic Orthopedic Surgery - Overview - Mayo Clinic. [cited 2022 Jul 12]. https://www.mayoclinic.org/departments-centers/robotic-orthopedic-surgery/overview/ovc-20472153

18. St Mart JP, Goh EL. The current state of robotics in total knee arthroplasty. EFORT Open Rev. 2021;6(4):270–9.

19. Computer Navigation and Patient-specific Instrumentation in... : Sports Medicine and Arthroscopy Review [cited 2022 Jul 12]. https://journals.lww.com/sportsmedarthro/pages/articleviewer.aspx?year=2014&issue=12000&article=00002&type=Fulltext

20. Surgical Robot - an overview | ScienceDirect Topics. [cited 2022 Jul 12]. https://www.sciencedirect.com/topics/engineering/surgical-robot

21. Li C, Wang L, Perka C, Trampuz A. Clinical application of robotic orthopedic surgery: a bibliometric study. BMC Musculoskelet Disord. 2021;22(1):968. https://pubmed.ncbi.nlm.nih.gov/34809652/

22. Sousa PL, Sculco PK, Mayman DJ, Jerabek SA, Ast MP, Chalmers BP. Robots in the operating room during hip and knee arthroplasty. Curr Rev Musculoskelet Med. 2020;13(3):309–17.

23. Facca S, Hendriks S, Mantovani G, Selber JC, Liverneaux P. Robot-assisted surgery of the shoulder girdle and brachial plexus. Semin Plast Surg. 2014;28(1):39–44.

24. Porcellini G, Tarallo L, Novi M, Spiezia F, Catani F. Technology applications in shoulder replacement. J Orthop Traumatol. 2019;20(1):27.

25. Darwood A, Hurst SA, Villatte G, Tatti F, El Daou H, Reilly P, et al. Novel robotic technology for the rapid intraoperative manufacture of patient-specific instrumentation allowing for improved glenoid component accuracy in shoulder arthroplasty: a cadaveric study. J Shoulder Elbow Surg. 2022;31(3):561–70.

26. Khor WS, Baker B, Amin K, Chan A, Patel K, Wong J. Augmented and virtual reality in surgery-the digital surgical environment: applications, limitations and legal pitfalls. Ann Transl Med. 2016;4(23):454.

27. Lohre R, Warner JJP, Athwal GS, Goel DP. The evolution of virtual reality in shoulder and elbow surgery. JSES Int. 2020;4(2):215–23.

28. Turhan B, Gümüş ZH. A brave new world: virtual reality and augmented reality in systems biology. Front Bioinform. 2022;2:873478.

29. Gomoll AH, O'Toole RV, Czarnecki J, Warner JJP. Surgical experience correlates with performance on a virtual reality simulator for shoulder arthroscopy. Am J Sports Med. 2007;35(6):883–8.

30. Casari FA, Navab N, Hruby LA, Kriechling P, Nakamura R, Tori R, et al. Augmented reality in orthopedic surgery is emerging from proof of concept towards clinical studies: a literature review explaining the technology and current state of the art. Curr Rev Musculoskelet Med. 2021;14(2):192–203.

31. Schlueter-Brust K, Henckel J, Katinakis F, Buken C, Opt-Eynde J, Pofahl T, et al. Augmented-reality-assisted K-wire placement for glenoid component positioning in reversed shoulder arthroplasty: a proof-of-concept study. J Pers Med. 2021;11(8):777.

32. Vávra P, Roman J, Zonča P, Ihnát P, Němec M, Kumar J, et al. Recent development of augmented reality in surgery: a review. J Healthc Eng. 2017;2017:4574172.

33. Mabrey JD, Reinig KD, Cannon WD. Virtual reality in orthopaedics: is it a reality? Clin Orthop Relat Res. 2010;468(10):2586–91.

34. Clarke E. Virtual reality simulation-the future of orthopaedic training? A systematic review and narrative analysis. Adv Simul (Lond). 2021;6(1):2.

35. Nyffeler RW, Werner CML, Gerber C. Biomechanical relevance of glenoid component positioning in the reverse Delta III total shoulder prosthesis. J Shoulder Elbow Surg. 2005;14(5):524–8.

36. Gregory TM, Sankey A, Augereau B, Vandenbussche E, Amis A, Emery R, et al. Accuracy of glenoid component placement in total shoulder arthroplasty and its effect on clinical and radiological outcome in a retrospective, longitudinal, monocentric open study. PLoS One. 2013;8(10):e75791.

37. Iannotti JP, Spencer EE, Winter U, Deffenbaugh D, Williams G. Prosthetic positioning in total shoulder arthroplasty. J Shoulder Elbow Surg. 2005;14(1 Suppl S):111S–21S.

38. Saragaglia D, Rubens-Duval B, Gaillot J, Lateur G, Pailhé R. Total knee arthroplasties from the origin to navigation: history, rationale, indications. Int Orthop. 2019;43(3):597–604.

39. Dallalana RJ, McMahon RA, East B, Geraghty L. Accuracy of patient-specific instrumentation in anatomic and reverse total shoulder arthroplasty. Int J Shoulder Surg. 2016;10(2):59–66.

40. Sadoghi P, Vavken J, Leithner A, Vavken P. Benefit of intraoperative navigation on glenoid component positioning during total shoulder arthroplasty. Arch Orthop Trauma Surg. 2015;135(1):41–7.

41. Nashikkar PS, Scholes CJ, Haber MD. Role of intraoperative navigation in the fixation of the glenoid component in reverse total shoulder arthroplasty: a clinical case-control study. J Shoulder Elbow Surg. 2019;28(9):1685–91.

42. Burns DM, Frank T, Whyne CM, Henry PD. Glenoid component positioning and guidance techniques in anatomic and reverse total shoulder arthroplasty: a systematic review and meta-analysis. Shoulder Elbow. 2019;11(2 Suppl):16–28.

43. Colasanti GB, Moreschini F, Cataldi C, Mondanelli N, Giannotti S. GPS guided reverse shoulder arthroplasty. Acta Biomed. 2020;91(4-S):204–8.

44. Kircher J, Wiedemann M, Magosch P, Lichtenberg S, Habermeyer P. Improved accuracy of glenoid positioning in total shoulder arthroplasty with intraoperative navigation: a prospective-randomized clinical study. J Shoulder Elbow Surg. 2009;18(4):515–20.

45. Rosenthal Y, Rettig SA, Virk MS, Zuckerman JD. Impact of preoperative 3-dimensional planning and intraoperative navigation of shoulder arthroplasty on implant selection and operative time: a single surgeon's experience. J Shoulder Elbow Surg. 2020;29(12):2564–70.

46. Giorgini A, Tarallo L, Novi M, Porcellini G. Computer-assisted surgery in reverse shoulder arthroplasty: early experience. Indian J Orthop. 2021;55(4):1003–8.

47. Verborgt O, Vanhees M, Heylen S, Hardy P, Declercq G, Bicknell R. Computer navigation and patient-specific instrumentation in shoulder arthroplasty. Sports Med Arthrosc Rev. 2014;22(4):e42–9.

48. Jahic D, Suero EM, Marjanovic B. The use of computer navigation and patient specific instrumentation in shoulder arthroplasty: everyday practice, just for special cases or actually teaching a surgeon? Acta Inform Med. 2021;29(2):130–3.

49. Gannon NP, Wise KL, Knudsen ML. Advanced templating for total shoulder arthroplasty. JBJS Rev. 2021;9(3) https://pubmed.ncbi.nlm.nih.gov/33735155/

50. Dearing JW. Applying diffusion of innovation theory to intervention development. Res Soc Work Pract. 2009;19(5):503–18.

51. Sherman WF, Wu VJ. Robotic surgery in total joint arthroplasty: a survey of the AAHKS membership to understand the utilization, motivations, and perceptions of total joint surgeons. J Arthroplast. 2020;35(12):3474–3481.e2.

The Subscapularis-Sparing Approach to Total Shoulder Arthroplasty

Corinne Sommi, Michael J. O'Brien, Felix H. Savoie III, and William F. Sherman

41.1 Introduction

Total shoulder arthroplasty (TSA) has become a highly effective option for many painful shoulder conditions as it not only alleviates pain but also restores joint function [1]. Patients experience significant, lasting improvements in studies of long-term implant survivorship and patient outcomes [1–4]. Results of surgical treatment are, however, largely dependent on the integrity of the rotator cuff or at least a repairable cuff. If a rotator cuff tear is suspected, a preoperative MRI is indicated for evaluation. The range of motion of the affected shoulder must also be considered prior to surgical intervention as the amount of loss of passive external rotation can dictate the best method of subscapularis reflection and repair. Techniques to mobilize the subscapularis include tenotomy (intra-tendinous incision), lesser tuberosity osteotomy with anatomic repair, lateral tendinous release with medial advancement, and z lengthening [5].

The most common approach for shoulder arthroplasty is the deltopectoral approach described by Neer [6]. The advantages of the deltopectoral approach include preservation of the deltoid origin and insertion as well as the extensible nature of the approach for exposure [5]. Drawbacks to this approach include the need for posterior deltoid retraction as excessive posterior deltoid retraction can hinder glenoid exposure with risk to the cephalic vein, deltoid, or brachial plexus [5]. The deltopectoral approach with subscapularis takedown represents a standard approach to the glenohumeral joint with predominantly good outcomes reported in the literature [1].

After both tenotomy and lesser tuberosity osteotomy, the subscapularis is prone to failure and dysfunction [7–12]. This is apparent by lack of active terminal internal rotation [11].

The impact of subscapularis insufficiency includes instability that may lead to glenoid loosening and revision surgery with a high failure and complication rate, especially in the active patient [13]. Subscapular insufficiency is a known complication after takedown with insufficiency rates as high as 56% seen on CT postoperatively [5]. Miller et al. completed a retrospective review of 41 patients who had undergone total shoulder replacement performed between 1995 and 2000 and found that 66% of postoperative patients had subscapularis deficits, such as the patients' ability to tuck in a shirt [11]. Ninety-one percent of

C. Sommi (✉)
Department of Orthopaedics, Tulane University School of Medicine, New Orleans, LA, USA
e-mail: csommi@tulane.edu

M. J. O'Brien · F. H. Savoie III · W. F. Sherman
Department of Orthopaedic Surgery, Tulane University School of Medicine,
New Orleans, LA, USA
e-mail: mobrien@tulane.edu; fsavoie@tulane.edu; Swilliam1@tulane.edu

© ISAKOS 2023
A. D. Mazzocca et al. (eds.), *Shoulder Arthritis across the Life Span*,
https://doi.org/10.1007/978-3-031-33298-2_41

these patients experienced significant strength differences when comparing the operative limb to contralateral limb [11]. Schiebel et al. performed a study in 2007 investigating MRI results after arthroscopic vs open shoulder stabilizations and found that 70% of primary open stabilizations and 91% of revision stabilizations in young patients had subscapularis dysfunction and atrophy in the postoperative period [14].

Other causative factors in subscapularis dysfunction include poor tissue quality, inappropriate physical therapy, and excessive tension due to oversize arthroplasty components [11]. The health of the subscapularis tendon may also be a contributor to pain and functional impairment in the postoperative state as in addition to failure of the reattachment of the tendon, neurologic atrophy and fatty infiltration of the muscle belly can occur [5, 15, 16]. Postoperative fatty atrophy of the subscapularis can occur after both subscapularis tenotomy and lesser tuberosity osteotomy [3]. It is undetermined if fatty infiltration occurs secondary to the original takedown during the procedure or if the majority of the damage occurs during retraction or lengthening of the muscle and tendon, leading to nerve damage and later fatty infiltration.

Various techniques of subscapularis takedown and reattachment have attempted to decrease the trauma to and increase the healing potential of the subscapularis with a failure rate incidence reported in up to 40% of patients [4, 7–12].

Montgomery and Jobe utilized a technique to avoid taking down the subscapularis tendon during capsulolabral repair by splitting the subscapularis and repairing it with suture anchors [17]. However, there remains concern for the tendency of subscapularis detachment. Techniques were investigated with the goal of a mini-open approach that would allow shoulder replacement without taking down the entire tendon. After multiple cadaver dissections by Savoie et al., a new technique was created for taking down only the inferior 30% to 50% of the subscapularis tendon and preserving the more critical upper part attached to the lesser tuberosity [18]. The authors conducted a prospective case series to evaluate this subscapularis-sparing approach. Fifty patients underwent humeral head replacement surgery through an upper subscapularis-sparing approach and postoperatively underwent magnetic resonance imaging, ultrasound evaluation, and clinical evaluations. All patients were followed for at least 2 years postoperatively. Savoie et al. found that all postoperative patients had subscapularis strength equal to the contralateral arm as measured by lift-off, belly-press, and bear hug tests. Not only were clinical exam findings comparable to the healthy extremity, but the average postoperative upper extremity scores such as the American Shoulder and Elbow Surgeons rating scale demonstrated statistically significant improvement from preoperative scores. In terms of postoperative imaging, all patients had an intact subscapularis tendon attachment without atrophy in the muscle belly as evaluated by either magnetic resonance imaging or ultrasound.

41.2 Operative Technique

The technique described by Savoie et al. was originally described in 2015 [18].

Patients are positioned in the beach chair position and placed under general anesthesia in combination with an interscalene block. Prophylactic antibiotics are to be administered prior to incision. A 5–7 cm vertical incision is made utilizing a standard deltopectoral approach. The long head of the biceps is located at the top of the pectoralis major tendon, followed through the rotator interval, which is released, and the biceps is released off the superior labrum. The bicep is tenodesed to the pec major tendon at this time. The subscapularis tendon is identified, and a split is made in the lower muscle tendon raphe approximately 1/2 to 2/3 inferior to the superior border of the tendon (Fig. 41.1a and b). An electrocautery is then used to follow a line straight down the humerus on the medial ridge of the biceps, grooved down to the pectoralis major insertion. The inferior 1/3 to 1/2 of the subscapularis is elevated off the humerus from the raphe inferiorly in a subperiosteal manner (Fig. 41.2a and b). It is quite important to continue the release medially under and around any inferior humeral spurs, all the way posteriorly under the teres minor insertion. As the soft tissues are

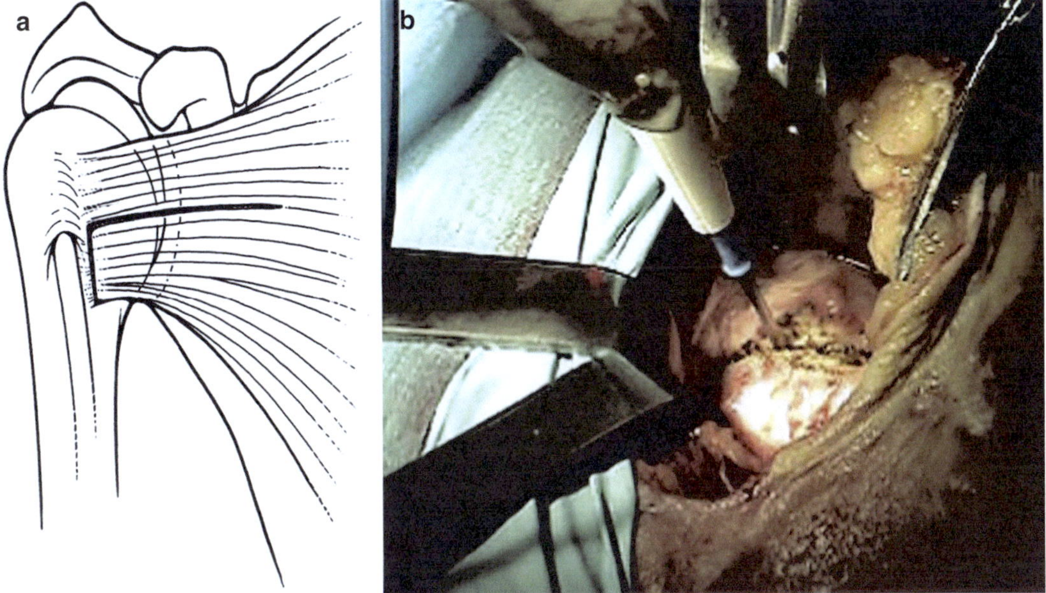

Fig. 41.1 (**a**) An illustration of the initial horizontal approach. (**b**) An anatomical view of the horizontal split

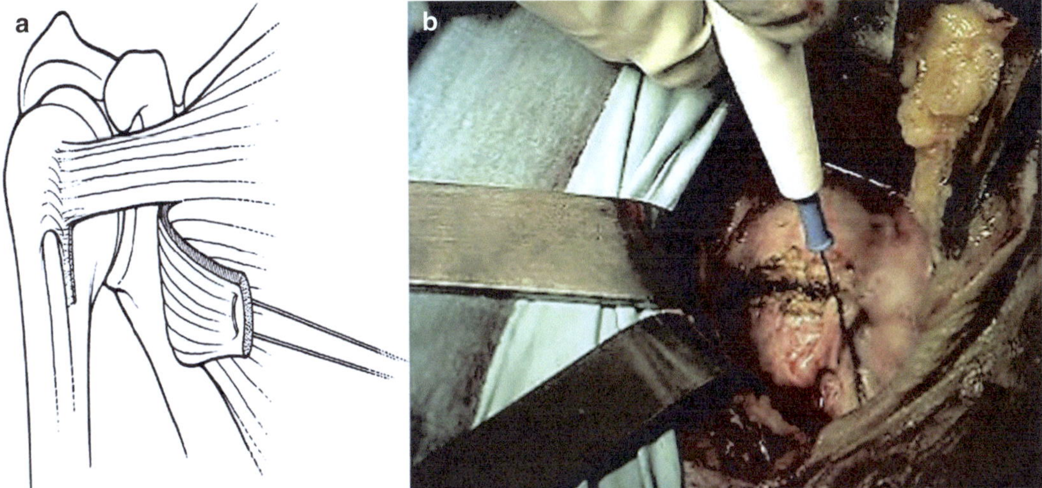

Fig. 41.2 (**a**) An illustration of the reflected lower half of the subscapularis is shown here. (**b**) The longitudinal part of the incision is taken inferiorly following the medial ridge of the bicipital groove

released, the arm is continually and slowly externally rotated and abducted to allow exposure of the inferior humeral head. Once the dissection reaches the posterior aspect of the humerus, a Cobb retractor is used to "flip" the upper subscapularis muscle over the superior aspect of the humeral head as the arm is continued to be abducted and externally rotated and the humeral head dislocated from the glenoid. A Chandler retractor is placed medially and a Hohmann retractor superiorly to protect the soft tissues and completely expose the humeral head (Fig. 41.3a and b). All inferior osteophytes are removed to allow adequate sizing of the implant. The humeral head may be either reamed for surface-type replacement or cut for humeral head replacement. In this approach, it is relatively easy to recreate the patient's normal version due to the exposure of the humerus. The glenoid can be evaluated either via this subscapularis win-

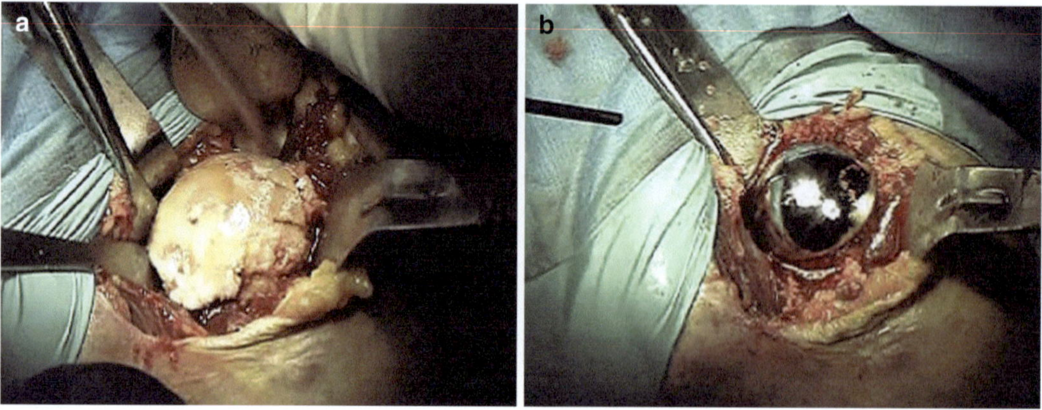

Fig. 41.3 (**a**) The inferior flap is continued medially, exposing the degenerative humeral head. (**b**) The replaced humeral head is visualized

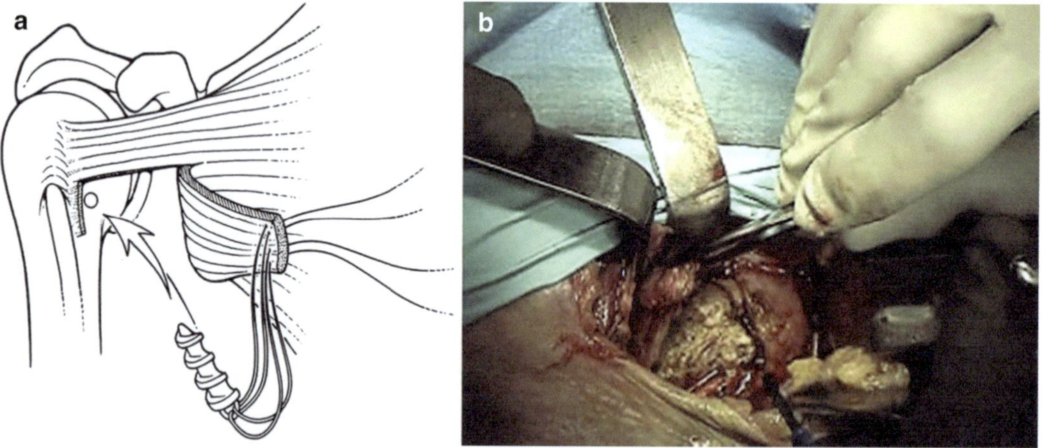

Fig. 41.4 (**a**) The humerus is reduced; the preserved superior flap is visualized and the lower subscapularis prepared for repair. (**b**) Anatomic view of the left shoulder showing the intact upper subscapularis tendon post humeral head reduction

dow (our preference) or via the interval split as described by Lafosse and also by Zuckerman [19]. We usually do the glenoid first, and then the humerus is replaced according to the surgeon's preference, either stemless or standard stem. Once the replacement is completed, the humeral head is reduced back into the glenoid space, allowing the intact superior ½ to 2/3 of the subscapularis to remain in place. The preserved upper subscapularis tendon is easily visualized (Fig. 41.4a and b). The lower subscapularis tendon is repaired with either a large nonabsorbable suture or using a double-loaded suture anchor and a double-row repair technique (Fig. 41.5a and b) as well as interrupted polydioxanone sutures (PDS, J& J Ethicon) to reinforce the repair, both in the split raphe and at the distal tendon insertion. All patients were placed into a sling with an abduction pillow in the operating room prior to awakening from anesthesia.

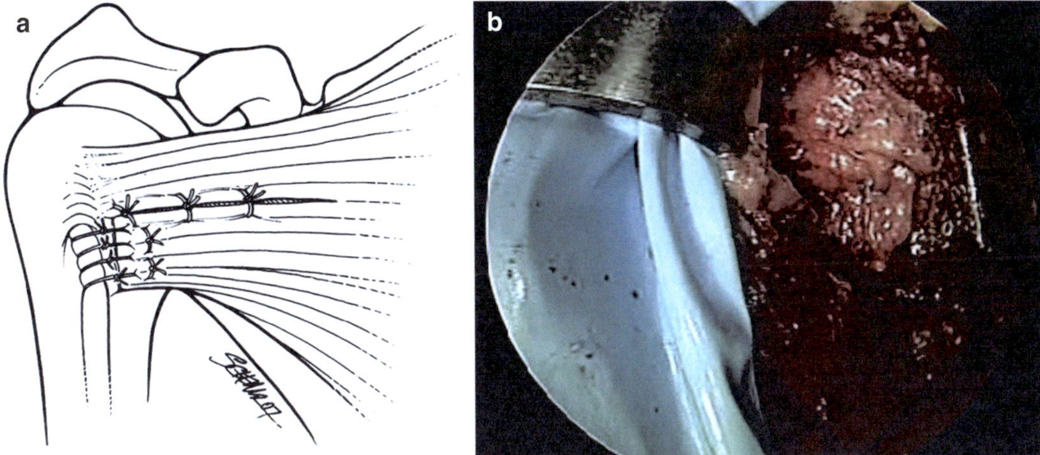

Fig. 41.5 (**a**) An illustration of the completed repair is presented. (**b**) The repaired lower half of the subscapularis is visualized

41.3 Postoperative Care

Radiographs are taken in the recovery room confirming proper implant positioning, with no malposition due to limiting the exposure by preserving the subscapularis muscle. Postoperatively, passive range of motion and active external rotation exercises are started at 1 week and active internal range of motion exercises started at 3 weeks with discontinuation of the sling. Physical therapy can be progressed as tolerated beginning at 4 weeks with most patients resuming gym workouts at that time. Even with this aggressive rehabilitation program, patients can preserve and maintain subscapularis function.

41.4 Discussion

Subscapularis takedown provides excellent exposure to the shoulder joint during TSA; however the subscapularis tendon-sparing approach has excellent clinical results and outcomes as well. The subscapularis-sparing approach however is clearly technically more difficult, especially in the stiffer, non-flexible shoulders [14]. The actual incidence of subscapular rupture after open surgical takedown and subsequent repair is not published in the literature. Throughout this discussion, it is important to recall that an intact subscapularis may not be necessary to achieve patient satisfaction with TSA.

Jackson et al. performed a case series investigating subscapularis healing rates after tenotomy used during TSA [20]. The authors found that of 15 patients in the study, 7 had a complete tear of the repaired subscapularis tendon based on ultrasound. These patients experienced significantly decreased strength with internal rotation testing and decreased Disabilities of the Arm, Shoulder, and Hand (DASH) scores. However, subscapularis tear did not correlated with pain or patient-reported outcomes. Other pathologic possibilities leading to subscapularis dysfunction include devascularization or denervation of the subscapularis from release or stretch of the cuff while trying to give the patient normal offset [20].

Jobe developed the subscapularis split technique for open capsule-labral procedures in an attempt to maintain the functional integrity of the entire rotator cuff including the subscapularis, particularly in athletes [17]. During TSA, subscapularis complete takedown classically has been thought of as necessary to achieve appropriate exposure though known to potentially create subscapularis failure. Multiple surgical techniques have been described to avoid postoperative detachment or failure of the repaired subscapularis tendon including lesser tuberosity osteotomy, varying suture patterns, and soft tissue reinforcement techniques [2, 4, 14, 21–25]. For example, Lafosse et al. proposed TSA through the rotator interval without detaching any of the subscapularis [19]. However, the authors were unable to remove inferior humeral spurs through the rotator interval [19]. Gerber also found good results in terms of postoperative subscapularis function with lesser tuberosity osteotomy [9, 14]. Despite these advances to prevent and treat subscapularis failure, it continues to be a source of instability, weakness, pain, and early failure in shoulder arthroplasty [10, 11, 14, 16, 26].

The subscapularis-sparing approach demonstrated by Savoie et al. was created to avoid subscapularis repair failures and fatty infiltration while letting patients undertake an accelerated rehabilitation program [18]. An initial dissection that later was discarded centered on approaching the shoulder from the axilla during the development of the technique by Savoie et al. This approach was deemed unsafe due to the excessive traction that could be placed on the axillary nerve during retraction. The finalized approach was to use one of the muscle tendon raphes present in the subscapularis as an entry point. Using the muscle tendon raphe of the subscapularis enables the surgeon to preserve the upper half of the subscapularis while gaining full exposure to the humeral head. The upper portion of the subscapularis provides 70% or more of the strength and function of the subscapular muscle-tendon unit and therefore is of utmost importance to maintain its integrity. The inferior subscapularis interval and approach to the shoulder may allow surgeons to remove the inferior humeral head spurs, perform a capsular release, and give access to the glenoid.

To summarize, key technical points in the approach include the following: (1) open the rotator interval by following the biceps tendon superiorly; (2) the initiating point for the inferior split is along the medial ridge of the bicipital groove; (3) the entire flap is then elevated as a unit subperiosteally around the humerus to the posterior aspect of the humeral shaft inferior to the humeral spurs to maintain soft tissue protection of the axillary nerve. The lower half could be repaired with an anchor(s) or with suture.

In conclusion, respecting and maintaining the superior half of the subscapularis gives patients a faster postoperative rehabilitation to build back function while decreasing unwanted poor outcomes associated with subscapularis atrophy or detachment.

Acknowledgments All authors assisted in the proofreading and preparation of this manuscript.

References

1. Deshmukh AV, Koris M, Zurakowski D, Thornhill TS. Total shoulder arthroplasty: long-term survivorship, functional outcome, and quality of life. J Shoulder Elbow Surg. 2005;14(5):471–9.
2. Defranco MJ, Higgins LD, Warner JJ. Subscapularis management in open shoulder surgery. J Am Acad Orthop Surg. 2010;18(12):707–17.
3. Lapner PL, Sabri E, Rakhra K, Bell K, Athwal GS. Healing rates and subscapularis fatty infiltration after lesser tuberosity osteotomy versus subscapularis peel for exposure during shoulder arthroplasty. J Shoulder Elbow Surg. 2013;22(3):396–402.
4. Walch G, Boileau P. Shoulder arthroplasty. Berlin: Springer; 1998.
5. De Wilde L, Boileau P, Van der Bracht H. Does reverse shoulder arthroplasty for tumors of the proximal humerus reduce impairment? Clin Orthop Relat Res. 2011;469(9):2489–95.
6. Neer CS II. Replacement arthroplasty for glenohumeral osteoarthritis. JBJS. 1988:70.
7. Armstrong A, Lashgari C, Teefey S, Menendez J, Yamaguchi K, Galatz LM. Ultrasound evaluation and clinical correlation of subscapularis repair after total shoulder arthroplasty. J Shoulder Elbow Surg. 2006;15(5):541–8.
8. Gerber C, Hersche O, Farron A. Isolated rupture of the subscapularis tendon. J Bone Joint Surg Am. 1996;78(7):1015–23.
9. Gerber C, Yian EH, Pfirrmann CA, Zumstein MA, Werner CM. Subscapularis muscle function and structure after total shoulder replacement with lesser tuberosity osteotomy and repair. J Bone Joint Surg Am. 2005;87:1739–45.
10. Miller BS, Joseph TA, Noonan TJ, Horan MP, Hawkins RJ. Rupture of the subscapularis tendon

after shoulder arthroplasty: diagnosis, treatment, and outcome. J Shoulder Elbow Surg. 2005;14(5):492–6.

11. Miller SL, Hazrati Y, Klepps S, Chiang A, Flatow EL. Loss of subscapularis function after total shoulder replacement: a seldom recognized problem. J Shoulder Elbow Surg. 2003;12(1):29–34.

12. Qureshi S, Hsiao A, Klug RA, Lee E, Braman J, Flatow EL. Subscapularis function after total shoulder replacement: results with lesser tuberosity osteotomy. J Shoulder Elbow Surg. 2008;17(1):68–72.

13. Scalise JJ, Ciccone J, Iannotti JP. Clinical, radiographic, 233 and ultrasonographic comparison of subscapularis tenotomy and lesser tuberosity osteotomy for total shoulder arthroplasty. J Bone Joint Surg Am. 2010;92(7):1627–34.

14. Scheibel M, Habermeyer P. Subscapularis dysfunction following anterior surgical approaches to the shoulder. J Shoulder Elbow Surg. 2008;17(4):671–83.

15. Scheibel M, Nikulka C, Dick A, Schroeder RJ, Popp AG, Haas NP. Structural integrity and clinical function of the subscapularis musculotendinous unit after arthroscopic and open shoulder stabilization. Am J Sports Med. 2007;35(7):1153–61.

16. Sperling JW, Potter HG, Craig EV, Flatow E, Warren RF. Magnetic 255 resonance imaging of painful shoulder arthroplasty. J Shoulder Elbow Surg. 2002;11(4):315–21.

17. Montgomery WH 3rd, Jobe FW. Functional outcomes in athletes after modified anterior capsulolabral reconstruction. Am J Sports Med. 1994;22(3):352–8.

18. Savoie FH 3rd, Charles R, Casselton J, O'Brien MJ, Hurt JA 3rd. The subscapularis-sparing approach in humeral head replacement. J Shoulder Elbow Surg. 2015;24(4):606–12.

19. Lafosse L, Schnaser E, Haag M, Gobezie R. Primary total shoulder arthroplasty performed entirely thru the rotator interval: technique and minimum two-year outcomes. J Shoulder Elbow Surg. 2009;18(6):864–73.

20. Jackson JD, Cil A, Smith J, Steinmann SP. Integrity and function of the subscapularis after total shoulder arthroplasty. J Shoulder Elbow Surg. 2010;19(7):1085–90.

21. Ahmad CS, Wing D, Gardner TR, Levine WN, Bigliani LU. Biomechanical evaluation of subscapularis repair used during shoulder arthroplasty. J Shoulder Elbow Surg. 2007;16(3 Suppl):S59–64.

22. Caplan JL, Whitfield B, Neviaser RJ. Subscapularis function after primary tendon to tendon repair in patients after replacement arthroplasty of the shoulder. J Shoulder Elbow Surg. 2009;18(2):193–6; discussion 197–8

23. Giuseffi SA, Wongtriratanachai P, Omae H, Cil A, Zobitz ME, An KN, Sperling JW, Steinmann SP. Biomechanical comparison of lesser tuberosity osteotomy versus subscapularis tenotomy in total shoulder arthroplasty. J Shoulder Elbow Surg. 2012;21(8):1087–95.

24. Krishnan SG, Stewart DG, Reineck JR, Lin KC, Buzzell JE, Burkhead WZ. Subscapularis repair after shoulder arthroplasty: biomechanical and clinical validation of a novel technique. J Shoulder Elbow Surg. 2009;18(2):184–92; discussion 197–8

25. Lapner PL, Sabri E, Rakhra K, Bell K, Athwal GS. Comparison of lesser tuberosity osteotomy to subscapularis peel in shoulder arthroplasty: a randomized controlled trial. J Bone Joint Surg Am. 2012;94(24):2239–46.

26. Scheibel M, Tsynman A, Magosch P, Schroeder RJ, Habermeyer P. Postoperative subscapularis muscle insufficiency after primary and revision open shoulder stabilization. Am J Sports Med. 2006;34(10):1586–93.

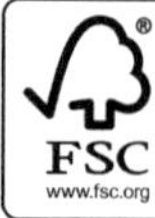